Pathology of the Liver and Biliary Tract

WILEY SERIES IN SURGICAL PATHOLOGY

Editor: *Steven G. Silverberg, M.D.*

SURGICAL PATHOLOGY OF THE UTERUS
Steven G. Silverberg, M.D.

PATHOLOGY OF THE LIVER
AND BILIARY TRACT
Boris H. Ruebner, M.D., and Carolyn K. Montgomery, M.D.

Pathology of the Liver and Biliary Tract

BORIS H. RUEBNER, M.D.
Professor
Department of Pathology
School of Medicine
University of California, Davis
Pathologist
University of California Davis Medical Center
Sacramento, California

CAROLYN K. MONTGOMERY, M.D.
Associate Professor in Residence
Department of Anatomic Pathology
School of Medicine
University of California, San Francisco
Assistant Chief, Department of Anatomic Pathology
Veterans Administration Medical Center
San Francisco, California

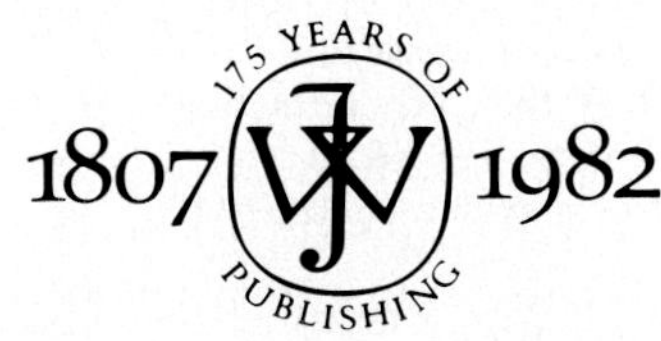

A WILEY MEDICAL PUBLICATION
JOHN WILEY & SONS
New York • Chichester • Brisbane • Toronto • Singapore

Library of Congress Cataloging in Publication Data:

Ruebner, Boris H.
Pathology of the liver and biliary tract.

(Wiley series in surgical pathology) (A Wiley
medical publication)
Includes index.

1. Liver—Diseases. 2. Biliary tract—Diseases.
I. Montgomery, Carolyn K. II. Title. III. Series.
IV. Series: Wiley medical publication. [DNLM:
1. Biliary tract diseases. 2. Liver diseases.
WI 700 R918p]

RC846.9.R83 616.3'6075 81-19849
ISBN 0-471-02453-8 AACR2

Printed in the United States of America

10 9 8 7 6 5 4 3 2 1

To
Susan, Sally, and Anthony
B.H.R.

Margaret and "Engine Jim"
C.K.M.

and
to those who stimulated and sustained
our interest in hepatology:
Dame Sheila Sherlock, M.D., Hans Popper, M.D.,
Peter Schener, M.D., and Rudi Schmid, M.D.

Preface

Our aim has been to provide a practical, problem-oriented approach to the pathologic diagnosis of hepatic and biliary disorders. We hope that it will be useful in the day-to-day practice of pathologists and that it will also be consulted by physicians and surgeons when they have to care for patients with such ailments.

This book begins with a discussion of the indications for obtaining different types of hepatic specimens and the process by which a pathologic diagnosis is made. Most chapters are oriented toward clinicopathologic entities, such as hepatitis, alcoholic liver disease, fatty liver, granulomas, cholestasis, space-occupying lesions, and drug-induced liver disease. Pediatric hepatic pathology, including storage disorders, is also discussed, and chapters on the gallbladder and biliary tract are included. The pathologic features of the various conditions are described, often with tables included for differential diagnosis. Our approach has not been encyclopedic. References are, therefore, provided for more detailed discussions of individual topics. Frequently, a disorder is referred to in more than one chapter. To minimize duplication we have inserted cross references to the more detailed descriptions wherever necessary. Careful consideration has been given to the roles of electron microscopy, immunopathology, and chemistry in reaching a diagnosis. In selecting illustrations, our aim has been to depict those morphologic lesions that are seen most frequently, or that have particular diagnostic importance.

We are most grateful to those of our colleagues in this country and abroad who provided us with material for illustrations. We believe that their generosity has greatly enhanced the usefulness of this book. Several of our colleagues, particularly S. W. French, M.D., Liisa Russell, M.D., and Rick Baier, M.D., have read the manuscript and provided constructive criticisms. Ms. Eileen Ginsberg of John Wiley was most helpful during the production stage. Any comments from readers will be most welcome.

B.H.R.
C.K.M.

Contents

1 A General Approach to Hepatic Pathology 1

2 Hepatitis 33

3 Hepatic Injury Produced by Infectious Agents and Miscellaneous Diseases 60

4 Granulomatous Diseases of the Liver 77

5 Alcoholic Liver Injury 95

6 Fatty Liver 106

7 Hyperbilirubinemia and Cholestasis 117

8 Hyperbilirubinemia and Cholestasis in Infancy 141

9 Metabolic Diseases Associated with Hepatocellular Necrosis 157

10 Diseases with Abnormal Hepatic Storage Products 173

11 Hepatic Pigments 188

12 Vascular Lesions of the Liver 196

13 Fibrosis, Nodules, and Cirrhosis 211

14 Space-Occupying Lesions of the Liver 233

15 Liver Injury Induced by Drugs and Other Chemicals 287

16 The Gallbladder 312

17 The Bile Ducts 333

Index 363

Pathology of the Liver and Biliary Tract

1
A General Approach to Hepatic Pathology

DIFFERENT TYPES OF SPECIMEN

The amount of information that can be obtained from a liver biopsy and the clinical value of this information depend to a considerable extent on the specimen itself. Significant considerations are choice of the most suitable type of specimen (needle or wedge), the manner in which it is obtained (percutaneously, at laparoscopy or laparotomy), and the anatomic relationship of the specimen to the lesions. Most specimens of liver received in the surgical pathology laboratory are obtained by blind percutaneous aspiration needle biopsy, although needle biopsy specimens can also be obtained through a laparoscope. A combination of laparoscopy with biopsy permits experienced operators to describe the surface of the liver and to select the specimen from area(s) they consider most likely to provide maximum information. The relative usefulness of needle biopsy specimens of hepatic lesions encountered at laparotomy compared with the more common surgical wedge biopsy specimen has been debated. Inspection and palpation of the liver assist the surgeon in selecting the most appropriate specimen; either type of material has its advantages and disadvantages, which will be discussed below. Larger samples are obtained surgically when space-occupying lesions are resected or at debridement for trauma.

Needle Biopsy

Percutaneous needle biopsy of the liver is a well-established diagnostic tool that, in most cases, should be employed as the first step in morphologic diagnosis (1). Wider use of percutaneous neecle biopsy by surgeons as well as other physicians sometimes obviates the need for surgical intervention (2). The selection of patients and the technique of aspiration have been clearly described by Sherlock (3), Menghini (4), and Walters and Paton (1), among others. Fine needle aspiration produces cytologic smears that can be employed more frequently in the future (5,6a,6b). Brushing of tumors at laparoscopy has also been recommended (6b).

The site of biopsy deserves some consideration before puncture. A standard intercostal biopsy in the right anterior axillary line is indicated if a patient suspected of having a hepatic disorder does not have a focal lesion. The tissue obtained by an adequate needle biopsy weighs 50–200 mg, compared with an adult liver weight of approximately 1500 g (3). This method, therefore, samples only a very small proportion of the liver. Nevertheless, there is little doubt that in diffuse hepatic diseases, such as acute viral hepatitis, alcoholic hepatitis, or chronic passive congestion, needle biopsy specimens measuring 15 mm or longer are representative of the principal histopathologic changes in the entire liver (7,8). In fact, specimens measuring 5 mm may be adequate (8). The length of the cylindrical needle biopsy specimen ensures that most of the tissue is not from the vicinity of the capsule, thereby avoiding one of the problems of wedge biopsy. By contrast, the narrowness of the tissue obtained sometimes makes it difficult histologically to identify complete lobules, which can pose a disadvantage in histologic interpretation. Needle biopsy, especially if less than 15 mm in length, is not as reliable in the diagnosis of patchy hepatic lesions, such as chronic active hepatitis, cirrhosis, neoplasms, or granulomas (7,8). Stepsections are mandatory if such lesions are suspected but not found on the first cuts. If a space-occupying lesion is suspected, the biopsy needle should be directed to the site most likely to be positive (9). If there is a large palpable nodule, this should be the target. Similarly, for a lesion on a scan, multiple scintiscans or CT scans should be used to localize the lesion and determine the direction of approach. The same is true if there appears to be a lesion involving one hepatic duct or one hepatic vein. It is in such situations that a combination of laparoscopy with biopsy should be seriously considered if an experienced operator is available. The recently introduced method of obtaining a biopsy through a hepatic vein catheter permits the use of needle biopsies, even in patients with a hemorrhagic tendency.

Wedge Biopsy

Surgical wedge biopsies are undertaken for diagnosis if a previous needle biopsy has not given adequate information, particularly if primary biliary cirrhosis, macronodular cirrhosis, or malignancy are suspected, but not confirmed. In some cases, preliminary needle biopsy should be omitted, especially if the patient has a hemorrhagic diathesis and hepatic vein biopsy is not available. Wedge biopsies can also be obtained if laparotomy is performed for diagnostic purposes, as in fever of unknown origin and in jaundice when the biliary tract is explored for possible obstruction. Another indication for wedge biopsy is the elucidation of unexpected focal or diffuse hepatic abnormalities encountered during abdominal surgery. Diffuse pallor and nodularity, for instance, suggest fatty change and cirrhosis, respectively. Adequate wedge biopsy specimens weigh 0.5–1 g, making it possible to obtain a microscopic sample of a much larger proportion of the liver than is possible with needle biopsies. The likelihood of finding focal lesions such as granulomas or metastatic tumors, is thus increased considerably. The subcapsular location of such specimens can give rise to difficulties in interpretation because of variation in the structure of the liver immediately beneath the capsule. A considerable amount of fibrous tissue may be present in this zone in otherwise normal livers. Islands of parenchyma that appear to be isolated and superficially suggestive of cirrhosis are occasionally seen in the immediate subcapsular zone. Some pathologists have been so disturbed by such changes that they prefer to interpret needle biopsy specimens taken from the liver at surgery to the more usual wedge specimens. Our observations agree with those of Petrelli and Scheuer (10), who found these changes to be limited to a depth of 2 mm below the capsule and did not consider these appearances a serious source of difficulty. Certainly, their observations reinforce the need for the surgeon to take wedge biopsy specimens of adequate size, that is, at least to a depth of 1 cm. Wedge biopsies permit better appreciation of certain microscopic features, for example, lobular architecture and lesions of the larger portal bile ducts. Wedge biopsy specimens also provide a larger sample for biochemical estimations than can be obtained by needle biopsy. Needle biopsy specimens may be taken during laparotomy in addition to wedge biopsies in order to obtain sampling from areas more remote from the capsule than can be obtained by a wedge biopsy. Needle biopsies at laparotomy can also provide a sampling of more widely distributed areas than can be obtained by a single wedge biopsy. Routine needle biopsy of the liver in all patients undergoing upper abdominal operations has been recommended (11).

Resection

Larger specimens are resected surgically for the diagnosis and treatment of space-occupying hepatic lesions and lacerations. The latter range from specimens only slightly larger than diagnostic wedge specimens to resections of hepatic segments, lobes (12), or even entire livers, before hepatic transplantation.

INSPECTION AND DESCRIPTION OF THE SPECIMEN

General Description

For a needle biopsy, it is usually sufficient to record the length of the biopsy cylinder. Whereas it is desirable to record the weight of needle biopsy specimens, it is an essential step in the case of wedge and larger biopsy specimens. Careful examination of every specimen is mandatory. Although examination can be accomplished with the naked eye, a dissecting microscope is helpful. Good lighting of the dissecting surface is essential. Specimens should be viewed not only by direct, but by transmitted light as well.

The capsular surface is easily identified in wedge biopsy specimens and in surgically resected specimens. Normally smooth and glistening, granularity or nodularity suggests cirrhosis. The capsule usually cannot be identified in needle biopsy specimens. Cirrhosis can sometimes be recognized, however, in such specimens by the observation of brownish cirrhotic nodules held together by paler fibrous connective tissue. Generally, though, the hepatic tissue obtained by needle biopsy from cirrhotic patients tends to crumble into irregular fragments. A fragmented needle biopsy specimen, therefore, should always raise the suspicion of cirrhosis.

The color of the cut surface of surgically resected and needle biopsy specimens is normally a uniform brown or tan. The regular arrangement of normal portal triads and central veins is generally recognizable on careful inspection. A pale, yellowish, greasy appearance indicates a fatty liver, which can be confirmed if the specimen floats in watery fixatives, such as buffered neutral formalin. A greenish appearance indicates cholestasis, either extra- or intrahepatic. The green coloration becomes more striking after exposure of the tissue to air or to formalin-containing fixatives. Under both conditions, bilirubin is oxidized to biliverdin, which is more intensely green. The green staining of cholestasis often has a finely punctate appearance, because the cholestasis is generally most pronounced in centrilobular zones. The dark red appearance of congestive cardiac failure and of the Budd-Chiari syndrome is also more pronounced in the centrilobular zones, forming the so-called nutmeg pattern. A diffuse rusty brown color suggests hemosiderosis. In hemochromatosis, cirrhosis may be present in addition to the brown pigmentation. Diffuse chocolate or black coloration suggests the Dubin-Johnson syndrome. We recommend that every fresh specimen received in the surgical pathology laboratory be examined under ultraviolet light so as not to overlook a diagnosis of porphyria cutanea tarda, which causes the liver to emit a purple fluorescence. A Woods light can be used, or alternatively, frozen sections or imprints of the fresh unfixed biopsy specimen can be viewed microscopically under an ultraviolet microscope. This procedure must be done promptly in order to protect the specimen from undue exposure to ambient light (13). Fluorescence is also found in protoporphyria and in some cases of porphyria variegata (Chapter 9). The liver in amyloidosis is often said to appear abnormally pale and translucent. Unfortunately, we have never found this helpful in making a gross diagnosis.

Focal Lesions

Multiple small diffusely scattered foci of white or yellowish discoloration measuring approximately 1–2 mm in diameter suggest neoplastic lesions, particularly leukemia or lymphoma, granulomas, or necrosis. Lymphomatous infiltration tends to be whitish and may have a regular distribution throughout the specimen because of localization in the portal areas. This pattern is particularly true of lymphatic leukemia. Granulomas usually appear as irregularly distributed small white or gray infiltrates. They are generally seen best by transillumination. Irregular yellowish foci suggest hepatic necrosis, particularly of viral origin, such as herpes simplex infection.

Larger space-occupying lesions may almost completely replace the normal hepatic parenchyma in a needle biopsy specimen. Such specimens are quite unlike normal liver in both color and consistency. The tissue obtained may vary from whitish and firm in the case of a scirrhous carcinoma to purple and soft in the case of vascular lesions. Because of the contrast between the lesion and the uninvolved part of the liver, space-occupying lesions are easier to describe in wedge specimens and in hepatic resection specimens. Firm, homogeneous, white lesions are suggestive of neoplasia, particularly metastases or primary bile duct carcinoma. Hepatocarcinomas may be hemorrhagic but are not uncommonly brown or green because of cholestasis. A variegated hemorrhagic appearance is suggestive of necrosis in a malignant tumor. The border between the lesion and the rest of the hepatic parenchyma should always be examined carefully. An irregular border with infiltration into the parenchyma is suggestive of malignancy, whereas the presence of a capsule at the periphery of the lesion favors a benign process. Penetration of the lesion to the serosa is of serious significance, because it suggests peritoneal involvement. A shaggy periphery with a necrotic center, often containing pus, suggests an abscess. Such lesions are sometimes encapsulated. Granulomas are whitish-gray with an irregular border, fibrotic or calcified. Yellowish liquid material in the center of such lesions is characteristic of caseation. Caseation is rare in hepatic granulomas. However, if present, caseation strongly suggests a diagnosis of tuberculosis or fungal infection. Caseation has also been described in brucellosis (14). Pale wedge-shaped lesions with a hemorrhagic border suggest infarcts, whereas lesions that are diffusely hemorrhagic are suggestive of hepatocellular or vascular neoplasms, trauma, or peliosis hepatis. Tears in the hepatic parenchyma with or without adherent thrombi are indicative of trauma. Cystic lesions are suggestive of a congenital or parasitic etiology. The hepatic parenchyma surrounding space-occupying lesions is frequently compressed and may show centrilobular congestion or cholestasis. Although such changes can be striking in a biopsy close to a lesion, it should not necessarily be assumed that the liver away from the lesion will show the same changes.

Anatomic Relationships

Larger specimens excised for diagnosis or treatment of space-occupying lesions should be described with an emphasis on the appearance and measurements of the lesions and on the anatomic relationships of the lesions to the hepatic landmarks. In order to describe such specimens correctly and obtain the appropriate blocks, an understanding of the surgical anatomy of the liver is required. The true anatomic division of the liver into lobes and lobules is more closely related to the internal distribution of vessels and ducts than to any external landmark, such as the falciform ligament, conventionally taken to divide the liver into right and left lobes. According to more recent views (14a), the true left lobe of the liver is much larger than conventionally described (Fig. 1). As they enter the hilum, the hepatic artery, portal vein, and the common hepatic duct divide into two separate systems serving the true right and left lobes. The line of division between the two lobes, the principal plane, extends in an oblique anteroposterior direction from the bed of the gallbladder to the hepatic fossa of the inferior vena cava. This plane bisects the caudate lobe. About equal in mass, the right and left lobes function almost like separate paired organs, and there is essentially no intrahepatic communication between the two systems. The division of the right lobe into segments has little surgical importance. However, the left lobe is divided into a medial and a lateral segment by the plane of the falciform ligament. The medial segment includes the quadrate lobe and part of the caudate lobe. Riedel's lobe is a downward prolongation of the right lobe often adherent to the mesocolon. Hypoplasia of entire lobes may occur (15).

Occasionally, ectopic hepatic tissue is found entirely detached from the liver in the abdominal (16) or thoracic (17,18) cavities. Such ectopia can be congenital (16) or the result of trauma sustained several years earlier (19). Ectopic hepatic tissue may be fibrotic when the rest of the liver is normal, but it can also be involved in hepatic diseases (20).

The level at which the right and left hepatic ducts join to form the common hepatic duct varies from just outside the liver to a distance of 3 cm or more. The

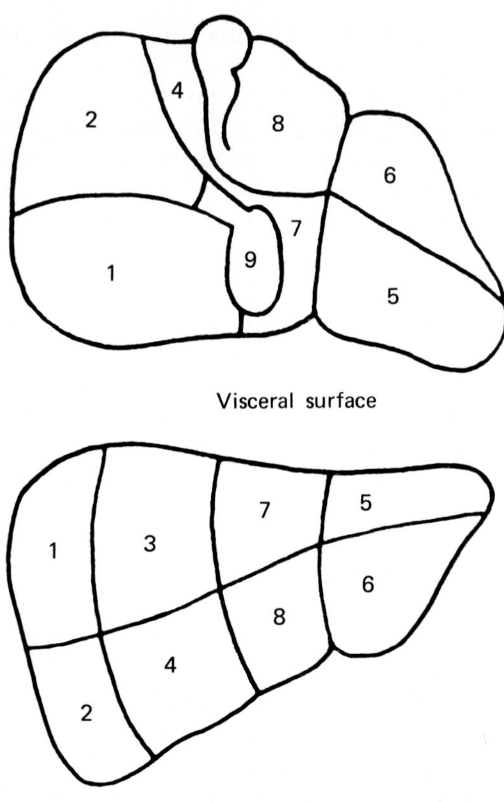

Figure 1. Diagrammatic representation of the division of the liver into subsegments. The relative sizes of the subsegments shown are those most frequently found. The right lobe is composed of subsegments 1, superior posterior; 2, inferior posterior; 3, superior anterior; and 4, inferior anterior. The left lobe is composed of subsegments 5, superior lateral; 6, inferior lateral; 7, superior medial; and 8, inferior medial (quadrate lobe). Number 9 is the caudate lobe. (Modified from Gupta, ref. 14.)

junction can even be intrahepatic, particularly in the presence of hepatomegaly (21). The cystic duct usually joins the common duct distal to the junction, but can join the right hepatic duct. Another anomaly involves a major segmental duct, most frequently from the posterior segment of the right lobe, joining the common hepatic duct. Anomalous divisions of the portal vein also occur (22). The hepatic arterial system is quite variable. Origin of the right hepatic artery from the superior mesenteric artery instead of the celiac artery is the commonest vascular anomaly. Biliary vascular bundles composed of portal vein, hepatic artery, and bile duct supply each of the segments described in the preceding discussion. The caudate lobe is unique in that it can receive branches from either or both right and left lobar systems.

There are three major hepatic veins—the left, the middle, and the right—located in the interlobar and intersegmental planes. The left and middle hepatic veins usually join to form a short stalk before entering the inferior vena cava. The right vein enters the inferior vena cava separately. The left hepatic vein drains the left lateral segment only. The middle vein lies in the interlobar plane and drains approximately one-third of the liver, that is, the medial segment of the left lobe and most of the anterior segment of the right lobe. The right hepatic vein drains the posterior segment and part of the anterior segment of the right lobe. A series of four or five small, but surgically important, paired hepatic veins pass directly from the inferior or posterior surface of the liver into the vena cava. One pair drains from the right and one from the left. Multiple small veins also drain from the caudate lobe into the diaphragmatic portion of the inferior vena cava. These small hepatic veins tend to remain patent in patients who have the Budd-Chiari syndrome, in whom occlusions of the major hepatic veins are generally found. It is for this reason that the caudate lobe tends to be somewhat protected from the pathologic changes in the Budd-Chiari syndrome. The caudate lobe can actually undergo hypertrophy in such patients (23).

After partial hepatectomy, an inflow and an outflow supply must be preserved for the remaining hepatic tissue. Thus, if a right hepatectomy is performed, the liver is transected in a plane to the right of the middle hepatic vein (23a). For an extended right hepatectomy, the liver is transected in a plane to the right of the falciform ligament, thereby removing the right lobe and the medial segment of the left lobe. For a left hepatectomy, the liver is transected in a plant to the left of the middle hepatic vein. For an extended left hepatectomy, the liver is transected on the right side of the principal plane, and the entire left lobe and a medial portion of the right lobe are removed. If a left lateral segmental resection is performed, the liver is transected in a plane to the left of the falciform ligament, thereby preserving the umbilical fissure and with it the left branches of the portal vein, hepatic artery, and bile duct that supply or drain the medial segment of the left lobe (12,24). A middle wedge resection or central hepatic resection consists of removing part of the liver located anterior to the hilum and including part of the anterior portion of the right lobe and part of the medial segment of the left lobe as well as the gallbladder.

GENERAL PRINCIPLES OF SPECIMEN HANDLING

In deciding to perform a liver biopsy, the physician should also decide whether routine handling is expected to be adequate. Routine handling consists of the production of paraffin sections and can include fixation of blocks for possible electron microscopic examination. If the operator believes that special methods might be indicated, this possibility should be discussed with the pathologist. A decision to employ special fixatives or methods, such as immunopathology, enzyme histochemistry, electron microscopy, biochemistry, or microbiology, should be made jointly by the operator and the pathologist. If this decision has been arrived at before obtaining the biopsy specimen, the pathologist will have made available to the operator the fixatives, other material, and technical help required. If the appearance of the specimen suggests special handling to the operator, the specimen should be taken immediately to the pathologist in a clean, and preferably sterile, container without fixative. After discussion of diagnostic possibilities, the pathologist can then arrange for appropriate processing. There is no doubt that there is no single correct way in which to handle a specimen. Ultimately, each laboratory has to use the methods best adapted to its needs and resources. We present here the methods we have found to work in our own laboratories.

Processing for Light Microscopy

Fixation and Preparation of Paraffin Blocks

Needle biopsy specimens are obtained most commonly using either a Menghini needle (4) or one of its modifications. Menghini's method is both quick and safe. Its main disadvantage is that in patients with fibrosis, the failure rate is high and the specimen obtained generally small or fragmented (3). With the Vim-Silverman needle, a larger specimen is obtained. This method is more successful in cirrhosis. Distortion and compression along the edges of the specimen are often severe, however. Menghini specimens are aspirated into a syringe containing normal saline. The tip of the needle is then placed into saline in a flat-bottomed glass receptacle, and only then is aspiration stopped and the specimen expelled. The Vim-Silverman needle is also attached to a syringe during aspiration, but the syringe contains no fluid.

A satisfactory needle biopsy specimen has been defined as 1–4 cm in length and weighing 50–200 mg (3). Depending on the length of the specimen, up to 0.5 cm of the liver biopsy cylinder can be cut off with a sharp razor blade, diced into small 1-mm^3 cubes, and put into modified Karnovsky's or McDowell's fixative (p. 13). If indicated, this portion can be processed for electron microscopic examination. The rest of the specimen is placed on a strip of thin paper before fixation, a practice that tends to keep the specimen flattened and in one piece during processing. The paper strip and the attached biopsy specimen are placed into 10% phosphate buffered formalin (25) for 3–10 hours. The biopsy is then dehydrated in graded alcohols, cleared in benzene, taken off its paper strip, and embedded in paraffin. Other investigators prefer different fixatives, such as Carnoy's. We employ special fixatives if storage diseases, particularly the glycogenoses or mucopolysaccharidoses, are suspected and for histochemistry of some enzymes. The advantage in using phosphate-buffered formaldehyde glutaraldehyde for routine fixation is that this fixative allows acceptable ultrastructural preservation, even after prolonged storage of tissue in the fixative as well as after routine processing with paraffin embedment. If electron microscopy is desirable, tissue can be excised from the paraffin block, rehydrated, and prepared for ultrastructural study. The fixative is dependably stable at room temperature for 1 week and for 2–3 months if stored at 4°C.

Wedge biopsy specimens of the liver should be cut at right angles to the capsule such that the capsule forms the base of a triangular block, each side of which measures approximately 1 cm. Blocks are selected to include both lesions and grossly uninvolved parenchyma. They are cut to a thickness of 1–2 mm. For electron microscopic study, cubes of approximately 1-mm thickness are cut and placed in fixative as described for needle biopsies. Tissue for light microscopic analysis is processed in the same way as material obtained by needle biopsy, but fixation should be somewhat longer. Care is taken to embed the blocks flat with the capsule along one edge.

Larger specimens should be cut into slices 0.5–1 cm in width. Several blocks should be taken to include grossly visible lesions and their relationship to the surrounding uninvolved liver and capsule. Blocks through apparently uninvolved liver should also be taken, both at the margin of resection and, if possible, some distance from the lesions. Blocks should also be obtained through any thickened, dilated, or obstructed ducts, and through any abnormal appearing vessels. One should sample ducts and vessels draining a lesion. Fixation is as described above for wedge and needle specimens. Sections should also be taken through any lymph nodes, such as those of the hilum (26), supplied with the specimen. If the gallbladder is included in the specimen, it should be described and processed as outlined in the discussion of the biliary tract (Chapter 16).

Microtomy and Staining

Paraffin sections are cut on a microtome at 5μm and stained by hematoxylin and eosin, by a silver method for reticulum, by Gomori's trichrome for collagen, and by Perl's stain for hemosiderin. Two sections may be left unstained for special stains. For example, if granulomas are found, Ziehl-Nielson's stain for acid-fast bacilli and a silver methenamine stain for fungi are used. Diastase-labile material, positive by the periodic acid-Schiff (PAS) reaction, is specific for glycogen. Unfortunately, the preservation of glycogen in formalin-fixed material is erratic. Preservation is better in paraffin sections of alcohol-fixed tissue or in fresh frozen sections. Diastase-resistant PAS-positive material and a positive mucicarmine stain indicate a mucin.

Recuts of the block may be required if more than two additional special stains are required, or if focal lesions such as granulomas or tumor are suspected on clinical or histopathologic grounds. If this is the case, serial sections are cut through the entire block and retained. Only a proportion, such as every fifth or tenth section, are mounted and stained with hematoxylin and eosin. If lesions are found, special stains may be indicated and can be done on adjacent sections. Recuts are also indicated in chronic persistent hepatitis to exclude focal piecemeal necrosis. If the latter is found, a diagnosis of chronic active hepatitis should be considered. If alpha-1-antitrypsin deficiency is suspected clinically or in neonatal hepatitis, in cirrhosis without a definite etiology, and when hyaline inclusions are found in hematoxylin and eosin sections, a PAS stain with diastase digestion should be done to demonstrate the PAS-positive inclusions characteristic of alpha-1-antitrypsin deficiency. If the patient's serum is positive for hepatitis B antigen, if ground-glass cells are seen by light microscopy, or if the histology suggests acute or chronic hepatitis, one of the empirical stains for HB_sAg should be done (27,28). We find the orcein method stain most satisfactory. Orcein stains elastic fibers (p. 120) and copper-binding protein (p. 120) as well. Immunohistologic staining with peroxidase-labeled antibody (see below) is desirable to confirm the diagnosis of alpha-1-antitrypsin deficiency or hepatitis B infection. The orcein staining method used in our laboratory is as follows:

1. Fix tissue in buffered formalin, embed it in paraffin, and cut 5μm sections.
2. Place deparaffinized sections in potassium permanganate for 15 minutes. (it is important to have good oxidation for contrast).
   Potassium permanganate, 0.5 g
   Distilled water, 95 ml
   3% H_2SO_4, 5 ml

3. Place in 2.0 oxalic acid until colorless (about 10 minutes).
4. Wash in tap water.
5. Wash in distilled water.
6. Stain in orcein for 4–6 hours at room temperature (6 hours preferred).
   Orcein (British Drug Houses or National Aniline), 1 g
   70% alcohol, 100 ml
   Concentrated HCl, 1 ml
   Adjust pH to 1–2
7. Differentiate in 1% HCl in 70% ethanol.
8. Dehydrate; then mount.

Plastic Sections

One or 2-μm-thick sections embedded in a water-soluble resin have become more popular in recent years (29,29a). Such sections provide better optical resolution and faster processing at somewhat higher cost.

Processing of Frozen Sections for Histologic Diagnosis and Histochemistry

Rapid diagnosis continues to be the principal purpose of frozen section examination of liver specimens in the surgical pathology laboratory. However, frozen sections can be used for many other purposes, such as fat stains, immunohistochemistry, and enzyme histochemistry. Frozen tissue is also required for chemical investigations and virologic studies. It is, therefore, most desirable to deep-freeze part of any liver specimen other than needle biopsy specimens received in the surgical pathology laboratory, on a routine basis. Of course, this is possible only when unfixed specimens are sent to the surgical pathology laboratory. Specimens should be sent immediately from the operating room to the laboratory in a clean, preferably sterile, container.

Blocks of fresh, unfixed tissue can be frozen and cut immediately in a cryostat at 5–10 μm. For immunohistochemistry and enzyme histochemistry, better results are obtained if the tissue is quick-frozen in liquid nitrogen or in isopentane cooled with dry ice and cut immediately, or at most, within 48 hours. Sections are placed on glass slides, to which they generally adhere well. For some of the more complicated stains, we have found gelatin coating of slides useful. Gelatin acts as an adhesive and tends to prevent sections from becoming detached from the slides (30). Sections are stained with hematoxylin and eosin in the same way as other rush-frozen sections. We have noted that bile pigment is frequently better preserved in rush-frozen hematoxylin and eosin sections than in permanent paraffin sections. Glycogen also tends to be better preserved in frozen sections stained with the PAS reaction than in formalin-fixed paraffin sections stained by the same method.

For fat stains, formalin-fixed tissue is cut on a cryostat. Fixed sections adhere less well than do unfixed sections. Therefore, gelatin coating of glass slides before staining is recommended to prevent sections from getting detached during staining (30). Oil-red-O and Sudan IV are generally reliable. Positive and negative controls are particularly desirable with fat stains. Osmium tetroxide fixation also results in the staining of most lipids (30A). Such tissue can be paraffin embedded, cut, and stained with hematoxylin and eosin without extraction of the lipids. If Reye's syndrome is suspected, it is recommended that frozen sections of unfixed tissue be stained with undiluted Giemsa stain for 30 seconds and be mounted in water (31).

Enzyme histochemistry, widely employed in the study of experimental liver injury, has, thus far, found relatively little application in diagnostic histopathology (32–34). However, this may change, particularly with respect to the identification of hepatic neoplasms, and perhaps of premalignant changes, as well as for diagnosis of certain storage diseases. Oxidative enzymes, such as succinic dehydrogenase, TPNH diaphorase, DPNH diaphorase, and glucose-6-dehydrogenase, are demonstrated by incubation with tetrazolium salts, such as nitro-BT or tetranitro-BT (35,36). Glucose-6-phosphatase is demonstrated on similar material by incubation with lead phosphate (35). For adenosine triphosphatase, cryostat sections are fixed in buffered neutral formalin. Alternatively, blocks fixed overnight in Baker's neutral formalin can be employed. Sections are stained by a modified Gomori lead salt method (35). For acid and alkaline phosphatase (33,34), simultaneous azo dye coupling methods using naphthol AS-TR and AS-BI, respectively, can be used after fixation of cryostat slides in acid-buffered acetone (37). Alternatively, a modified Gomori lead salt technique can be used on formalin-fixed cryostat sections or on sections obtained from blocks fixed overnight in Baker's neutral formalin (33,34). For electron histochemistry, the tissue is minced into small fragments and then briefly fixed in 2% buffered glutaraldehyde. After washing in buffer, the tissue is incubated with lead salts as described earlier for glucose-6-phosphatase, acid phosphatase, alkaline phosphatase, and ATPase. For details on light microscopic histochemistry, we have found Barka and Anderson's description (38) useful. Pearse (39) covers light microscopic histochemistry in greater detail and is recommended as a source for electron microscopic histochemical methods.

Processing for Immunohistology

Hepatitis B. Conventionally, demonstration of hepatitis antigens and antibodies in tissues requires the use of unfixed frozen sections and fluorescence microscopy. A study employing unfixed cryostat sections of rapidly frozen liver and indirect immunofluorescence for the Australia or hepatitis B surface (HB_sAg) and core (HB_cAg) antigens was that of Gudat et al. (40). Arnold et al. (41) used frozen sections and direct immunofluorescence to localize the hepatitis B e-antigen (HB_eAg). Another recent study (42) employed frozen sections and antibodies labeled with peroxidase. The hepatitis B antigens have been shown to be relatively resistant to routine fixatives and are preserved quite well in paraffin sections (43–45), clearly a great advantage in routine practice because tissue blocks can be easily stored, the size of the blocks can be larger, and there is no hazard of laboratory infection. Good histologic quality is easy to achieve, and retrospective studies are possible. Freezing equipment and procedures are not required. In paraffin sections fluorescence is almost as intense as in frozen sections, and localization of the antigen is more precise (45). Instead of labeling antibodies with fluorescein, they can be labeled with peroxidase, which does not require a fluorescent microscope. Of these two immunologic staining reactions, some workers prefer the fluorescein tracer at the light microscopic level (43). Background fluorescence interfering with immunofluorescence can be reduced by digestion of the sections with pronase (43). However, peroxidase is rapidly becoming the method of choice (44, 46–48). Indirect immunostaining is generally preferred for the peroxidase method (49). Fixation in buffered formalin is generally adequate, if restricted to the time required for optimum fixation (49). There is little doubt that these immunologic methods are more sensitive and more specific in demonstrating the hepatitis B antigens than are Shikata's empirical methods (27). However, both free horseradish peroxidase and peroxidase conjugated to an antibody other than hepatitis B have an affinity for HB_sAg, which can give false-positive reactions for such antigens (50).

In chronic hepatitis B, intranuclear IgG capable of fixing complement in vitro has been demonstrated by direct immunofluorescence (51). This type of complement fixation appears to indicate a poor prognosis (52). Immunoglobulin G (IgG) has also been demonstrated by immunofluorescence on the cell membranes of hepatocytes isolated from biopsies of patients with chronic hepatitis (53–55). In demonstrating sections of immunoglobulin by the peroxidase method, Zenker's fixative or commercial B5 fixative (preferably at half-strength) may be preferable to buffered formalin (49).

Alpha-fetoprotein. Just as in the case of hepatitis B antigens, a variety of methods have been employed in demonstrating the presence of alpha-fetoprotein (AFP). Purtilo and Yunis (56) used fresh-frozen tissue sectioned at 5 μm and fixed in 95% ethanol. Indirect immunofluorescence was used. Husby et al. (57) used the same method, except for cold acetone fixation. Nayak et al. (58) were successful in demonstrating the presence of AFP in paraffin sections of ethanol-fixed tissue. These workers used both indirect immunofluorescence and immunoperoxidase techniques, preferring the immunoperoxidase technique. Formalin-fixed paraffin embedded tissue is adequate, and, therefore, most convenient (49,59).

Alpha-1-Antitrypsin. The PAS-positive droplets found in the livers of patients with alpha-1-antitrypsin deficiency have been shown to contain alpha-1-antitrypsin. As in the case of hepatitis B and of alpha-fetoprotein, the indirect immunoperoxidase method is rapidly becoming the method of choice in confirming the identity of these droplets (49,59,60).

PROCESSING FOR TRANSMISSION ELECTRON MICROSCOPY

Scanning electron microscopy was introduced into hepatology only very recently, in particular to study the bile canaliculi. However, its usefulness for diagnosis has not yet been established. It is most desirable to fix a part of every specimen for transmission electron microscopy as soon as the biopsy has been performed. It is important to use a new, or at least a very sharp, razor blade to prepare blocks of the appropriate size for electron microscopy. Blocks should be cubes approximately 1 mm in diameter modified. Karnovsky's fixative is widely used (61). This consists of 2% w/v paraformaldehyde and 2.5% v/v glutaraldehyde in 0.06 M phosphate buffer at pH 7.2. Another fixative is McDowell's universal formaldehyde-glutaraldehyde mixture (61a). This is prepared by mixing together:

1.16 g $NaH_2^-PO_4^-H_2^-0$
0.27 g NaOH
88 ml distilled H_20
10 ml 38–40% formaldehyde (Fisher F-79)
2 ml 50% glutaraldehyde (Fisher biologic grade G151) pH adjusted to 7.2

This fixative should be stored at 4° C, at which it is stable for at least 3 months. Tissue sections are fixed by immersion at room temperature and should not exceed 1 mm^3. The minimum fixation time for 1-mm^3 sections is 3 hours. Tissues can remain in the fixative without changing the solution for at least 6 months with little deterioration of ultrastructural preservation. The availability of a specimen properly fixed for electron miscroscopy greatly increases the range of options for the pathologist.

Once the pathologist who studied the routine light microscopic preparations is familiar with the clinical problem, he or she might decide that further processing of tissue fixed for electron microscopy is not worth the expense entailed. Such a specimen can then be discarded. Alternatively, the pathologist might decide that the specimen should be embedded for possible future use, embedded and sectioned at 1-μm thickness, or embedded and studied by electron microscopy. This decision must be made by the individual pathologist with due regard to the clinical problem, as well as to the available facilities. If a decision is made to proceed with processing a specimen, it is dehydrated and embedded in an epoxy resin. We use Spurr's resin (62). One micron thick sections are then cut on an ultramicrotome and stained with a mixture of equal parts 1% methylene blue in 1% borax and 1% azure II for light microscopic orientation (63). The latter is a very important step. Occasionally, the section will show enough detail to make electron microscopy unnecessary, for example, if it is desirable to elucidate the nature of certain clear spaces in hepatocytes in sections prepared for routine light microscopy. If, in 1-μm-thick plastic sections stained in this way, green droplets are observed, it can then be considered confirmed that the droplets contain fat. Sectioning at 8°C has been recommended for this purpose (64). The principal use of these 1-μm sections, however, is to provide an intermediate step between routine light microscopy and electron microscopy. One-μm sections are used to check whether the lesions found by light microscopy are present in the material fixed for electron microscopy and to permit the electron microscopist or technician to trim the block such that it contains the lesion and as little as possible of apparently normal liver. One-μm sections also make it possible for the experienced observer to eliminate blocks and parts of blocks that have too many artifacts. Once a block has been trimmed, ultrathin sections are cut on an ultramicrotome and stained in 4% uranyl acetate in 70% ethanol for 5–7 minutes followed by lead citrate (65). These thin sections are then viewed and photographed in an electron microscope.

TISSUE HANDLING FOR CHEMICAL INVESTIGATIONS

For enzyme assays, fresh unfixed liver tissue is washed free from blood, homogenized, and analyzed as soon as possible. For most other chemical measurements, fresh unfixed specimens should be placed in a deep freeze, and kept at −70°C as soon as possible after they are obtained. Snap-freezing in pentane and dry ice, or in liquid nitrogen, is desirable. Chemical assays can then be done at one's convenience. Quite a variety of biochemical methods, even some requiring subcellular fractionation, are now sufficiently sensitive for use on needle biopsy specimens (66,66a), including the following methods for lipids: total lipids (67), triglycerides, fatty acids, cholesterol, cholesterol esters, and phospholipids (68,69). Methods have also been developed for glycogen and enzymes related to carbohydrate metabolism, such as phosphorylase, amylo-1, 6-glucosidase, acid α-glucosidase, and glucose-6-phosphatase (68). Lysosomal enzymes can also be studied, including β galactosidase, N-acetyl β glucosaminidase, β glucuronidase, acid phosphatase, and α-mannosidase (68,70,71). Prolyl hydroxylase is an indicator of collagen synthesis (72–74). Incorporation of ^{14}C-proline into hydroxyproline can also be measured (73). Cytochrome P450 (75) and several mixed-function oxidase enzymes (76–78) can also be studied. Of enzymes related to bilirubin metabolism, uridine diphosphoglucose (UDPG) transferase can be measured (79).

The chemical measurement of hepatic copper in the diagnosis of Wilson's disease (80) is important, because the histochemical methods are often considered not very quantitative. However, Irons et al. (81) recently claimed that the rhodanine method is satisfactory for screening purposes. Chemical measurement of nonhemin iron is desirable in the diagnosis of hemochromatosis (68). It is not essential, however, because staining for hemosiderin gives an adequate indication of the degree of iron storage.

There is no unanimity as to the reference base in terms of which of these various parameters should be expressed. Dry weight, protein, and DNA have all been used (82). Normal iron is 100 mg/100 g dry liver. In hemochromatosis, it is well above this level. Normal copper is about 3 mg/100 g, whereas in Wilson's disease it is more than 25. Normal lipid is 5% of wet liver (83). Normal triglycerides are 100 mg/g protein, or 65 mg% dry weight. Needle biopsy can yield sufficient material for these assays.

TISSUE HANDLING FOR MICROBIOLOGY

The normal human liver is sterile, with respect to anaerobic and aerobic bacteria, fungi, and viruses. Not only should abscesses and caseous granulomas be investigated microbiologically, but other, not obviously neoplastic, space-occupying lesions as well. Since this cannot be done on fixed specimens, it is preferable that unfixed surgical specimens be submitted immediately to the surgical pathology laboratory in sterile containers. There, the decision is made whether to study a specimen microbiologically. If it is decided that the lesion might be the result of an infection, part of the lesion, including its wall and contents, should be taken under sterile conditions and submitted to the microbiology laboratory for smears and culture for aerobes, anaerobes, mycobacteria, and fungi. If schistosomiasis mansoni is suspected, about 3 mm fresh tissue should be cut off a needle biopsy specimen, squeezed to translucency in glycerol, and examined under a low-power microscope (84). Routine paraffin sections should also be prepared. The walls and contents of cysts should be studied microscopically for parasites and ova, both in the fresh state as well as in routine paraffin sections. If the gross picture is suspicious, or if ova or parasites are seen, suitable animals should be inoculated for parasites. In clinical practice, viruses and viral antibodies are usually studied in serum specimens. Therefore, hepatic biopsy specimens are not often submitted for viral culture. However, this is occasionally desirable, particularly in patients with viral hepatitis. The possibility that viral culture may be required, like the possibility that chemical investigations may be needed, is an other good reason for routinely storing part of all liver biopsy specimens in a sterile container at −70°C, at least until evaluated light microscopically. At that time, an informed decision can be made as to whether to proceed with viral isolation or biochemical studies.

GENERAL PRINCIPLES OF HISTOLOGIC DESCRIPTION AND INTERPRETATION

The principal objective of pathologic examination is to help arrive at a diagnosis on which patient management can be based. Secondary objectives are to assess the severity of a disease or to assess progress on therapy. We have found it desirable to approach a pathologic diagnosis in two clearly defined steps. The first of these is an objective gross and microscopic description and diagnosis without knowledge of the clinical history, except for age and sex of the patient (85). This first step may result in a definite etiologic diagnosis, as in the case of neoplasms or other space-occupying lesions. In many cases it results in a probable diagnosis. In some cases two or three possible diagnoses are suggested. Occasionally, only nonspecific changes are seen and a descriptive histologic diagnosis is all that is possible. Observer variation can be reduced by a special interest and experience in hepatic pathology (86).

The second step in reaching a pathologic diagnosis begins with a review of the patient's clinical data obtained from the form accompanying the specimen or from one of the physicians concerned with the care of the patient. Any available previous biopsies are reviewed as well. Additional data usually permit pathologists to confirm the probable histologic diagnosis or to choose the most likely of possible alternative diagnoses. In some cases, particularly a proportion of those patients suspected of being alcoholics, the clinical and pathologic data will appear contradictory. Such cases should be discussed by clinician and pathologist as soon as the specimen has been examined. Both should reconsider their data and be prepared to change their diagnosis. In addition, regular clinicopathologic correlation conferences are desirable at which patients and their biopsy specimens are discussed by clinicians and pathologists. At these conferences specimens with clear-cut diagnoses, as well as difficult and debatable cases, should be shown. Such conferences are of immediate benefit to the patients discussed and play an important role in the continuing education of physicians. Even after this entire sequence has been followed, no specific etiologic diagnosis may be possible in some cases. The diagnosis then should consist of a brief descriptive summary of the histopathologic findings coupled with an indication of their severity. This should be followed by a note outlining various possible diagnoses and additional investigations that might be useful. If the specimen is inadequate in size or poorly prepared, this should be stated and a repeat specimen requested.

Overall Morphology

First, a hematoxylin and eosin-stained section should be inspected with the naked eye; any distinct landmarks, such as the capsule, large portal triads, and central veins, should be noted (Figs. 2–4). Next, inspection of the section with a magnifying glass or inverted microscope eyepiece is desirable to enable the pathologist to study these features in greater detail. However, this step can be omitted if the overall architecture is carefully studied with a low-power microscopic objective. For this, a 2.5× objective is optimal, but a 4× objective is adequate.

The liver is composed of many small subunits arranged in a honeycomb pattern. The most commonly employed concept of the basic subunit is that of the hepatic lobule (Fig. 5). According to this concept, each lobular subunit consists of a hepatic vein branch in its center and several portal triads on its periphery. From this concept follows the customary, but somewhat arbitrary, division of the lobule into central, midzonal, and peripheral zones (the more usual but less accurate term is periportal). A concept alternative to the hexagonal lobule is that of Rappaport's acinus (Fig. 5) (87,87a). According to this concept, the portal triad is at the center. Rappaport's zone I has the best blood supply, whereas zones II and III are progressively less well supplied with oxygen and nutrients. The hepatic acinus is not merely a lobule in reverse. Its subdivisions differ in shape from those of the lobule. Although Rappaport's acinus probably represents a more physiologic subunit than does the traditional lobule, the lobular concept continues to be found generally more convenient by histopathologists. The lobular concept permits pathologists to classify most zonal hepatic lesions if several lobules are available. Since the width of the midzone is not easy to define, we rarely use the category midzonal. Lesions are classified as central if they tend to occupy the central half of the lobule and if at least some are adjacent to central veins. The term pericentral is used if a lesion (e.g., fibrosis) surrounds a central vein. Lesions that tend to occupy the outer half of the lobules and that touch at least some portal triads are termed peripheral. Lesions that have destroyed entire groups of lobules are classified as massive, whereas those that have partially destroyed adjacent lobules are classified as submassive. Focal lesions are those that are peppered at random through the parenchyma. The proportion of lobules involved and the size of the lesions will vary according to the severity of the disease.

There is a distinct variation between the central and peripheral zones with respect to some chemical and histochemical reactions. Glycogen tends to be preserved predominantly in central zones in conditions of partial starvation (88).

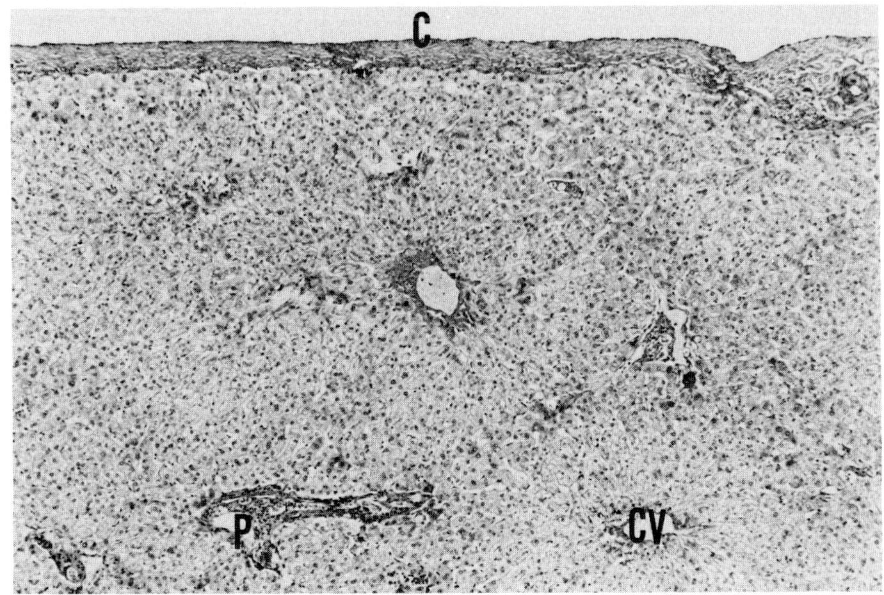

Figure 2. Low-power light microscopic view of the liver. C = Capsule of the liver; CV = central vein; P = portal triad. (Hematoxylin and eosin, ×70.)

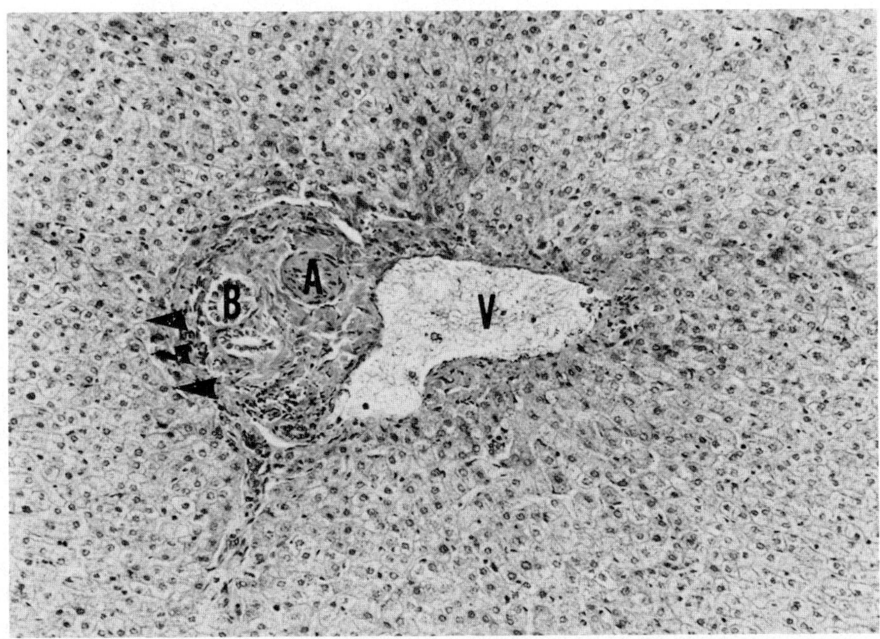

Figure 3. Higher power view of portal triad. Note the limiting plate (arrowheads). A = Hepatic artery; B = bile duct; V = portal vein. (Hematoxylin and eosin, ×140.)

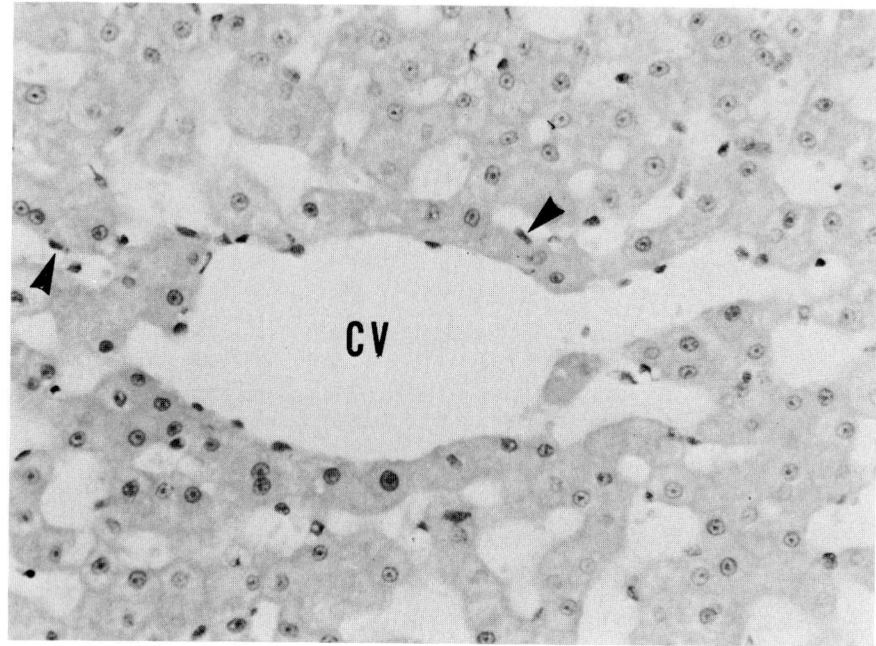

Figure 4. Higher power view of central vein (CV) and sinusoids, which appear empty and are lined by sinusoidal lining cells with elongated nuclei (arrowheads). (Hematoxylin and eosin, ×350.)

Succinic dehydrogenase and glucose-6-phosphatase tend to be more active in the lobular periphery. Hemosiderin tends to have a peripheral distribution, whereas lipofuscin tends to be central. In most conditions, bile plugs also are more predominantly found in a central location (89).

The first step in studying a liver biopsy specimen under low power is to establish whether the lobular architecture is intact. This involves subjective judgments about the distance between portal triads and central veins, as well as the amount of fibrovascular connective tissue in portal triads and adjacent to central veins. The hematoxylin and eosin stain is often adequate to answer these questions. However, stains for reticulin and collagen are desirable and may be essential if there are mild alterations from normal. Stains for collagen and reticulin are both helpful in assessing the portal triads. Normally, the smaller triads contain relatively little collagen, and excessive periportal or pericentral fibrosis is easily assessed, particularly in collagen stains. However, the histopathologist must keep in mind that the larger portal triads might normally contain considerable amounts of collagen. Polarized light is also helpful in studying hepatic collagen. When viewed in this manner, the collagen fibers of the portal triads are coarser than those in scars and surround the structures of the portal triads in a characteristic pattern. The reticulum stain (Fig. 6) is especially helpful if bridging necrosis or lobular collapse is suspected in hematoxylin and eosin-stained sections. Undue approximation of reticulin fibers in segments of lobules, or entire

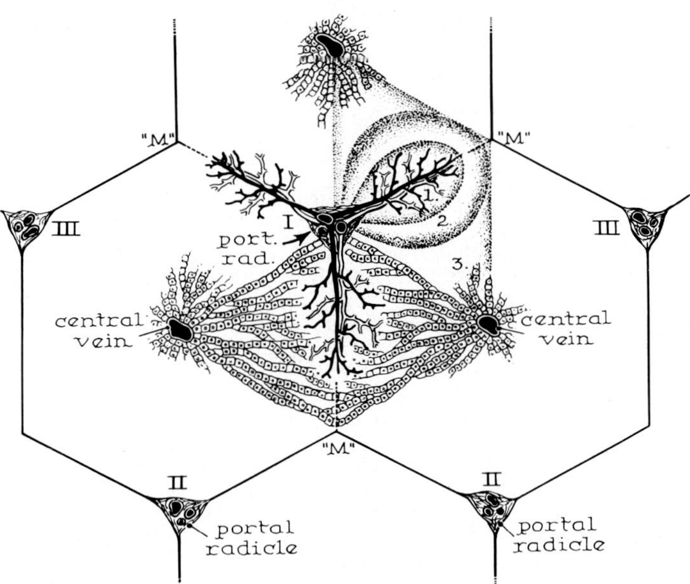

Figure 5. Diagram illustrating both the lobular and acinar concepts of hepatic structure. Two hexagonal lobules are shown, each having a central vein and three portal radicles at its periphery. Two diamond-shaped acini are also demarcated. Zones 1, 2, and 3 are shown in one of the acini. Zone 1 has the best blood supply and contains branches of the hepatic artery and portal vein. (Reproduced from Ham's *Anatomy*, ref. 87.)

lobules coupled with negative stains for collagen (trichrome) and elastic fibers (orcein) (90) suggest recent hepatocellular necrosis due to dropout of hepatocytes. In wedge biopsy specimens, thickening of the capsule with some subcapsular formation of fibrous septa and islands of hepatocytes are occasionally seen. This appearance must be interpreted with caution. If the fibrosis involves only lobules in close proximity to the capsule, then these subcapsular alterations must be considered to be without pathologic significance (10).

The Portal Triads

Most portal triads contain branches of portal vein, hepatic artery, and bile duct in roughly equal proportions (Fig. 3). A significantly decreased or increased proportion of any of these is abnormal and calls for an explanation. For instance, in adults a decrease in the number of bile ducts to a mean of 0.5 per portal triad or less suggests primary biliary cirrhosis (91). In infants, a value of 0.4 or less suggests intrahepatic atresia (92). Occasionally, clusters of dilated bile ducts, sometimes containing bile plugs, are seen in portal triads. These bile ducts are embedded in a dense collagenous stroma and have been called bile duct hamartomas or Meyenburg's complexes (Chapter 14). The term bile duct adenoma seems less appropriate. Very scanty lymphocytes are normally found throughout

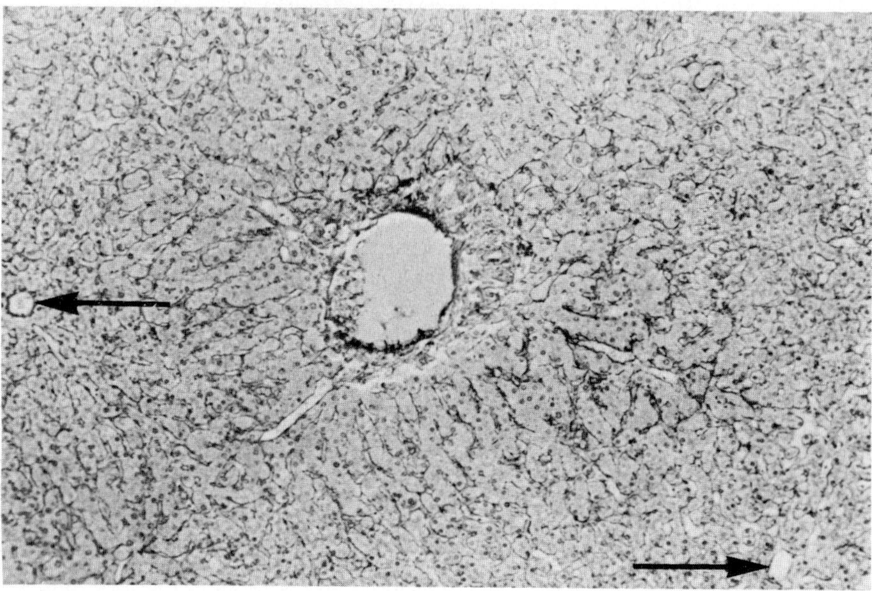

Figure 6. The reticulum framework of the liver is clearly demonstrated. A portal triad is seen in the center. Central veins (arrows) are also seen. Delicate reticulin fibers can be seen throughout the lobule separating liver cell plates from one another. (Reticulum stain, ×85.)

the portal triads. Occasionally this infiltration is fairly conspicuous. If, however, no other abnormalities are seen, such infiltrates appear to have little pathologic significance. In addition to branches of the portal vein, hepatic artery, and bile ducts, the portal triads also contain some generally inconspicuous lymphatics.

The Lobule

The central veins are normally thin-walled, delicate structures that communicate directly with the sinusoids (Fig. 4). The parenchymal cells are rounded in outline, rather than angular and arranged in plates, most of which run radially between portal triads and central veins. After age 5 years, these plates are only one cell wide. Before age 5, the plates may be multilayered (93). The bile canaliculi are slitlike spaces visible in the normal liver only in electron micrographs (Fig. 7). The canaliculi are interposed in a chickenwire-like pattern between the parenchymal cells. At the periphery of the lobules, the canaliculi join the ductules (also called cholangioles or ducts of Hering); these, in turn, join the portal bile ducts. In normal triads the ductules are very short and are therefore generally inconspicuous. Ductular proliferation, often quite striking, occurs in response to various types of injury. Unfortunately, it is not specific for any particular etiology. In addition to the radial plates of hepatocytes, there is usually one plate surrounding the portal triads. This has been called the limiting plate (Fig. 3). Pathologic alterations affect the hepatocytes of this plate particularly, but not exclusively, in chronic active hepatitis.

The sinusoids are located between the hepatic plates, lined principally by two types of cells. Both have elongated nuclei. The histiocytic Kupffer cells have more cytoplasm than do the flattened fenestrated endothelial cells (94, 95). The distinction between these two types of lining cells is often difficult by light microscopy and may require electron microscopic or even electron histochemical study. By light microscopy, these sinusoidal lining cells are closely adjacent to the hepatocytes. By electron microscopy, however, they are separated from the hepatocytes, not by a basement membrane, but by the space of Disse (Fig. 7) (95a). Kupffer cells and endothelial cells with perforations form a continuous layer, but are not attached to each other by desmosomes. In the space of Disse there are also scattered lipocytes or Ito cells (96). Their function is uncertain; it is thought they may play a part in collagen deposition. A fourth type of cell, the pit cell, has also been described (94,95). Clusters of hemopoietic stem cells, predominantly red blood cell precursors, extramedullary hemopoiesis, may also be seen in the space of Disse. This is a normal finding in fetuses and newborns, but is pathologic at older ages. Extramedullary hemopoiesis may be seen not only in the space of Disse, but also surrounding portal triads (Fig. 8).

Histologic Differences Between Biopsies and Autopsies

The overall hepatic lobular architecture in biopsies is identical to that seen at autopsy. However, in hematoxylin and eosin stained sections of biopsy specimens, the hepatic parenchymal cells appear larger and paler than in corresponding autopsy material. This is probably a consequence of their greater glycogen content. The glycogen can generally be demonstrated by staining sections adjacent to those stained with hematoxylin and eosin by the PAS reagent, both with and without prior digestion with diastase. This demonstrates glycogen as diastase labile material. Unfortunately, the preservation of glycogen in formalin-fixed, routinely processed sections is erratic. Glycogen is generally decreased and may sometimes be lost completely during tissue preparation. The space of Disse is more conspicuous in autopsy than in biopsy material, possibly because of the greater shrinkage of hepatocytes in autopsy material. The space of Disse can, however, be visualized easily by electron microscopy. Inflammatory infiltrates appear to be more conspicuous in biopsy specimens than in autopsy material, perhaps because inflammatory cells autolyze rather rapidly. Centrilobular hepatic necrosis, common in autopsy specimens, is less often seen in biopsy specimens, probably because it is a preterminal lesion.

Histologic Differences Between Surgical Wedge and Needle Biopsy Specimens

There are also differences between surgical wedge and needle biopsy specimens. Some of these, such as the difficulties of interpretation which may be caused in wedge biopsy specimens by subcapsular fibrosis, have already been discussed (see above). Another finding in surgical biopsy specimens is a patchy infiltration by neutrophils, with inconspicuous damage to the parenchymal cells (Fig. 9). The

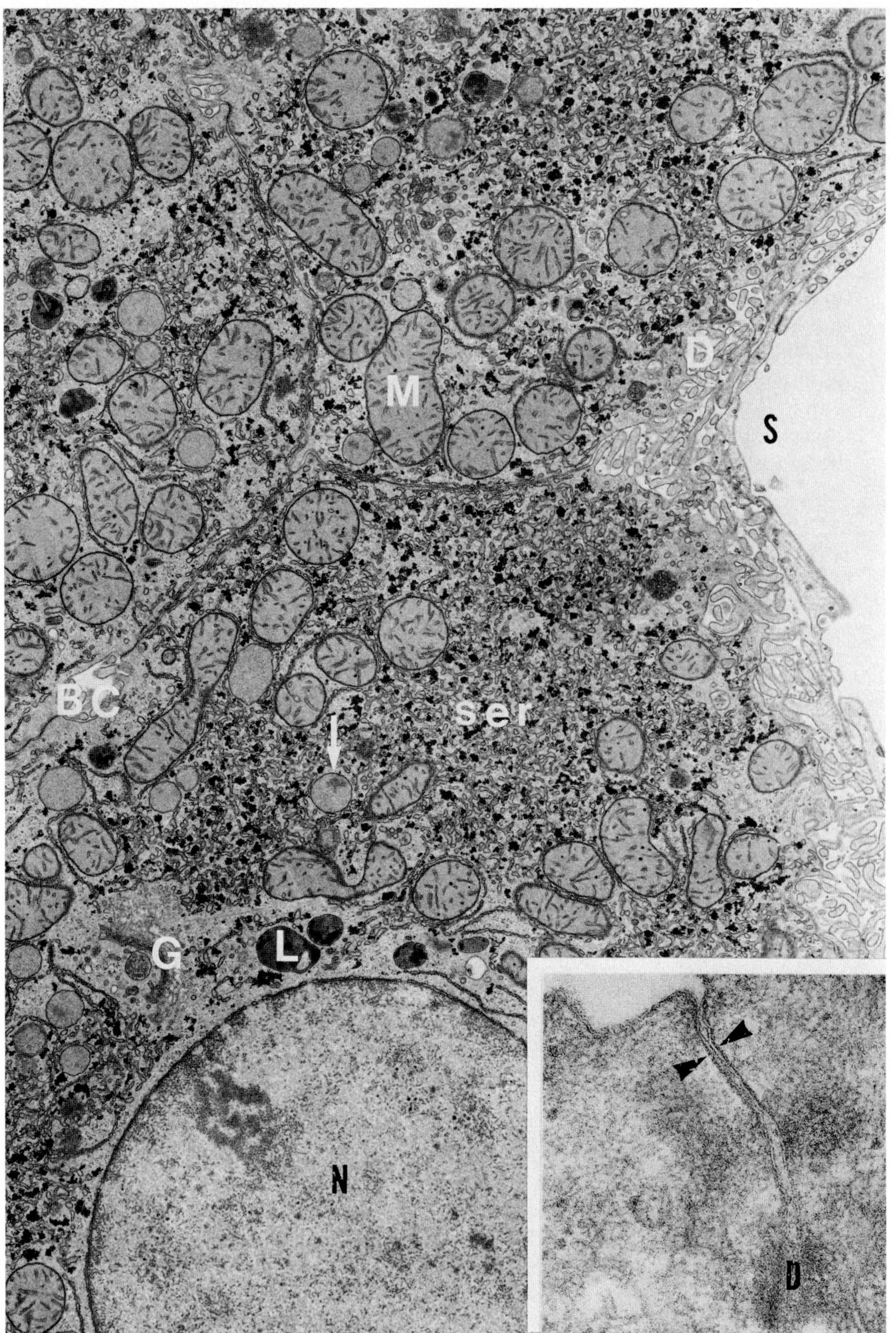

M
D
S
BC
ser
G
L
N
D

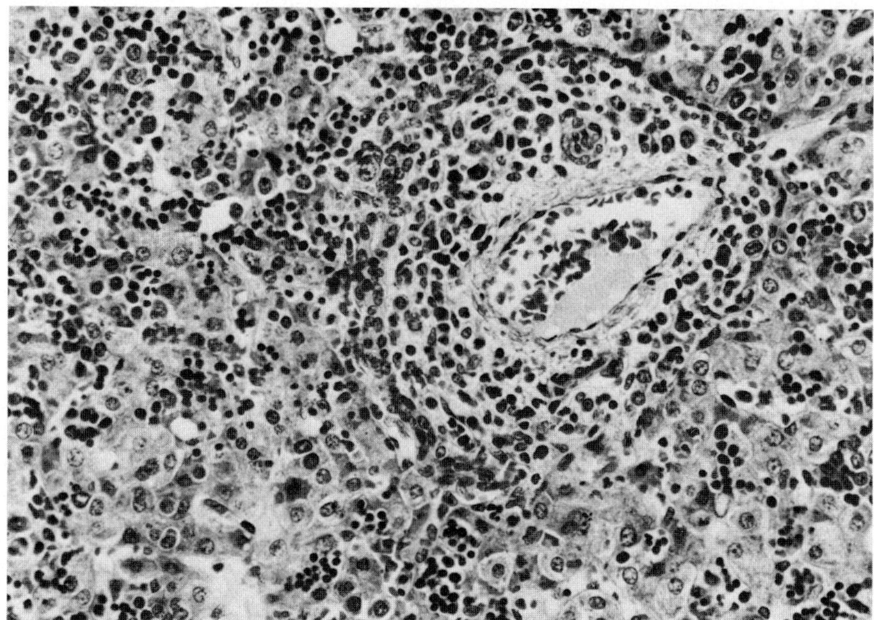

Figure 8. Extramedullary hemopoiesis in the liver of a premature infant. The sinusoids and the portal triad in the right center are diffusely infiltrated by immature hemopoietic cells. (Hematoxylin and eosin, ×250.)

leukocytes may be especially prominent immediately beneath the capsule. This type of neutrophil infiltration is not seen in needle biopsy specimens and is produced by surgical handling of the liver. It can be largely avoided if the surgon takes a wedge biopsy specimen as soon as practical during a laparotomy. Similar changes are seen in victims of recent abdominal trauma. This lesion has to be distinguished from neutrophil infiltration seen in alcoholic liver disease (Chapter 5) and bacterial hepatitis (Chapter 3).

Nuclear Enlargement and Inclusions

Most of the nuclei of hepatocytes in adults are (96a) diploid and appear relatively uniform (97,98). In older patients, a larger proportion of tetraploid and even octaploid nuclei may be found. This leads to greater variation in nuclear size, with some giant, irregularly shaped hyperchromatic nuclei. It is not quite

---

Figure 7. Low-power transmission electron micrograph of portions of three rat liver cells. Note the bile canaliculus (BC), centrally located between adjacent hepatocytes, nucleus (N), smooth endoplasmic reticulum (SER), lysosomes (L), Golgi complex (G), mitochondria (M), microbodies (arrow), sinusoid (S), microvilli in the space of Disse (D). (×12,500.) The inset (×150,000), shows the merging of the outer leaflets of two hepatocyte plasma membranes, thereby forming a tight junction (arrowheads). A few short profiles of microfilaments can be seen in the pericanalicular cytoplasm. Desmosomes (D). (Contributed by A. L. Jones, M.D., ref. 95.)

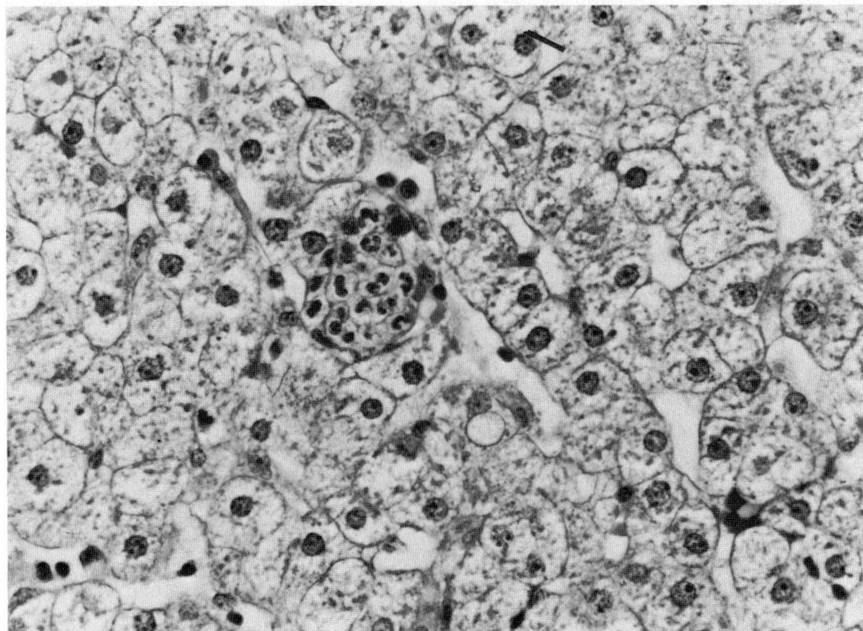

Figure 9. Wedge biopsy specimen obtained at laparotomy. Foci of neutrophils are seen without any other lesions. (Hematoxylin and eosin ×425.)

clear whether it is always possible to distinguish this aging change from nuclear dysplasia, which is thought to be a premalignant change (Chapter 14) (99). Intranuclear inclusions have been long recognized by light microscopy but have been more clearly identified since the advent of electron microscopy. The commonest type of intranuclear inclusion is composed of glycogen and is located most commonly in peripheral zones. By light microscopy, this type of inclusion usually has a clear, punched-out appearance. It is seen most commonly in diabetics and also occurs in glycogen storage disease and Wilson's disease (Fig. 10). However, it may also be seen in many other conditions, and sometimes even in apparently normal livers. It is therefore of little help in diagnosis. Because of the difficulty of preserving glycogen, it is often not easy to confirm the presence of glycogen in these vacuoles. Cowdrey's type A intranuclear inclusions are typical of certain viral infections, such as herpes and coxsackie (Chapter 3). These inclusions appear purple in hematoxylin-stained sections and are typically separated from the nuclear membrane by a clear space, or halo. The inclusions are Feulgen positive and must be distinguished from the rather nonspecific Cowdrey type B inclusions. Type B inclusions are pale pink, in hematoxylin and eosin-stained sections and lack a halo. These inclusions are Feulgen negative. Electron microscopy suggests that they actually consist of cytoplasmic organelles which have herniated into the nucleus. The ingestion of lead or bismuth may result in the formation of inclusions resembling Cowdrey's viral type A inclusions. However, unlike viral inclusions, they are acid fast, PAS positive, and Feulgen negative. The renal tubules are more susceptible to the development of these inclusions than the liver.

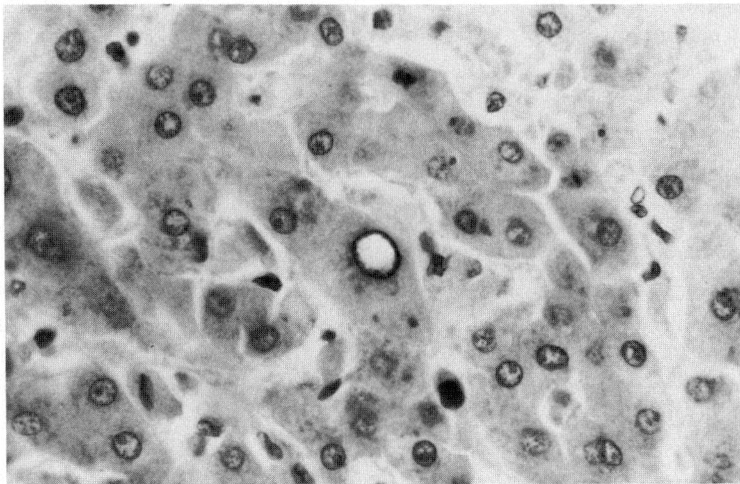

Figure 10. Glycogen nucleus. An enlarged, empty-appearing nucleus containing glycogen is shown in the center of the field. (Hematoxylin and eosin, ×540.)

The Cytoplasm of Hepatocytes

Hepatocytes generally possess quite abundant amphophilic cytoplasms. Their appearance varies greatly, particularly in pathologic conditions, but to some extent in apparently normal livers. The cytoplasm stains somewhat less intensely along the cell periphery. Generalized pallor of hepatocytes, especially in 1-μm sections of tissue embedded for electron microscopy, has been considered to be due to mild hydropic degeneration, but may represent an artifact of fixation (100). More definite pallor and swelling of hepatocytes (ballooning) are well recognized as a form of hepatocellular injury, particularly in viral hepatitis (Chapter 2). A somewhat similar change occurs in cholestasis when groups of hepatocytes containing bile pigment undergo swelling, the so-called feathery degeneration (Chapter 7). It is sometimes difficult to distinguish hydropic swelling from fatty metamorphosis, particularly of the small droplet type. This distinction is made definitively either by frozen sections stained with fat stains, such as Sudan IV or Giemsa (31), or by studying 1-μm-thick sections of tissue embedded for electron microscopy by light microscopy (Chapter 6). This method of preparation usually preserves lipids well and gives them the appearance of greenish droplets. Another type of light hepatocyte is the so-called ground-glass cell, which has abundant pale eosinophilic cytoplasm (Chapter 2). This change is a light microscopic equivalent of proliferated smooth endoplasmic reticulum and is seen in patients treated with certain drugs or infected with hepatitis B (101–103). Similar inclusions may be seen in certain storage disorders. Those in glycogenosis type IV and Lafora's disease (Chapter 10) resemble groundglass hepatocytes, but the inclusions are somewhat more refractile. Those in the other storage disorders are usually more pale staining or empty appearing. Pale globular amyloid bodies have also been described (Chapter 10).

Just as light cells may represent an artifact, so dark cells have been claimed to be artifactual. These are cells, which are otherwise quite normal in their cytoplasmic ultrastructure (100). Certainly distinct hyalinization of hepatocytes (deep pink staining and loss of cytoplasmic basophilia) is a true degenerative change seen particularly, but by no means only, in hepatocellular necrosis due to viruses. Light microscopic cytoplasmic hyalinization may be produced by a variety of ultrastructural lesions (104). One distinct form is the rounded acidophilic (Councilman) body (Chapter 2). Hyaline droplets within hepatocytes may be PAS positive. In such patients, a diagnosis of alpha-1-antitrypsin deficiency should be considered, particularly if the droplets are predominantly periportal (Chapter 9). However, similar droplets may be seen in patients who do not have this condition. These droplets are generally predominantly pericentral, are negative when stained for alpha-1-antitrypsin and are positive for IgG (105). They are probably secondary lysosomes. PAS-negative hyaline bodies in the cytoplasm are most commonly Mallory's hyalin or swollen mitochondria and suggest alcoholic liver disease, particularly in the presence of other histologic changes suggestive of this condition (Chapter 5) (106,107). Mallory's hyalin is an intracellular eosinophilic or slightly purplish material that typically forms ropelike structures twisting around the nucleus. Swollen mitochondria are round or oval structures. Deeply eosinophilic granular hepatocytes (oncocytes) are seen in a great variety of hepatic diseases, particularly hepatitis B and cirrhosis. Oncocytes are densely packed with mitochondria and stain with phosphotungstic acid hematoxylin (108,108a). Calcification of hepatocyte cytoplasm is seen occasionally and is probably related to hepatocellular degeneration (dystrophic calcification).

Hepatic Pigments

Several types of yellowish-brown granular pigment can be seen in the liver by light microscopy, the three principal ones being bile (Chapters 7 and 8), hemosiderin, and lipofuscin (Chapter 11). These pigments can generally be distinguished in formalin-fixed, paraffin-embedded hematoxylin and eosin-stained sections. In addition, performance of the Prussian blue reaction for hemosiderin is usually desirable when a hepatic pigment is found. Occasionally, special stains for bilirubin and lipofuscin, or even electron microscopy to identify a pigment such as lipofuscin and the pigment of the Dubin Johnson syndrome, may also be indicated. Bilirubin, as well as the other pigments, is better preserved in frozen section than in routine sections of paraffin blocks. Frozen sections are, therefore, strongly recommended to demonstrate and identify pigments (109). Bile pigment is not demonstrable histologically in the normal liver. In most cases of cholestasis, whether extra- or intra-hepatic, bile pigment is seen predominantly in central zones (Chapters 7 and 8) (89). It may be present in two forms: as yellowish-brown granules, predominantly in hepatocytes, and as cylindrical plugs in bile canaliculi. Canalicular bile plugs have a characteristic morphology in hematoxylin and eosin-stained sections. Granules of bile pigment, on the other hand, are difficult to identify without special stains. The presence of bilirubin is confirmed by histochemical oxidation to a green pigment (biliverdin) performed by one of a variety of methods. This reaction is usually, but not always, positive on material known to be composed of bile pigment. Sections stained for bile therefore have to be interpreted somewhat cautiously.

Scanty hemosiderin granules normally may be seen in parenchymal cells. Hemosiderin in Kupffer cells and in bile ducts is probably not a normal finding (Chapter 11). Hemosiderin is predominantly located in the hepatocytes at the periphery of the lobules. It is located in pericanalicular lysosomes and therefore has a characteristic intracellular distribution. Refractile yellowish-brown granules can be proved to be hemosiderin by the Prussian blue reaction. This reaction also converts a variable proportion of any bile pigments that might also be present to green biliverdin, particularly if the hydrochloric acid employed in the procedure is freshly made up.

Lipofuscin is normally present in hepatocytes (Chapter 11). Although considered a wear-and-tear pigment, it may be found even in infants. Lipofuscin granules are yellowish-orange, and unlike hemosiderin, are preferentially localized in central zones. Lipofuscin, like hemosiderin, is located in lysosomes and has a similar distribution within hepatocytes. Lipofuscin is actually a group of pigments that are heterogeneous histochemically (39) and morphologically by electron microscopy. They stain negatively with the Prussian blue reaction for hemosiderin and with stains for bilirubin. Lipofuscin is usually positive when stained by fat stains in frozen sections, and sometimes even in sections of paraffin-embedded material, indicating that it may be a form of ceroid. Lipofuscin is usually PAS positive, even after diastase digestion, and is often acid fast.

Morphometry

Up to the present, histology and histopathology have been essentially descriptive and qualitative. Attempts to introduce a more quantitative approach are now being made by many investigators. In light microscopy, measurements are being performed by micrometers, graticules, or by projection (98,110,111). Such methods have been employed particularly in the measurement of nuclear size, and in the study of ploidy and of parenchymal cell necrosis. After the work of Weibel and Loud, morphometric analysis has been applied to electron micrographs. Most of this work has been on experimental material. The mean proportions of the volume of various cellular organelles (volumetric density) and the density of the membranes (membrane surface density) have now been estimated in human subjects (112). It has also been shown that needle biopsies can provide enough material for such studies (113–115). Light microscopic morphometry can be done with a fairly simple apparatus and should take relatively little more time and effort than required for conventional descriptive methods. Wider use of these methods will require that pathologists alter their attitudes. Electron microscopic morphometry requires more sophisticated technology and a greater number of prints than one would normally take. This has hampered the introduction of these methods into diagnostic electron microscopy.

REFERENCES

1. Walters JRF, Paton A: Liver biopsy. *Br Med J* 1:776, 1980.
2. Wilson J, Mason E, Lamis P, et al: Percutaneous needle biopsies of the liver. *Am Surg* 37(3):155, 1971.

3. Sherlock S: Needle biopsy of the liver: A review. *J Clin Pathol* 15:291, 1962.
4. Menghini G: One-second biopsy of the liver—problems of its clinical application. *N Engl J Med* 283:582, 1976.
5. Carney CN: Clinical cytology of the liver. *Acta Cytol* 19:244, 1975.
6. Sipponen P, Pikkarainen P, Vuori E, et al: Copper deposits in fine needle aspiration in primary biliary cirrhosis. *Acta Cytol* 24:203, 1980.
6a. Ho CS, McLoughlin M, Tao LC, et al: Guided percutaneous fine needle aspiration Biopsy of the liver. *Cancer* 47:1781, 1981.
6b. Lightdale CJ, Hajdu SI, Luisi CB: Cytology of the liver, spleen and peritoneum obtained by sheathed brush during laparoscopy. *Am J Gastroenterol* 74:21, 1980.
7. Layden TJ: Percutaneous needle biopsy specimens. *Arch Intern Med* 139:856, 1979.
8. Holund B, Poulsen H, Schlichting P: Reproducibility of liver biopsy diagnosis in relation to the size of the specimen. *Scand J Gastroenterol* 15:329, 1980.
9. Conn HO: Rational use of liver biopsy in the diagnosis of hepatic cancer. *Gastroenterology* 62:142, 1972.
10. Petrelli M, Scheuer PJ: Variation in subcapsular liver structure and its significance of wedge biopsies. *J Clin Pathol* 20:743, 1967.
11. Michel SL, Lipsky R, Morgenstern L: "Routine" liver biopsy in upper abdominal surgery. *Arch Surg* 112:959, 1977.
12. Joishy SK, Balasegaram M: Hepatic resection for malignant tumors of the liver. Essentials for a unified surgical approach. *Am J Surg* 139:360, 1980.
13. Lundvall O, Enerback L: Hepatic fluorescence in porphyria cutanea tarda studied in fine needle aspiration biopsy smears. *J Clin Pathol* 22:704, 1969.
14. Bastin R, Lapresle C, Dupont B, et al: Brucella hepatitis with caseous necrosis. *Med Chir Dig* 2:199, 1973.
14a. Gupta SC, Gupta CD, Arora AK: Subsegmentation of the human liver. *J Anat* 124:413, 1977.
15. Faintucy J, Machado MCC, Raia AA: Suprahepatic gall bladder with hypoplasia of the right lobe of the liver. *Arch Surg* 115:658, 1980.
16. Lieberman MK: Cirrhosis in ectopic liver tissue. *Arch Pathol Lab Med* 82:443, 1966.
17. Vercelli-Retta J: Fetal supradiaphragmatic accessory liver lobe. *Virchows Arch* [*Pathol Anat*] 378:259, 1978.
18. Organ CH, Hayes DF: Supradiaphragmatic right liver lobe and gallbladder. *Arch Surg* 115:989, 1980.
19. Lasser A, Wilson GL: Ectopic liver tissue mass in the thoracic cavity. *Cancer* 36:1823, 1975.
20. Gaber M: Accessory liver containing metastatic tumor. *Virchows Arch* [*Pathol Anat*] 385:361, 1980.
21. Bauer JA, Hellerer O: Characteristics of the shape of the porta hepatis in relation to the size of the liver. *MMW* 116(43):1881, 1974.
22. Ryncki PV: Anatomie chirurgicale du foie. Variations et évolution des techniques d'exérèse et de dérivation. *Helv Chir Acta* 41:543, 1974.
23. Tavill AS, Wood EJ, Kreel L, et al: The Budd-Chiari syndrome: Correlation between hepatic scintigraphy and the clinical, radiological, and pathological findings in nineteen cases of hepatic venous outflow obstruction. *Gastroenterology* 68:509, 1975.
23a. Joishy SK, Balasegaram M: Hepatic Resection for malignant tumors of the liver: Essentials of a unified surgical approach. *Am J Surg* 139:360, 1980.
24. Elias H, Sherrick JC: *Morphology of the Liver*. New York, Academic Press, 1969, p 295.
25. Carson FL, Martin JH, Lynn JA: Formalin fixation for electron microscopy: A re-evaluation. *Am J Clin Path* 59:365, 1972.
26. Hardy KJ, Wheatley IC, Anderson AIE, et al: The lymph nodes of the porta hepatis. *Surg Gynecol Obstet* 143:225, 1976.
27. Shikata T, Uzawa T, Yoshiwara N, et al: Staining methods of Australian antigen in paraffin section—Detection of cytoplasmic inclusion bodies. *Jpn J Exp Med* 44:25, 1974.

28. Deodhar KP, Tapp E, Scheuer PJ: Orcein staining of hepatitis B antigen in paraffin sections of liver biopsies. *J Clin Pathol* 28:66, 1975.

29. Chi EY, Smuckler EA: A rapid method for processing liver biopsy specimens for 2μ sectioning. *Arch Pathol Lab Med* 100:457, 1976.

29a. Zerpa H, Walik NJ, Arborgh BM: Application of routine and immunohistochemical staining methods to liver tissue embedded in a water soluble resin. *Liver* 1: 602, 1981.

30. Luna LG: *Manual of Histologic Staining Methods of the Armed Forces Institute of Pathology*, ed 3. New York, McGraw-Hill (Blakiston), 1968, p 28.

30a. Hall P, Gormley PM, Jarvis JR, et al: A staining method for the detection and measurement of fat droplets in hepatic tissue. *Pathology* 12:605, 1980.

31. Wigger HJ: Frozen section of liver in the diagnosis of Reye Syndrome. *Am J Surg Pathol* 101:271, 1977.

32. Petzhold H, Rogos R: Use of histochemical techniques for studying enzymes in biopsies for the diagnosis of liver disease. *Dtsch Z Verdau Stoffwechselkr* 34(5/6):301, 1974.

33. Hägerstrand I: Distribution of alkaline phosphatase activity in healthy and diseased human liver tissue. *Acta Pathol Microbiol Scand* [*A*] 83:519, 1975.

34. Hägerstrand I: Bile canalicular alkaline phosphatase in necropsy specimens of the liver and its relation to disease. *Acta Pathol Microbiol Scand* [*A*] 84:278, 1976.

35. Wachstein M, Meisel E, Falcon C: Enzymatic histochemistry in the experimentally damaged liver. *Am J Pathol* 40:219, 1962.

36. Ruebner BH, Hirano T: Viral hepatitis in mice. Changes in oxidative enzymes and phosphatases after murine hepatitis virus infection. *Lab Invest* 14:157, 1965.

37. Kaplow LS, Burstone MS: Acid buffered acetone as a fixative for enzyme histochemistry. *Nature* 200:690, 1963.

38. Barka T, Anderson PJ: *Histochemistry*. New York, Hoeber–Harper & Row, 1963.

39. Pearse AGE: *Histochemistry. Theoretical and Applied.* ed 3, Boston, Little Brown, 1968.

40. Gudat F, Bianchi L, Sonnabend W, et al: Pattern of core and surface expression in liver tissue reflects state of specific immune response in hepatitis B. *Lab Invest* 32:1, 1975.

41. Arnold W, Nielsen JO, Hardt F, et al: Localisation of e-antigen in nuclei of hepatocytes in HBsA-positive liver diseases. *Gut* 19:994, 1977.

42. Lamothe F, Laurencin-Piché J, Côté J, et al: Detection of surface and core antigens of hepatitis B virus in the liver of 164 human subjects. *Gastroenterology* 71:102, 1976.

43. Huang S, Minnassian H, More JD: Application of immunofluorescent staining on paraffin sections improved by trypsin digestion. *Lab Invest* 35:383, 1976.

44. Nayak NC, Sachdeva R. Dhar A, et al: Demonstration of hepatitis B virus surface component in human hepatocellular cancer cells. *Indian J Med Res* 69:161, 1979.

45. Ray MB, Desmet VJ: Immunofluorescent detection of hepatitis B antigen in paraffin-embedded liver tissue. *J Immunol Methods* 6:283, 1975.

46. Nayak NC, Sachdeva R: Localization of hepatitis B surface antigen in conventional paraffin sections of the liver. *Am J Pathol* 81:479, 1975.

47. Sumithran E: Methods of detection of hepatitis B surface antigen in paraffin sections of liver: A guideline for their use. *J Clin Pathol* 30:460, 1976.

48. Tapp E, Jones DM: HBsA and HBcAg in the livers of asymptomatic hepatitis B antigen carriers. *J Clin Pathol* 30:671, 1977.

49. Taylor CR: Immunoperoxidase techniques. *Arch Pathol Lab Med* 102:113, 1978.

50. Omata M, Liew CT. Ashcaval M, et al: Non-immunologic binding of horseradish peroxidase to hepatitis B surface antigen. *Am J Clin Pathol* 73:626, 1980.

51. Gerber MA, Sarno E, Vernace SJ: Immune complexes in hepatocytic nuclei of HB Ag-positive chronic hepatitis. *N Engl J Med* 294:922, 1976.

52. Rizetto M, Diana S, Bonino F, et al: Prognostic significance of in-vitro complement fixation in liver biopsy specimens from patients with acute viral hepatitis type B. *Lancet* 2:436, 1976.

53. Hopf U, zum Büschenfeld KHM, Arnold W: Detection of a liver-membrane autoantibody in HBsAg-negative chronic active hepatitis. *N Engl J Med* 294:578, 1976.
54. Tage-Jensen U, Arnold W, Dietrichson O, et al: Liver-cell-membrane auto-antibody specific for inflammatory liver diseases. *Br Med J* 1:206, 1977.
55. Hutteroth TH, zum Büschenfeld KHM: Clinical relevance of the liver-specific lipoprotein (LSP). *Acta Hepatogastroenterol* 25:243, 1978.
56. Purtilo DT, Yunis EJ; Alpha-fetoprotein. Its immunofluorescent localization in human fetal liver and hepatoma. *Lab Invest* 25:291, 1971.
57. Husby G, Strickland RG, Caldwell JL, et al: Localization of T and B cells and alpha-fetoprotein in hepatic biopsies from patients with liver disease. *J Clin Invest* 56:1198, 1975.
58. Nayak NC, Das PK, Bhuyan UN, et al: Localization of α-fetoprotein in human and rat fetal livers. An immunohistochemical method using horseradish peroxidase. *J Histochem Cytochem* 22:414, 1974.
59. DeLellis RA, Sternberg LA, Mann RB, et al: Immunoperoxidase technics in diagnostic pathology. *Am J Clin Pathol* 71:483, 1979.
60. Ray MB, Desmet VJ: Immunofluorescent detection of α_1-antitrypsin in paraffin embedded liver tissue. *J Clin Pathol* 28:717, 1975.
61. Karnovsky MJ: A formaldehyde-glutaraldehyde fixative of high osmolality for use in electron microscopy. *J Cell Biol* 27:137A, 1965.
61a. McDowell EM, Trump BF: Histologic fixatives suitable for diagnostic light and electron microscopy. *Arch Pathol Lab Med* 100:405, 1976.
62. Spurr AR: A low viscosity epoxy resin embedding medium for electron microscopy. *Ultrastruc Res* 26:31, 1969.
63. Richardson KC, Jarret L, Finke EH: Embedding in eopxy resins for ultrathin sectioning in electron microscopy. *Stain Technol* 35:313, 1960.
64. Peterson P: Lipid droplets in fatty liver: An electron microscopic study on ultrasections obtained by a new cutting technique. *Acta Pathol Microbiol Scand [A]* 82:225, 1974.
65. Venables JH, Coggeshall R: A simplified lead citrate stain for use in electron microscopy. *J Cell Biol* 25:407, 1965.
66. Peters TJ, Jenkins W, Dubowitz V: Subcellular fractionation studies on hepatic tissue from a patient with Pompe's disease (Type II/glycogen storage disease). *Clin Sci* 59:7, 1980.
66a. Peters TJ: Investigation of tissue organelles by a combination of analytical subcellular fraction-ation and enzymic microanalysis: A new approach to pathology. *J Clin Pathol* 34:1, 1981.
67. Billing BH, Conlon HJ, Hein DE, et al: The value of needle biopsy in the chemical estimation of liver lipids in man. *J Clin Invest* 32:214, 1953.
68. Lundquist A: Fine-needle aspiration biopsy of the liver. *Acta Med Scand* 520:1, 1971.
69. Eisele JW, Barker EA, Smuckler EA: Lipid content in the liver of fatty metamorphosis of pregnancy. *Am J Pathol* 81:545, 1975.
70. Peters TJ, Seymour CA: Acid hydrolase activities and lysosomal integrity in liver biopsies from patients. *Clin Sci Mol Med* 50(1):75, 1976.
71. Seymour CA, Neale G, Peters TJ: Lysosomal changes in liver tissue from patients with the Dubin-Johnson-Sprinz syndrome. *Clin Sci Mol Med* 52(3):241, 1977.
72. Mann SW, Fuller GC, Rodil JV, et al: Hepatic prolyl hydroxylase and collagen synthesis in patients with alcoholic liver disease. *Gut* 20:825, 1979.
73. Hahn EG, Martini GA: Clinical parameters of fibroplasia. *Ital J Gastroenterol* 12:41, 1980.
74. McPhie JL: Hepatic prolyl hydroxylase activity in human liver disease. *Acta Hepatogastroenterol* 27:277, 1980.
75. Gabrielle L, Leterrier F, Cristau P, et al: Determination of human liver cytochrome P-450 level by electron paramagnetic resonance of liver biopsies. *Clin Chim Acta* 60:147, 1975.
76. Schoene B, Fleischmann RA, Remmer H, et al: The cytochrome P-450 content and the activities of various microsomal enzymes in liver biopsy material from patients. *Gut* 72:760, 1971.

77. Boobis AR, Brodie MJ, Kahn GC, et al: Monooxygenase activity of human liver in microsomal fractions of needle biopsy specimens. *Br J Clin Pharmacol* 9:11, 1980.
78. Held H: Correlation between the activity of hepatic benzo (α) pyrene hydroxylase in human needle biopsies and the clearance of glymidine. *Acta Hepatogastroenterol (Stuttg)* 27:266, 1980.
79. Felsher B, Carpio N: Unconjugated hyperbilirubinemia and chronic persistent hepatitis. *Clin Res* 26:150A, 1978.
80. Sternlieb I: The development of cirrhosis in Wilson's disease. *Clin Gastroenterol* 4:367, 1975.
81. Irons R, Schenk E, Lee J: Cytochemical methods for copper. *Arch Pathol Lab Med* 101:298, 1977.
82. Stuart KL, Bras G, Patrick SJ, et al: Further clinical and investigative uses of liver biopsy. *Arch Intern Med* 101:67, 1958.
83. Hoyumpa AM Jr, Greene HL, Dunn GD, et al: Fatty liver: Biochemical and clinical consideration. *Dig Dis* 20:1142, 1975.
84. Kubasta M, Kubastova B: Liver biopsy in schistosomiasis mansoni. *Acta Univ Palackianae Olomucensis Fac Med* 42:35, 1966.
85. Baggenstoss AH: Morphologic and etiologic diagnoses from hepatic biopsies without clinical data. *Medicine* 45:435, 1966.
86. Theodossi A, Skene AM, Portmann B, et al: Observer variation in assessment of liver biopsies including analysis by Kappa statistics. *Gastroenterology* 79:232, 1980.
87. Rappaport AM: The microcirculatory acinar concept of normal and pathological hepatic structure. *Beitr Pathol* 157:215, 1976.
87a. Ham AW: *Anatomy*, et 7. Philadelphia, Lippincott, 1974, p 695.
88. Sasse D: Dynamics of liver glycogen. *Histochemistry* 45:237, 1975.
89. Dubin IN, Peterson L: An explanation for the centrolobular localization of intrahepatic bile stasis in acute liver diseases. *Am J Med Sci* 336(1):45, 1958.
90. Scheuer PJ, Maggi G: Hepatic fibrosis and collapse. Histological distinction by orcein staining. *Histopathology* 4:487, 1980.
91. Baggenstoss AJ, Foulk WT, Butt HR, et al: The pathology of primary biliary cirrhosis with emphasis on histogenesis. *Am J Clin Pathol* 42:259, 1964.
92. Alagille D: Intrahepatic neonatal cholestasis, in Javitt NB (ed): *Neonatal Hepatitis and Biliary Atresia,* NIH 79-1296. Washington, D.C., US Department of Health, Education, and Welfare, 1979, p 177.
93. Morgan JD, Hartoft WS: Juvenile liver. *Arch Pathol Lab Med* 71:86, 1961.
94. Wisse E: Ultrastructure and function of Kupffer cells and other sinusoidal cells in the liver, in Wisse E, Knook DL (eds): *Kupffer Cells and Other Liver Sinusoidal Cells.* Amsterdam, Elsevier-North Holland, Biomedical Press, 1977, p 33.
95. Wisse E: Observations on the fine structure and peroxidase cytochemistry of normal rat liver Kupffer cells. *Ultrastruct Res* 46:393, 1974.
95a. Jones AL, Schmucker DL, Renston PH: The architecture of bile secretion. A morphological perspective of physiology. *Dig Dis* 25:610, 1980.
96. Bronfenmajer S, Schaffner F, Popper H: Fat-storing cells (lipocytes) in human liver. *Arch Pathol Lab Med* 82:447, 1966.
96a. Adler CP, Ringlage WP, Böhm N: DNA content and cell number in heart and liver of children. *Path Res Pract* 172:25, 1981.
97. Klinge O, Ross W, Struder E: Das Karyogramm normaler und verfetteter Lebern des Menschen. *Virchows Arch [Pathol Anat]* 366:203, 1975.
98. Ranek L, Keiding N, Jensen ST: A morphometric study of normal human liver cell nuclei. *Acta Pathol Microbiol Scand [A]* 83:467, 1975.
99. Anthony PP, Vogel CL, Barker LF: Liver cell dysplasia: A premalignant condition. *J Clin Pathol* 26:217, 1973.
100. Ganote CE, Moses HL: Light and dark cells as artifacts of liver fixation. *Lab Invest* 18:740, 1968.

101. Thomsen P, Poulsen H, Petersen P: Different types of ground glass hepatocytes in human liver biopsies: Morphology, occurrence and diagnostic significance. *Scand J Gastroenterol* 11:113, 1976.

102. Vazquez JJ, Pardo-Mindan J: Liver cell injury (bodies similar to Lafora's) in alcoholics treated with disulfiram (antabuse). *Histopathology* 3:377, 1979.

102a. Thomson P, Reinicke V: Ground glass inclusions in liver cells in an alcoholic treated with cyanamide (Dispan). *Liver* 1:67, 1981.

103. Hadziyannis S, Gerber MA, Vissoulis C, et al: Cytoplasmic hepatitis B antigen in "ground-glass" hepatocytes of carriers. *Arch Pathol Lab Med* 96:327, 1973.

104. Cossel L: Der lichtmikroskopische Befund der globularen hyalinen Körper in der menschlichen Leber und seine elektronen-mikroskopische Aquivalente. *Zentralbl Allg Pathol and Pathol Anat* 123:479, 1979.

105. Reintoft I: Alpha-1-antitrypsin globules in livers from a mediocolegal autopsy material. *Acta Pathol Microbiol Scan [A]* 81:447, 1979.

106. Iseri OA, Gottlieb LS: Alcoholic hyalin and megamitochondria as separate and distinct entities in liver disease associated with alcoholism. *Gastroenterology* 60:1027, 1971.

107. Goldberg SJ, Mendenhall CL, Connell AM, et al: "Non-alcoholic" chronic hepatitis in the alcoholic. *Gastroenterology* 72:598, 1977.

108. Lefkowitch JH, Arborgh BAM, Scheuer PJ: Oxyphilic granular hepatocytes, mitochondrion rich liver cells in hepatic diseases. *Am J Clin Pathol* 74:432, 1980.

108a. Gerber MA, Thung SN: Hepatic oncocytes. Incidence, staining characteristics and ultrastructural features. *Amer J Clin Pathol* 75:498, 1981.

109. Glenner G: Simultaneous demonstration of bilirubin, hemosiderin and lipofusin in tissue sections. *Am. J Clin Pathol* 27:1, 1957.

110. Scott J, Opolon P, Etève J, et al: Liver biopsy and prognosis in acute liver failure. *Gut* 14:927, 1973.

111. Gazzard BG, Portmann B, Murray-Lyon IM, et al: Causes of death in fulminant hepatic failure and relationship to quantitative histological assessment of parenchymal damage. *QJ Med* XLIV(176):615, 1975.

112. Jezequel AM, Koch M, Orlandi F: A morphometric study of the endoplasmic reticulum in human hepatocytes. *Gut* 15:737, 1974.

113. Rohr HP, Luthy J, Gudat F, et al: Stereology of liver biopsies from healthy volunteers. *Virchows Arch [Pathol Anat]* 371(3):251, 1976.

114. Roessner A, Kolde G, Stahl K, et al: Ultrastructural morphometric investigations of normal human liver biopsies. *Acta Hepatogastroenterol* 25:119, 1978.

115. Hess FA, Gnägi HR, Weibel ER, et al: Morphometry of dog liver: Comparison of wedge and needle biopsies. *Eur J Clin Invest* 3:451, 1973.

2
Hepatitis

Although the term hepatitis implies inflammation of the liver, it is generally used as a synonym for hepatocellular injury associated with inflammation. Whether the hepatocellular injury or the inflammation is primary continues to be a matter of dispute in different types of hepatitis.

ACUTE HEPATITIS

In most patient populations, a large proportion of those with acute hepatocellular injury evidenced by anorexia, nausea, abdominal discomfort, and abnormal liver function tests suffer from acute viral hepatitis. Jaundice is frequently present as well. However, certain infections (Chapter 3) and drugs (Chapter 15), may mimic the clinical, and less commonly, the histopathologic features of acute viral hepatitis quite closely. If the diagnosis of uncomplicated acute viral hepatitis is made with confidence on clinical grounds, biopsy confirmation is often omitted. Nevertheless, the histologic picture of "acute lobular hepatitis" (1) seen characteristically in acute viral hepatitis, remains the standard pattern with which other types of hepatocellular injury are compared.

Acute Viral Hepatitis

When a biopsy is performed in acute viral hepatitis, the histologic picture is generally well established (1–4a). Truly early pathologic changes are, therefore, rarely seen in biopsy specimens (5). Proliferation of sinusoidal lining cells and mitotic figures in hepatocytes have been reported. We have also seen focal hepatocellular necrosis with a polymorphonuclear response. The pathologic changes of established viral hepatitis affect most severely the cells in the lobules, rather than those of the portal areas. The pattern of changes includes lesions of hepatocytes, sinusoidal lining cells, and ductular cells combined with a characteristic inflammatory response. Viewed individually, none of these changes is specific. When considered together, however, acute lobular hepatitis, most likely of viral origin, can be diagnosed histopathologically with considerable confidence in the great majority of cases. Despite considerable effort, it remains impossible to distinguish with assurance, in individual cases, the histopathologic changes produced by hepatitis A, hepatitis B, and hepatitis non-A non-B (5). However, hepatitis A, which can be diagnosed by immunofluorescence (6) and electron microscopy (6a), is relatively mild, without any bridging necrosis (7) or tendency to chronicity, and is reported to be predominantly periportal (8). Marked cholestasis may be seen in this type (9). Poulson's bile duct lesion (Fig. 19) (10) and fatty change (9) have been reported to suggest non-A non-B hepatitis. Ultrastructural alterations have also been reported in this disease. (10a). Immunohistochemistry for HB_sAg and HB_cAg is only occasionally positive in acute type B viral hepatitis (11). Orcein stains are usually negative (12,13). Patients with acute hepatitis B whose biopsy specimens show ground glass cells (see p. 51) or other hepatocytes positive for HB_sAg seem to be at an increased risk for chronic hepatitis (13a).

Hepatocellular Alterations

The most striking microscopic alteration in acute viral hepatitis is a disturbance of the normal, orderly arrangement of the hepatic plates. This disturbance is usually termed "lobular disarray" and is quite obvious with the medium-power objective of the light microscope, and possibly even on low power (Fig. 1). When viewed with the high-power objective, it becomes clear that lobular disarray is the result of a great variety of histologic lesions that, while frequently most severe in the central zones (Fig. 2), affect the liver diffusely. These alterations are a mixture of degenerative and regenerative hepatocellular changes associated with alterations in the sinusoidal lining cells and mononuclear inflammatory cell infiltration. The hepatocytes undergo two basic types of degeneration that appear to be the result of cellular changes in opposite directions (14).

The first lesion is hydropic swelling or ballooning degeneration, characterized by enlarged hepatocytes with rounded countours, which appear empty along the cell periphery (Fig. 3). Distinct vacuoles generally cannot be made out in the swollen cells. Special stains show that this cytoplasmic appearance is not the result of fatty change or glycogen accumulation. Residual small wisps of normal appearing cytoplasm may be seen adjacent to the nucleus, the canalicular membrane, or the sinusoidal border. The severity of hydropic change is extremely variable, so that there are striking differences in cell size and shape, even between adjacent hepatocytes. The swelling may be barely perceptible, and presumably reversible, or extremely severe. The nuclei also may vary greatly in size and shape. Severely affected cells tend to have enlarged or swollen nuclei. However, they remain located centrally in the cell. The swelling appears to generally be the result of dilatation of the rough endoplasmic reticulum (Fig. 4).

The second basic morphologic type of degeneration is intense cytoplasmic eosinophilia or hyalinization, as seen most typically in the acidophilic bodies originally described by Councilman in yellow fever (Figs. 5, 6). Acidophilic bodies are rounded, hyalinized, generally shrunken hepatocytes extruded from the liver cell plates into the sinusoids. They are more prominent in viral hepatitis than in other types of acute hepatic injury. Like the other individual histologic changes described here, however, acidophilic bodies are by no means specific for viral hepatitis. The acidophilia is probably at least partly the result of a decrease in ribosomes, and the shrinkage is most likely due to cellular dehydration. The nuclei of these cells tend to be pyknotic and may be absent altogether. Acidophilic degeneration of hepatocytes still located in the hepatic plates is detected only rarely.

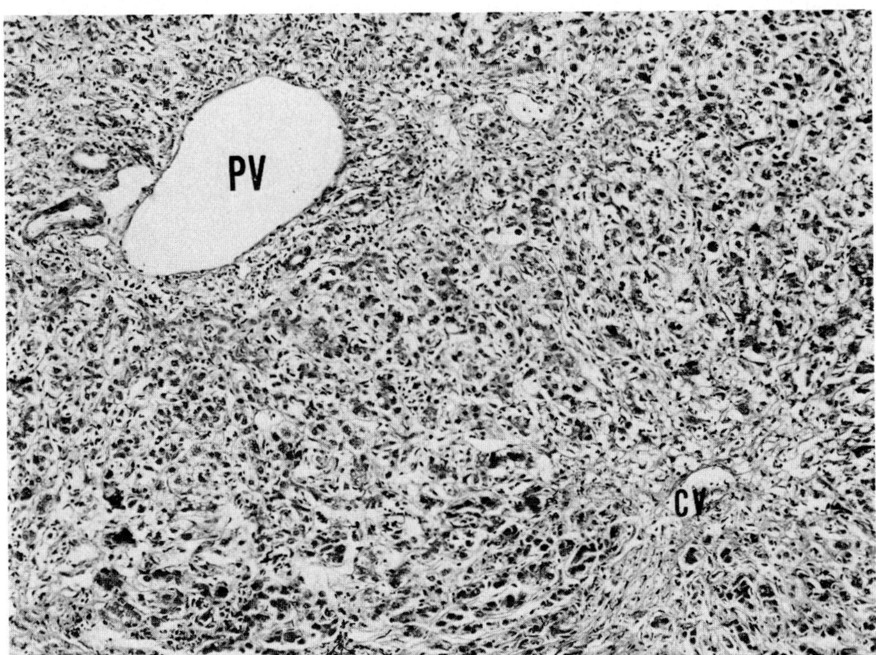

Figure 1. Biopsy specimen from patient with acute viral hepatitis. A portal vein (PV) is seen in the left upper corner and a central vein (CV) in the right lower corner. Some inflammatory cells have accumulated in the portal triad. Note dropout of hepatocytes in the vicinity of the central vein. Considerable irregularity ("disarray") of the hepatocyte plates running from the central vein to the portal triad is evident. (Hematoxylin and eosin, ×100.)

Fatty change is rare in acute viral hepatitis, except in non-A non-B hepatitis (7), and suggests an alcoholic or drug etiology. The histologic diagnosis of viral hepatitis in an alcoholic without the help of viral serology, immunohistochemistry, or electron microscopy remains difficult, if not impossible.

Gaps in the normally continuous hepatocyte plates are common in acute viral hepatitis. These are the result of dropout of single or small groups of hepatocytes as a consequence of necrosis. However, hepatocytes actually undergoing necrosis other than acidophilic bodies are seen only rarely. Large heptocytes with relatively basophilic cytoplasm are often present, particularly in the vicinity of portal triads. These cells sometimes show mitotic figures and may be binucleated or even multinucleated, probably representing an attempt at regeneration. Bile thrombi in canaliculi (Chapter 7), particularly in central zones, are the histologic hallmark of cholestasis and are seen in about half the biopsy specimens from patients with viral hepatitis. A pseudoglandular or pseudoacinar arrangement of hepatocytes surrounding a central lumen often containing a bile thrombus is also seen quite commonly (Chapter 7). Bile pigment may also be found in the form of granules in hepatocytes or in Kupffer cells, where it is sometimes aggregated into clumps. However, it is rare to find granules of bile pigment in the absence of canalicular bile plugs. A granular pigment unassociated with bile plugs should,

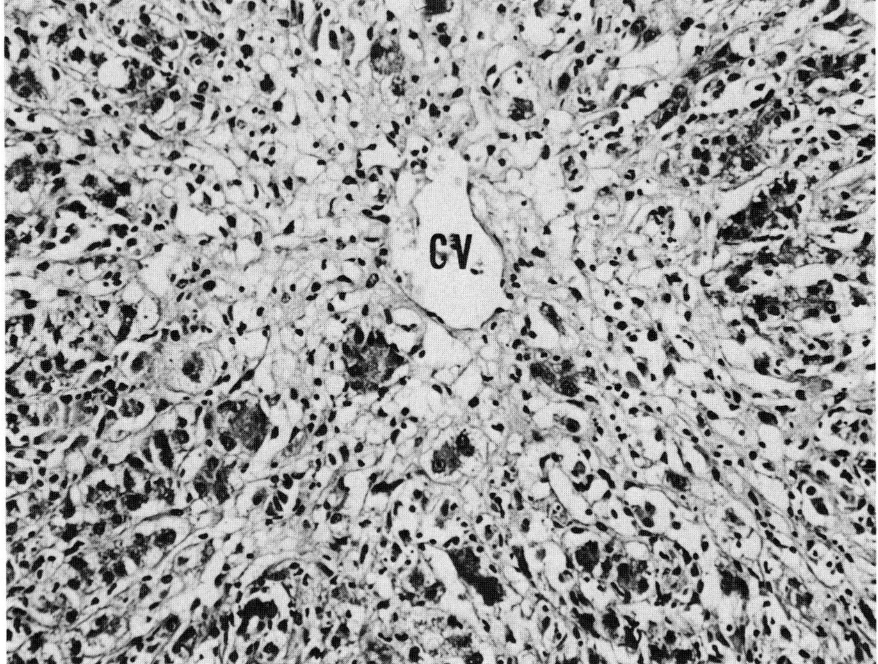

Figure 2. Biopsy specimen from patient with acute viral hepatitis. A central vein (CV) and the central part of a lobule are shown. Note marked drop-out of hepatocytes adjacent to the central vein. Therefore, few of the parenchymal cell plates approach the vicinity of the central vein. The hepatocytes in the plates show considerable disarray. (Hematoxylin and eosin, ×200.)

therefore, not be identified as bile without prussian blue and PAS stains to prove that the pigment is not hemosiderin or lipofuscin (Chapter 1).

Inflammatory Response

Within the hepatic lobule, the inflammatory response associated with widespread acute hepatocellular injury consists predominantly of lymphocytes and macrophages with few, if any, neutrophils. Whether the macrophages are activated Kupffer cells or newly arrived blood monocytes is difficult to determine. The inflammatory reaction is focally accentuated where there has been a dropout of hepatocytes. In these foci, there often are acidophilic bodies extruded from the liver cell plates to be taken up by Kupffer cells. There is also a diffuse Kupffer cell activation with a generalized increase in the number and size of the nuclei of the sinusoidal lining cells. The cytoplasm of the Kupffer cells is PAS positive, even after diastase digestion. Many Kupffer cells contain brown pigment (hemosiderin, bile, or lipofuscin) and nuclear or cytoplasmic debris. Phlebitis involving the walls of the central veins has been described as characteristic of viral rather than other etiologic types of acute hepatitis.

The second principal site of the inflammatory reaction associated with acute viral hepatitis is the portal triads. The inflammatory resonse affects all portal

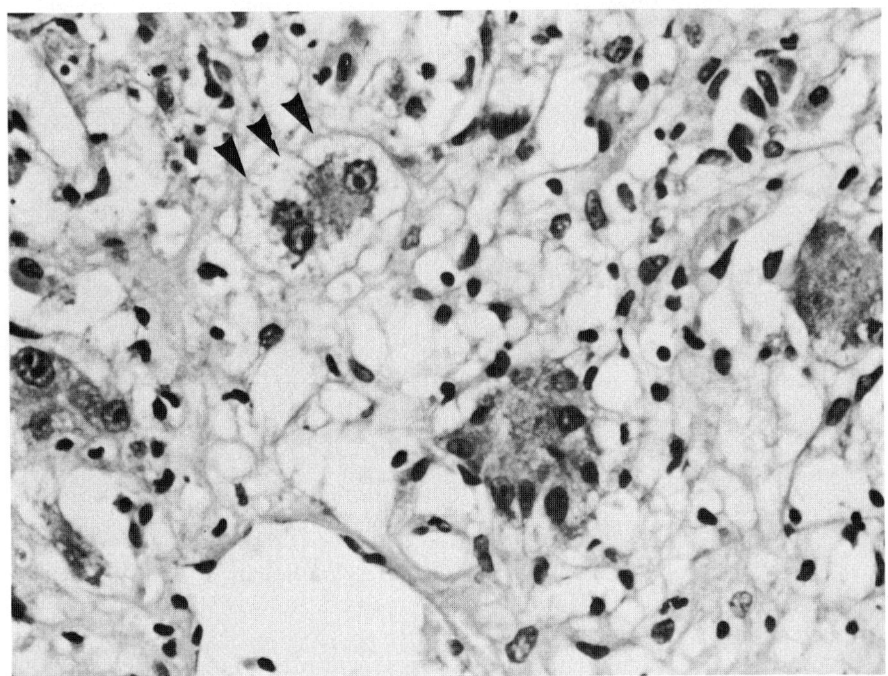

Figure 3. Higher-power view of same area shown in Figure 2. Two hepatocytes are undergoing hydropic swelling (arrowheads). (Hematoxylin and eosin, ×500.)

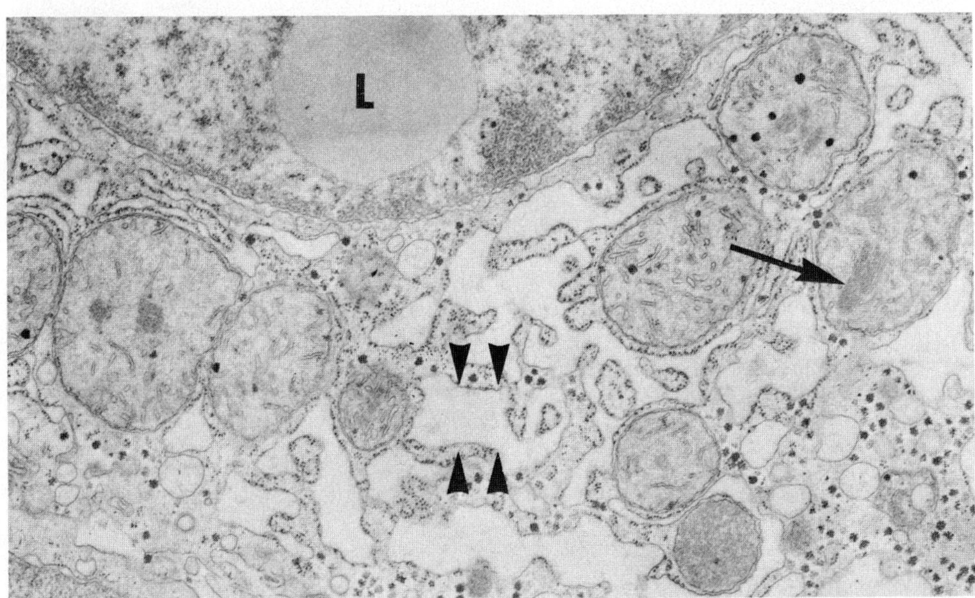

Figure 4. Electron micrograph of a biopsy specimen from a patient with acute viral hepatitis, showing dilation and degranulation of the rough endoplasmic reticulum (arrowheads). Several mitochondria contain paracrystalline inclusions (arrow). A lipid droplet is seen in the nucleus (L). (Lead citrate, ×20,000.)

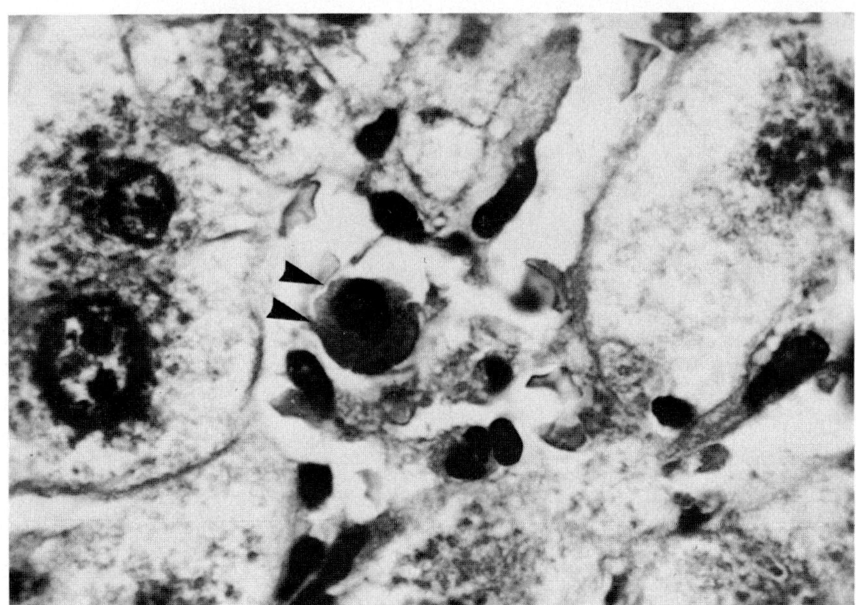

Figure 5. Biopsy specimen from patient with acute viral hepatitis. An acidophilic body (arrowheads) is seen in a sinusoid. The surrounding hepatocytes have undergone hydropic change. (Hematoxylin and eosin, ×1,150.)

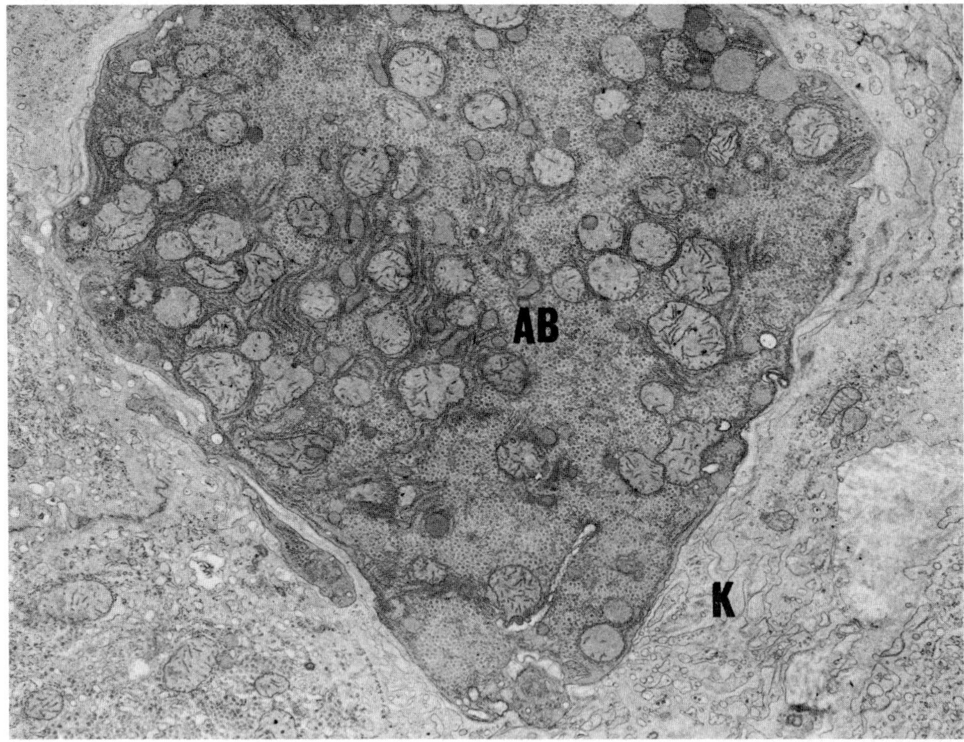

Figure 6. Electron micrographic of an acidophilic body still containing glycogen rosettes and rough endoplasmic reticulum. It is closely adjacent to a sinusoidal lining cell (K). (Lead citrate, ×8,100)

tracts ("universal triaditis" of Gall). The inflammatory cells consist principally of lymphocytes interspersed with macrophages, some of which contain brown pigment similar to that in the lobules. In general, this inflammatory response is virtually confined to the portal areas and extends only slightly, if at all, through the limiting plate into the lobules (Figs. 7, 8). Extension of the portal inflammation through the limiting plate into the lobules with true piecemeal necrosis (see section on chronic active hepatitis) may indicate an increased risk of progression to chronic hepatitis (13a, 15). Ductular proliferation is commonly seen in the portal areas and, unlike the inflammatory reaction in the lobule, the inflammatory response in the vicinity of the proliferated ductules often contains a considerable proportion of neutrophils. Damaged interlobular bile ducts mimicking those seen in primary biliary cirrhosis (PBC) are seen rarely (Fig. 19) (9). If such lesions are found, the differentiation of hepatitis from PBC may require consideration of the total histologic, clinical, and serologic picture.

Bridging Necrosis

Submassive confluent or bridging necrosis (15,16) is seen histologically in specimens of some patients with acute viral hepatitis. In these patients the dropout of liver cells is not limited to small scattered foci as in the average case of acute hepatitis, but involves entire bands (Figs. 9, 10). In terms of the conventional lobule, these extend from central to central, central to portal, or portal to portal areas, whereas in the Rappaport acinus they are located in zone III. In hematoxylin and eosin-stained sections, the inflammatory response accompanying bridging necrosis is generally more conspicuous than the necrosis itself. The inflammatory reaction has a composition similar to that seen in cases of standard severity. The presence of bridging necrosis is best confirmed by reticulin stains showing condensation of the reticulum framework (formation of passive septa as a result of parenchymal cell dropout). Portal to portal bridging is thought by some investigators to be a variant of piecemeal necrosis and less ominous than central–central or central–portal bridging (15). It has been suggested that an adequate biopsy specimen for the diagnosis of bridging necrosis be at least 2 cm in length and contain at least two or three bridges (17). In needle biopsies, however, these criteria can be difficult to fulfill. In such cases, bridging necrosis can only be suspected. In practice it can also be difficult to tell whether the bridges join central or portal areas. The clinical illness of patients with bridging necrosis is not necessarily unusually severe, but it is believed that in these patients it is more likely that massive hepatic necrosis with liver failure will develop or progress to chronic active hepatitis and cirrhosis. Prospective studies are needed to confirm this impression (13a,18,18a).

Massive Necrosis

Massive necrosis is seen in the most severe and frequently fatal fulminant form of hepatitis. Patients suffering from this type of hepatitis rarely have biopsies performed, and most descriptions of the histopathology are based on autopsies. However, the lesions of this type of hepatitis have been studied by biopsy, and the severity of the disease has been assessed morphometrically. The prognosis is poor if liver volume occupied by hepatocytes is reduced to 35% or less (19,20). In

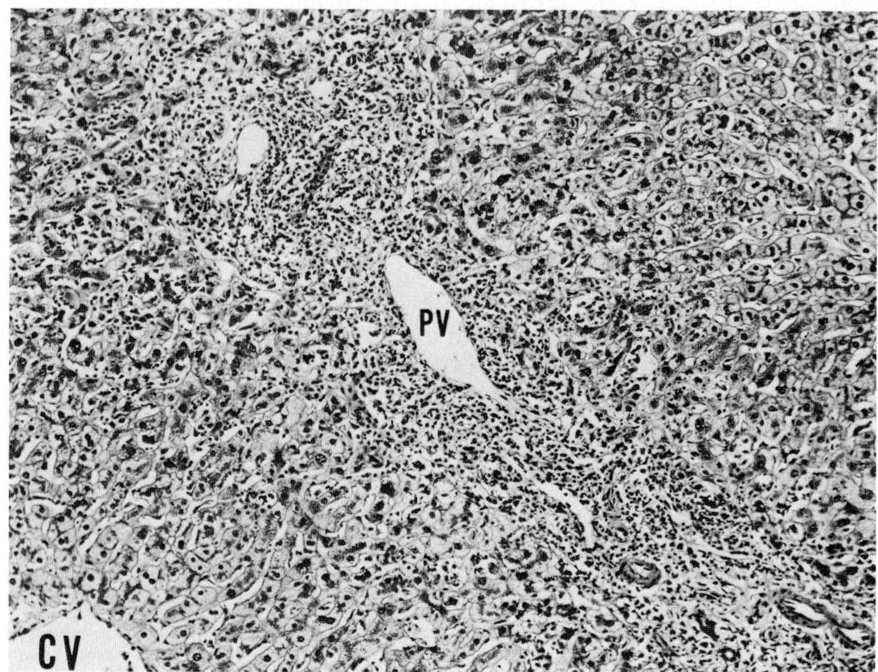

Figure 7. Liver biopsy specimen from patient with acute viral hepatitis. A portal vein (PV) is seen in the center and a central vein (CV) in the left lower corner, showing marked round cell infiltration of the portal triad surrounding the portal vein. (Hematoxylin and eosin, ×100.)

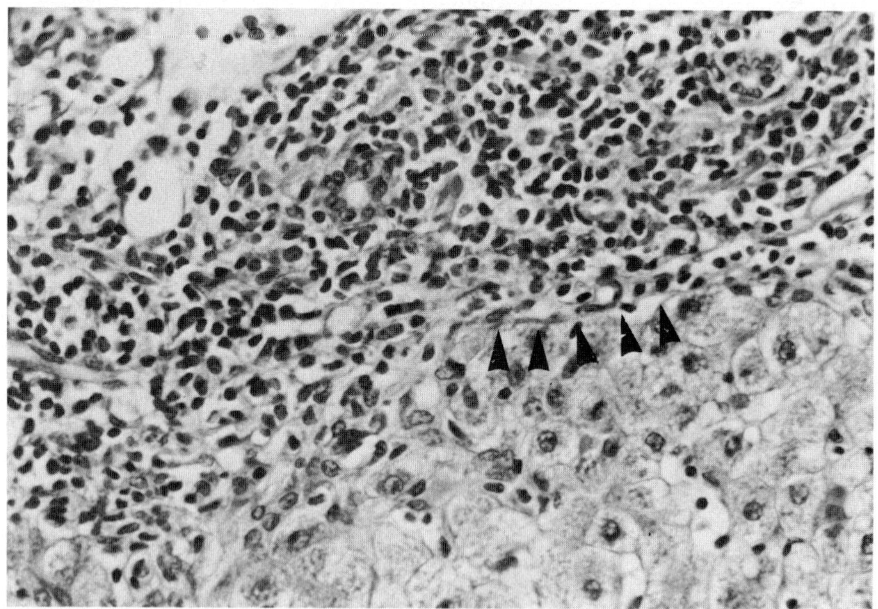

Figure 8. Higher-power view of a portal triad similar to that shown in Figure 7. Note the intense infiltration of the triad with chronic inflammatory cells. The limiting plate (arrowheads), however, is intact. (Hematoxylin and eosin, ×350.)

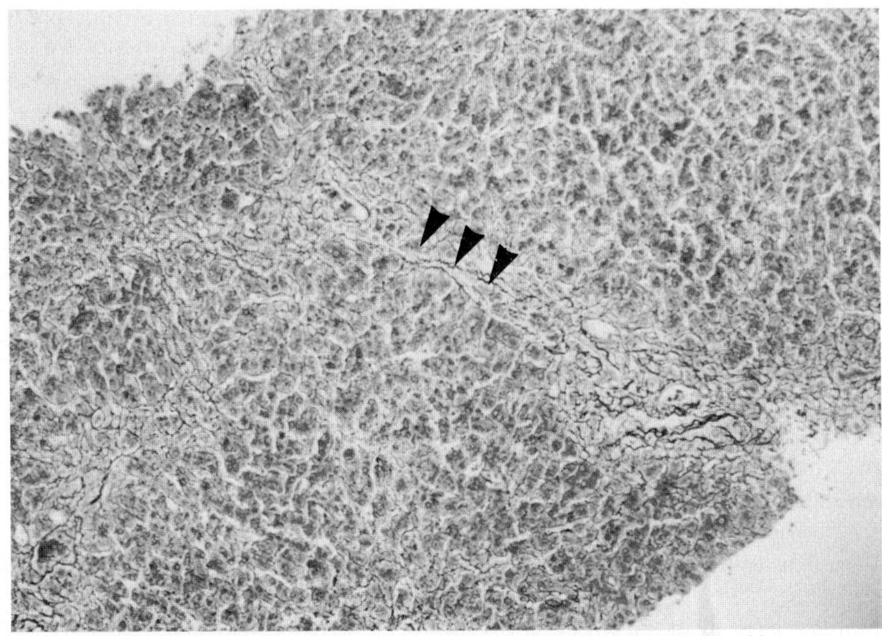

Figure 9. Bridging necrosis in acute hepatitis is indicated by dropout of hepatocytes and undue approximation of reticulin fibrils in a line between a portal triad and central vein (arrowheads). (Reticulin stain, ×85.)

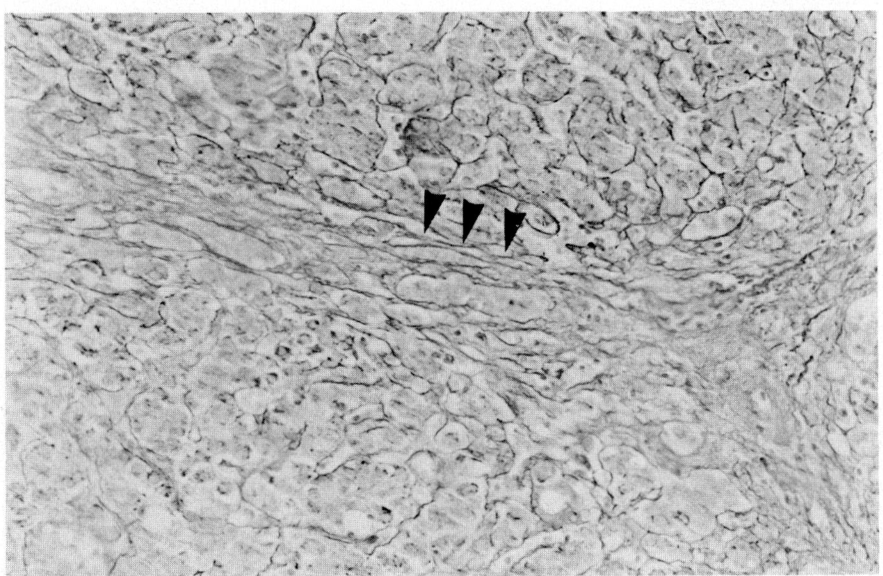

Figure 10. Higher-power view of a different area of bridging necrosis. Note approximation of reticulin fibrils (arrowheads). (Reticulin stain, ×200.)

fulminant hepatitis, the necrosis involves entire lobules, rather than parts of lobules, as in the case of submassive necrosis. Prominence of portal bile ducts and ductules is generally striking in these patients (Fig. 11). This finding may be the result of relative sparing of these structures or may be due to actual proliferation. The ductules are frequently surrounded by neutrophils and may contain bile plugs (3). However, the inflammatory reaction in the lobule remains predominantly mononuclear. Regenerative nodules (Chapter 13) may be seen if the disease has been present for several weeks.

After recovery from fulminant hepatitis, there is considerable collapse and distortion of the hepatic architecture and often some fibrosis (2). Hepatocellular necrosis and inflammation, however, are not conspicuous. Although histologic return to normal can take a year or more, chronic hepatitis and cirrhosis rarely supervene (21,22). During the early recovery phase, many patients undergo a stage of severe cholestasis that can be accompanied by bile lakes (Chapter 7), a finding customarily associated with extrahepatic obstruction (23). The recovery from hepatitis of ordinary severity is characterized by a gradual resolution of the histopathologic changes of acute viral hepatitis. The most persistent changes are focal proliferations of sinusoidal lining cells and persistent groups of enlarged macrophages (Fig. 12), usually containing lipofuscin or hemosiderin, or both, in the lobules, as well as in portal triads. Mitotic figures in hepatocytes are sometimes quite prominent at this stage. Slender, fibrous septa are occasionally seen extending into the lobules from portal triads.

Cholestatic Hepatitis

The diagnosis of cholestatic hepatitis has been used for patients whose major symptom is severe jaundice. Liver biopsy specimens in such cases show severe cholestasis, predominantly central. The histologic differentiation of extra- and intrahepatic cholestasis is discussed in Chapters 7 and 8. Hydropic swelling and pseudoglandular transformation of hepatocytes are striking in cholestatic hepatitis. Xanthomatous (feathery) transformation of hepatocytes, more commonly seen in extrahepatic obstruction and occasionally in primary biliary cirrhosis and drug-induced cholestasis (Chapter 15), has also been described in cholestatic hepatitis (3). The other histologic features of lobular hepatitis, such as acidophilic bodies, are generally present but tend to be less severe than in the standard type of viral hepatitis. The portal tract changes may mimic those seen in mechanical extrahepatic obstruction. The number of small bile ductules in portal tracts usually appears increased and the walls of the ductules may be infiltrated by neutrophils. The ductules might also be dilated and contain bile plugs. There may also be some portal fibrosis. Finding at least some of the typical lobular changes of hepatitis is in favor of cholestatic hepatitis, whereas proliferation of large bile ducts and periductal fibrosis are in favor of mechanical obstruction. Cholestatic hepatitis may have a prolonged course before recovery, so much so that Ishak (3) has coined the term "chronic cholestatic viral hepatitis." However, complete recovery is the rule in these patients, even though it can take up to 1 year. Cholestatic hepatitis seems to be relatively common in type A hepatitis (8).

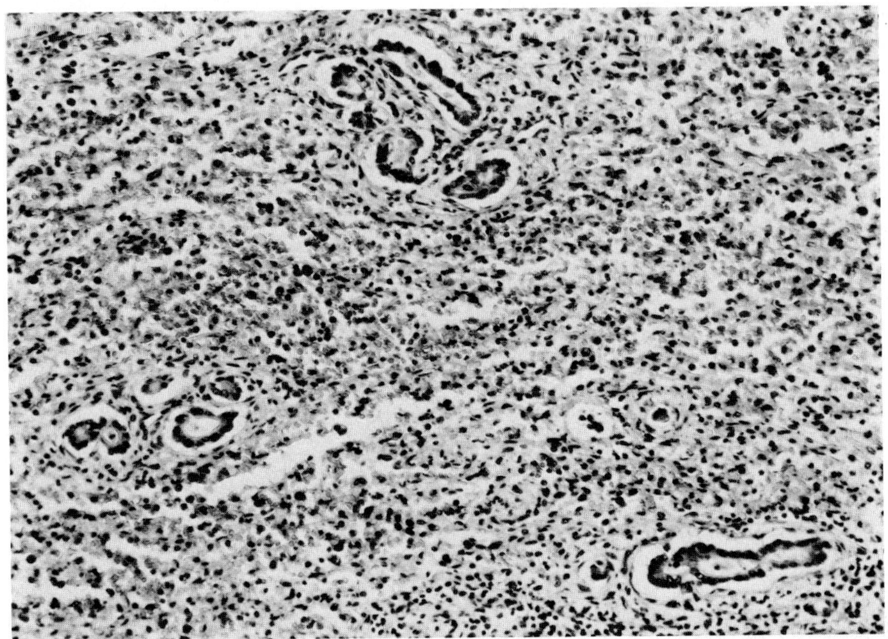

Figure 11. Massive hepatic necrosis, showing virtually no hepatocytes. Three groups of bile ducts, however, are spared and stand out prominently. (Hematoxylin and eosin, ×90.)

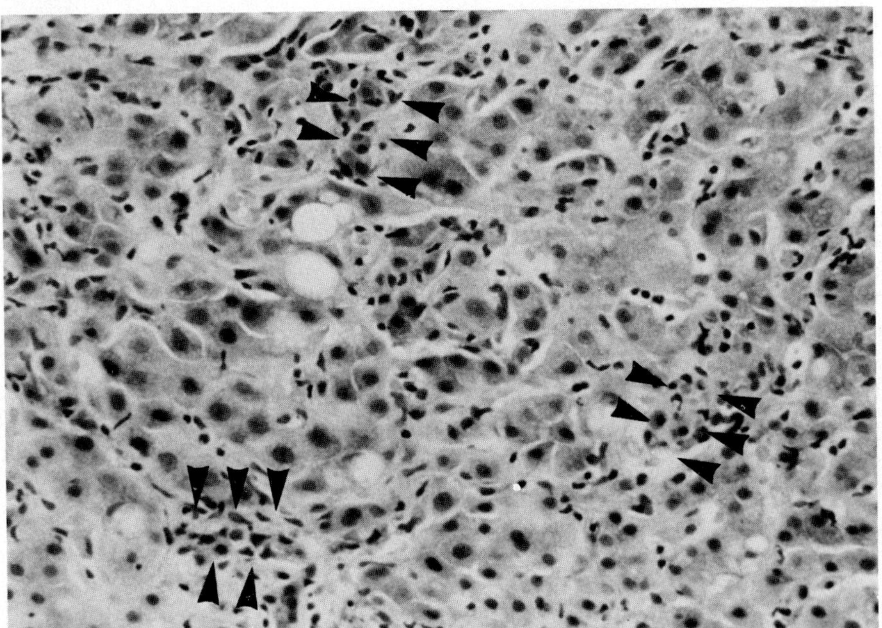

Figure 12. Biopsy specimen from a patient recovering from acute viral hepatitis, showing some lobular unrest. Several Kupffer cell aggregates are seen (arrowheads). Hematoxylin and eosin, ×55.)

CHRONIC HEPATITIS

The clinical picture of chronic hepatitis resembles quite closely that of acute hepatitis. The histologic features also cannot always be relied on to make this distinction (24). A generally accepted, if somewhat arbitrary, definition is that acute hepatitis usually lasts less than 6 months, whereas chronic hepatitis is usually not diagnosed until the illness has lasted at least 6 months. The histopathology of chronic hepatitis has been reviewed in several recent articles (1,4,15,17,25–27c). Chronic hepatitis most frequently is of viral or autoimmune etiology. However, drug-induced liver injury (Chapter 15), as well as Wilson's disease and possibly alpha-1-antitrypsin deficiency (Chapter 9), can assume the morphologic features of chronic hepatitis. Primary biliary cirrhosis and pericholangitis (Chapter 7) share morphologic features with chronic hepatitis. Apparently alcoholic hepatitis can, in rare instances, have the morphology of chronic active hepatitis (Chapter 5). Nonspecific reactive hepatitis (Chapter 3) may be indistinguishable from chronic persistent hepatitis morphologically. Chronic hepatitis in children may differ somewhat from the disease seen in adults (27c).

Chronic Lobular Hepatitis

Chronic lobular hepatitis is the diagnostic term used for patients who have the clinical and histopathologic features of acute viral hepatitis from 6 months up to several years (28,29). Histologically, this type of hepatitis appears to be a protracted form of acute hepatitis and has little in common with chronic persistent and chronic active hepatitis. Parenchymal cell ballooning, acidophilic bodies, and portal inflammation tend to be less striking than in acute viral hepatitis, although focal necrosis, Kupffer cell activation, and portal fibrosis are relatively pronounced (29). In one series all patients were negative for hepatitis B. Complete clinical and morphologic recovery was the rule (30).

Chronic Persistent Hepatitis

Chronic persistent or portal (1) hepatitis also is a benign, self-limiting condition that can wax and wane for years without leading to cirrhosis. It is characterized by conspicuous inflammatory infiltrates of the portal tracts, which, unlike those seen in acute viral hepatitis, may spare some portal triads almost completely. The infiltrates are composed of lymphocytes, macrophages, and occasional plasma cells, which rarely form follicular aggregates (Fig. 13). There may be a relatively mild degree of ductular proliferation. These small ductules can extend into the lobular parenchyma and can be surrounded by a cuff of inflammatory cells and thin septa of connective tissue. Patients with chronic persistent hepatitis who show such septa have been designated as a special group under the term "chronic septal hepatitis" (31). In chronic persistent hepatitis there may be some spillage of inflammatory cells through the limiting plate into the periphery of the lobule. However, the hepatocellular changes of piecemeal necrosis, described in the following section, are not seen in this type of chronic hepatitis or are minimal. Since piecemeal necrosis is a focal lesion, step sections to look for this lesion are indicated in all biopsies showing the appearance of chronic persistent

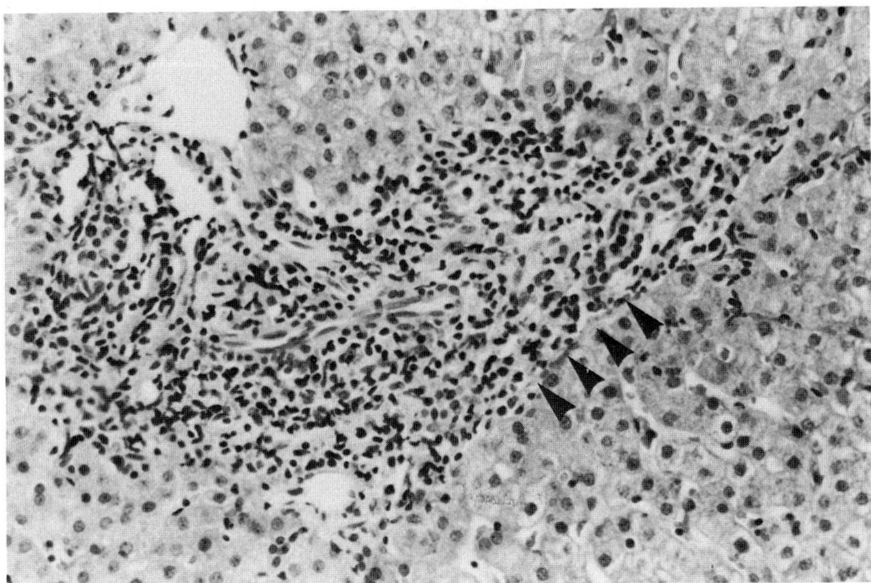

Figure 13. Chronic persistent hepatitis, showing marked portal round cell infiltration. The limiting plate between the portal triad and hepatic lobule (arrowheads), however, is intact. (Hematoxylin and eosin, ×55.)

hepatitis and containing only a few portal triads. Apart from scanty scattered acidophilic bodies and small foci of necrosis (Fig. 14) scattered through the lobules, the parenchymal cells are normal, and the lobular disarray characteristic of acute viral hepatitis is absent. In occasional patients having this disease, clinical exacerbations develop and then have morphologic changes identical with those of chronic lobular hepatitis. Apart from the duration of their illness and possibly a rather intense portal round cell infiltrate, there may be very little to distinguish biopsy specimens during such exacerbations from those of patients with classical acute viral hepatitis. A few patients with chronic persistent hepatitis progress to mild chronic active hepatitis, but cirrhosis apparently does not develop (32).

Chronic Active Hepatitis

Chronic active hepatitis has also been called chronic aggressive or chronic periportal hepatitis (1,5). This diagnosis implies the possible development of cirrhosis and suggests that steroid therapy should at least be considered. In chronic active hepatitis, the portal inflammatory infiltrate is similar in cellular composition to that of chronic persistent hepatitis. As in chronic persistent hepatitis, some portal triads may be spared, and lobular disarray is minimal. However, the infiltrates in the portal triads tend to be more intense than in chronic persistent hepatitis, and plasma cells may be more prominent. The portal inflammatory infiltrates may be organized into lymphoid follicles, sometimes with germinal centers. The term "plasma cell hepatitis" has been applied to those patients whose portal inflammatory infiltrate has a particularly high proportion of plasma cells. It is questionable as to whether this feature defines a clinically

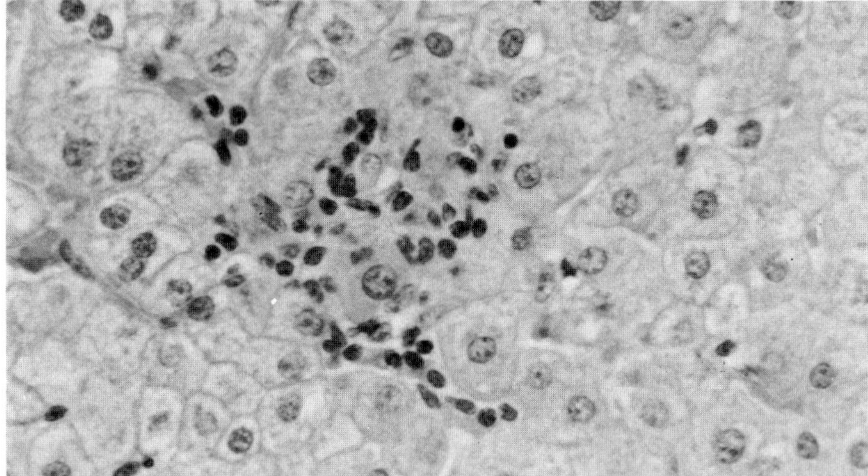

Figure 14. Chronic persistent hepatitis, showing a small focus of necrosis, with dropout of hepatocytes and infiltration by inflammatory cells in a lobule. (Hematoxylin and eosin, ×350.)

distinct subgroup of patients with chronic active hepatitis. However, plasma cell hepatitis appears to be more common in "lupoid hepatitis," a subgroup negative for hepatitis B but positive for antinuclear antibodies. The differentiation of "lupoid hepatitis" from systemic lupus erythematosus with hepatic involvement continues to be a subject of debate (33).

The histologic hallmark of chronic active hepatitis is piecemeal necrosis. This consists of infiltration of inflammatory cells from some portal areas into the lobule with erosion of the limiting plate (Figs. 15,16). Individual hepatocytes in the limiting plate or small groups of hepatocytes arranged in a pseudoacinar pattern are swollen (ballooned) and surrounded by inflammatory cells and reticulin fibers. Baggenstoss and collaborators (34) pointed out that bridging (submassive) necrosis (Figs. 9,10) or multilobular necrosis (Fig. 17), and fibrosis may be seen in association with chronic active hepatitis. Evidence of regeneration, as indicated by hepatic plates more than one cell thick (Fig. 18) and cirrhosis, most frequently macronodular (Chapter 13), may also be evident. Boyer (4) therefore subclassified this group of patients into those with piecemeal necrosis only, those with bridging necrosis and multilobular necrosis, in addition to piecemeal necrosis, and those with cirrhosis, as well as chronic active hepatitis. Baggenstoss et al. (34) graded the inflammatory response in chronic active hepatitis from + to +++. There is now widespread, but not universal, agreement that patients with bridging or multilobular necrosis have a greater tendency to progress to cirrhosis than is true of those patients who have piecemeal necrosis only (4,35). Lesions have been described in chronic, as well as acute hepatitis (36) involving the medium-size interlobular bile ducts and resembling those seen in primary biliary cirrhosis (Fig. 19) (9). These lesions appear to be characteristic of hepatitis non-A non-B. Multinucleated hepatocytic giant cells, like those seen in "neonatal giant cell hepatitis" (Chapter 8), are occasionally seen in adults with chronic hepatitis (37).

In practice, it can be difficult to diagnose chronic active hepatitis in biopsy

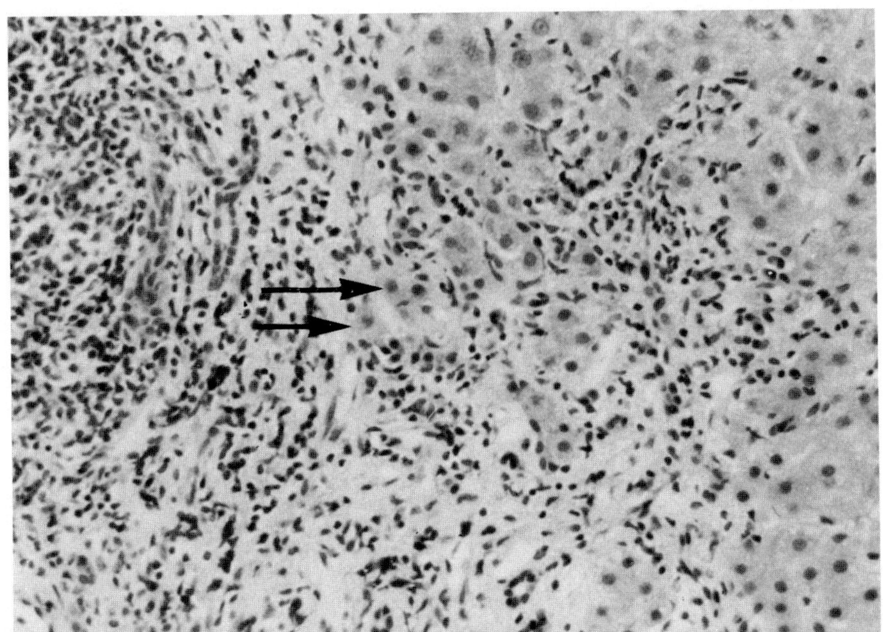

Figure 15. Chronic active hepatitis with piecemeal necrosis. Groups of inflammatory cells have invaded from the portal triad on the left through the limiting plate into the lobule. Individual hepatocytes or small groups of hepatocytes (arrows) in the region of the limiting plate are surrounded by inflammatory cells. (Hematoxylin and eosin stain, ×55.)

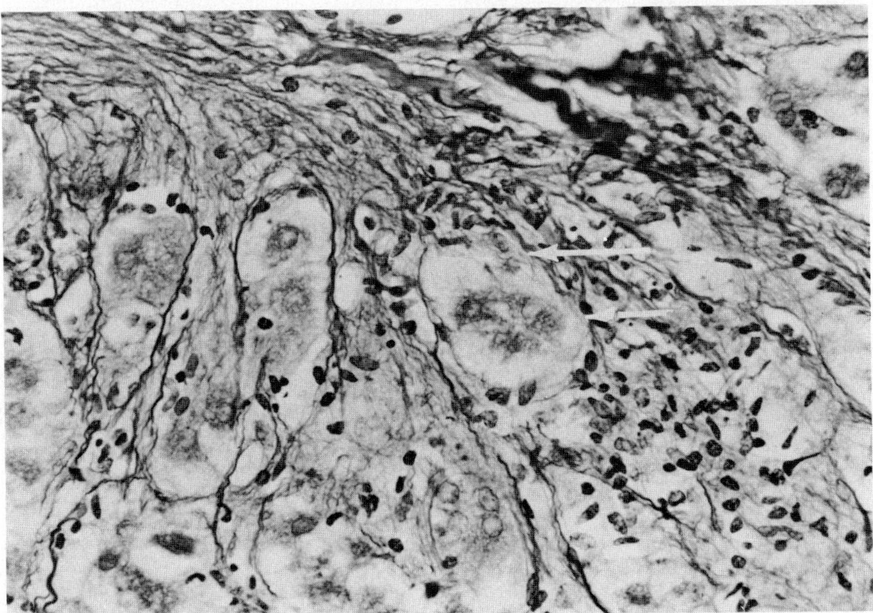

Figure 16. Higher-power view of piecemeal necrosis in a patient with chronic active hepatitis. The portal triad is in the upper part of the field. Ballooned individual hepatocytes and small groups of hepatocytes (arrows) in the region of the limiting plate are surrounded by inflammatory cells and reticulin fibers. (Reticulin stain, ×350.)

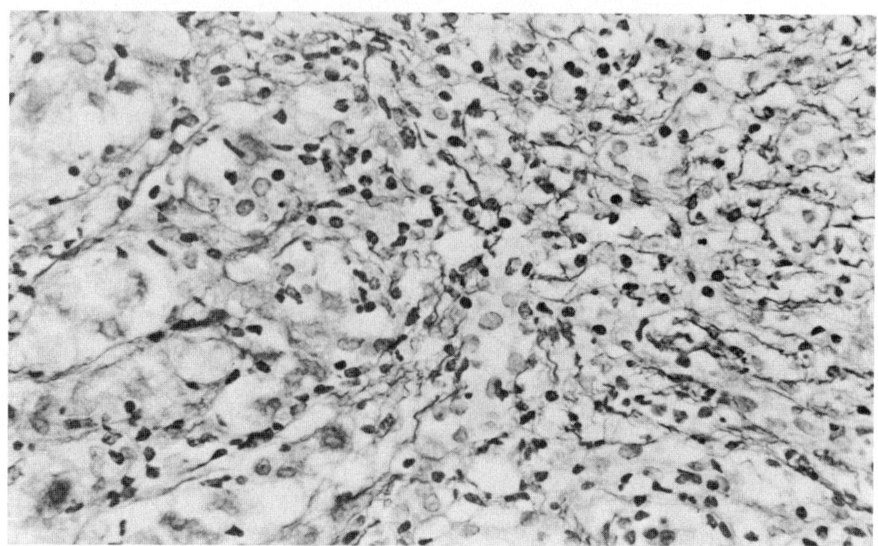

Figure 17. Biopsy specimen from patient with chronic active hepatitis. Extensive collapse of a lobule is indicated in the right half of the field, as evidenced by approximation of reticulin fibers, compared with the left half, which shows viable hepatocytes and a more normal reticulum pattern. (Reticulin stain, ×350.)

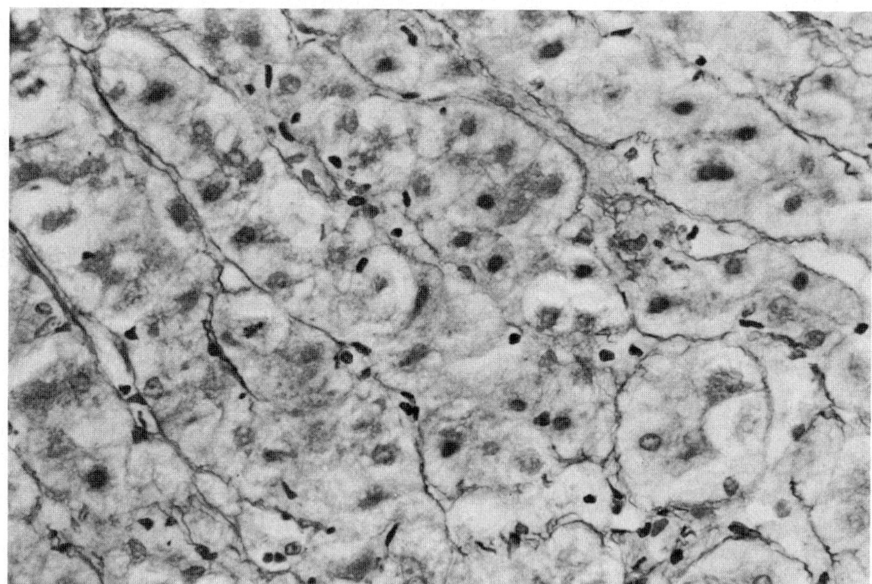

Figure 18. A different area from the same biopsy shown in Figure 17 shows liver cell plates, mostly two cells thick, suggesting regeneration. (Reticulin stain, ×350.)

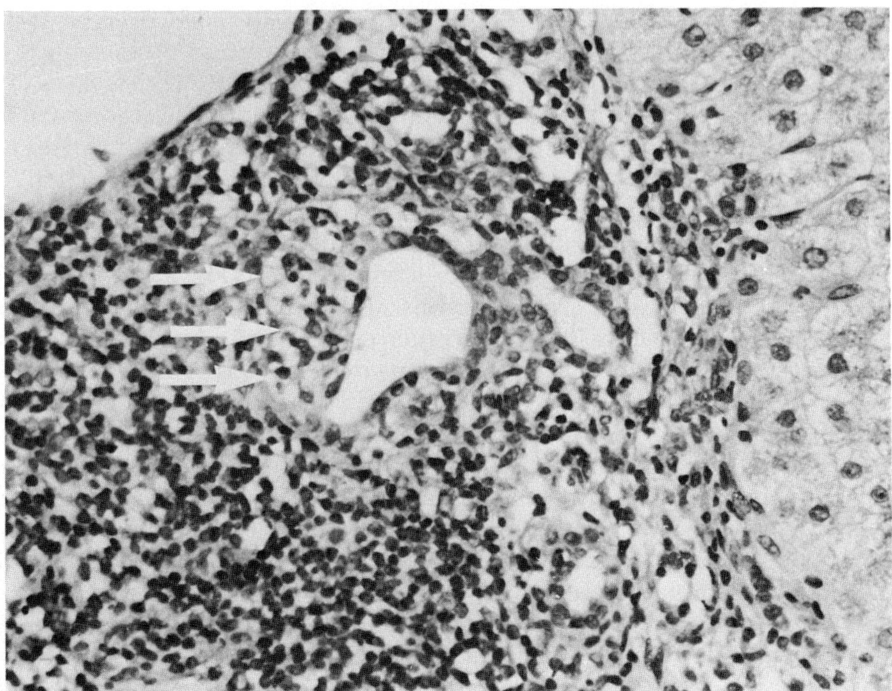

Figure 19. Chronic active hepatitis, showing a portal triad with chronic inflammatory cells and an abnormal bile duct with multilayered and vacuolated epithelium (arrows). (Hematoxylin and eosin, ×250.) (Contributed by H. Poulson, M.D.)

specimens of patients who still have the lobular features of acute viral hepatitis, or in those who have chronic active hepatitis with acute lobular exacerbation. Careful clinical follow-up with sequential biopsies may be required in such cases. The suggestion not to diagnose chronic active hepatitis until the disease has been present for at least 6 months is also of some help. Nevertheless, a diagnosis of chronic hepatitis can occasionally be made with a shorter clinical history, provided patients demonstrate the typical pathologic and biochemical findings of chronic hepatitis. Presumably, such patients have had a previous subclinical phase of the disease. Sequential biopsies are also valuable in following patients with chronic active and chronic persistent hepatitis. A scoring system for assessing histologic activity in serial biopsies has been described (37a). Chronic persistent hepatitis occasionally seems to be transformed into chronic active hepatitis (32), whereas chronic active hepatitis occasionally changes into chronic persistent hepatitis, particularly under steroid therapy. However, the principal reason for sequential biopsies in chronic active hepatitis is to monitor the possible development of fibrosis and cirrhosis. Because of the possibility of sampling error, some caution is indicated in drawing conclusions from sequential biopsies.

Immunopathology of Hepatitis

Routine light microscopy generally does not permit identification of the etiologic factor responsible in an individual case. Hepatitis caused by type B viral hepatitis has been investigated more thoroughly than has hepatitis associated with other causal factors. Morphologic clues available in the diagnosis of type B viral hepatitis include the occasional finding in hematoxylin and eosin-stained sections of hepatocytes with ground-glass cytoplasm (Figs. 20,21) (38) or "sanded nuclei" (39) or proof by immunohistochemistry or electron microscopy of the presence of hepatitis B antigens. Ground-glass hepatocytes are cells that tend to be enlarged, having a lightly eosinophilic cytoplasm resembling frosted glass. This change may affect the entire cytoplasm or only part of it (40,41). The ground-glass appearance in hepatitis B is the result of proliferation of the smooth endoplasmic reticulum interspersed with tubules of HB_sAg (Fig. 25). Ground-glass cells are very rare in acute viral hepatitis and are most plentiful in chronic carriers of HB_sAg who have little or no other morphologic evidence of hepatitis. Ground-glass hepatocytes can also be seen in chronic persistent or chronic active hepatitis, in cirrhosis, and even in hepatocarcinomas. Shikata et al. (13) introduced three empirical methods to stain the cytoplasm of ground-glass hepatocytes. Of these, the orcein (Fig. 21) and aldehyde fuchsin methods are most popular. The mechanism of these stains is thought to depend on disulfide bonds in the HB_sAg. Shikata's stains distinguish ground-glass cells associated with HB_sAg from similar cells, which may be the result of drug-induced proliferation of the smooth endoplasmic reticulum (Fig. 22). Although the Shikata stains are useful in practice, immunohistochemical identification of HB_sAg is more specific and more sensitive (42). Both Shikata's methods and immunohistochemistry have also shown that the HB_sAg may be present in cells that do not have the classic ground-glass cytoplasm. Some of these contain faintly basophilic cytoplasmic material. Irregularly shaped intranuclear inclusions (sanded nuclei) containing HB_cAg have now also been identified by light microscopy. These inclusions are finely granular and faintly eosinophilic without a limiting membrane (39). More specifically, HB_cAg particles have been localized both immunohistochemically (Fig. 23) and by electron microscopy (Fig. 24), predominantly, but not exclusively in the nucleus (43).

Differences have been described in the frequency, distribution and morphology of surface and core antigens of patients with different types of hepatitis B. Morphologic demonstration of these antigens is, therefore, helpful in the subclassification of hepatitis B, particularly in distinguishing between acute and chronic hepatitis (44,45). In acute hepatitis B, HB_sAg and HB_cAg are rarely demonstrable. In healthy carriers, islands of hepatocytes usually contain diffuse cytoplasmic HB_sAg without membranous localization and no HB_cAg (46,47). Positive cells amount to about 20% of hepatocytes (48). Similar results have been obtained in chronic persistent hepatitis and in cirrhosis with little activity (45,47). In chronic active hepatitis and active cirrhosis, nuclear HB_cAg and cytoplasmic HB_sAg are randomly distributed in almost equal amounts in about 1% of hepatocytes (48). Often, the HB_sAg does not occupy the entire cell but is localized principally along cell membranes (Fig. 25) (45,47,49,50). Patients with neonatal, vertically transmitted hepatitis B and immunosuppressed kidney transplant recipients have been found to have HB_cAg in every liver cell nucleus, with only focal appearance of cytoplasmic HB_sAg (47,51). Other investigations have found large amounts of both antigens in renal transplant recipients (51a). HB_eAg has been demonstrated particularly in chronic active and chronic persis-

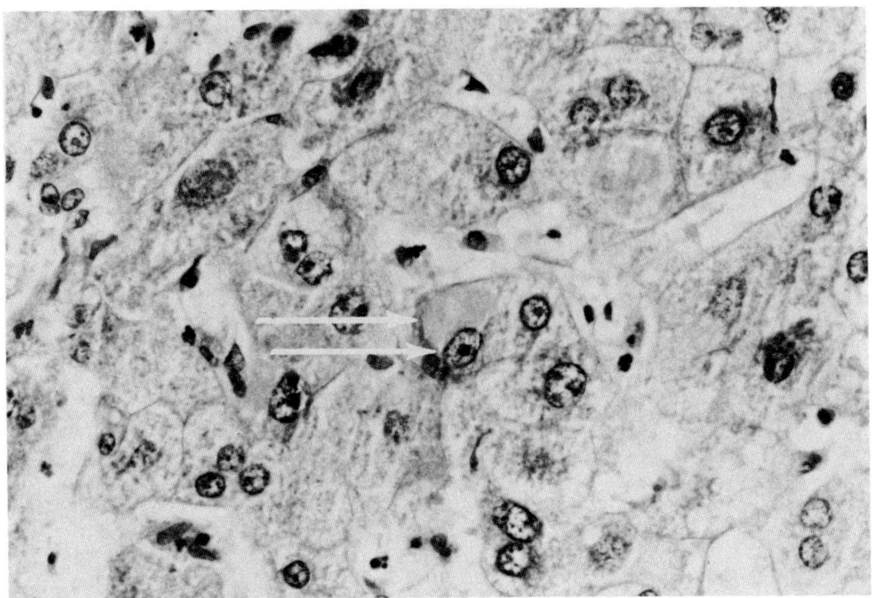

Figure 20. Chronic persistent hepatitis, showing a single hepatocyte with ground-glass cytoplasm (arrows). (Hematoxylin and eosin, ×425.)

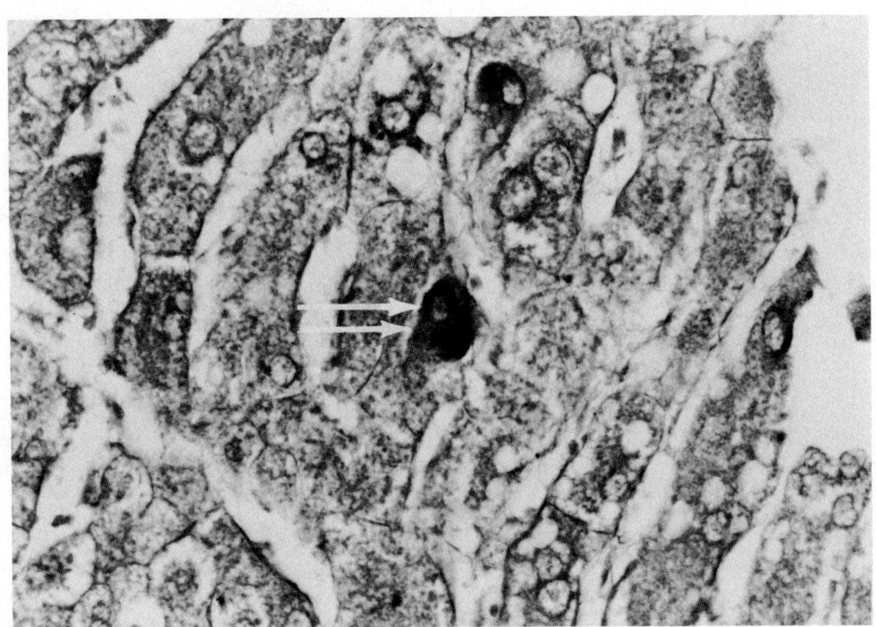

Figure 21. Section from same patient expressed in Figure 20, showing a ground-glass hepatocyte (arrows). (Orcein, ×425.)

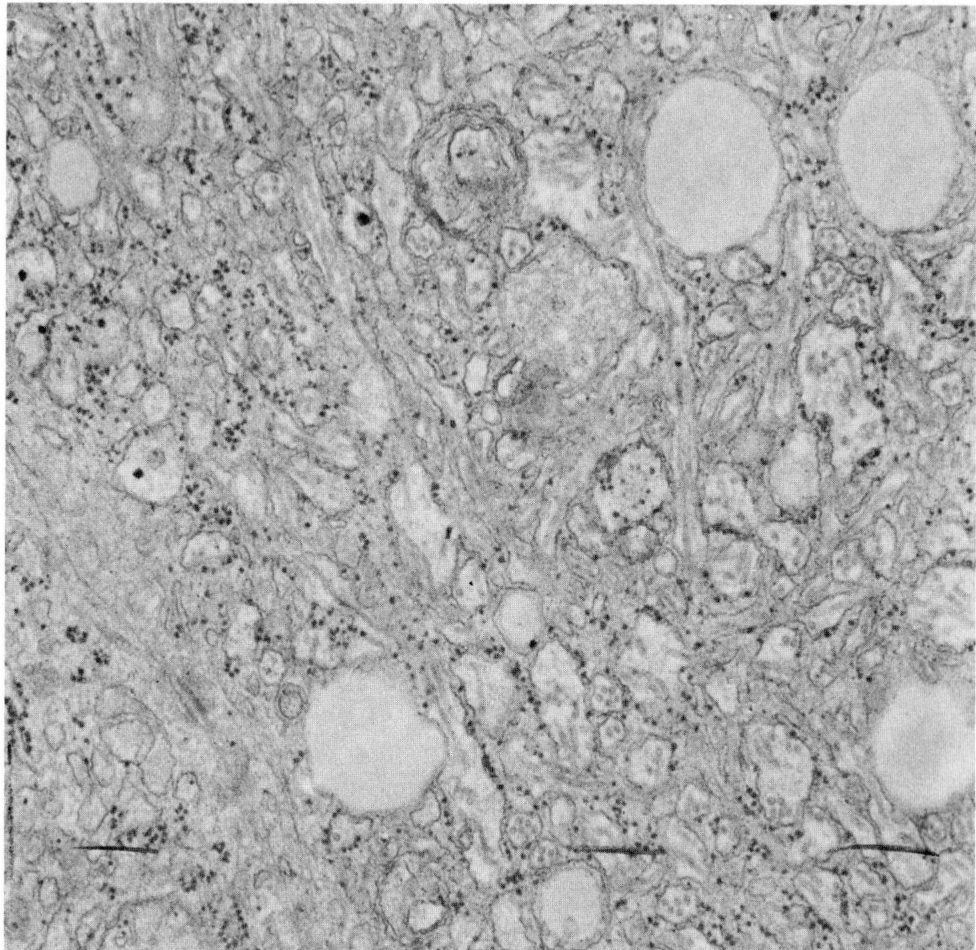

Figure 22. Carrier of HB_sAg. Electron micrograph shows part of the cytoplasm of a ground-glass hepatocyte, with numerous longitudinally and cross-sectioned tubules of HB_sAg in the endoplasmic reticulum. (×57,500.) (Contributed by R. De Vos M.D., and Professor Desmet.)

tent hepatitis in nuclei (52) and in the cytoplasm (48). The δ antigen appears to have a similar localization and significance (52A). The antigens of hepatitis B have also been carefully studied by electron microscopy (Figs. 24, 25) (45,48,50). Clearly, there is little relationship between the presence of hepatitis B antigens and hepatocellular necrosis. A possible exception is the correlation described between membranous localization (Fig. 25) of HB_sAg and piecemeal necrosis in chronic active hepatitis (46,50). For these reasons, the pathologic manifestations of hepatitis B have been attributed to immune responses of the host. Reactions against viral and host antigens at the cell surface have been postulated in acute and chronic viral hepatitis (48).

The evidence for cell-mediated cytotoxicity in chronic hepatitis includes an increase in activated T cells in the liver (53), although this is disputed (54), as well

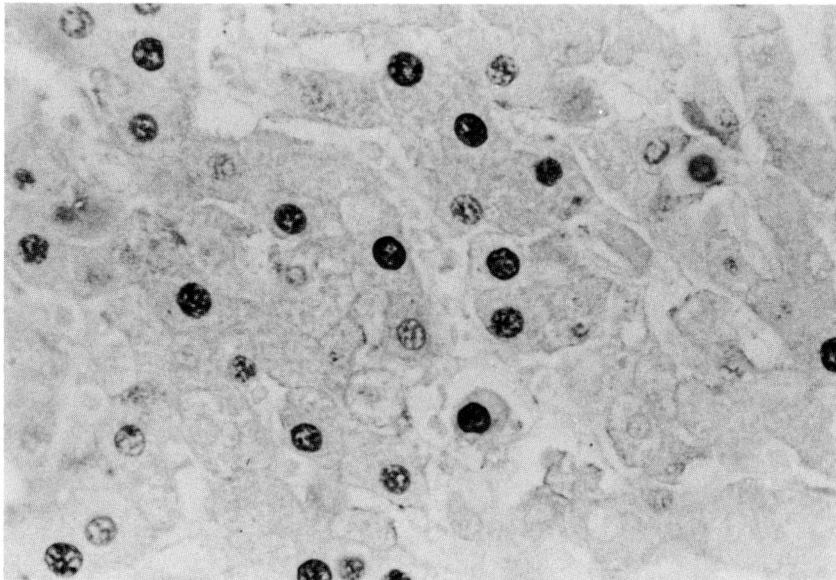

Figure 23. Liver of patient with chronic active hepatitis, showing presence of HB_cAg in many hepatocellular nuclei. (Paraffin section, anti-HB_c, PAS technique, ×250.) (Contributed by M. A. Gerber, M.D., ref. 44.)

as close contact between T lymphocytes and hepatocytes, which have HB_sAg at their surface and in the cytoplasm (55). Cell-mediated immunity appears to be particularly important in chronic active hepatitis and humoral immunity with antigen-antibody complexes in chronic persistent hepatitis (56). The evidence that humoral mechanisms may contribute to hepatocellular injury in chronic hepatitis also includes an increase in the proportion of B lymphocytes in hepatic infiltrates (54). Autoantibody production against hepatocyte surface membrane antigens is suggested by the binding of IgG to membranes. A granular IgG pattern has been demonstrated by immunofluorescence on the cell membranes of hepatocytes isolated from biopsy specimens of patients with chronic hepatitis B (57,58). Intranuclear IgG capable of fixing complement in vitro has also been observed. This reaction appears to indicate a poor prognosis (59,60). Nuclear IgG is generally found in patient who also have HB_cAg (61).

Hepatitis A has no tendency to become chronic and progress to cirrhosis. Hepatitis non-A non-B, however, has been shown to lead to chronic active hepatitis and cirrhosis (62,63), but the likelihood of this happening is uncertain (64). In the autoimmune type of chronic hepatitis unassociated with viral infection a linear pattern of gamma globulin deposition has been demonstrated by immunofluorescence on the membranes of hepatocytes isolated from such patients (57).

"Hippie Hepatitis"

Chronic hepatitis in abusers of intravenous drugs ("hippie hepatitis") can resemble morphologically, either chronic persistent or chronic aggressive hepatitis.

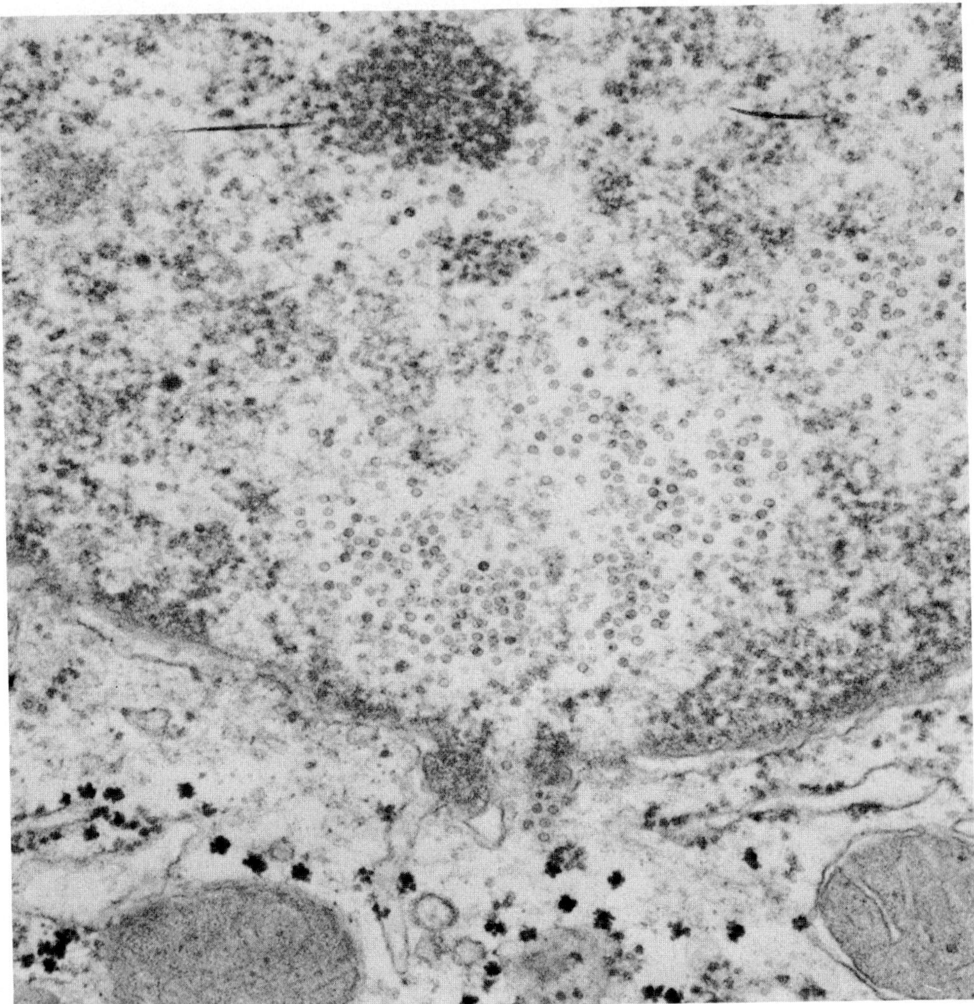

Figure 24. Patient with HBV-positive chronic active hepatitis. Electron micrograph shows numerous HB_cAg particles in the nucleoplasm, one HB_cAg particle in a nuclear pore, and a small group in distinct particles in the hyaloplasm nearby. (×71,000.) (Contributed by R. De Vos M.D., and Professor Desmet, ref. 45.)

Portal and intralobular inflammation are relatively severe and can take the form of dense portal and intralobular aggregates of lymphocytes or of lymphocytes and macrophages. Actual lymphoid follicles may be formed. Occasionally foreign-body giant cells or eosinophils are the predominant cell type (3). In about one-quarter of these patients, birefringent material in the form of small spicules and granules can be demonstrated in the macrophages of inflammatory aggregates in the portal tracts (Fig. 26) or in the lobules within Kupffer cells (65–67). Some of these patients can be shown serologically or morphologically (ground-glass hepatocytes, positive Shikata stains, or immunohistochemistry) to be infected with hepatitis B virus. The etiology of others remains unclear at the

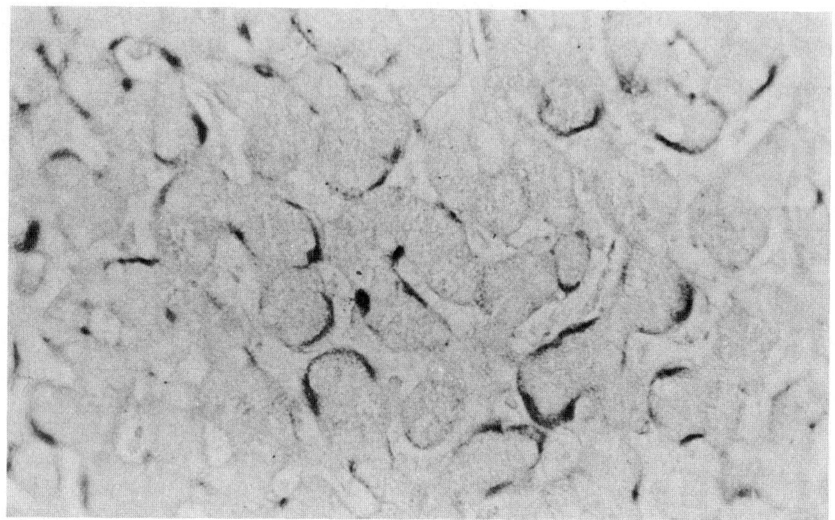

Figure 25. Liver of HB_sAg carrier with minor histologic changes. In this part of the section, HB_sAg is expressed mainly in the vicinity of the plasma membrane. (Paraffin section, anti-HB_s, PAS technique, ×250.) (Contributed by M. A. Gerber, M.D., ref. 44.)

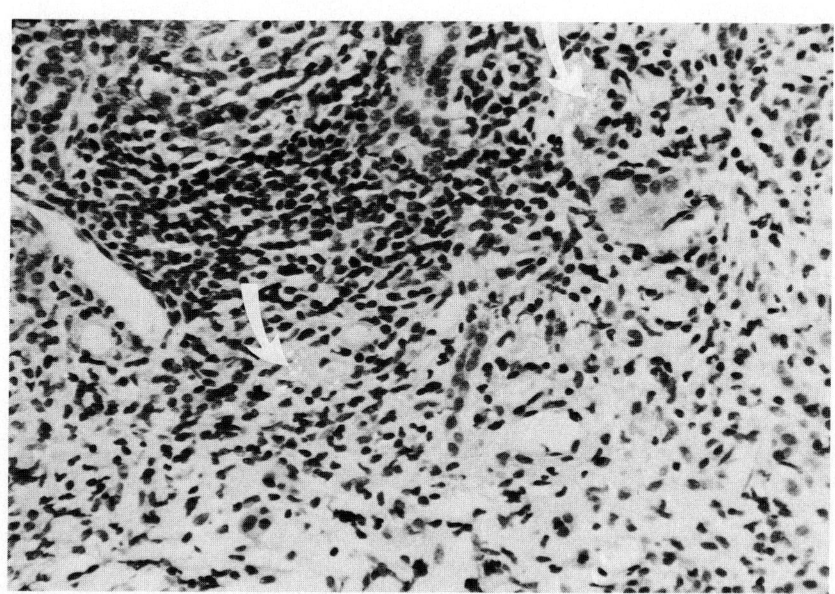

Figure 26. Biopsy specimen from a patient with chronic active, "hippie" hepatitis, showing spicules of birefringent material are seen in the vicinity of a portal triad with piecemeal necrosis. (Hematoxylin and eosin, ×190.) Partially polarized. (Contributed by R. Munn.)

present time. Their disease may be attributable to infection with non-A non-B hepatitis or produced by the talc or other foreign materials injected with the narcotics. Progression to cirrhosis in this group of patients may be less frequent than might be expected from the dramatic histologic picture which is often seen. In fact, there is often a tendency to improvement (68). Since correlation between clinical and histologic diagnosis in this group is poor, repeated biopsies are particularly valuable (69).

REFERENCES

1. Ludwig J: A review of lobular, portal and periportal hepatitis. *Hum Pathol* 8:269, 1977.
2. Peters RL: Viral hepatitis, a pathologic spectrum. *Am J Med Sci* 270:17, 1975.
3. Ishak KG: Light microscopic morphology of viral hepatitis. *Am J Clin Pathol* 65:787, 1976.
4. Boyer JL: The diagnosis and pathogenesis of clinical variants in viral hepatitis. *Am. J Clin Pathol* 65:898, 1976.

4a. Phillips WJ, Poucell S: Modern aspects of the morphology of viral hepatitis. *Human Path* 12:1060, 1981.

5. Popper H: Clinical pathologic correlation in viral hepatitis. *Am J Pathol* 81:609, 1975.
6. Mathiesen LR, Fauerholdt L, Moller AM, et al: Immunofluorescence studies for hepatitis A virus and hepatitis B surface and core antigen in liver biopsies from patients with acute viral hepatitis. *Gastroenterology* 77:623, 1979.

6a. Tanaka T, Tanaka I, Kogo M, et al: Morphologic findings of acute hepatitis A. *Acta Hep Jap* 22:494, 1981.

7. Ishak K: in Bianchi L, Gerock W, Sickinger K, et al (eds): *Virus and the Liver*, Falk Symposium No. 28. Lancaster, England, MTP Press, 1980, p. 120.
8. Popper H, Dienstag JL, Feinstone SM: Lessons from the pathology of hepatitis in chimpanzees, in Bianchi L, Gerock W, Sickinger K, et al (eds): *Virus and the Liver,* Falk Symposium No. 28. Lancaster, England, MTP Press, 1980, p 137.
9. Scheuer PJ, Texeira MR Jr, Weller IVD, et al: Pathology of acute hepatitis. *Gastroenterology* 79:1124, 1980.
10. Poulsen H, Christoffersen P: Abnormal bile duct epithelium in liver biopsies with histological signs of viral hepatitis. *Acta Pathol Microbiol Scand* [*A*] 76:383, 1969.

10a. De Wolf-Peeters C, De Vos R, Desmet VJ, et al: Human Non-A non-B hepatitis: ultrastructural alterations in hepatocytes. *Liver* 1:50, 1981.

11. Ray MB, Desmet VJ: Immunofluorescent detection of hepatitis B antigen in paraffin-embedded liver tissue. *J Immunol Methods* 6:283, 1975.
12. Deodhar KP, Tapp E, Scheuer PJ: Orcein staining of hepatitis B antigen in paraffin sections of liver biopsies. *J Clin Pathol* 475, 28:66, 1974.
13. Shikata T, Uzawa T, Yoshiwara N, et al: Staining methods of Australian antigen in paraffin section. *Jpn J Exp Med* 41:25, 1974.

13a. Houthoff HJ, Niermeijer P, Gids CH, et al: Hepatic morphologic findings and viral antigens in acute hepatitis B. *Virchows Arch Pathol Anat* 389:153, 1980.

14. Ruebner BH, Slusser R: Hepatocytes and sinusoidal lining cells in viral hepatitis. *Arch Pathol Lab Med* 86:1, 1968.
15. Bianchi L, DeGroote J, Desmet VJ, et al: Acute and chronic hepatitis revisited. *Lancet* 2:914, Oct 1968.
16. Boyer JL, Klatskin G: Pattern of necrosis in acute viral hepatitis. Prognostic value of bridging (subacute hepatic necrosis). *N Engl J Med* 283(20):1063, 1970.
17. Conn HO: Chronic hepatitis: Reducing an iatrogenic enigma to a workable puzzle. *Gastroenterology* 70:1182, 1976.

18. Nisman RM, Ganderson AP, Vlahevic ZR, et al: Acute viral heptatitis with bridging hepatic necrosis. An overview. *Arch Intern Med* 139:1289, 1979.

18a. Ware AJ, Cuthbert JA, Shorey J, et al: A prospective trial of steroid therapy in severe viral hepatitis. The prognostic significance of bridging. *Gastroenterology* 80:219, 1981.

19. Scotto J, Opolon P, Etève J, et al: Liver biopsy and prognosis in acute liver failure. *Gut* 14:927, 1973.

20. Gazzard BG, Portmann B, Murray-Lyon IM, et al: Causes of death in fulminant hepatic failure and relationship to quantitative histological assessment of parenchymal damage. *Q J Med* [New ser] XLIV(176):615, 1975.

21. Karvountzis GG, Redeker AG, Peters RL: Long term follow-up studies of patients surviving fulminant viral hepatitis. *Gastroenterology* 67:870, 1974.

22. Horney JT, Galambos JT: Liver physiology and disease. The liver during and after fulminant hepatitis. *Gastroenterology* 73:639, 1977.

23. Schmid M, Cueni B: Portal lesions in viral hepatitis with submassive hepatic necrosis. *Hum Pathol* 3:209, 1972.

24. Fauerholdt L, Asnaes S, Ranek L, et al: Significance of suspected "chronic aggressive hepatitis" in acute hepatitis. *Gastroenterology* 73(3):543, 1977.

25. Scheuer PJ: Chronic hepatitis: A problem for the pathologist. *Histopathology* 1:5, 1977.

26. Scheuer PJ: Liver biopsy in chronic hepatitis: 1968–78. *Gut* 19:554, 1978.

27. Boyer J: Prognostic determinants in chronic hepatitis B infection. *West J Med* 128:340, 1978.

27a. Gardiol D, Hofstetter JR, Fontolliet C, et al: The histological pattern of chronic active hepatitis—excluding cirrhosis—and their prognostic significance. *Acta Hepatogastroenterol (Stuttg)* 27:343, 1980.

27b. Lefkowitch J: Liver biopsy interpretation in chronic hepatitis. *Prog Surg Pathol* 3:221, 1981.

27c. Kadas I, Peley I: Experience with liver biopsy in chronic hepatitis in children. *Zbl Allg Pathol* 125:208, 1981.

28. Popper H, Schaffner F: The vocabulary of chronic hepatitis. *N Engl J Med* 284:1154, 1972.

29. Gardiol D, Rivier E: Chronic lobular hepatitis. *Schweiz Med Wochenschr* 104(41):1450, 1974.

30. Wilkinson SP, Portmann B, Cochrane AMG, et al: Clnical course of chronic lobular hepatitis. *Q J Med* 188:421, 1978.

31. Gerber MA, Vernace S: Chronic septal hepatitis. *Virchows Arch* [*Pathol Anat*] 363:303, 1974.

32. Chadwick RG, Galizzi J, Lyssiotis HT, et al: Chronic persistent hepatitis; hepatitis B virus markers and histological follow-up. *Gut* 20:372, 1979.

33. Runyan BA, La Breque DR, Anuras S: The spectrum of liver disease in systemic lupus erythematosus. Report of 33 histologically proved cases and review of the literature. *Am J Med* 69:187, 1980.

34. Baggenstoss AH, Soloway RD, Summerskill WHJ, et al: Chronic active liver disease. The range of histologic lesions, their response to treatment, and evolution. *Hum Pathol* 3:183, 1972.

35. Dietrichsen O, Zoffmann H, Christoffersen P, et al: Acute hepatitis: A prognostic study with observation time up to 37 years. *Acta Med Scand* 202:271, 1977.

36. Christoffersen OD, Faber V, Poulsen H: The occurrence and significance of abnormal bile duct epithelium in chronic aggressive hepatitis. *Acta Pathol Microbiol Scand* [*A*] 80:294, 1972.

37. Richey J, Rogers S, Van Thiel DH, et al: Giant multinucleated hepatocytes in an adult with chronic active hepatitis. *Gastroenterology* 73(3):570, 1977.

37a. Knodell RG, Ishak KG, Black WC, et al: Formulation and application of a numerical scoring system for assessing histological activity in asymptomatic chronic active hepatitis. *Hepatology* 1:431, 1981.

38. Hadziyannis S, Gerber MA, Vissoulis C, et al: Cytoplasmic hepatitis B antigen in "gound-glass" hepatocytes of carriers. *Arch Pathol Lab Med* 96:327, 1973.

39. Bianchi L, Gudat F: Sanded nuclei in hepatitis B. *Lab Invest* 35:1, 1976.

40. Borchard F, Gussmann V: Detection of HBsAg containing cells in liver biopsies by different stains and classification of positively reacting ground-glass hepatocytes. *Virchows Arch* [*Pathol Anat*] 384:245, 1979.

41. Thomsen P, Poulsen H, Petersen P: Different types of gound glass hepatocytes in human liver biopsies: Morphology, occurrence and diagnostic significance. *Scand J Gastroenterol* 11:113, 1976.

42. Clausen P, Thomsen P: Demonstration of hepatitis B-surface antigen in liver biopsies. *Acta Pathol Microbiol Scand* [*A*]86:383, 1978.

43. Gudat F, Bianchi L: Evidence for phasic sequences in nuclear HBcAg formation and cell membrane-directed flow of core particles in chronic hepatitis B. *Gastroenterology* 73:1194, 1977.

44. Gerber MA, Thung SN: The localization of hepatitis viruses in tissues. *Int Rev Exp Pathol* 20:49, 1979.

45. De Vos R, Ray MB, Desmet VJ: Electron microscopy of hepatitis B virus components in chronic active liver disease. *J Clin Pathol* 32:590, 1979.

46. Ray MB, Desmet VJ, Bradburne AF, et al: Differential distribution of hepatitis B surface antigen and hepatitis B core antigen in the liver of hepatitis B patients. *Gastroenterology* 71:462, 1976.

47. Gudat F, Bianchi L, Sonnabend W, et al: Pattern of core and surface expression in liver tissue reflects state of specific immune response in hepatitis B. *Lab Invest* 32:1, 1975.

48. Yamada G, Feinberg LE, Nakane PK: Hepatitis B. Cytologic localization of virus antigens and the role of the immune response. *Hum Pathol* 9:93, 1978.

49. Trevisan A, Realdi G, Alberti A, et al: Relationship between membrane-bound immunoglobulin and viral antigens in liver cells from patients with hepatitis B virus infection. *Gastroenterology* 77:209, 1979.

50. Huang S, Neurath AR: Immunohistologic demonstration of hepatitis B viral antigens of liver with reference to its significance in liver injury. *Lab Invest* 40:1, 1979.

51. Bianchi L, Gudat F: Immunopathology of Hepatitis B, in Popper H, Schaffner F (eds): *Liver Diseases.* New York, Grune & Stratton, 1979, vol VI, p 371.

51a. Amat D, Camilleri JP, Feldmann G, et al: Hepatocyte localization of hepatitis B core and surface antigens in renal transplant recipients. *Vir. Arch Pathol Anat* 391:153, 1981.

52. Arnold W, Nielsen JO, Hardt F, et al: Localisation of e-antigen in nuclei of hepatocytes in HBsAG-positive liver disease. *GUT* 19(12):994, 1977.

52a. Stocklin E, Gudat F, Krey G, et al: δ Antigen in hepatitis B: Immunohistology of frozen and paraffin embedded liver biopsies and relation to HBV infection. *Hepatology* 1:238, 1981.

53. Sanchez-Tapias J, Thomas HC, Sherlock S: Lymphocyte populations in liver biopsy specimens from patients with chronic liver disease. *Gut* 18:472, 1977.

54. Fargion D, Sangalli G, Ronchi G, et al: Evaluation of T and B lymphocytes in liver infiltrates of patients with chronic active hepatitis. *J Clin Pathol* 32:344, 1979.

55. Karasawa T, Shikata T: Necrosis of the hepatocyte with hepatitis B surface antigen. *Arch Pathol Lab Med* 101:280, 1977.

56. Thomas HC: Cellular immunity to the hepatitis B virus, in Bianchi L, Gerock W, Sickinger K, et al (eds): *Virus and the Liver*, Falk Symposium 28. Lancaster, England, MTP Press, 1980.

57. Hopf U, zum Büschenfeld KHM, Arnold W: Detection of a liver-membrane autoantibody in HBsAg-negative chronic active hepatitis. *N Engl J Med* 294:578, 1976.

58. Hutteroth TH, zum Büschenfeld KHM: Clinical relevance of the liver-specific lipoprotein (LSP). *Acta Hepatogastroenterol (Stuttg)* 25:243, 1978.

59. Gerber MA, Sarno E, Vernace SJ: Immune complexes in hepatocytic nuclei of HB Ag-positive chronic hepatitis. *N Engl J Med* 294:922, 1976.

60. Rizetto M, Diana S, Bonino F, et al: Prognostic significance of in-vitro complement fixation in liver biopsy specimens from patients with acute viral hepatitis type B. *Lancet* 2:436, 1976.

61. Gudat F, Bianchi L, Finch M, et al: Nuclear fluorescence of liver cells for IgG in viral hepatitis B: significance and relation to hepatitis B-core and anti-hepatitis B-core formation. *Klin Wochenschr* 55:329, 1977.

62. Iwarsen S, Lindberg J, Lundin P: Progression of hepatitis non-A, and non-B to chronic active hepatitis. (Clinical follow-up of two cases.) *J Clin Pathol* 32:351, 1979.

63. Knodell RG, Conrad ME, Ishak KG: Development of chronic liver disease after acute non-A non-B post-transfusion hepatitis: Role of alphaglobulin prophylaxis in its prevention. *Gastroenterology* 72:902, 1977.

64. Berman M, Alter HJ, Ishak KG, et al: Chronic sequelae of non-A, non-B hepatitis. *Ann Intern Med* 91:1, 1979.

65. Min KW, Gyorky F, Cain GD: Talc granulomata in liver disease in narcotic addicts. *Arch Pathol Lab Med* 98:331, 1974.

66. Buschmann RJ, Mir J: Electron microscopic identity of talc in the liver of a narcotic addict. *Hum Pathol* 10:736, 1979.

67. Groth DH, MacKay GR, Crable JV, et al: Intravenous injection of talc in a narcotics addict. *Arch Pathol Lab Med* 94:171, 1972.

68. Cherubin CE, Stenger RE, Strauss R: Chronic liver disease in asymptomatic narcotic addicts. *Ann Intern Med* 76:391, 1972.

69. Seef LB, Zimmerman HJ, Wright EC, et al: Hepatic disease in asymptomatic parenteral drug abusers: A Veterans Administration collaborative study. *Am J Med Sci* 270:41, 1975.

3
Hepatic Injury Produced By Infectious Agents and Miscellaneous Diseases

NONSPECIFIC REACTIVE HEPATITIS

Liver biopsies are frequently performed as part of the diagnostic workup of patients who have hepatomegaly, abnormal liver function test, fever of undetermined origin, or some other finding suspicious of hepatic involvement. Biopsies are indicated in patients known or suspected to have a malignant neoplasm, granulomatous disease, specific infection, or inflammatory bowel disease. Biopsy specimens obtained from such patients may enable the pathologist to make a specific diagnosis such as carcinoma, or to narrow down the diagnostic possibilities to such categories as granulomatous disease or certain viral infections. However, in many patients, a nonspecific morphologic picture is seen that has been called nonspecific reactive hepatitis (1), but that perhaps should be called focal, nonspecific, hepatic necrosis. There is a considerable range of variation in the type and severity of the morphologic changes. Most striking are areas of focal hepatocellular necrosis involving single hepatocytes or small groups of cells with the formation of acidophilic bodies or hydropic degeneration. Dropout of injured hepatocytes is often more easily observed than necrosis. These foci are infiltrated by macrophages, lymphocytes, and less frequently by neutrophils; the portal tracts may show a similar cell population. Piecemeal necrosis and cholestasis are absent. Slight or moderate fatty change and some irregularity in the arrangement of hepatic plates may be seen. This morphologic picture may or may not be associated with hepatic lesions more characteristic of a specific disease. Therefore, this diagnostic term suggests that further etiologic clues, such as granulomas or metastatic tumors (2), should be sought. Occasionally they are found in step sections or in repeat biopsies, either because of more fortunate sampling, or because of progression of the disease. The histologic findings in nonspecific reactive hepatitis actually resemble those of chronic persistent hepatitis (Chapter 2). However, fatty change may be more striking, and the infiltrates tend to be less dense. Moreover the clinical course is not marked by exacerbations of nausea, vomiting, malaise, and cholestasis over a period of-months or years. If no specific morphologic changes can be found, a diagnosis may be possible on the basis of clinical, radiologic, biochemical, or microbiologic findings. Drug-induced hepatocellular injury, for instance, may be diagnosed if the clinical findings are consistent.

HEPATIC LESIONS IN VIRAL INFECTIONS

Viral infections other than hepatitis A, B, or non-A non-B should always be considered in the presence of focal necroses randomly distributed throughout the lobule, particularly if the necrotic foci are larger than those seen in nonspecific reactive hepatitis. Grossly, these areas are usually yellowish white or hemorrhagic and measure 0.1–0.5 cm in diameter. In contradistinction to viral hepatitis, cellular unrest outside these foci is generally quite mild. The hepatocytes in the necrotic foci most commonly have undergone acidophilic hyaline necrosis with pyknosis, karyorrhexis, or loss of their nuclei. Hydropic degeneration or dropout of necrotic cells may also be seen. Occasionally the necrotic foci are large or confluent, or both (Fig. 1), which can result in submassive hepatic necrosis. In such cases, differentiation from severe infectious hepatitis and from drug-induced submassive necrosis may depend on the demonstration of viral inclusions, immunohistology, electron microscopy, virus isolation from tissues or blood, or the demonstration of serum antibodies.

Adenovirus Infection

Adenovirus hepatitis is relatively rare and is usually seen in children (3) and in immunodepressed adults (4). The histologic picture consists of focal necrosis and resembles that described for herpes hepatitis (Fig. 1). Typical Cowdry type A, Feulgen-positive, intranuclear inclusions are seen that, by light microscopy, resemble those seen in patients with herpes hepatitis (Fig. 2). The inclusions may be surrounded by a rather characteristic halo, which is a shrinkage artifact. Careful light microscopy of the inclusions may, and electron microscopy undoubtedly will, make possible a diagnosis of adenovirus infection (Fig. 3) (3). This can be confirmed by immunohistology, culture of the liver, or by serum antibody estimations.

Herpes Infection

Herpes simplex hepatitis is usually part of a severe generalized infection, particularly in children and immunosuppressed adults (5–7b). Morphologic diagnosis is suggested by characteristic hepatic histopathologic findings. Punched-out foci of necrosis (Fig. 4) are surrounded by hepatocytes containing amphophilic Cowdry type A intranuclear inclusions, staining positively for DNA by the Feulgen method and indicative of an intranuclear DNA virus (Fig. 5). The surrounding hepatocytes may appear normal or may show severe degenerative changes. Identification of the virus as a member of the herpes group is performed by electron microscopy of the liver; species identification as herpes

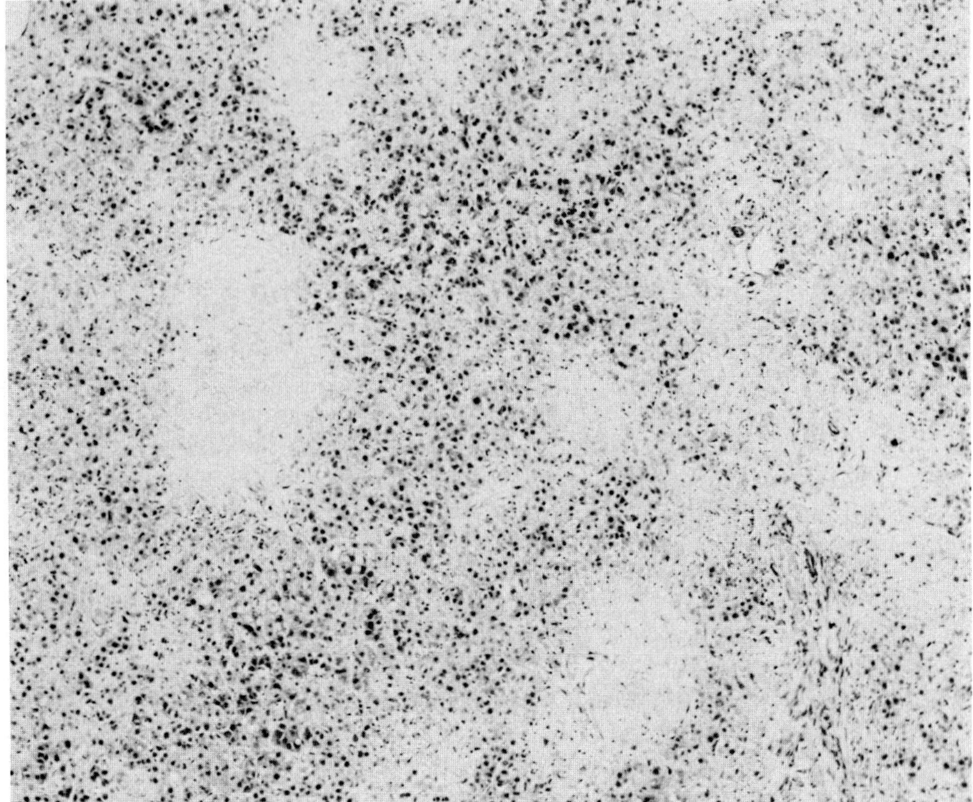

Figure 1. Adenovirus infection. Low-power view shows several irregularly distributed areas of necrosis scattered throughout the liver. Some necrotic foci are confluent. There is no significant inflammatory response. (Hematoxylin and eosin, ×16.) (Contributed by K. Aterman, M.D., ref. 3.)

simplex is confirmed by immunohistochemistry, by culture of the liver, or by the characteristic antibody rise in the serum.

Varicella-zoster has also been reported to cause fatal massive hepatic necrosis (7b).

Infectious Mononucleosis

In infectious mononucleosis, mild hepatic involvement is not uncommon, as evidenced clinically by some elevation of the transaminases and bilirubin. This elevation is usually short-lived, but can last several weeks, and recovery is usually complete. Irreversible hepatic failure has been described in very few cases (8–10). Histologically, cases of average severity show marked widening of the portal tracts by infiltration with mononuclear cells, chiefly lymphocytes (11). In severe cases, the portal infiltrates may extend into the periportal sinusoids and may have an atypical cytology (Fig. 6). Both the cytology and distribution of these

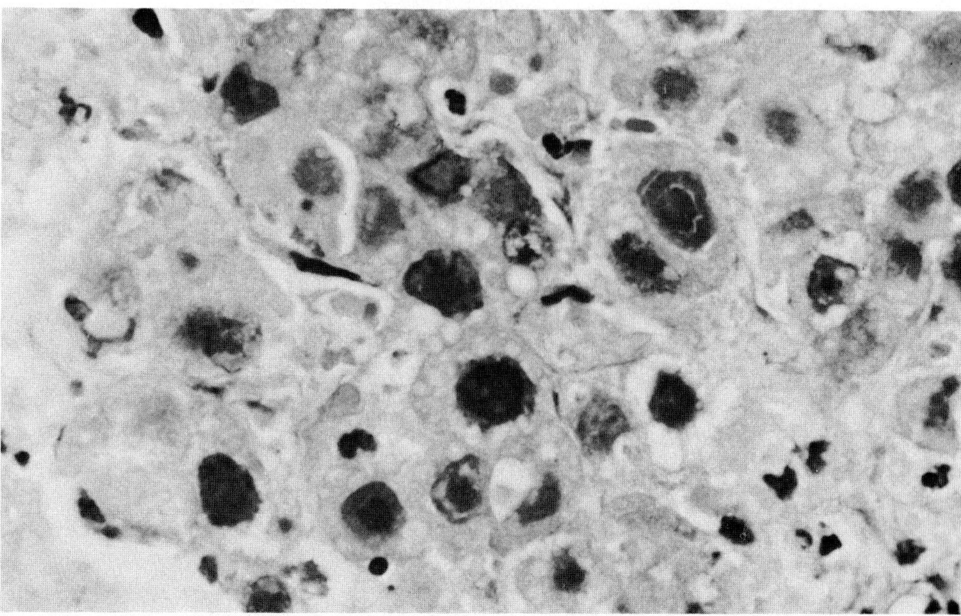

Figure 2. Adenovirus infection. Higher-power view of hepatocytes on the periphery of a necrotic focus shows many intranuclear inclusions. The margin of the necrotic area can be seen at the left border. (Hematoxylin and eosin, ×800.) (Contributed by K. Aterman, M.D., ref. 3.)

cells may mimic leukemia or granulomas. In distribution and severity, the inflammatory reaction may resemble "hippie hepatitis." However, birefringent material cannot be demonstrated (Chapter 2). The hepatocellular changes are usually relatively mild, resembling those seen in a mild viral hepatitis, with ballooning and acidophilic bodies, or in focal nonspecific hepatitis. Cholestasis may be present. Extensive hepatocellular necrosis is generally seen in fatal cases, often associated with disseminated fibrin thrombi (9). Herpes-like intranuclear inclusions have been described (8), considered as probably related to the Epstein-Barr virus, the etiologic agent in this disease. We have also seen lipogranulomas resembling those of Q fever (p. 68) and epithelioid granulomas (p. 88). Diagnosis is confirmed by the characteristic blood smear and positive Paul-Bunnell test. Cytomegalovirus infection and phenyl butazone should be considered as possible etiologic agents in those cases that have a negative serology.

Cytomegalovirus Infection

Cytomegalovirus hepatitis occurs as part of cytomegalic inclusion disease in children and also in adults, particularly those with lymphoma or leukemia. The histopathologic changes resemble those described earlier as characteristic of viral infection other than viral hepatitis. Granulomas may be observed in this infection (Chapter 4). Large cells with large Feulgen-positive intranuclear Cowdry type A inclusions and cytoplasmic inclusions positive both by the PAS reaction, as well as the Feulgen stain, are diagnostic of this disease (Fig. 7). They may be

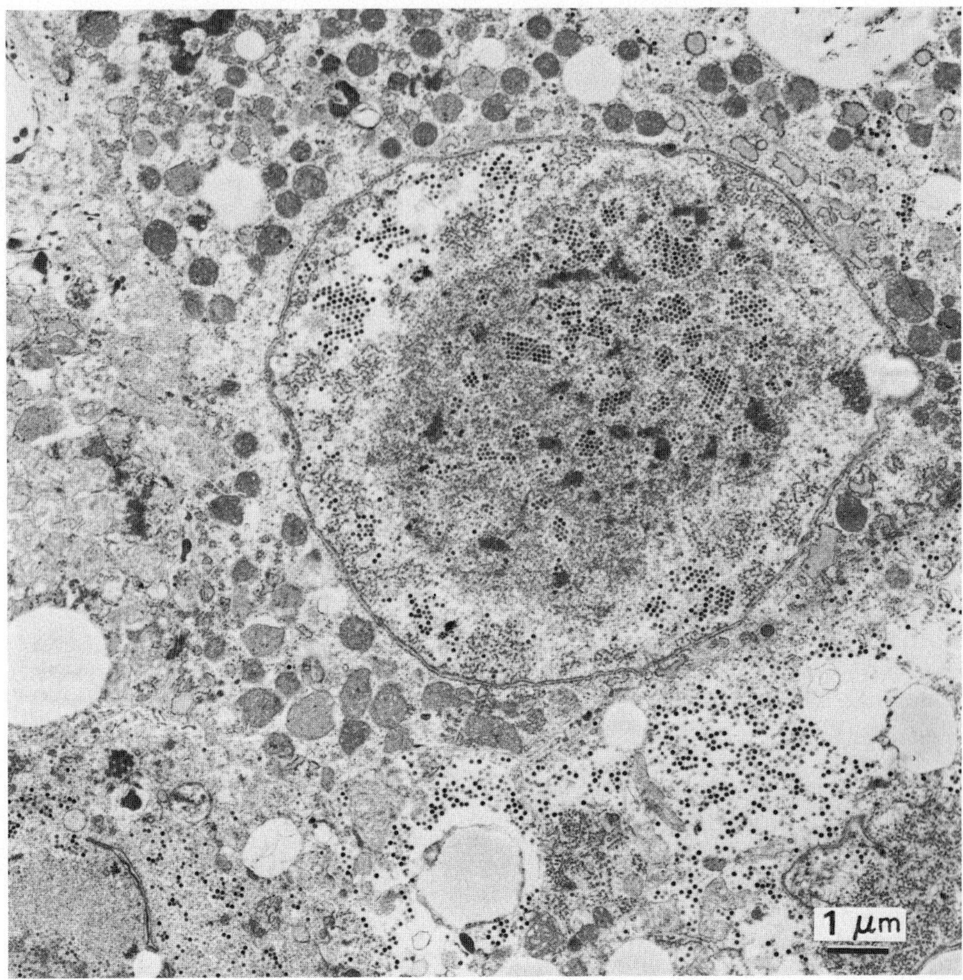

Figure 3. Adenovirus particles in a hepatocyte. Electron micrograph shows virus particles in the nuclei and also in the cytoplasm. (×8,730.) (Contributed by K. Aterman, M.D., ref. 3.)

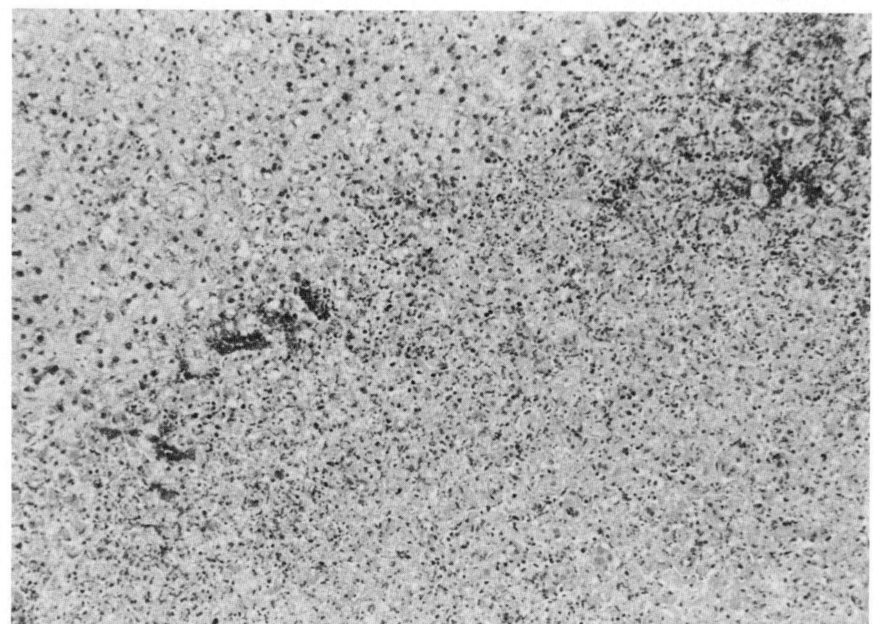

Figure 4. Herpes simplex. Low-power view of a large necrotic focus on the lower right. Surviving hepatocytes are seen on the upper left. (Hematoxylin and eosin, ×34.)

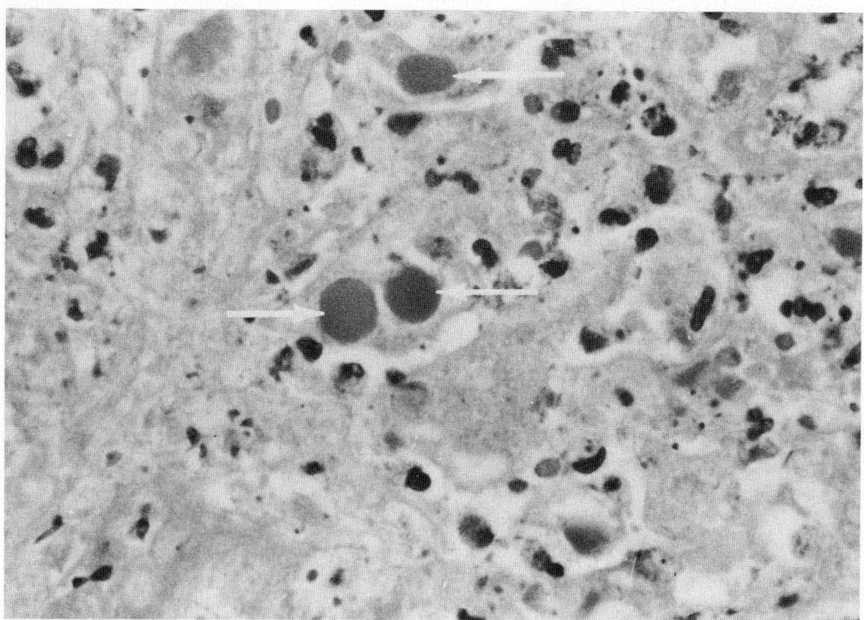

Figure 5. Herpes simplex. Higher-power view of necrotic focus shown in Figure 4, showing three intranuclear inclusions (arrows) among pyknotic nuclear debris. (Hematoxylin and eosin, ×545.)

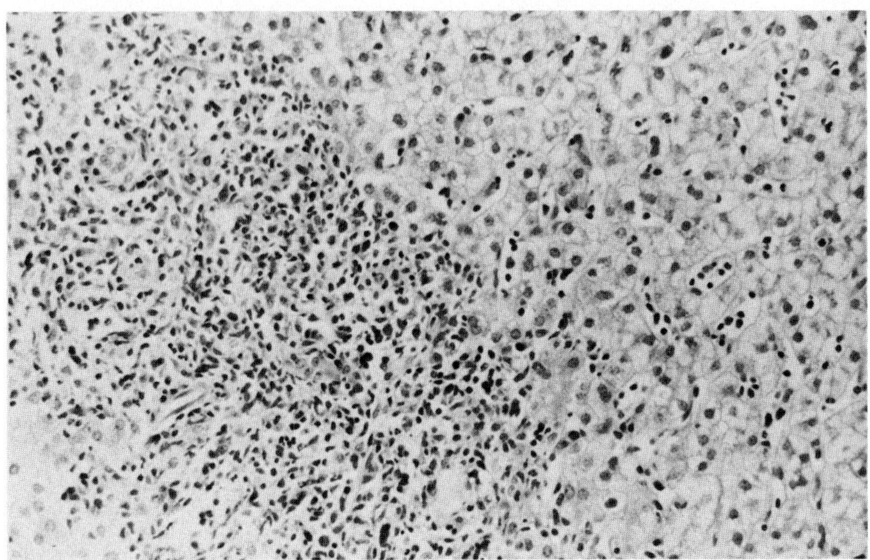

Figure 6. Infectious mononucleosis, showing marked infiltration of a portal triad, with somewhat pleomorphic chronic inflammatory cells. A few of these cells have spilled through the limiting plate into the periportal sinusoids. Only minimal hepatocellular changes are seen. (Hematoxylin and eosin, ×55.)

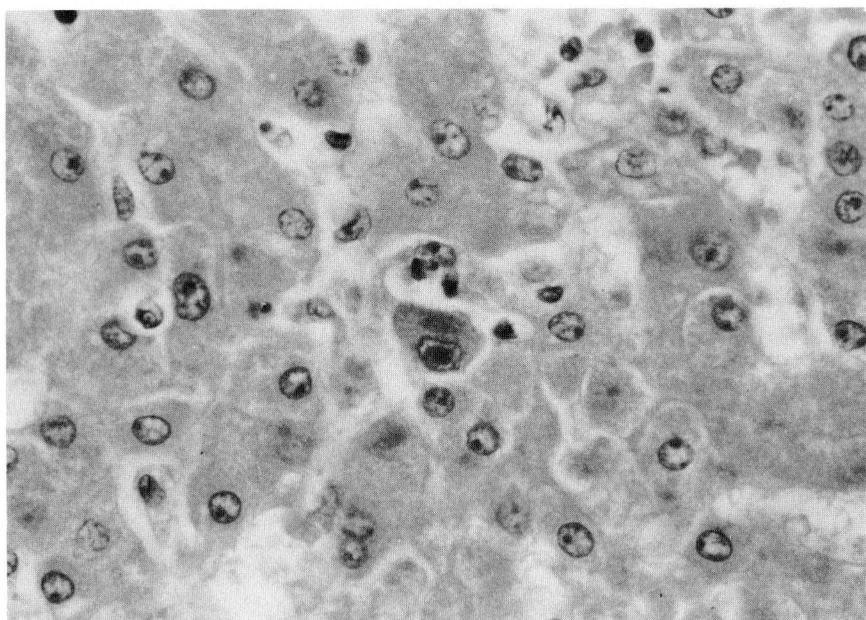

Figure 7. Cytomegalovirus infection, showing a typical intranuclear inclusion in the center of the field. The infected hepatocyte also has a rather less distinct cytoplasmic inclusion. No significant hepatocellular necrosis is seen here. (Hematoxylin and eosin, ×545.)

found in biliary epithelial cells, as well as in hepatocytes and may produce a clinicopathologic picture resembling graft versus host disease (see p. 73) (12,13). Other patients, clinically and pathologically, have a mononucleosis-like picture. In such patients, typical inclusions may be difficult or impossible to find. The diagnosis, therefore, has to be made by serum antibody levels or by the demonstration of characteristic intranuclear inclusions in cytologic preparations of urine or bronchial washings.

Coxsackie Virus

Coxsackie virus infection in newborns and some adults may become generalized and involve the liver. The hepatic lesions consist of dropout of individual hepatocytes and focal necrosis with a polymorphonuclear infiltrate. The picture therefore is that of a nonspecific reactive hepatitis (14). Characteristic cytoplasmic inclusions may be demonstrated by electron microscopy. The diagnosis can be confirmed by isolating the virus from the liver or blood or by a rise in serum antibody titers.

Yellow Fever

Yellow fever is one of the earliest and best studied viral infections of the liver. In fact, acidophilic bodies were first described in this disease by Councilman. The histopathology of yellow fever may vary from that of a nonspecific reactive hepatitis (p. 60) to severe multifocal or even submassive necrosis (15). Unlike acute viral hepatitis, focal fatty change is a common accompaniment. It used to be said that the necrosis in yellow fever preferentially affects the midzones of lobules. However, more recent descriptions have not stressed this midzonal localization (15). The microscopic features of yellow fever, therefore, are compatible with this disease and suggestive, but not diagnostic of it. The diagnosis has to be confirmed by virus isolation or serology.

Marburg Virus

Marburg virus hepatitis is a severe viral illness observed relatively rarely in persons who had contact with monkeys, either during animal experimentation or in the monkey's natural habitat (16). In mild cases, single-cell necrosis is all that can be observed (17). In more severe cases, larger areas of focal necrosis develop that can coalesce. The necrotic cells may be phagocytosed with subsequent reticulum collapse. Ballooning of hepatocytes occurs relatively late, and fatty change often develops in surviving hepatocytes. Cholestasis apparently has not been reported. Histiocytes and round cells infiltrate the portal tracts. Recovery, if it occurs, is usually complete and neither fibrosis nor cirrhosis have developed. Characteristic pleomorphic viral particles are seen in hepatocytes by electron microscopy. A diagnosis can also be made by the presence of serum antibodies. Ebola virus infections resembles Marburg virus infections clinically, pathologically, and virologically (16).

Other Viral Infections

Lassa fever is an acute febrile disease having a hemorrhagic diathesis and high mortality. The causative agent has been placed into the recently defined arenavirus group, which also includes the agents of Bolivian and Argentinian hemorrhagic fevers (16). Dengue and Kyasanur forest fever also produce a similar clinical and pathologic picture. Irregularly scattered foci of hepatocellular necrosis varying from single cells to small groups of cells and larger foci with bridging have been described (18,19). Hydropic swelling of hepatocytes and acidophilic bodies may be seen, but the inflammatory reaction is relatively mild and nonspecific. Fatty change of variable severity occurs. Electron microscopy shows characteristic 120-nm arenavirus particles in hepatocytes, as well as in bile canaliculi. The virus can be isolated from tissues or serum and antibodies demonstrated in the blood. Rift valley fever is a mosquito-borne arbovirus infection of sheep and cattle. Man is usually infected by contact with sick animals. Hemorrhages and jaundice indicate a poor prognosis (16). Hepatic necrosis tends to be periportal.

RICKETTSIAL HEPATITIS

Q fever is a generalized infection caused by *Rickettsia burnetti.* Hepatomegaly is common in this disease, although jaundice is not, and alkaline phosphatase levels tend to be elevated. The hepatic lesion consists of focal necroses with an inflammatory response which is variable. Groups of polymorphonuclear leukocytes, eosinophils, and round cells or actual granulomas (Chapter 4) composed of histiocytes or epithelioid cells are present. Central lipid vacuoles in these lesions are common (20). A close association of focal necrosis with polymorphs and fatty change has been described as lipogranulomas characteristic of this infection (Fig. 8). However, we have observed apparently identical lesions when Q fever titers were negative. The earliest lesion in Q fever is said to be a characteristic eosinophilic necrosis of the sinusoidal walls. Later abnormal prominence of sinusoidal lining cells may develop, giving a "string of beads" appearance. Mononuclear infiltration of the portal tract is usually also seen. The lesions may persist for more than a year and may progress to portal fibrosis and cirrhosis (21). The diagnosis is confirmed by a rise in serum antibody titers.

In Boutonneuse fever, another rickettsial hepatitis, the symptoms and signs are similar to those of Q fever, except for frequent elevations of the transaminase enzymes. The histologic lesions also resemble those of Q fever. Hepatic involvement is also seen in Rocky Mountain spotted fever produced by *R. rickettsii* (22). The most striking histologic features were portal inflammation, portal vasculitis, and cholestasis. Mild hepatocellular necrosis and erythrophagocytosis are also seen.

BACTERIAL HEPATITIS

Bacterial infection and actinomycosis should be considered in patients with prolonged fever of unknown origin sometimes associated with jaundice, particularly

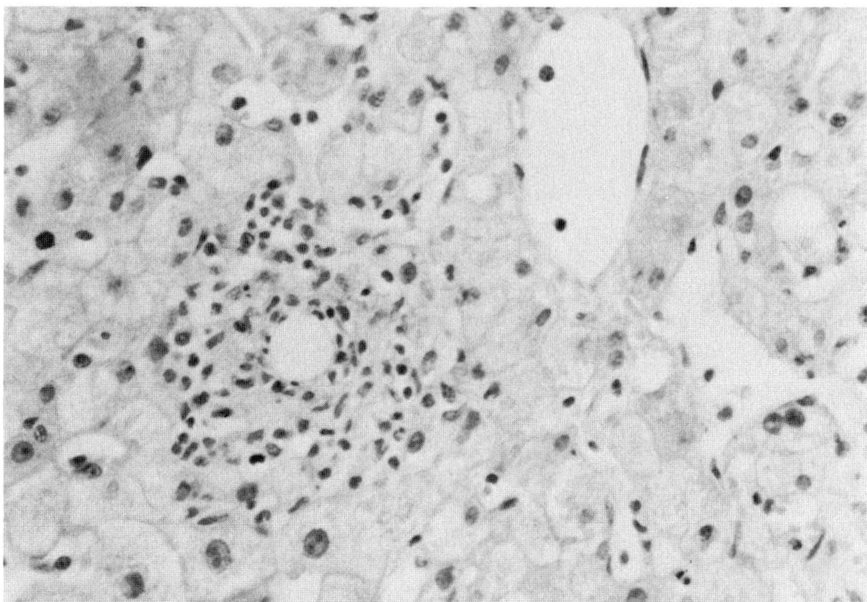

Figure 8. Q fever, showing characteristic necrotic focus containing a lipid droplet surrounded by neutrophils and round cells. (Hematoxylin and eosin, ×214.)

in immunologically deficient patients (23–25,25a). Since the hepatic pathologic changes may be only those of focal nonspecific hepatitis or of focal polymorph infiltration, multiple cultures of biopsies are mandatory in making such a diagnosis. Similar histologic changes are seen in scarlet fever (26). The characteristic organisms of Whipple's disease have been seen in the liver by electron microscopy (27). "Surgical polymorphs" in wedge biopsies (Chapter 1) and alcoholic liver disease (Chapter 5) have to be considered before making a diagnosis of bacterial hepatitis. Abscesses are most frequently the result of pylephlebitis, cholangitis, or staphylococcal septicemia and will be dealt with in the chapters on space-occupying lesions (Chapter 14) and biliary obstruction (Chapters 7 and 8).

Syphilis

Syphilis affects the liver differently at different stages of the disease. In congenital syphilis, hepatocytes are isolated from each other by a diffuse fibrous reaction accompanied by acute and chronic inflammatory cells. Microgummas may also be seen. Treponemal organisms are usually said to be easily demonstrable by the Warthin-Starry silver stain. Recently 1-μm-thick epoxy-resin-embedded sections or electron microscopy have been strongly recommended to demonstrate the presence of the organisms (28). In early syphilis, hepatic involvement seems to occur in about 10% of cases (29). The problem is to distinguish hepatic damage produced by *Treponema pallidum* from coincident viral hepatitis, which is common in the same population. Some patients with viral hepatitis can easily be diagnosed because their serum is positive for HB_sAG. In patients with hepatic involvement caused by early syphilis, mild elevations of transaminase enzymes, bilirubin, and serum alkaline phosphatase are found (29,30). The histologic changes consist of prominence of Kupffer cells or nonspecific reactive hepatitis, but may be more extensive (31). Necrotic foci involving only one or two cells may be anywhere in the lobule, but localization around the central vein appears to be most suggestive of syphilis (29). The inflammatory infiltrate surrounding the foci of necrosis consists of neutrophils, eosinophils, lymphocytes and macrophages. Granulomatous hepatitis has been reported (29a). Inflammatory cells may also be found in the vicinity of portal veins (29b). Treponemes in the liver of these cases are scanty and, therefore, probably best demonstrated by silver impregnation, such as Warthin-Starry (28,29,29b). Tertiary hepatic syphilis is now very rare, resulting in gummas and coarse scarring (hepar lobatum).

Enteric Infection

In typhoid or paratyphoid fever, hepatomegaly and jaundice with mild elevations of SGOT and SGPT occur in about 10–20% of patients. The pathologic basis of these chemical abnormalities is focal hepatic necrosis with infiltration of the lesions and the portal tracts by round cells and macrophages. The lesions have been dignified by the term "typhoid nodules," but actually they are rarely distinguishable from nonspecific reactive hepatitis (32, 33). The diagnosis has to be made by serology or by isolation of the organism from blood or feces.

Weil's Disease

Weil's disease, caused by organisms of the genus *Leptospira*, is a severe, often fatal, infection characterized by fever, jaundice, hepatomegaly, renal insufficiency, and hemorrhages of the skin and mucosal surfaces. Transaminase elevations are slight, and focal hepatic necrosis inconspicuous. This is surprising in view of the severity of the bile retention as assessed clinically and histologically (34). A mild portal inflammatory reaction is also usually present. The diagnosis is made by serology or by isolation of the organism from blood or feces.

PROTOZOAL INFECTIONS

Leishmaniasis involves the reticuloendothelial system, including spleen and Kupffer cells (Fig. 9) (34a,b,c). Hepatic involvement is generally mild, both clinically and pathologically (34d).

Biopsy specimens of the liver from patients with malaria, whether caused by *Plasmodium vivax* or *P. falciparum,* show few abnormalities. Sinusoidal congestion and prominence of Kupffer cells containing brown malarial pigment (Chapter 11) are the most conspicuous changes (35). Fatty change has also been reported (35a).

Toxoplasmosis clinically and pathologically may mimic infectious hepatitis and is a cause of "neonatal hepatitis" (Chapter 8). The histologic picture may be that of nonspecific reactive hepatitis or granulomatous hepatitis (36). The diagnosis is best confirmed by immunofluorescence on liver biopsy specimens (37).

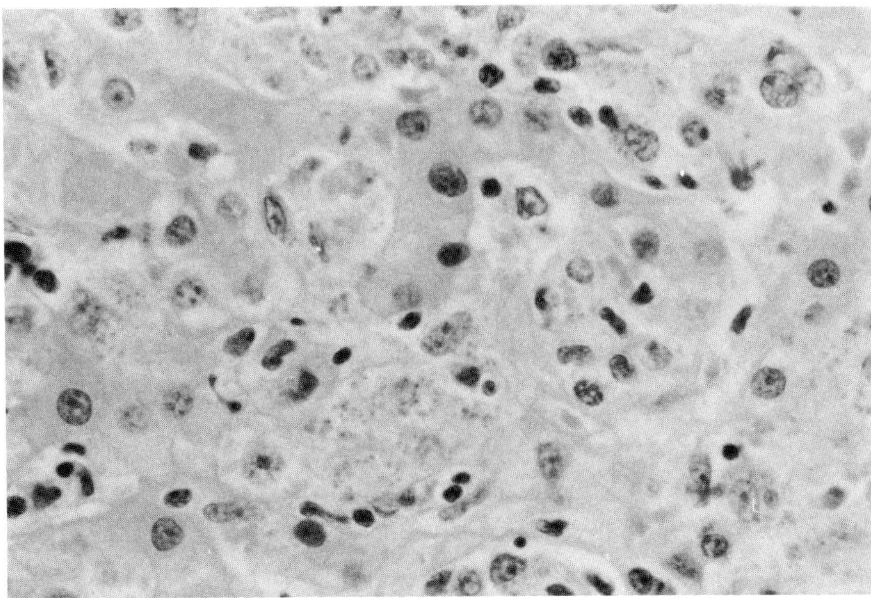

Figure 9. Leishmaniasis, showing characteristic groups of granules representing organisms in Kupffer cells. (Hematoxylin and eosin, ×545.)

RHEUMATIC DISEASES

Arthritis is a recognized complication of hepatitis B. In patients with rheumatoid arthritis primary biliary cirrhosis is a rare development (Chapter 7) (38). Much more frequently, rheumatoid arthritis may be accompanied by hepatomegaly with modest elevations of transaminase enzymes and serum bilirubin, as well as retention of bromsulphalein. Histologic alterations are nonspecific, essentially those of nonspecific reactive hepatitis. There may also be prominence of Kupffer cells (39,40). Rheumatic fever, polymalgia rheumatica and temporal arteritis may also be accompanied by hepatic dysfunction, particularly elevation of the alkaline phosphatase. Nonspecific reactive hepatitis with marked fatty change and massive infiltration of the portal spaces with lymphocytes have been described. The focal inflammatory aggregates have been considered to be granulomas (41,42,42a). Giant cell arteritis involving the hepatic artery has been observed (42b).

ECLAMPSIA

Preeclampsia is accompanied by rather characteristic foci of acidophilic necrosis adjacent to the portal zones (Fig. 10) (43). In severe cases these foci may be quite large. The presence of fibrinogen, IgG, IgM, and C_3 has been demonstrated by immunofluorescence in the foci and in adjacent sinusoids (44). Rupture of these foci may give rise to catastrophic intra-abdominal hemorrhage.

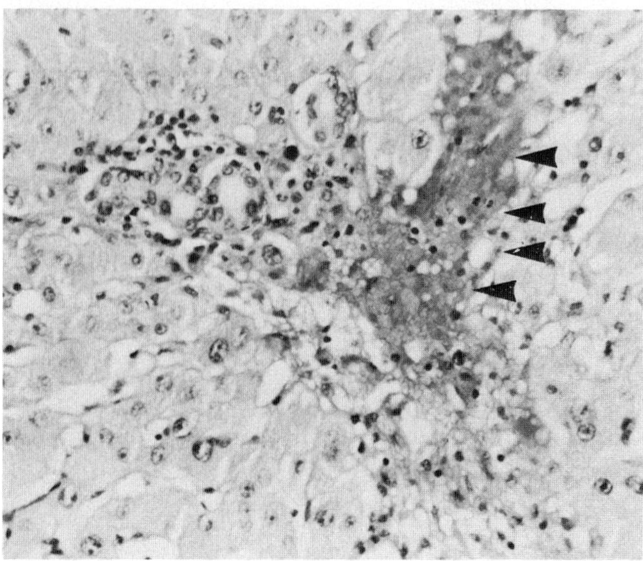

Figure 10. Preeclampsia, showing a characteristic focus of fibrinoid necrosis (arrowheads) in the vicinity of a portal triad (Hematoxyin and eosin, ×214.)

THERMAL INJURY

In patients with burns, the hepatocellular alterations are usually mild and consist of focal fatty change, slight activation of Kupffer cells, and some irregularity in size and shape of hepatocyte nuclei. Centrilobular necrosis is seen relatively rarely (45).

In heat stroke, the most striking change is centrilobular confluent necrosis involving up to one-third of the lobule. The liver cells in these areas disappear rapidly and sinusoidal lining cells are conspicuous in the areas of necrosis. Along the periphery of these necrotic zones, there is conspicuous hydropic swelling of hepatocytes. Surviving hepatocytes show considerable variation in size and shape of the nuclei, as well as mitotic figures. Areas of single cell necrosis (acidophilic bodies) are scattered through the lobules and there is prominence of Kupffer cells, many of which contain brown pigment (46). Bile thrombi are conspicuous. Portal inflammation is slight and consists of neutrophils, lymphocytes, and macrophages. PAS-negative hyaline droplets have been described in the hepatocytes (47,48). Because of its striking centrilobular localization, the picture resembles that produced by hepatotoxins, such as *amanita phalloides*, or sensitizing drugs, such as halothane (Chapter 15), rather than the histologic picture of viral hepatitis.

NEOPLASIA

Hepatic dysfunction associated with malignant neoplasms always raises the possibility of metastatic spread; this possibility should be investigated as outlined in the chapter on space-occupying hepatic lesions (Chapter 14). Inability to find such lesions may be due to sampling error, particularly if the lesions are small. However, occasionally malignant neoplasms that have not yet metastasized to the liver may give rise to hepatic dysfunction, an example of which is the syndrome of carcinoma of the kidney, with increased alkaline phosphatase, prolonged prothrombin time, altered serum proteins, and retention of bromsulphalein. Histologic study of these livers exhibits a nonspecific reactive hepatitis (p. 60) of varying severity, characterized by mild ballooning of hepatocytes with scattered acidophilic necrotic cells or dropout of hepatocytes and their replacement by polymorphonuclears, mononuclear inflammatory cells, and macrophages. Kupffer cells are diffusely prominent and show striking aggregates, even in areas in which no necrosis may be detected. Portal tracts show moderately severe infiltration by polymorphonuclear leukocytes, round cells, and macrophages. After nephrectomy, there may be normalization of the biochemical changes, and presumably of the histologic changes (49–51).

In patients with acute leukemia, the clinicopathologic picture of acute viral hepatitis or nonspecific reactive hepatitis may develop, not necessarily attributable to the chemotherapy (52).

GRAFT-VERSUS-HOST REACTION

The graft-versus-host reaction (GVHR) is frequently associated with clinical and morphologic signs of hepatic involvement. However, since these patients usually have other serious problems, particularly immunosuppression and susceptibility to infections, there is some doubt as to the specificity of the lesions that have been described (53). Portal lymphoid infiltrates, hyaline necrosis of periportal hepatocytes, and foci of hepatocellular necrosis within the liver lobules appear to be closely related to early GVHR (12). A striking necrosis of portal bile ducts (12) and periportal cholestasis (54) is also seen in GVHR (Chapter 7).

HEMODIALYSIS AND TRANSPLANTATION

Liver dysfunction and histologic evidence of hepatic injury are common in this group of patients (55). This may take the form of non-specific reactive hepatitis, viral infections, particularly hepatitis B and non A non B, cytomegalovirus, herpes, or adenovirus or of a reaction to foreign material (p. 78). Reactions to immunosuppressive drugs (Chapter 15) or the graft versus host reaction may also occur.

REFERENCES

1. Popper H, Schaffner F: *Liver Structure and Function*. New York, McGraw-Hill, 1957, p 406.
2. Dirschmid K: Biopsy findings of liver parenchyma in the presence of metastasis. *Zentralbl Allg Pathol* 121(3):225, 1977.

3. Aterman K, Embil J, Easterbrook KB, et al: Liver necrosis, adenovirus Type 2 and thymic dysplasia. *Virchows Arch [Pathol Anat]* 360:155, 1973.
4. Carmichael GP Jr, Zahradnik JM, Moyer GH, et al: Adenovirus hepatitis in an immunosuppressed adult patient. *Am J Clin Pathol* 71:352, 1979.
5. Anuras A, Summers R: Fulminant herpes simplex hepatitis in an adult: Report of a case in renal transplant recipient. *Gastroenterology* 70:425, 1976.
6. Elliott WC, Houghton DC, Bryant RE: Herpes simplex type 1 hepatitis in renal transplantation. *Arch Intern Med* 140:1656, 1980.
7. Eron L, Kosinski K, Hirsch MS: Hepatitis in an adult caused by herpes simplex virus Type 1. *Gastroenterology* 71:500, 1976.

7a. Orenstein JM, Castadot MJ, Wilens SL: Fatal herpes hepatitis associated with pemphigus vulgaris and steroids in an adult. *Hum Pathol* 5:489, 1974.

7b. Ross JS, Lee Fanning W, Beautyman W, et al: Fatal massive hepatic necrosis from varicella zoster hepatitis. *Am J. Gastroenterol* 74:423, 1980.

8. Chang MY, Campbell WG: Fatal infectious mononucleosis. *Arch Pathol Lab Med* 99:185, 1975.
9. Pelletier LL Jr, Borel DM, Romig DA, et al: Disseminated intravascular coagulation and hepatic necrosis: Complications of infectious mononucleosis. *JAMA* 235(11):1144, 1976.
10. Harries JT, Ferguson AW: Fatal infectious mononucleosis with liver failure in two sisters. *Arch Dis Child* 43:480, 1968.
11. Brun C, Madsen S, Olsen S: Infectious mononucleosis with hepatic and renal involvement. *Scand J Gastroenterol* 5:89, 1970.
12. Beschorner WE, Pino J, Boitnott JK, et al: Pathology of the liver with bone marrow transplantation. Effects of busulfan, carmustine, acute graft versus host reaction and cytomegalovirus infection. *Am J Pathol* 99:369, 1980.
13. Henson DE, Grimley PM, Strano AJ: Postnatal cytomegalovirus hepatitis. *Hum Pathol* 5:93, 1974.
14. Gregor GR, Geller SA, Walker GF, et al: Coxsackie hepatitis in an adult, with ultrastructural demonstration of the virus. *Mt Sinai J Med* 42:575, 1975.
15. Smetana HF: Yellow fever, 60 years later. *Milit Med* 128(4):306, 1963.
16. Zuckerman AJ, Simpson DIH: Exotic virus infections of the liver. *Prog Liver Dis* 6:425, 1979.
17. Bechtelsheimer H, Korb G, Gedigk P: The morphology and pathogenesis of Marburg hepatitis. *Hum Pathol* 3:255, 1972.
18. Buckley SM, Casals J: Pathobiology of Lassa fever. *Int Rev Exp Pathol* 78:97, 1978.
19. Winn WC, Monath TP, Murphy FA, et al: Lassa virus hepatitis. *Arch Pathol Lab Med* 99:599, 1975.
20. Bernstein M, Edmondson HA, Barbour BH: The liver lesion in Q fever. *Arch Intern Med* 116:491, 1965.
21. Turck WPG, Howitt G, Turnberg LA, et al: Chronic Q fever. *Q J Med* (New ser) XLV 178:193, 1976.
23. Meade RH III: Primary hepatic actinomycosis. *Gastroenterology* 78:355, 1980.
24. Weinstein L: Bacterial hepatitis: A case report on an unrecognized cause of fever of unknown origin. *N Engl J Med* 299:1052, 1978.
25. Zimmerman HJ, Fang M, Utili R, et al: Jaundice due to bacterial infection. *Gastroenterology* 77:362, 1979.

25a. Wray BW, Middleton HM, Mills LR, et al: Recurrent purulent triaditis with congenital x-linked Agammaglobulinemia. *Am J Gastro* 75, 140, 1981.

26. Kocak N, Ozsoylu S, Ertugrul M, et al: Liver damage in scarlet fever: Descriptions of two affected children. *Clin Ped* 15:462, 1976.
27. Misra PS, Lebwohl P, Laufer H: Hepatic and appendiceal Whipple's disease with negative jejunal biopsies. *Am J Gastro* 75:302, 1981.
28. Brooks SE, Hanchard B, Terry S, et al: Hepatic ultrastructure in secondary syphilis. *Arch Pathol Lab Med* 103:451, 1979.

29. Feher J, Somogyi T, Timmer M, et al: Early syphilitic hepatitis. *Lancet* 2:896, Nov 1975.

29a. Morrison EB, Norman DA, Wingo CS: Simultaneous hepatic and renal involvement in acute syphilis. Case report and review of the literature. *Dig Dis* 25:875, 1980.

29b. Romell J, Rybak B, Dave P: Spirochetal vasculitis and bile ductular damage in early syphilis. *Am J Gastroenterol* 74:352, 1980.

30. Sobel HJ, Wolf EH: Liver involvement in early syphilis. *Arch Pathol Lab Med* 93:565, 1972.

31. Tiliakos N, Shamma'a JA, Nasrallah SM: Syphilitic hepatitis. *Am J Gastroenterol* 73:60, 1980.

32. Ramachandran S, Godfrey JJ, Perera MVF: Typhoid hepatitis. *JAMA* 230:236, 1974.

33. Ayhan A, Gokoz A, Kartazadag S, et al: The liver in typhoid fever. *Am J Gastroenterol* 59:141, 1973.

34. Arean VM: The pathologic anatomy and pathogenesis of fatal human leptospirosis (Weil's disease). *Am J Pathol* 40:393, 1962.

34a. Daneshbrod K: Visceral Leishmaniasis (Kala Azar) in Iran. A pathologic and electron microscopic study. *Am J Clin Pathol* 57:156, 1981.

34b. Pampiglione S, La Placa M, Schlick G: Studies on Mediterranean Leishmaniasis. I. An outbreak of visceral Leishmaniasis in northern Italy. *Trans Roy Soc Trop Med Hyg* 68:349, 1974.

34c. Pampiglione S, Manson Bahr PEC, Giungi F, et al: Studies on Mediterranean Leishmaniasis. II. Asymptomatic cases of visceral Leishmaniasis. *Trans Roy Soc Trop Med Hyg* 68:447, 1974.

34d. Barrier J, Grolleau JY, LeBodic MF, et al: Adult kala azar with jaundice and immunologic abnormalities. *Gastroenterol Clin Biol* 5:847, 1981.

35. DeBrito T, Barone AA, Faria RM: Human liver biopsy in *P. falciparum* and *P. vivax malaria. Virchows Arch* [*Pathol Anat*] 348:220, 1969.

35a. Ghishan FK, Myers MG, Younszai K: Hepatic fatty metamorphosis in latent exoerythrocytic malaria. *Gastroenterology* 74:532, 1980.

36. Weitberg AB, Alper JC, Diamond I, et al: Acute granulomatous hepatitis in the course of acquired toxoplasmosis. *Med Int* 300:1093, 1979.

37. Vischer TL, Bernheim C, Engelbrecht E: Two cases of hepatitis due to *Toxoplasma gondii. Lancet* 2:919, Oct 1967.

38. Ellman MH, Weis MJ, Spellberg MA: Liver disease in rheumatoid arthritis. *Am J Gastroenterol* 62:46, 1974.

39. Mills PR, MacSween RNM, Dick WC, et al: Liver disease in rheumatoid arthritis. *Scott Med J* 25:18, 1980.

40. Schaller J: The liver and arthritis. *J Pediatr* 79:139, 1971.

41. Gossman HH, Dolle W, Korb G, et al: Alterazione epatiche nell' arterite a cellule giganti. *Minerva Med* 71:475, 1980.

42. Kosolcharoen P, Magnin GE: Liver dysfunction and polymyalgia rheumatica. A case report. *J Rheumatol* 3(1):50, 1976.

42a. Kuntz HD, Oellig WP, Thiel H: Granulomatous liver changes in acute rheumatic fever. *Med Klin* 76:504, 1981.

42b. Ogilvie AL, James PD, Toghill PJ: Hepatic artery involvement in Polymyalgia arteritica. *J Clin Pathol* 34:769, 1981.

43. Antia, FP, Bharadwaj TP, Watsa MC, et al: Liver in normal pregnancy, preeclampsia, and eclampsia. *Lancet* 2:776, Oct 1958.

44. Arias F, Mancilla-Jimenez R: Hepatic fibrinogen deposits in pre-eclampsia. *N Engl J Med* 295:578, 1976.

45. Chlumský J, Dobiás J, Vrabec R, et al: Liver changes in burns, as seen in the clinical morphologic picture. *Acta Hepatogastroenterol (Stuttg)* 23:118, 1976.

46. Langlinais PC, Panke TW: Intrasinusoidal bodies in the livers of thermally injured patients. *Arch Pathol Lab Med* 103:499, 1979.

47. Bianchi L, Ohnacker H, Beck K, et al: Liver damage in heatstroke and its regression. *Hum Pathol* 3:237, 1972.

48. Wills EJ, Findlay JM, McManus JPA: Effects of hyperthermia therapy on the liver. *J Clin Pathol*

29:1, 1976.

49. Utz D, Warren M, Gregg J, et al: Reversible hepatic dysfunction association with hypernephroma. *Mayo Clin Proc* 45:161, 1970.
50. Strickland RC, Schenker S: The nephrogenic hepatic dysfunction syndrome. A review. *Am J Dig Dis* 22(1):49, 1977.
51. Delpre G, Ilie B, Papo J, et al: Hypernephroma with nonmetastatic liver dysfunction (Stauffer's syndrome) and hypercalcemia. *Am J Gastroenterol* 72:239, 1979.
52. Armitage J, Burns C, Kent T: Liver disease complicating the management of acute leukemia during remission. *Cancer* 41:737, 1978.
53. Woodruff JM, Hansen JA, Good RA, et al: The pathology of the graft versus host reaction (GVHR) in adults receiving bone marrow transplants. *Transplant Proc* 8:675, 1976.
54. Rothko K, Moore GW, Hutchins GM: Analysis of cause of death following bone marrow transplantation. A clinicopathologic study of forty three patients. *Lab Invest* 42:146, 1980.
55. Fennell RS III, Andres JM, Pfaff WW, et al: Liver disease in children and adolescents during hemodialysis and after renal transplantation. *Pediatrics* 67:855, 1981.

4
Granulomatous Diseases of the Liver

DEFINITION

The term *granuloma* is difficult to define, and this has led to some disagreement as to which diseases are associated with hepatic granulomas. Probably the most useful definition of a granuloma is a clustering of inflammatory cells including macrophages, lymphocytes, and plasma cells (1). Epithelioid cells and giant cells of both the foreign body and Langhans' types are also often seen in granulomas. There is no difficulty about diagnosing a granuloma when one sees a group of epithelioid cells with or without giant cells. Our minimal requirement for diagnosing a granuloma is an organized collection of macrophages with or without round cells. The distinction between such a granuloma and the groups of round cells, seen in some hepatic diseases such as focal nonspecific reactive hepatitis, is often difficult and perhaps arbitrary. In fact, granulomas are often accompanied by lesions that have all the histologic characteristics of focal nonspecific reactive hepatitis (Chapter 3). In such cases, sampling error can determine whether a diagnosis of granuloma is possible or whether a provisional diagnosis of focal nonspecific hepatitis is all that can be made.

SUBTYPES

Within the broad spectrum of granulomas, several morphologic subtypes, such as tubercles, foreign-body granulomas, and lipogranulomas, can be defined. Subclassification of a granuloma can be diagnostically useful. Special stains for acid-fast bacilli and fungi, as well as polarization microscopy, are usually indicated. Even then, the etiology of hepatic granulomas cannot often be established on histologic grounds alone. Cultures or chemical investigations of the biopsy specimen are frequently indicated as well. Blood cultures and serology, as well as skin tests, are helpful in many cases. The term "granulomatous hepatitis" has been used not only for specimens with granulomas accompanied by nonspecific reactive hepatitis, but also for granulomas accompanied by little or no inflammation. Granulomatous hepatitis has been reviewed by several investigators (2–6).

Tubercles

Tubercles are composed of epithelioid cells and are frequently associated with Langhans' giant cells (Figs. 1–3, 12). The epithelioid cells are almost always surrounded by lymphocytes, sometimes interspersed with plasma cells. Tubercles are particularly characteristic of tuberculosis, sarcoidosis, and fungal infections, but can be seen in many other conditions, such as drug sensitivity (Chapter 15). Although caseation is rare in hepatic tubercles, it occurs in tuberculosis, fungal infections, and brucellosis, but not in sarcoidosis. Some central necrosis may, however, be seen in sarcoidosis.

Foreign-Body Granulomas

Foreign-body granulomas are the result of the accumulation of various foreign materials in the liver with a macrophage response (Figs. 4–7). The granulomas are composed of histiocytes and often contain foreign-body giant cells. These cells tend to differ from Langhans' giant cells in a more irregular or centralized arrangement of their nuclei. A practical method for the chemical identification of particulate and crystalline material was recently described (7). Such material is seen in narcotics addicts (Fig. 8) (see "hippie hepatitis," Chapter 2). Lesions consist of aggregates of macrophages of varying sizes, some with foamy cytoplasm, other resembling epithelioid cells. The macrophages may be surrounded by round cells, but there is little tendency to fibrosis. When these lesions are viewed under polarized light, small doubly refractile needle-shaped crystals are seen measuring 5–12 μm in length and probably representing talc granules (8) injected intravenously with drugs (Fig. 8) (see also chapter 2). Occasionally, such histiocytes contain PAS-positive granules with a Maltese-cross appearance under polarized light, typical of starch granules (6). Refractive, but nonpolarizable particles surrounded by foreign body giant cells have been reported in hemodialysis patients (8a,b). These aggregates of histiocytes and round cells may be seen in the portal triads, as well as within the lobular Kupffer cells. Fragments from degenerating prosthetic heart valves may also give rise to Kupffer cell foreign body granulomas (8c). In anthracosilicosis, histiocytic granulomas or fibrous nodules containing silica crystals can be seen in the liver, particularly near central veins (9,10).

Lipogranulomas

The term *lipogranuloma* has been employed for two different entities. Both types are composed of macrophages and have a close relationship to lipids. One type of lipogranuloma (6,11) consists of foamy macrophages, usually with interspersed foreign-body giant cells, generally located not in the lobule, but in the vicinity of central veins (Fig. 9). These granulomas are probably related to the ingestion of mineral oil, particularly in the form of laxatives containing paraffin (11,12). This type of lipogranuloma could also be classified as a foreign-body granuloma and is unrelated to fatty metamorphosis of the hepatocytes. Appreciable hepatic damage is rarely associated with these lesions (13). A second type of lipogranuloma is seen only within the lobules and only in the presence of hepatocellular steatosis (Fig. 10) (14). Lipogranulomas of this type consist of

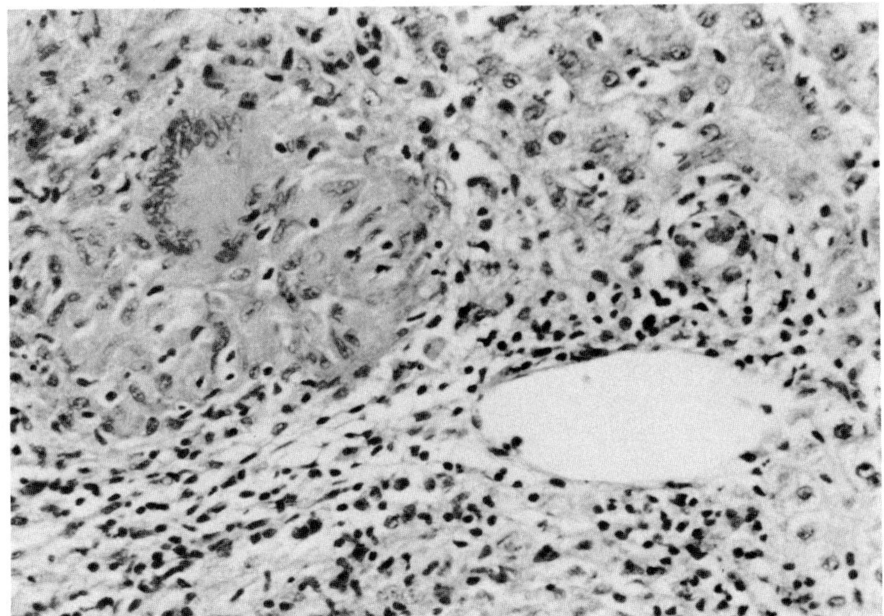

Figure 1. Active tuberculosis, showing a tubercle composed of epithelioid cells and a Langhans' giant cell in a portal triad. Note lack of caseation. (Hematoxylin and eosin, ×250.)

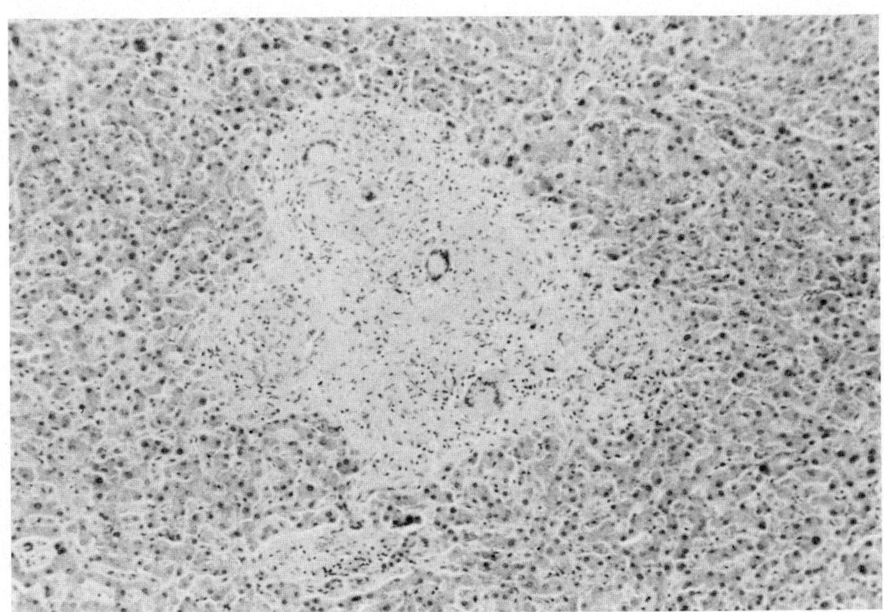

Figure 2. Active tuberculosis, showing a tubercle composed of Langhans' cells embedded in necrotic debris with chronic inflammatory cells. (Hematoxylin and eosin, ×85.)

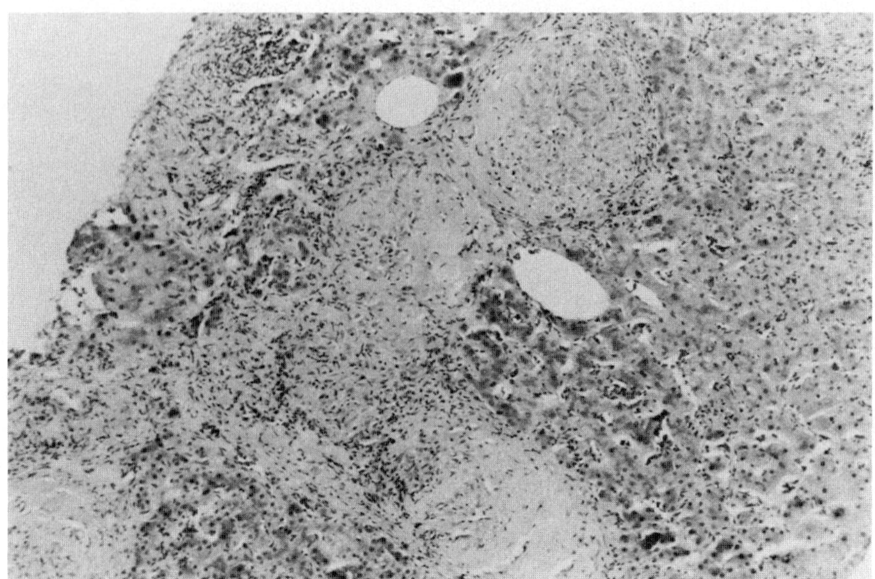

Figure 3. Sarcoidosis, exhibiting some tubercles with characteristic peripheral fibrosis and (centrally) surviving Langhans' giant cells. (Hematoxylin and eosin, ×85.)

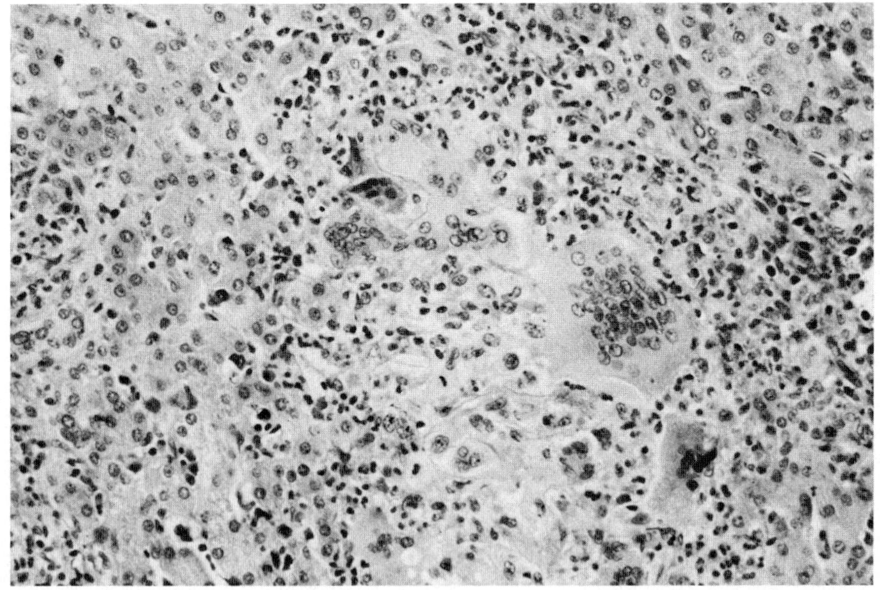

Figure 4. Foreign-body granuloma in a patient with toxocaral infection. No parasites or debris can be seen in this granuloma. The inflammatory reaction consists predominantly of foreign-body giant cells. (Hematoxylin and eosin, ×215.)

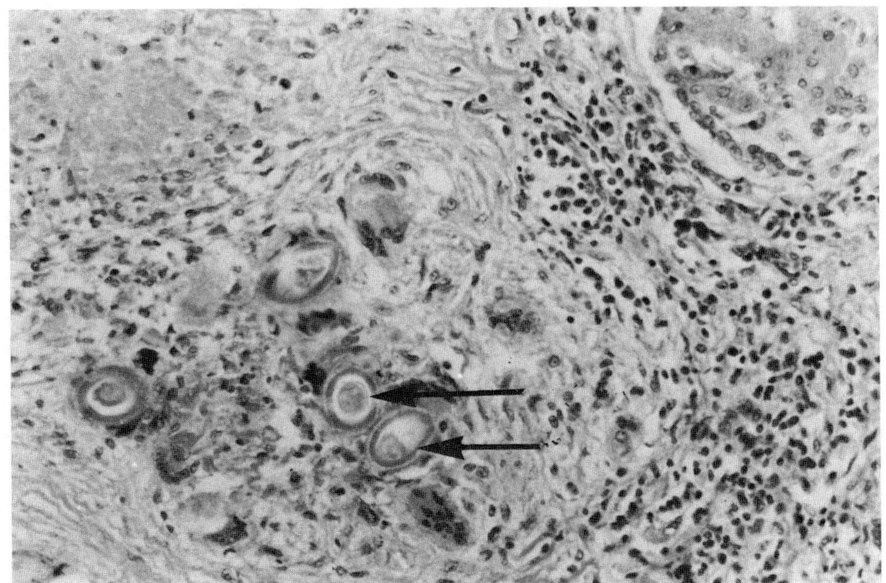

Figure 5. Capillaria hepatica in a child, in whom the organisms have given rise to a foreign-body giant cell reaction as well as hepatic fibrosis. (Hematoxylin and eosin, ×215.)

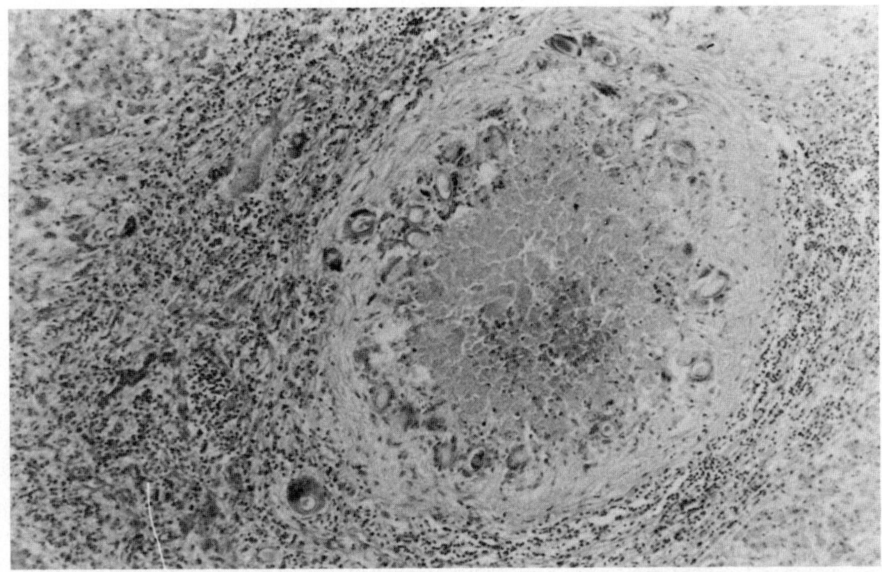

Figure 6. Capillaria hepatica in a child. A mass of organisms have formed a granuloma with central necrosis. The granuloma is surrounded by fibrous tissue. (Hematoxylin and eosin, ×85.)

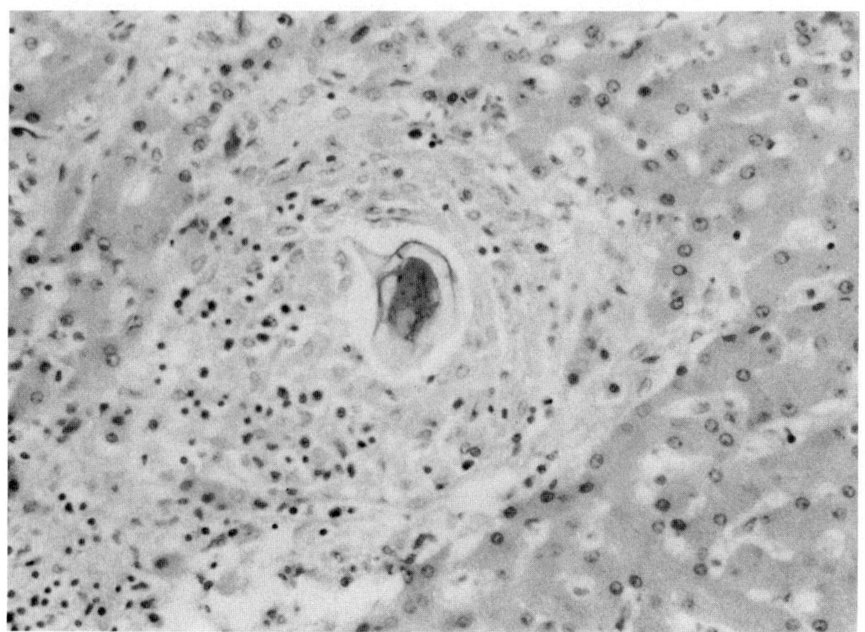

Figure 7. *Schistosoma mansoni* infection, demonstrating a typical ovum with a lateral spine is seen in a portal granuloma. (Hematoxylin and eosin, ×215.)

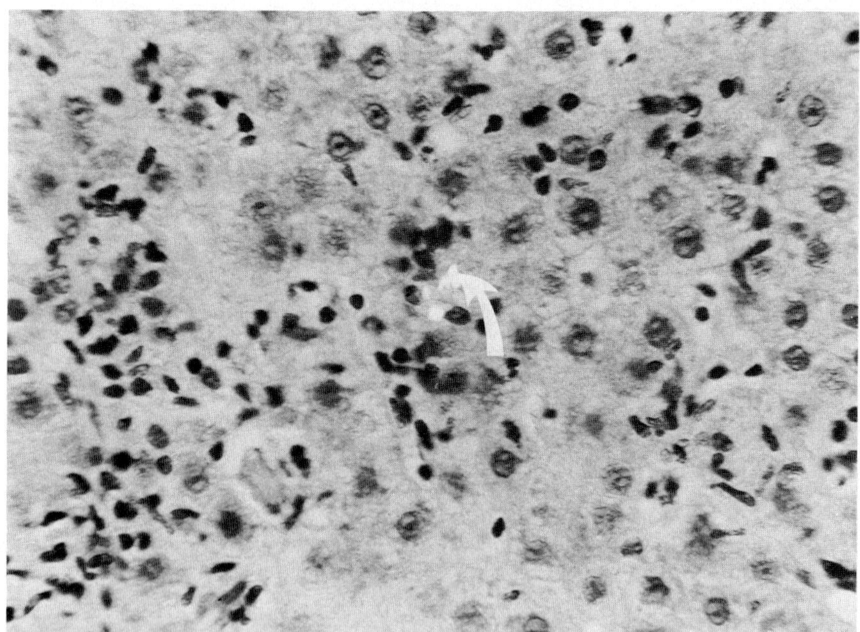

Figure 8. Biopsy specimen from a patient with "hippie hepatitis". Spicules of birefringent material are seen in the hepatic lobule and surrounded by a small group of macrophages partially polarized. (Hematoxylin and eosin, ×300). (Contributed by R. Munn.)

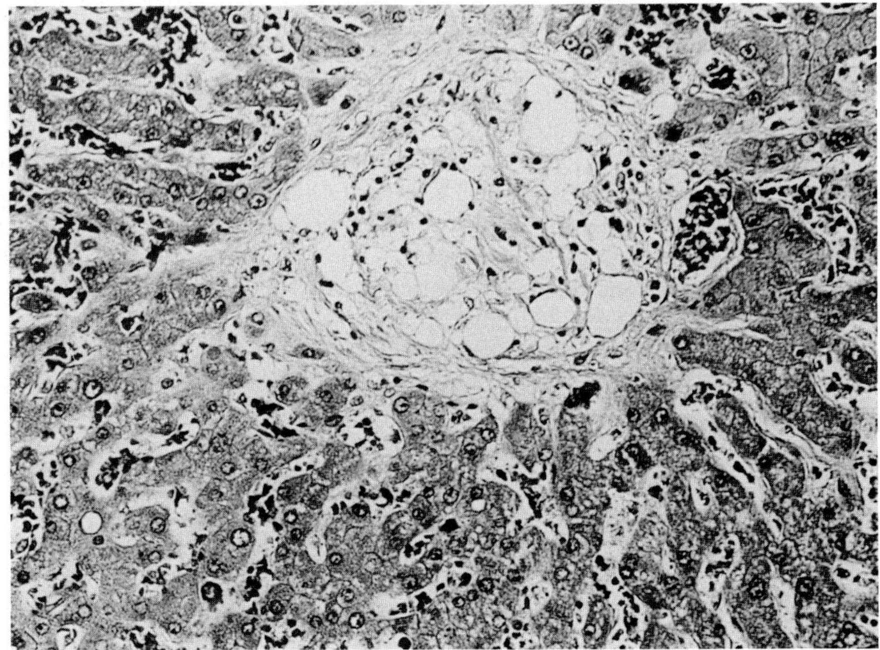

Figure 9. Lipogranuloma in a liver without fatty change. An oil granuloma composed of histiocytes containing lipid droplets is seen close to a central vein. (Hematoxylin and eosin.) (Contributed by H. Dincsoy, M.D.)

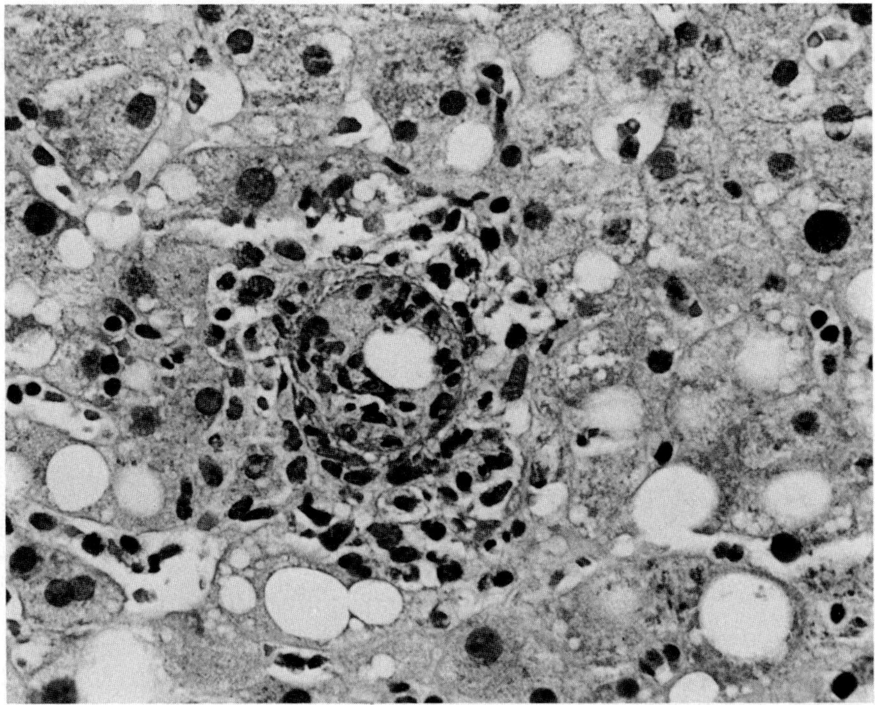

Figure 10. Lipogranuloma in the fatty liver of an alcoholic without cirrhosis. Note macrophages and round cells surrounding a lipid droplet. (Hematoxylin and eosin, ×250.) (Contributed by H. Poulson, M.D.)

nodules of macrophages surrounding one or more lipid droplets (15). Lipogranulomas of this type usually have a distinctive appearance, but are occasionally difficult to distinguish from epithelioid cell granulomas in a fatty liver. Paraffin sections are generally adequate to differentiate the foamy lipid-containing macrophages, usually seen in this lesion, from the nonlipid containing epithelioid cells of tubercles. Fat stains may, in rare cases, be required for this differentiation. Lipogranulomas associated with fatty metamorphosis are most common in alcoholics (16) (Chapter 5), particularly in patients with alcoholic hepatitis, but are also seen in patients treated for obesity by intestinal bypass. Somewhat similar lesion may also be seen in Q fever (Chapter 3) (17). It is possible that these lipogranulomas heal by fibrosis and are precursors of scarring, and even of cirrhosis.

SIGNIFICANCE OF GRANULOMAS

The finding of hepatic granulomas does not necessarily imply an underlying systemic granulomatous disease (6). Even in tuberculous patients, tubercles may be virtually limited to the liver. The density of hepatic granulomas is quite variable. Quantitative assessment of granulomas has, therefore, been suggested (14). Because of this great variation in density, sampling error has to be kept in mind when granulomatous hepatitis is suspected, but not confirmed histologically. Step sections at multiple levels are mandatory in such cases. Some of these sections should be left unstained, so that appropriate special stains can be performed later. Granulomas may resolve completely, as is usual in sarcoidosis or tuberculosis, or may heal with fibrosis starting at the periphery of the granuloma, as happens occasionally in sarcoidosis. Granulomas, due to *Capillaria hepatica*, may also cause fibrosis and cirrhosis (18).

CLINICAL FEATURES

The clinical manifestations of granulomatous hepatitis depend to a considerable extent on the etiology of the granulomas (5). Fever, fatigue, chills, abdominal pain, and weight loss are quite common (19). Hepatomegaly and splenomegaly are often present. Laboratory findings indicative of hepatic involvement may be absent or may suggest predominantly cholestatic or hepatocellular disease. In patients with cholestasis, jaundice and alkaline phosphatase elevation are usually present. Serum transaminase enzymes and serum cholesterol also are usually mildly elevated (3a). In the hepatocellular group, jaundice and alkaline phosphatase elevations are less pronounced. By contrast, serum transaminase levels are usually significantly elevated. Portal hypertension may be associated with granulomatous hepatitis, even in the absence of fibrosis or cirrhosis (20).

ETIOLOGIC FACTORS

In most series of granulomatous hepatitis, tuberculosis, fungal infections, and sarcoidosis account for the great majority of cases (2,3a,4,5). However, the proportion of drug-induced granulomas seems to be increasing (Chapter 15). In these diseases, the lesions are typically well-developed epithelioid cell granulomas, many of which contain Langhans'-type giant cells. Occasionally, especially in patients with overwhelming infections, the granulomas are composed only of histiocytes. Whereas granulomas tend to be somewhat preferentially localized in the periportal zones, they can occur anywhere in the lobule. The etiologic factors mentioned above are particularly likely if tubercles are accompanied by little or no inflammation (4). Individual etiologic factors are enumerated in Table 1 and discussed below.

Mycobacterial Infections

Mycobacterial infections, like infections caused by fungi and *Brucella*, are usually associated with classic tubercles consisting of epithelioid cells and Langhans' giant cells (Figs. 1,2) and may be associated with caseation. However, caseation is not often seen in the liver. Acid-fast bacilli are usually recognized most easily in tubercles with caseation or necrosis. They can either be seen in the amorphous areas of necrosis or in the epithelioid and giant cells lining the necrotic zones (2). In overwhelming infections, the lesions contain many acid-fast bacilli, but the granulomatous response may be poorly developed, and many lesions have the appearance of non-specific focal necrosis and chronic reactive hepatitis. In one series acid-fast bacilli were identified in 45% of liver biopsy specimens of patients with miliary tuberculosis, but only 18% of specimens from patients with non-miliary tuberculosis (2). The finding of acid-fast bacilli enables one to make a diagnosis of mycobacterial infection, most likely human tuberculosis. However, the definitive identification of the causative organism depends on its cultural identification. Noncaseating epithelioid granulomas without detectable acid-fast bacilli, negative when cultured for tubercle bacilli, have been found in patients treated with bacille Calmette Guérin (BCG) immunotherapy for tumors (21–22a). Granulomatous hepatitis produced by atypical mycobacteria cannot be distinguished morphologically from that produced by *Mycobacterium tuberculosis* (23,24) and requires cultural identification of the organism. Hepatic involvement is quite common in leprosy. Leprosy bacilli are somewhat less acid-fast than are *M. tuberculosis*, and this difference in staining can be employed as a differentiating feature using Fite's stain. Epithelioid cell tubercles with very few organisms, if any, are seen in the tuberculoid form of leprosy, while foam-cell granulomas teeming with mycobacteria are seen in lepromatous leprosy (25).

Other Bacterial Infections

Brucellosis and tularemia are commonly associated with hepatic tubercles; caseation has been described in brucellosis (26). Diagnosis of these infections is made by culture of the specimen and by serology. Histiocytic hepatic granulomas have been described in granuloma inguinale (27) and melioidosis (28). Tertiary syphilis may be associated with gummas and hepar lobatum, but these are now rarely seen.

Table 1. Reported Causes of Granulomatous Hepatitis

- I. Infections
  - A. Bacterial
    - 1. Mycobacteria (2,3a,5)
      - a. *M. tuberculosis* (2,5)
      - b. BCG treatment (21–22a)
      - c. Atypical mycobacteria (5)
      - d. Leprosy (25)
    - 2. Gram-negative bacteria
      - a. Brucellosis (26,45)
      - b. Tularemia (5)
      - c. Granuloma inguinale (27)
      - d. Melioidosis (28)
    - 3. Spirochetes (syphilis) (5,45a)
  - B. Fungal
    - 1. Histoplasmosis (46)
    - 2. Coccidioidomycosis (47,48)
    - 3. North American blastomycosis (5)
    - 4. South American blastomycosis (5,49)
    - 5. Aspergillosis (5)
    - 6. Actinomycosis (5)
    - 7. Nocardiosis (5)
    - 8. Cryptococcosis (5)
    - 9. Candidiasis (5,5b)
  - C. Rickettsial
    - 1. Q fever (17,32,32a)
    - 2. Psittacosis (33)
  - D. Viral
    - 1. Acute viral hepatitis (4,6)
    - 2. Cytomegalovirus (31,50)
    - 3. Varicella (30)
    - 4. Lymphogranuloma (5)
    - 5. Influenza B (5)
    - 6. Infectious mononucleosis (6)
  - E. Parasitic
    - 1. Lingulatia serrata (51)
    - 2. Ascaris canis (5)
    - 3. Toxocara canis and catti (5)
    - 4. Ancylostoma caninum (5)
    - 5. Strongyloides stercoralis (34)
    - 6. Schistosoma mansoni (6,35)
    - 7. Capillaria hepatica (18)
    - 8. Amebiasis (36,37)
    - 9. Toxoplasmosis (52)
    - 10. Fasciola hepatica (53)
- II. Foreign body granulomas
  - A. "Hippie hepatitis" (8)
  - B. Hemodialysis (8a,8b)
  - C. Heart valve fragments (8c)
  - D. Starch granuloma (6)
  - E. Paraffin lipogranuloma (11,13)
  - F. Cement granuloma (54)
  - G. Anthracosilicosis (9,10)

Table 1. (Continued)

III. Hypersensitivity
A. Drugs (Chapter 15) (5a)
B. Metals
1. Berylliosis (6)
2. Copper (38)
C. Autoimmune (rheumatic) disorders
1. Erythema nodosum (5)
2. Allergic granulomatosis (39)
3. Wegener's granulomatosis (5)
4. Polymyalgia rheumatica (40)
5. Temporal arteritis (6,55)
6. Rheumatic fever (55a)
IV. Hepatic diseases
A. Primary biliary cirrhosis (Chapter 7) (6)
B. Cholangitis (6)
C. Chronic active hepatitis (4,6)
D. Alcoholic liver disease (16)
E. Cirrhosis (4,6)
F. Lipogranulomas with fatty liver (14)
G. Obesity with bypass (56,57)
H. Porphyria cutanea tarda (58)
V. Diseases of uncertain etiology
A. Sarcoidosis (2,20,29,59)
B. Crohn's disease (41)
C. Granulomatosis of infancy (5)
D. Congenital immunologic deficiency (60)
E. Etiocholanone fever (5)
F. Eosinophilic gastroenteritis (61)
F. Neoplasms, particularly Hodgkin's disease (6,42)
VI. Granulomas of unknown Etiology (3b,19,44)

Sarcoidosis

Sarcoidosis is a likely etiology when special stains and cultures do not show either fungi or acid-fast bacilli. True caseation does not occur in sarcoidosis but mild central necrosis may. Asteroid and Schaumann's bodies are characteristic of this disease. Unfortunately, they may be seen in other granulomatous diseases as well. Diffuse fibrosis and even cirrhosis may develop in a small proportion of patients with sarcoidosis. In such patients the granulomas may be surrounded by thick collagen bundles (Fig. 3). Granulomas tend to become less conspicuous as cirrhosis develops (29).

Viral Infections

Hepatitis and hepatic necrosis produced by viruses have been described in chapters 2 and 3. Hepatic granulomas are an unusual response to viral infections but have been documented on a few occasions. Epithelioid cell granulomas have been reported in acute viral hepatitis (4,6), but must be rare and appear to be without prognostic significance. A granulomatous response with foci of epithelioid cells and giant cells has also been documented in case reports of patients with varicella (30) and cytomegalovirus infections (31). In infectious mononucleosis, hepatic infiltration occurs with atypical mononuclear cells. Hepatic granulomas have been reported in these patients (6).

Rickettsiae

Rickettsial infections, such as Q fever (17,32,32a) and psittacosis (33), produce a great variety of hepatic lesions. Most commonly, the lesions resemble nonspecific reactive hepatitis (Chapter 3). However, Q fever may produce a rather characteristic type of lipogranuloma (Chapter 3, Fig. 8) with a central lipid droplet and fibrinoid material or more classic granulomas with occasional giant cells (32a).

Fungi

Fungi may cause hepatic granulomas resembling those of tuberculosis. Unlike sarcoidosis, they occasionally caseate. This is particularly true of coccidioidomycosis (Fig. 11). A diagnosis of fungal infection can, in many cases, be made by demonstrating organisms in histologic sections. The larger fungi, such as coccidioidomycosis, blastomycosis, aspergillosis, and candidiasis, are often seen in hematoxylin and eosin-stained sections. However, special stains (e.g., methenamine silver, PAS) are very helpful. Since histoplasma organisms are only 2–3 μm in diameter, they can easily be overlooked, even with special stains. On the other hand, small calcospherules in old granulomas may be mistaken for histoplasma. Candidiasis of the liver usually produces abscesses with acute inflammation, but granulomas resembling sarcoidosis have been reported. Fungal infection can certainly be diagnosed histologically, but specific identification of the fungus generally requires culture. Serology and skin reactions often can contribute to making a diagnosis.

Parasites

Parasitic infections may give rise to foreign-body type granulomas (Figs. 4–6) or to tubercles with Langhans' giant cells and epithelioid cells (Fig. 12). Visceral larva migrans may also present clinically as a space-occupying lesion. The disease may be produced by larvae of a variety of parasites including toxocara, lingulatia (tongue worm), ascaris, ancylostoma, and strongyloides. The lesions consist of amorphous acellular eosinophilic, sometimes calcified, debris within which fragments of a necrotic wormlike parasite may be found. Identification of the organisms is often difficult but may sometimes be made on the basis of the detailed morphology of the larvae. Granulomas may be found in portal tracts and in lobules, consisting of necrotic fragments, macrophages, giant cells, eosinophils, and occasionally neutrophil granulocytes (Fig. 4). Focal fatty change and mild cholestasis may also be seen (34). In capillaria hepatica there is an intense foreign-body reaction surrounding the ova (Figs. 5,6). If the infection is sufficiently heavy, cirrhosis may supervene in a few years (18). In schistosomiasis mansoni, a dense inflammatory reaction is seen in portal triads composed of macrophages, epithelioid cells, giant cells, round cells, and eosinophils (Figs.

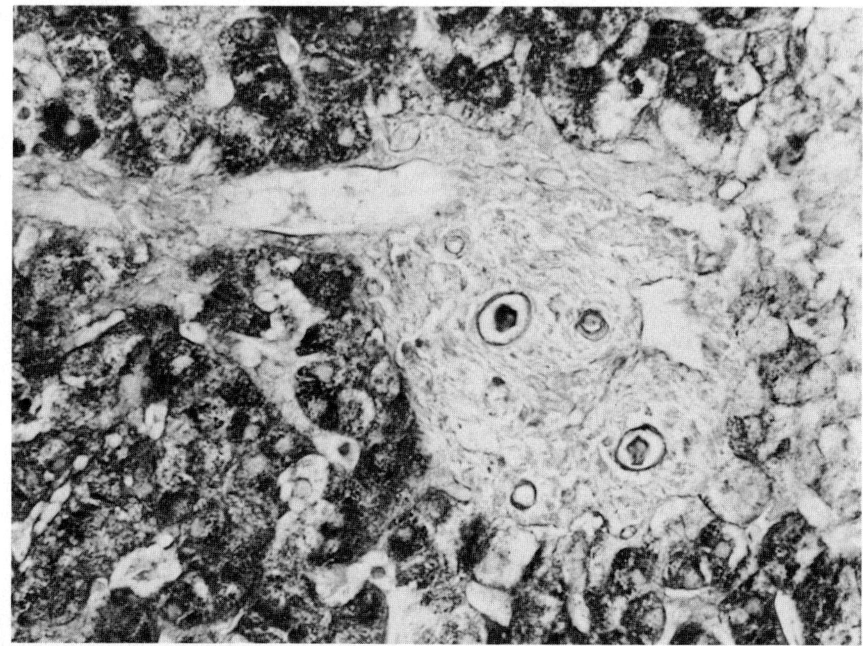

Figure 11. Coccidioidomycosis, displaying several spherules in a portal triad. (Methenamine silver, ×350.)

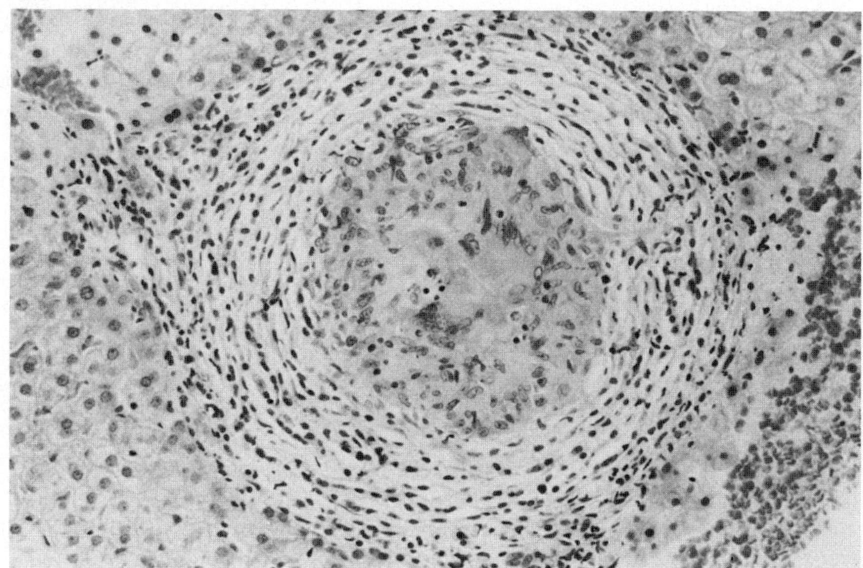

Figure 12. Tubercle composed of Langhans' giant cells and epithelioid cells in a patient with schistosomiasis in the same case examined in Figure 7. No organisms can be seen in this granuloma. (Hematoxylin and eosin, ×215.)

7,12)(35). Quite frequently, the characteristic ova are seen in the infiltrate and sometimes in portal veins (Fig. 7). After many years periportal fibrosis, the so-called pipe-stem cirrhosis (35a), develops. The existence of amebic hepatitis is controversial. Granulomatous hepatitis as a response to amebiasis has been reported (36). Certainly amebic abscesses can have a granulomatous reaction in their walls (37).

Heavy Metals

Chronic beryllium poisoning produces a granulomatous reaction resembling sarcoidosis. This reaction is thought to be a hypersensitivity phenomenon (6). Copper poisoning has also been found to be associated with histiocytic and epithelioid cell granulomas (38). Copper has been demonstrated histochemically in the granulomas. This is very different from Wilson's disease, in which the copper is found predominantly in hepatocytes.

Autoimmune Disease

Granulomatous hepatitis has been reported in some of these diseases and is thought to be of autoimmune etiology, such as erythema nodosum (5), Wegener's granuloma (5), allergic granulomatosis (39), and polymyalgia rheumatica (40).

Hepatic Diseases

The hepatic disease most commonly associated with granulomas is primary biliary cirrhosis. The granulomas in this condition may be tubercles composed of epithelioid cells, often with Langhans' giant cells, or they may be of the foreign-body histiocytic type. They are almost invariably located in portal tracts (Chapter 7). The diagnosis of primary biliary cirrhosis has to be made on the basis of the other changes characteristic of that disease, particularly the typical alterations of portal bile ducts. Epithelioid cell granulomas have also occasionally been reported in chronic active hepatitis, pericholangitis, and cirrhosis (4,6) as well as in fatty liver, particularly in morbid obesity after jejunoileal bypass (Fig. 13) (56,57). Lipogranulomas may be seen in patients with a fatty liver, particularly alcoholics (14).

Inflammatory Bowel Disease

Hepatic epithelioid cell granulomas may occur in Crohn's disease (41) and less frequently, in ulcerative colitis. Differentiation of hepatic Crohn's disease from such diseases as sarcoidosis must be made by the demonstration of the characteristic intestinal lesions.

Systemic Granulomatous Diseases

Hepatic granulomas may be seen in fatal granulomatosis of infancy and childhood (5). Etiocholanone fever also is said to be associated with hepatic granulomas (5).

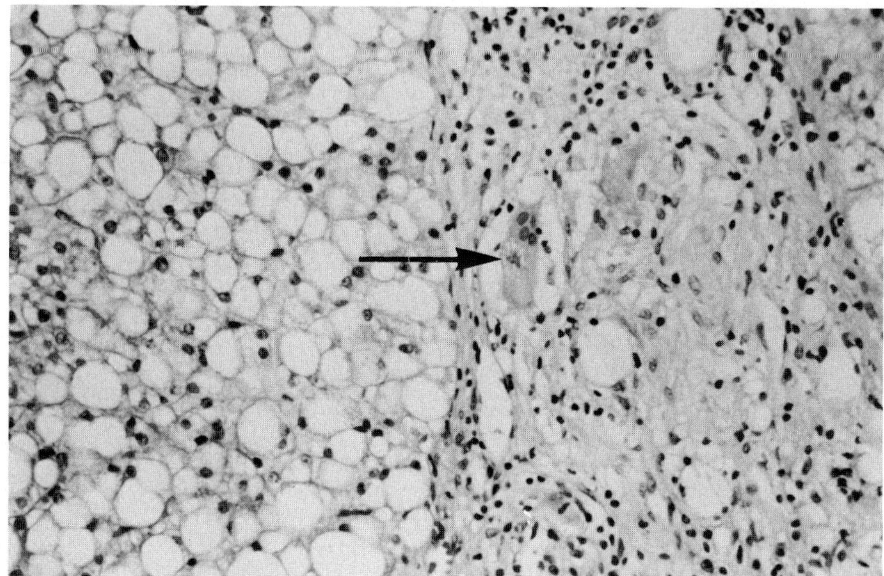

Figure 13. Patient with fatty liver and portal fibrosis after bypass for morbid obesity. A granuloma is seen in a fibrotic portal triad. One of the giant cells composing the granuloma contains an asteroid body (arrow). (Hematoxylin and eosin, ×85.)

Neoplasms

Patients with malignant neoplasms may have clinical evidence of hepatic involvement in the absence of primary or metastatic hepatic tumors. Sometimes the hepatic lesions are those of nonspecific reactive hepatitis, but occasionally granulomas are found. Granulomas can also be found in patients with Hodgkin's disease who are being staged surgically (Chapter 14), but can also occur in patients with carcinoma (42). Granulomatous hepatitis in such patients may be unaccompanied by clinical signs or symptoms of hepatic involvement. Such granulomas are apparently of no clinical significance, and it is, therefore, very important not to confuse them with actual hepatic involvement by Hodgkin's disease or carcinoma.

Drugs

Granulomatous hepatitis has been described as a rare complication of a number of drugs but may be increasing in frequency (5a). The granulomas may be composed of epithelioid cells or may be histiocytic. Giant cells may be present. In addition, the granulomas contain varying proportions of lymphocytes, plasma cells, and neutrophils. Eosinophils are prominent, particularly in early drug-induced granulomas, but are rare in either tuberculosis or sarcoidosis (5a). Caseation is not seen in drug-related granulomas, nor can acid-fast bacilli or fungi be demonstrated. Drug-induced hepatic granulomas, such as those produced by halothane, are often accompanied by lesions resembling nonspecific reactive hepatic necrosis (Chapter 3) or by lesions resembling viral hepatitis (Chapter 2), even massive hepatic necrosis (43). A listing of drugs associated with granulomatous hepatitis is given in Table 1, Chapter 15.

Granulomas of Unknown Etiology

After considering all these possibilities, no cause can be established for about 20% of hepatic granulomas in most series (5). No doubt the size of this category depends on the intensity with which these patients are investigated. It seems most likely that the great majority of patients in this group do in fact suffer from one of the conditions described above but this likelihood has not been proved. Cautious treatment with antibacterial drugs for possible tuberculosis and/or steroids for sarcoidosis may, therefore, be indicated in such cases. Granulomatous hepatitis of unknown etiology involving the small portal and hepatic vein radicles and associated with portal hypertension has been reported (44).

REFERENCES

1. La Via MF, Hill RB: *Principles of Pathobiology*, ed 2. New York, Oxford U. Press, 1975, p 133.
2. Alexander JF, Galambos, T: Granulomatous hepatitis. The usefulness of liver biopsy in the diagnosis of tuberculosis and sarcoidosis. *Am J Gastroenterol* 59:23, 1973.

3a. Mir-Madjlessi SH, Farmer RG, Hawk WA: Granulomatous hepatitis. A review of 50 cases. *Am J Gastroenterol* 60:122, 1973.

3b. Mir-Madjlessi SH, Farmer RG, Hawk WA: Spectrum of hepatic manifestations of granulomatous hepatitis of unknown etiology. *Am J Gastroenterol* 60:221, 1974.

4. Iversen K, Christoffersen P, Poulsen H: Epithelioid cell granulomas in liver biopsies. *Scand J Gastroenterol* 7:61, 1970.
5. Guckian J, Perry J: Granulomatous hepatitis—an analysis of 63 cases and review of the literature. *Ann Intern Med* 65(5):1081, 1966.

5a. McMaster KR, Hennigar GR: Drug-induced granulomatous hepatitis. *Lab Invest* 44:61, 1981.

5b. Jones JM: Granulomatous hepatitis in patients with acute leukemia. *Ann Int Med* 94:475, 1981.

6. Klatskin G: Hepatic granulomata: Problems in interpretation. *Mt Sinai J Med* 44(6):798, 1977.

6a. Kuntz HD, Dellig WP, Thiel H, et al: Granulomatous liver changes in acute rheumatic fever. *Med Klin* 76:504, 1981.

7. Crocker PR, Doyle DV, Levison DA: A practical method for the identification of particulate and crystalline material in paraffin-embedded tissue specimens. *J Pathol* 131:165, 1980.
8. Groth DH, Mackay GR, Crable JV, et al: Intravenous injection of talc in a narcotics addict. *Arch Pathol Lab Med* 94:171, 1972.

8a. Leong ASY, Disney AP, Gove DW: Spallation and migration of silicone from blood-pump tubing in patients on hemodyalisis *New Engl J Med:* 306:135, 1982.

8b. Krempien B, Bommer J, Ritz E: Foreign body giant cell reaction in lungs, liver and spleen. A complication of long term hemodialysis. *Vir Arch Pathol Anat* 392:73, 1981.

8c. Ridolfi RL, Hutchins GM: Detection of ball valve variance in prosthetic heart valves by liver biopsy. *Johns Hopkins Med J* 134:131, 1974.

9. Carmichael GP, Targoff C, Pintar K, et al: Hepatic silicosis. *Am J Clin Pathol* 73:720, 1980.
10. Dirschmid K, Kiesler J: Morphology of the liver in anthracosilicosis. *Leber Magen Darm* 10:115, 1980.
11. Boitnott J, Margolis S: Saturated hydrocarbons in human tissue. III. Oil droplets in the liver and spleen. *Johns Hopkins Med J* 128:65, 1970.
12. Dincsoy HP, Weesner R: Lipogranulomas (LG) in human livers without fatty change. *Gastroenterology* 79:1013, 1980.
13. Blewitt RW, Bradbury K, Greenall MJ, et al: Hepatic damage associated with mineral oil deposits. *Gut* 18:476, 1977.
14. Christoffersen P, Brendstrup O, Juhl E, et al: Lipogranulomas in human liver biopsies with fatty change. *Acta Pathol Microbiol Scand* 79A:150, 1971.

15. Petersen P, Christoffersen P: Ultrastructure of lipogranulomas in human fatty liver. *Acta Pathol Microbiol Scand* 87:45, 1979.
16. Bruguera M, Bordos JM, Rodés J: Asymptomatic liver disease in alcoholics. *Arch Pathol Lab Med* 101:644, 1977.
17. Bernstein M, Edmondson HA, Barbour BH: The liver lesion in Q fever. *Arch Intern Med* 116:491, 1965.
18. Calle S: Parasitism by capillaria hepatica. *Pediatrics* 27:648, 1961.
19. Shee CD, Cremer B: Idiopathic granulomatous hepatitis and abdominal pain. *Postgrad Med J* 56:342, 1980.
20. Mistilis SP, Green JR, Schiff L: Hepatic sarcoidosis with portal hypertension. *Am J Med* 36:470, 1964.
21. Bodurtha A, Kim YH, Laucius JF, et al: Hepatic granulomas and other hepatic lesions associated with BCG immunotherapy for cancer. *Am J Clin Pathol* 61:747, 1974.
22. D'Alessandri R, Khakoo R: Granulomatous hepatitis in a healthy adult following BCG injection into a plantar wart. *Am J Gastroenterol* 68:392, 1977.
22a. Flippin T, Mukherji B, Dayal Y: Granulomatous hepatitis as a late complication of BCG immunotherapy. *Cancer* 46:1759, 1980.
23. Koenig MH, Collins RD, Heyssel RM: Disseminated mycobacteriosis caused by Battey type mycobacteria. *Ann Intern Med* 64:145, 1966.
24. Wood LE, Buhler DV, Pollak H: Human infection with the "yellow" acid bacillus, a report of 15 additional cases. *Am Rev Tuberc* 73:917, 1956.
25. Chen TSN, Drutz DJ, Whelan GE: Hepatic granulomas in leprosy. *Arch Pathol Lab Med* 100:182, 1976.
26. Bastin R, Lapresle C, Dupont B, et al: Brucella hepatitis with caseous necrosis. *Med Chir Dig* 2:199, 1973.
27. Lyford J III, Johnson RW Jr, Blackman S, et al: Pathologic findings in a fatal case of disseminated granuloma inguinale with miliary bone and joint involvement. *Johns Hopkins Med J* 79:349, 1946.
28. Borchardt KA, Stansifer P, Albano PM: Osteomyelitis due to pseudomonas pseudomallei. *JAMA* 196:660, 1966.
29. Maddrey WC, Johns CJ, Boitnott JK, et al: Sarcoidosis and chronic hepatic disease: A clinical and pathologic study of 20 patients. *Medicine* 49(5):375, 1970.
30. Eshchar J, Reif L, Waron M, et al: Hepatic lesion in chickenpox: A case report. *Gastroenterology* 64(3):462, 1973.
31. Reller LB: Granulomatous hepatitis associated with acute cytomegalovirus infection. *Lancet* 1:20, 1973.
32. Turck WPG, Howitt G, Turnberg LA, et al: Chronic Q fever. *Q J Med* 1976.
32a. Pellegrin M, Delsoe G, Auvergnat JC, et al: Granulomatous hepatitis in Q fever. *Human Pathol* 11:51, 1980.
33. Cornog JL, Hanson CW: Psittacosis as a cause of miliary infiltrates of the lung and hepatic granulomas. *Am Rev Resp Dis* 98:1033, 1968.
34. Poltera AA, Katsimbura N: Granulomatous hepatitis due to strongyloides stercoralis. *J Pathol* 113:241, 1974.
35. Carter RA, Shaldon S: The liver in schistosomiasis. *Lancet* 2:1003, 1959.
35a. Dunn MA, Kamel R: Hepatic Schistosomiasis. *Hepatology* 1:653, 1981.
36. Doxiades T, Candrevotis N, Yiotsas ZD, et al: Chronic amebic hepatitis. Clinical and experimental observations. *Arch Intern Med* 111:219, 1963.
37. Aikat BK, Bhusnurmath SR, Pal AK, et al: Amoebic liver abscess—A clinicopathological study. *Indian J Med Res* 67:381, 1978.
38. Pimentel J, Menezes A: Liver disease in vineyard sprayers. *Gastroenterology* 72:275, 1977.
39. Sokolov RA, Rachmaninoff N, Kaine HD: Allergic granulomatosis. *Am J Med* 32:131, 1962.
40. Long R, James 0: Polymyalgia rheumatica and liver disease. *Lancet* 1:77, 1974.

41. Maurer H, Hughs R, Folley J, et al: Granulomatous hepatitis associated with regional enteritis. *Gastroenterology* 53:301, 1967.

42. Saunders J: Lymph node and hepatic granulomata associated with carcinoma. *Br Med J* 1:437, 1976.

43. Dordal E, Glagov. S, Orlando R, et al: Fatal halothane hepatitis with transient granulomas. *N Engl J Med* 283:357, 1970.

44. Nakanuma Y, Ohta G, Doishita K, et al: Granulomatous liver disease in the small hepatic and portal veins. *Arch Pathol Lab Med* 104:456, 1980.

45. Williams E: Brucellosis and the British farmer. *Lancet* 1:604, 1970.

45a. Morrison EB, Norman DA, Wingo CS: Simultaneous hepatic and renal involvement in acute syphilis. Case report and review of the literature. *Dig Dis* 25:875, 1980.

46. Lanza F, Nelson R, Somayaji B: Acute granulomatous hepatitis due to histoplasmosis. *Gastroenterology* 58(3):392, 1970.

47. Craig JR, Hillberg RH, Balchum OJ: Disseminated coccidioidomycosis. *West J Med* 122:171, 1975.

48. Knapp WA, Seeley TT, Ruebner BH: Fatal coccidioidomycosis. Report of two cases. *Calif Med* 116:86, 1972.

49. Texeira F, Gayotto LC, DeBrito T: Morphological patterns of the liver in South American blastomycosis. *Histopathology* 2:231, 1978.

50. Clarke J, Craig RM, Saffro R, et al: Cytomegalovirus granulomatous hepatitis. *Am J Med* 66:264, 1979.

51. Mendeloff J: Healed granulomas of the liver due to tongue worm infection. *Am J Clin Pathol* 43:433, 1965.

52. Weitberg AB, Alper JC, Diamond I, et al: Acute granulomatous hepatitis in the course of acquired toxoplasmosis. *N Engl J Med* 300:1093, 1979.

53. Acosta-Ferreira W, Vercelli-Retta J, Falconi LM: Fasciola hepatica human infection. *Virchows Arch [Pathol Anat]* 383:319, 1979.

54. Pimentel JC, Menezes AP: Pulmonary and hepatic granulomatous disorders due to the inhalation of cement and mica dusts. *Thorax* 33(2):219, 1978.

55. Litwack KD, Bohan A, Silverman L: Granulomatous liver disease and giant cell arteritis. Case report and literature review. *J Rheumatol* 4(3):307, 1977.

56. Sweet RM, Smith CL, Berkseth EO, et al: Jejunoileal bypass surgery and granulomatous disease of the kidney and liver. *Arch Intern Med* 138:626, 1978.

57. Banner BF, Banner AS: Hepatic granulomas following ileal bypass for obesity. *Arch Pathol Lab Med* 102:655, 1978.

58. Cortes JM, Oliva H, Paradinas FJ, et al: The pathology of the liver in porphyria cutanea tarda. *Histopathology* 4:471, 1980.

59. Lehmuskallio E, Hannuksela M, Halme H: The liver in sarcoidosis. *Acta Med Scand* 202:289, 1977.

60. Vesin P, Grumbach R, Cattan D: Hyperplasie histiocytaire bénigne granulomatose hépatique et carence immunitaire. *Med Chir Dig* 5:265, 1976.

61. Everett GD, Mitros FA: Eosinophilic gastroenteritis with hepatic eosinophilic granulomas. *Am J Gastroenterol* 74:519, 1980.

5
Alcoholic Liver Injury

Clinically manifest liver injury in alcoholics generally occurs only after several years of alcohol abuse. A history of alcoholism is often denied; all that may be known about these patients is that they complain of symptoms, such as vomiting, abdominal pain, hematemesis, or melena. Jaundice, hepatic failure, and sudden death may also occur (1–4) but are seen in only a small proportion of cases. The hepatic histopathology in biopsy specimens from alcoholic patients is variable. As in viral hepatitis, none of the individual features is pathognomonic. Still, the total constellation of pathologic changes in alcoholics is often highly characteristic (4a,4b,4c). In a few patients the morphologic picture of alcoholic liver disease is apparently seen in nonalcoholics, most of whom are obese, middle-aged, white women (5–7a). The histology of the liver in patients with an ileojejunal bypass for morbid obesity (8), after intestinal resection (9,10), and in diabetics (11) may also mimic that of alcoholic liver disease.

Fatty Change and Hydropic Swelling

The commonest microscopic abnormality in alcoholics is fatty change (Fig. 1), which is present in about 90% of patients (12), but the proportion of involved hepatocytes may vary from less than 20 to 75% or more. The severity of involvement of the individual hepatocytes is also quite variable. Generally, the lipid droplets within hepatocytes are quite large, displacing the nucleus toward the periphery of the cell. The shape of hepatocytes is round rather than polygonal. In experimental animals (13) and probably in patients as well, the fatty change seems to be somewhat more marked in central zones. Uncomplicated fatty liver is generally asymptomatic and probably has little tendency to progress to cirrhosis. However, it may be associated with sudden death (4).

Hydropic swelling of the hepatocytes in paraffin sections stained with hematoxylin and eosin superficially resembles fatty metamorphosis. However, instead of containing clearly defined empty droplets, the cytoplasm is faintly vesicular or granular, and nuclei tend to remain central. This change is also most marked in centrilobular zones, but may be focal, and is often associated with Mallory's hyalin (Fig. 1) and dropout of small groups of hepatocytes.

Cytoplasmic Inclusions

Mallory bodies ("alcoholic hyalin") are refractile, eosinophilic, or slightly purplish intracytoplasmic inclusions. Christoffersen (14) distinguished two types

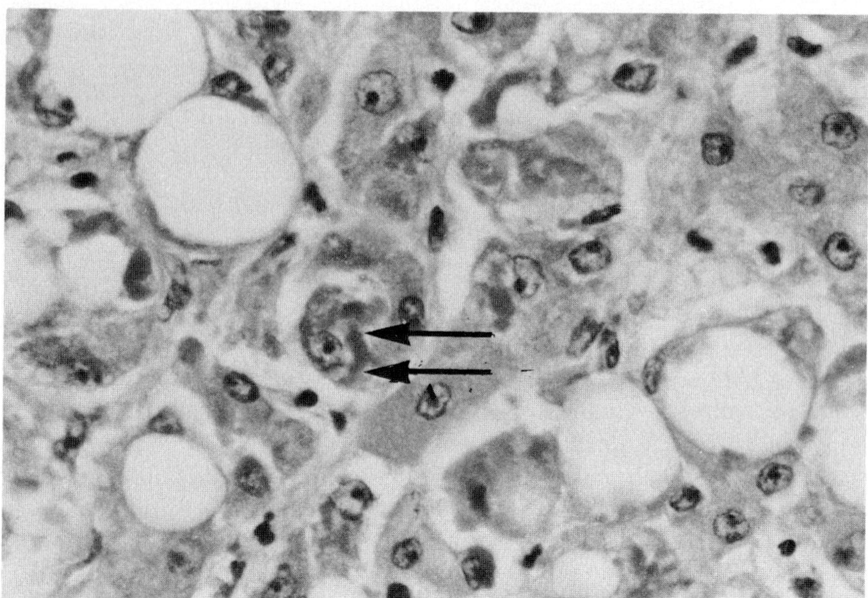

Figure 1. Alcoholic hepatitis. Mallory's hyalin (arrows) is seen in several hepatocytes that also have hydropic cytoplasm and prominent nucleoli. Fatty change is present in some of the other hepatocytes. (Hematoxylin and eosin, ×545.)

of Mallory bodies by light microscopy. One consisted of highly eosinophilic rope-like structures 2–3 μm in diameter, twisting and curling, horse shoe or crescent fashion, around the nuclei of individual hepatocytes (Fig. 1). Larger, more irregular masses, relatively pale centrally, also occur. Both the crescent-shaped and irregular masses were included in Christoffersen's type 2 hyalin. Christoffersen's type 1 bodies are roughly spherical, measuring 2–3 μm in diameter. They stain less intensely than do type 2 and occur singly or in small aggregates. In alcoholics, Mallory bodies may be found in a high proportion of hepatocytes throughout the lobule. A system of quantitating Mallory bodies was also introduced by Christoffersen (14). Less than $1/mm^2$ = +, 1–5 = ++, and more than 5 = +++. Mallory bodies are not specific for alcoholic liver injury. They are usually abundant in Indian childhood cirrhosis (Chapter 9). Mallory bodies are not uncommon in Wilson's disease, primary biliary cirrhosis, and in other cholestatic hepatic diseases (15), in which, however, they are usually seen in only a few periportal hepatocytes. Mallory bodies have even been reported in Weber-Christian disease (16). Because of this lack of specificity, the term Mallory body, after its discoverer, seems preferable to alcoholic hyalin. Stains that can be useful in helping distinguish Mallory bodies from other intracellular hyaline structures are the negative PAS reaction coupled with a positive reaction to certain stains, such as Luxol-fast blue (14). Mallory bodies have to be distinguished particularly from megamitochondria (see below). By electron microscopy Mallory bodies have a highly characteristic fibrillar structure and three electron microscopic subtypes have been described (17). Type 1 consists of parallel filaments, type 2 of randomly oriented fibrils (Fig. 2) and type 3 of

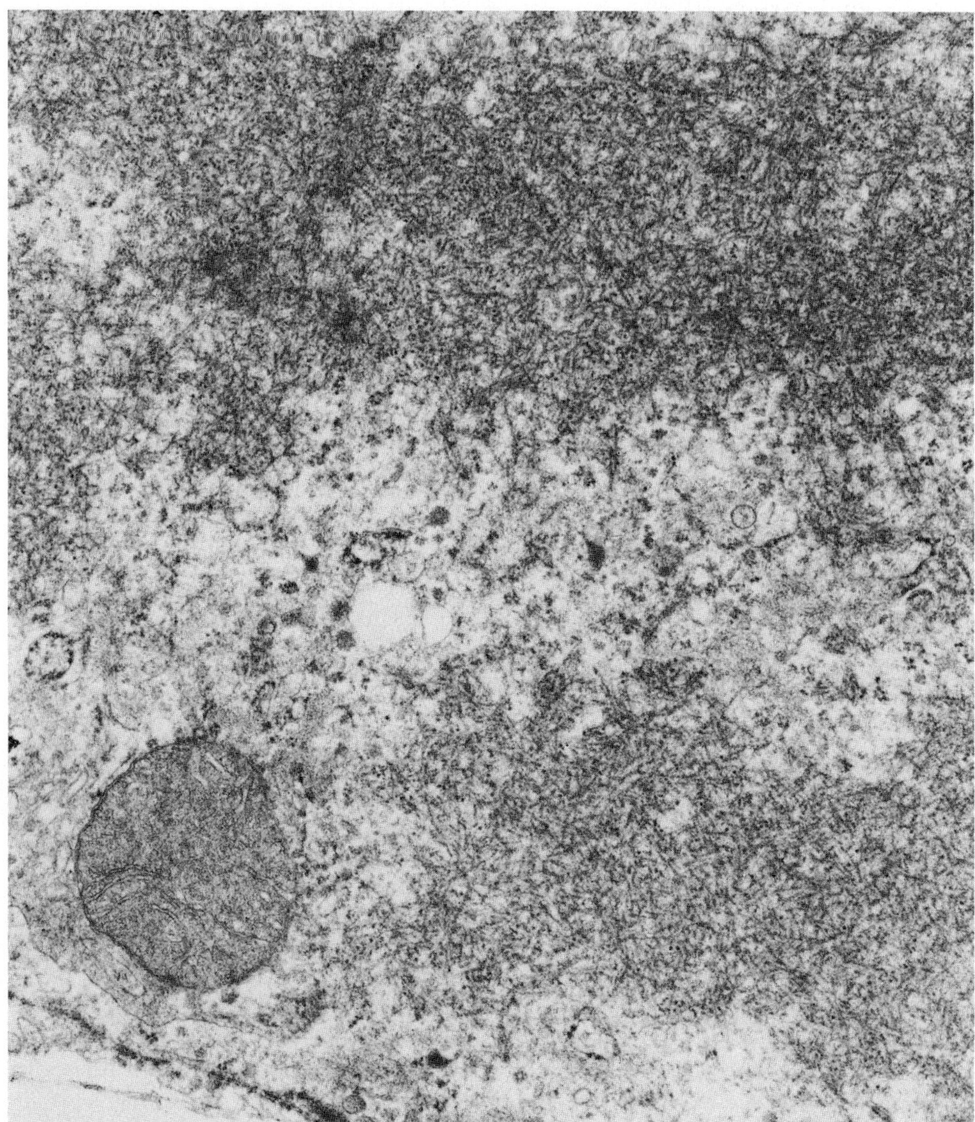

Figure 2. Randomly oriented (type 2) fibrils of Mallory's hyalin in a hepatocyte. (Contributed by S. W. French, M.D.) (×20,000.)

granular material with only scattered fibrils. It is now generally accepted that Mallory's hyalin is composed of intermediate-type filaments (18,18a). Hematoxylin and eosin-stained sections are generally adequate in identifying Mallory's hyalin, particularly the classic type 2 of Christoffersen. In identifying the less typical type 1 of Christoffersen, electron microscopy is desirable and sometimes essential. If specific sera are available, immunohistochemistry can be employed (18,18a).

Roughly spherical or oval, relatively pale eosinophilic hyalin bodies resembling red blood cells are occasionally seen in the hepatocytes of alcoholics (Fig. 3). In

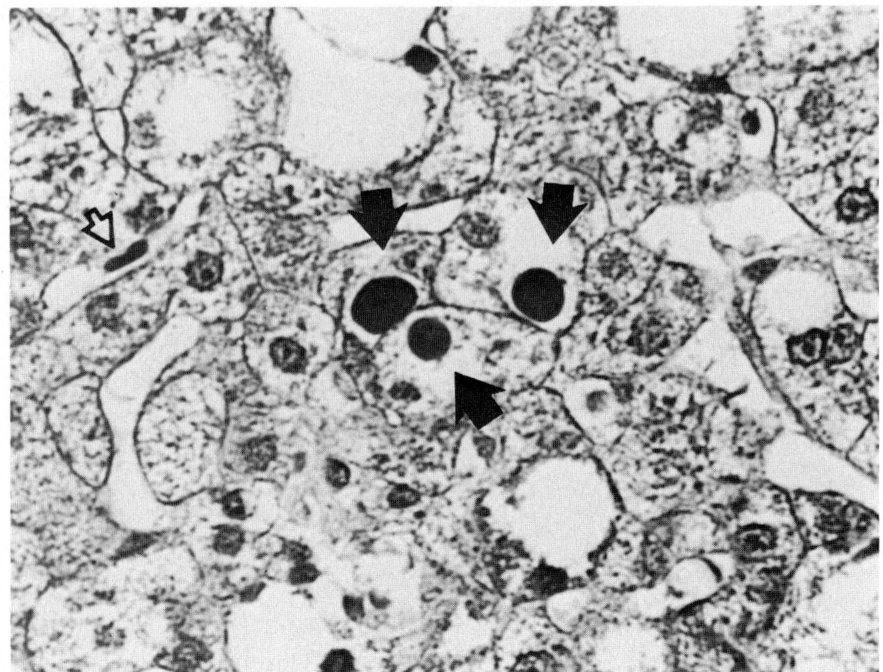

Figure 3. Alcoholic liver disease. Several hepatocytes contain round megamitochondria (solid arrows) resembling red blood cells (hollow arrow), but staining somewhat differently and intracellular in location. (Masson trichrome, ×700.) (Contributed by H. Yokoo, M.D., ref. 20.)

hematoxylin and eosin-stained sections these structures differ not only in shape from Mallory bodies, but also in their paler and more uniform staining. In trichrome-stained sections, they are red. Like Mallory's hyalin, these bodies are PAS negative. Electron microscopy has clearly shown that they are abnormally large mitochondria and are unrelated to Mallory's hyalin (Fig. 4) (19,20). We have hardly ever seen megamitochondria by light microscopy in biopsy specimens that were not from alcoholics. With electron microscopy, however, megamitochondria would appear to be a nonspecific finding (21–23).

Inflammatory Response

Focal polymorph infiltration is commonly seen in liver biopsy specimens from alcoholics (Fig. 5). In some series, this lesion is even more common than fatty change (14). Groups of polymorphs may be seen scattered among apparently healthy hepatocytes and hepatocytes showing fatty change or hydropic swelling. However, more characteristically, groups of polymorphs are seen in foci of necrosis or in areas of cellular dropout, and particularly surrounding hepatocytes containing Mallory's hyalin.

The inflammatory reaction may include mild to moderate prominence of the Kupffer cells, as well as of the perisinusoidal fat storing (Ito) cells or lipocytes (24). Lymphocytes and occasional plasma cells may also be seen in the lobules. Lipogranulomas of the type seen in fatty livers (Chapter 4, Fig. 10) consist of

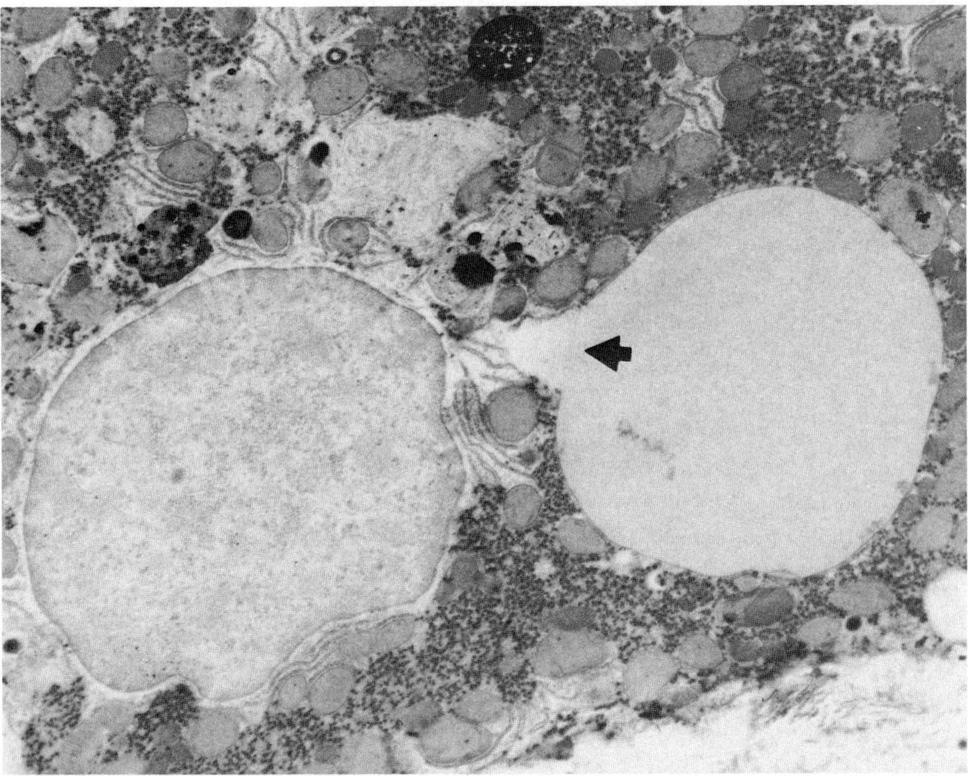

Figure 4. Hepatocyte contains a large, round megamitochondrion adjacent to the nucleus. Several cristae are seen at the limiting membrane of the mitochondrion, which is focally disrupted (arrow). (Electron micrograph, ×8,700.) (Contributed by H. Yokoo, M.D., ref. 20.)

lipid droplets surrounded by lymphocytes, histiocytes, and often eosinophils (25). They may occur singly or in groups and may be located anywhere in the lobule. They are seen in a significant proportion of biopsy specimens from alcoholics. A lesion resembling chronic active hepatitis has been described in alcoholics (26). We have also seen such cases. Unusual features were a lobular inflammatory response containing more neutrophils than is usual in chronic active hepatitis, as well as scanty Mallory's hyalin. Portal inflammation is usually present and consists of round cells, macrophages, neutrophils or, rarely, plasma cells or eosinophils. The intensity of the portal inflammation and ductular proliferation tend to be relatively mild, except in some cases of cholestasis, which may show marked ductular proliferation as well as a marked periductular neutrophil reaction. Biopsy specimens from such patients may mimic extrahepatic obstruction. However, in alcoholics the larger bile ducts are less often involved and true cholangitis is rare.

Cholestasis and Hemosiderosis

Bile thrombi are seen in only a minority of biopsy specimens. Conspicuous cholestasis (Chapter 7) is seen in a small proportion of patients with alcoholic

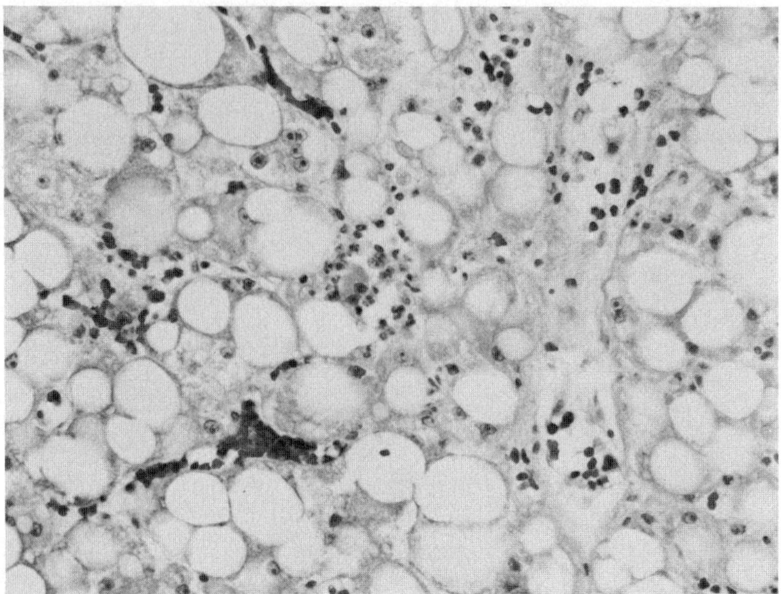

Figure 5. Alcoholic hepatitis. Fatty change with focal dropout of hepatocytes and patchy neutrophil infiltration. (Hematoxylin and eosin, ×400.)

liver injury (2,27). A few acidophilic bodies are occasionally seen. The amount of hemosiderin in specimens from alcoholics seems to vary greatly in different areas of the world. In some alcoholics, iron deposition may mimic in severity that seen in hemochromatosis (28), while in many others little stainable iron can be demonstrated. Most likely, these differences depend on the iron content of the alcoholic beverage consumed, although a variety of other mechanisms may play a part.

Alcoholic Hepatitis

Alcoholics with hepatic symptomatology generally tend to have Mallory's hyalin or focal polymorph infiltration, or both, in addition to fatty change. It is now generally believed that these patients are the ones most liable to progress to cirrhosis. This progressive alcoholic liver disease has been termed alcoholic hepatitis or steatonecrosis-Mallory body type (29). Alcoholic hepatitis has been variously defined by previous authors. An early definition equated the presence of Mallory bodies with alcoholic hepatitis (30). More recently, Mallory bodies and polymorphonuclear neutrophil infiltration were required (31). Later still, fatty metamorphosis, necrosis, and Mallory bodies were considered characteristic (29). Galambos in 1972 (32) required portal edema and inflammation with invasion of the limiting plate, central necrosis, and polymorph infiltration. Birschbach et al. (33) believed that steatonecrosis with Mallory bodies tended to be clinically more severe than steatonecrosis without Mallory bodies. Elkhauser et al. (34) hold similar opinions. For some years now we have made a presumptive diagnosis of alcoholic hepatitis if two of the following three were present:

Mallory bodies, large droplet fatty change, and focal polymorph infiltration. However, we recognize that in a few cases these criteria will fail us. "Surgical polymorphs" seen in wedge biopsy specimens (Chapter 1, Fig 9) may be accompanied by fatty change, but not by Mallory bodies. Similarly, fatty change may accompany surgical trauma and bacterial infections (Chapter 3), both of which may be associated with neutrophils. Distinction of these reactions from alcoholic hepatitis is generally possible if one remembers that (*1*) such polymorphs tend to aggregate around sinusoids, (*2*) they tend to be arranged in layers under the capsule, and (*3*) the adjacent parenchyma usually appears healthy. In particular there is, at most, mild fatty change and no fibrosis. In order to minimize this problem, it is recommended that wedge biopsy specimens be taken early in the course of laparotomy. Sinusoidal fibrosis surrounding individual hepatocytes is quite characteristic, although certainly not diagnostic, of alcoholic liver injury. We have thus found megamitochondria and sinusoidal fibrosis useful as supporting criteria in the diagnosis of alcoholic hepatitis.

Fibrosis

An increase in connective tissue, including both collagen and reticulin, can be demonstrated histologically in the majority of biopsy specimens from alcoholics. Elevation of hepatic prolyl hydroxylase activity is a useful chemical indicator of active hepatic fibrogenesis (35). Excessive connective tissue tends to be deposited in the portal tracts, especially surrounding ductules and in the walls of the central veins (Fig. 6) (36) and in the sinusoidal space of Disse (12). Sometimes the portal tracts (2), and at other times the central veins, appear to be more severely involved. As it increases in quantity, the connective tissue tends to obliterate sinusoids and to encircle individual hepatocytes and small groups of hepatocytes. Sclerosing hyaline necrosis is a term coined by Edmondson and co-workers (31) for a form of noncirrhotic alcoholic liver injury in which the central veins become preferentially involved by necrosis, inflammation and fibrosis (Figs. 7,8) (37). This may progress to occlusion of the central veins by scar tissue. This form of liver injury may progress to cirrhosis (Chapter 13) and has a poor prognosis.

Progression to Cirrhosis

There can be no doubt that cirrhosis develops in a considerable proportion of severe alcoholics, usually after 10 or more years. However, unanimity has not been reached as to the intermediate steps between uncomplicated fatty liver and cirrhosis. Many investigators believe that alcoholic hepatitis is a necessary precursor lesion in the development of cirrhosis. However, Karasawa and Chedid (37) believe that sclerosing hyaline necrosis plays this part. Van Waes and Lieber-(36), on the basis of their studies in alcoholic patients as well as in baboons, believe that sclerosis around central veins is important in this respect. Lipogranulomas (Chapter 4, Fig 10) (25) may also play a role and possibly the chronic active hepatitis described in alcoholics (Chapter 2) (26). Further studies are clearly required to elucidate the intermediate steps in the histogenesis of cirrhosis in alcoholics. Cirrhosis is discussed in Chapter 13.

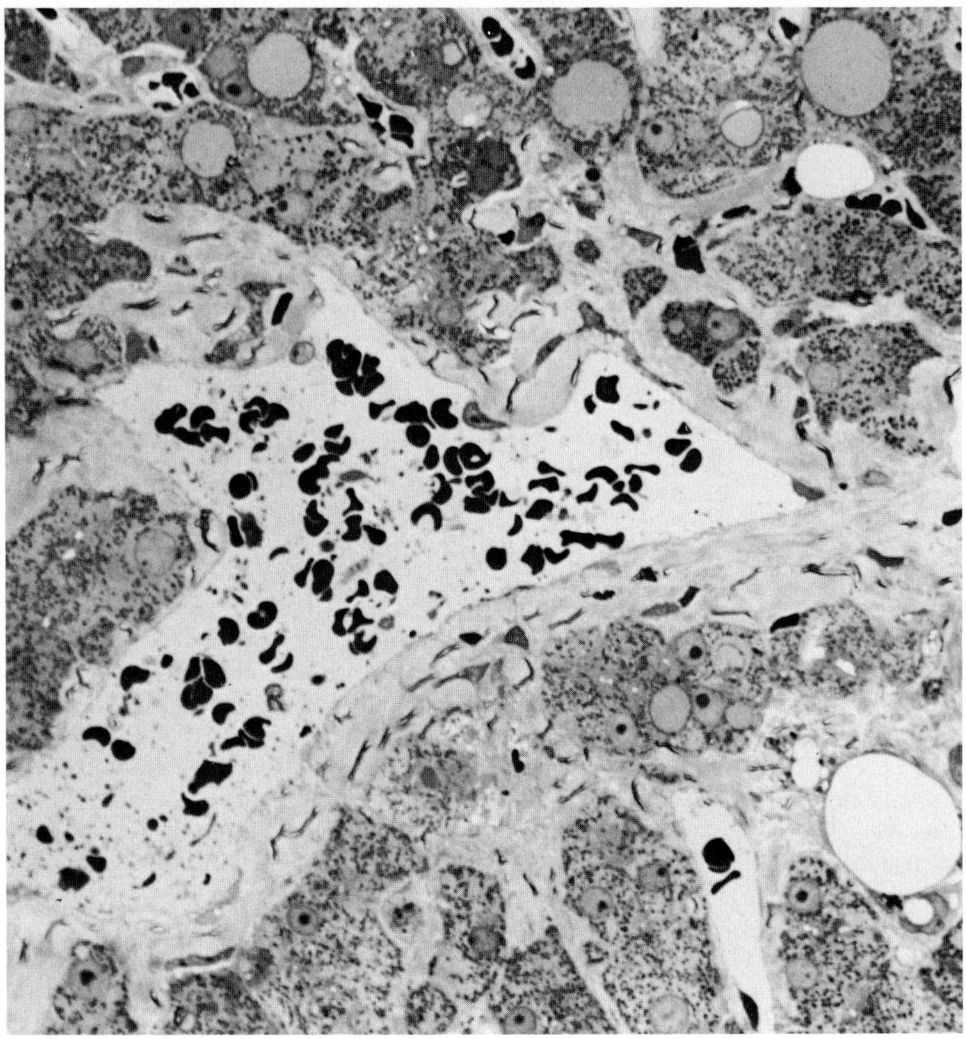

Figure 6. Sclerosis of central vein and surrounding some centrilobular hepatocytes in early alcoholic hepatitis (1-μm-thick section stained with toluidine blue, ×560.) (Contributed by T. Okanue, M.D.)

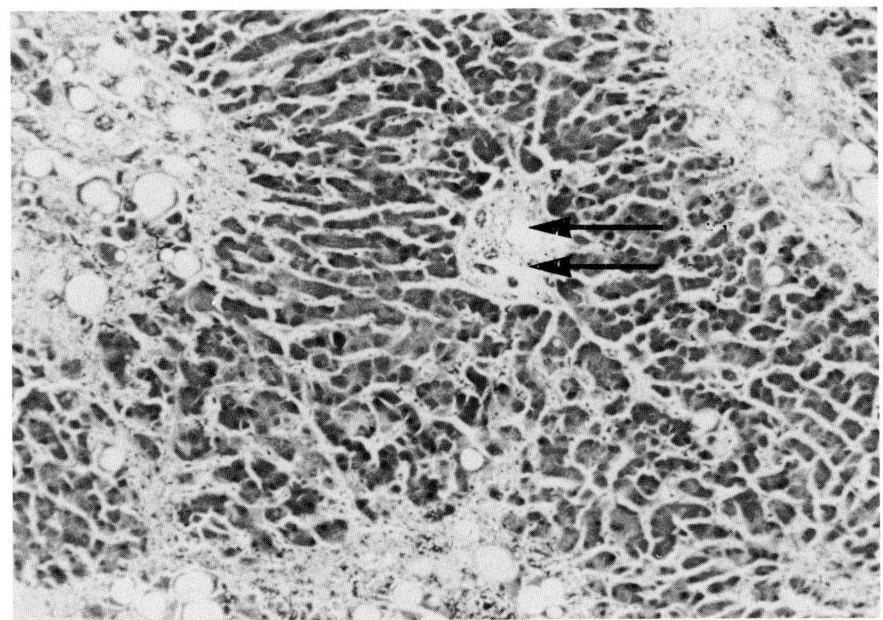

Figure 7. Central hyaline sclerosis. Note fibrosis and fatty change in centrilobular zones at the periphery. No central veins can be discerned. The portal area in the center of the photograph (arrows) is relatively normal. (Hematoxylin and eosin, ×85.)

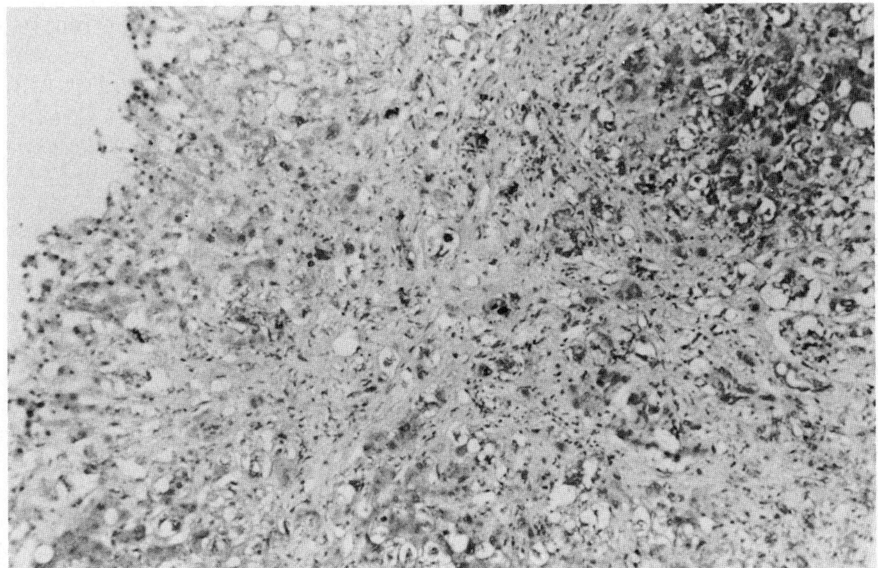

Figure 8. Severe central hyaline sclerosis, showing marked central fibrosis, which often surrounds individual hepatocytes and groups of hepatocytes. No central veins can be seen. (Hematoxylin and eosin, ×34.)

Fetal Alcohol Syndrome

In the fetal alcohol syndrome, hepatic dysfunction was recently described. This histologic picture does not resemble that of acute alcoholic liver disease, but it is nonspecific and variable. Central fibrosis and bile duct proliferation have been reported (38,39).

REFERENCES

1. Perrillo RP, Griffin R, DeSchryver-Kecskemeti K, et al: Alcoholic liver disease presenting with marked elevation of serum alkaline phosphatase. A combined clinical and pathological study. *Dig Dis* 23(12):1061, 1978.
2. Morgan MY, Sherlock S, Scheuer PJ: Acute cholestasis, hepatic failure, and fatty liver in the alcoholic. *Scand J Gastroenterol* 13:209, 1978.
3. French SW, Burbige EJ: Alcoholic hepatitis: clinical, morphologic, pathogenetic and therapeutic aspects. *Prog Liver Dis* 6:557, 1979.
4. Randall B: Sudden death and hepatic fatty metamorphosis. *JAMA* 243:1723, 1980.

4a. Edmondson HA: Pathology of alcoholism. *Am J Clin Pathol* 74:725, 1980.

4b. Baptista A, Bianchi L, de Grote J, et al: Alcoholic liver disease. Morphologic manifestations. Review by an international group. *Lancet* 1:707, 1981.

4c. Boitnott JK, Maddrey WC: Alcoholic liver disease: I. Interrelationships among histologic features and the histologic features of Prednisolone therapy. *Hepatology* 1:599, 1981.

5. Adler M, Schaffner F: Fatty liver hepatitis and cirrhosis in obese patients. *Am J Med* 67:811, 1979.
6. Ludwig J, Viggiano TR, McGill DB, et al: Non-alcoholic steatohepatitis. Mayo Clinic experiences with a hitherto unnamed disease. *Mayo Clin Proc* 55:434, 1980.
7. Miller DJ, Ishimaru H, Klatskin G: Non-alcoholic liver disease mimicking alcoholic hepatitis and cirrhosis. *Gastroenterology* 77:A27, 1979.

7a. Nasrallah SM, Wills CE, Galambos JT: Hepatic morphology in obesity. *Dig Dis* 26:325, 1981.

8. Galambos JT: Jejunoileal bypass and nutritional liver injury. *Arch Pathol Lab Med* 100:229, 1976.
9. Peura DA, Strohmeyer FW, Johnson LF: Liver injury with alcoholic hyalin after intestinal resection. *Gastroenterology* 79:128, 1980.
10. Craig RM, Neumann T, Jeejeebhoy CN, et al: Severe hepatocellular reaction resembling alcoholic hepatitis with cirrhosis after massive bowel resection and total parenteral nutrition. *Gastroenterology* 79:131, 1980.
11. Falchuk KR, Fiske SC, Haggit RC, et al: Pericentral hepatic fibrosis and intracellular hyalin in diabetes mellitus. *Gastroenterology* 78:535, 1980.
12. Edmondson HA, Peters RL, Frankel HH, et al: The early stage of liver injury in the alcoholic. *Medicine* 46:119, 1967.
13. Ruebner BH, Brayton MA, Freedland RA, et al: Production of a fatty liver by ethanol in Rhesus monkeys. *Lab Invest* 27:71, 1972.
14. Christoffersen P: Light microscopical features in liver biopsies with Mallory bodies. *Acta Pathol Microbiol Scand* [*A*] 80:705, 1972.
15. Denk H, Franke WW, Kerjaschki D, et al: Mallory bodies in experimental animals and man. *International Review of Experimental Pathology*. 1979, 20, p 78.
16. Kimura H, Kako M, Yo K, et al: Alcoholic hyalin (Mallory bodies) in a case of Weber Christian disease: Electron microscopic observations of liver involvement. *Gastroenterology* 78:807, 1980.
17. Yokoo H, Minick OT, Kent K: Morphologic variants of alcoholic hyalin. *Am J Pathol* 69:25, 1972.

18. French SW: The Mallory body: structure, composition and pathogenesis. *Hepatology* 1:76, 1981.

18a. Denk H, Franke W, Dragosisc B, et al: Pathology of cytoskeleton of liver cells: Demonstration of Mallory bodies (alcoholic hyalin) in murine and human hepatocytes by immunofluorescence microscopy using antibodies to cytokeratin polypeptides from hepatocytes. *Hepatology* 1:9, 1981.

19. Iseri OA, Gottlieb LS: Alcoholic hyalin and megamitochondria as separate and distinct entities in liver disease associated with alcoholism. *Gastroenterology* 60:1027, 1971.

20. Yokoo H, Singh SK, Hawasli AH: Giant mitochondria in alcoholic liver disease. *Arch Pathol Lab Med* 102:213, 1978.

21. Petersen P: Abnormal mitochondria in hepatocytes in human fatty liver. *Acta Pathol Microbiol Scand [A]* 85(3):413, 1977.

22. Feldmann G, Maurice M, Husson JM, et al: Hepatocyte giant mitochondria: An almost constant lesion in systemic scleroderma. *Virchows Arch [Pathol Anat]* 374(3):215, 1977.

23. Chedid A, Jao W, Port J: Megamitochondria in hepatic and renal disease. *Am J Gastroenterol* 73:319, 1980.

24. Balázs M, Várkonyi S, Pinté RA: Electron microscopic study of alcoholic liver disease with special attention to the changes of mesenchymal cells of the liver. *Exp Pathol (Jena)* 14:340, 1977.

25. Christoffersen P, Braendstrup O, Juhl E, et al: Lipogranulomas in human liver biopsies with fatty change. *Acta Pathol Microbiol Scand [A]* 79:150, 1971.

26. Goldberg SJ, Mendenhall CL, Connell AM, et al: "Non-alcoholic" chronic hepatitis in the alcoholic. *Gastroenterol* 72:598, 1977.

27. Glover SC, McPhie JL, Brunt PW: Cholestasis in acute alcoholic liver disease. *Lancet* 2:1305, Dec 1977.

28. McDonald RA: Haemochromatosis. *Lancet* 1:1157, May 1966.

29. Harinasuta U, Chomet B, Ishak K, et al: Steatonecrosis-Mallory body type. *Medicine* 46(2):141, 1967.

30. Zimmerman HJ: The evolution of alcoholic cirrhosis: clinical, biochemical and histologic correlations. *Med Clin North Am* 39:241, 1955.

31. Edmondson HA, Peters RL, Reynolds TB, et al: Sclerosing hyaline necrosis of the liver in the chronic alcoholic: A recognizable clinical syndrome. *Ann Intern Med* 59:646, 1963.

32. Galambos JT: Natural history of alcoholic hepatitis. III. Histological changes. *Gastroenterology* 63:1026, 1972.

33. Birschbach HR, Harinasuta U, Zimmerman HJ: Alcoholic steatonecrosis. Prospective study of prevalence of Mallory bodies in biopsy specimens and comparison of severity of hepatic disease in patients with and without this histologic feature. *Gastroenterology* 66:1195, 1974.

34. Eckhauser FE, Appelman HD, O'Leary TJ, et al: Hepatic pathology as a determinant of prognosis after portal decompression. *Am J Surg* 139:105, 1980.

35. Mann SW, Fuller GC, Rodic JV, et al: Hepatic prolyl hydroxylase and collagen synthesis in patients with alcoholic liver disease. *Gut* 20:825, 1979.

36. Van Waes L, Lieber CS; Early perivenular sclerosis in alcoholic fatty liver: An index of progressive liver injury. *Gastroenterology* 73:646, 1977.

37. Karasawa T, Chedid A: Sclerosing hyaline necrosis in non-cirrhotic chronic alcoholic hepatitis. *Am J Clin Pathol* 66(5):802, 1976.

38. Habbick BF, Casey R, Zaleski WA, et al: Liver abnormalities in three patients with fetal alcohol syndrome. *Lancet* 1:580, 1979.

39. Moller J: Hepatic dysfunction in patient with fetal alcohol syndrome. *Lancet* 1:605, 1979.

6
Fatty Liver

Mild fatty change is a common accompaniment of a great variety of hepatic and systemic disorders. This chapter deals with morphologically significant fatty change (fatty metamorphosis or steatosis) involving 10% or more of the hepatocytes. Fatty change may be more common in people over the age of 60 (1). Biochemically it may be defined as an accumulation of lipid, principally triglycerides, exceeding 5% of the wet liver weight (2,3). Grossly, fatty livers appear pale or yellowish. Histologically, a considerable proportion of hepatocytes contain punched-out empty vacuoles in hematoxylin and eosin-stained sections that can be proved to contain lipid by appropriate methods (Chapter 1). Edmondson et al. (4) graded fatty change using 1+ for fatty change involving up to 25% of hepatocytes, 2+ for 25–50%, 3+ for 50–75%, and 4+ for more than 75%.

SMALL- AND LARGE-DROPLET FAT

It is convenient to distinguish two morphologic types of fatty liver (5). In the common type, large droplets displace the nuclei toward the periphery of the cell. The diameters of these hepatocytes are two to three times normal (Fig. 1,2). Rupture of contiguous cells may lead to the formation of even larger lipid droplets. In the rare small-droplet type (Figs. 3,4), the hepatocytes are only moderately enlarged by small lipid vacuoles diffusely dispersed throughout the cytoplasm and barely discernible even by high-power light microscopy. The nuclei remain in a central location. In the absence of other histologic changes, large-droplet fatty change is not diagnostic of any specific disease state (Table 1). Small-droplet fatty change suggests Reye's syndrome, fatty liver of pregnancy, tetracycline toxicity, or possibly cholesterol ester storage disease. The lobular localization of fatty change is relatively seldom diagnostically useful. In patients with obesity, particularly after jejunoileal bypass, fatty change tends to be centrilobular. In kwashiorkor, it tends to be predominantly periportal.

CLINICOPATHOLOGIC CORRELATIONS

Clinically significant lipid accumulation, regardless of etiology, is associated with hepatomegaly. Apart from this, however, the clinical mode of presentation may differ markedly. Some etiologic factors, such as obesity, usually produce a fatty

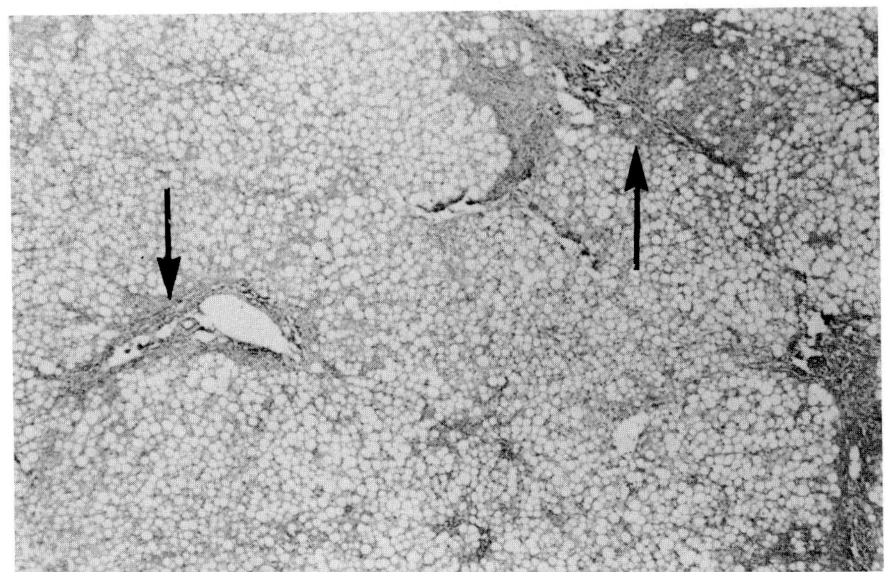

Figure 1. Marked large-droplet fatty change in a patient who had a jejunoileal bypass performed for morbid obesity. Mild-to-moderate periportal fibrosis (arrows) is also present. (Hematoxylin and eosin, ×34.)

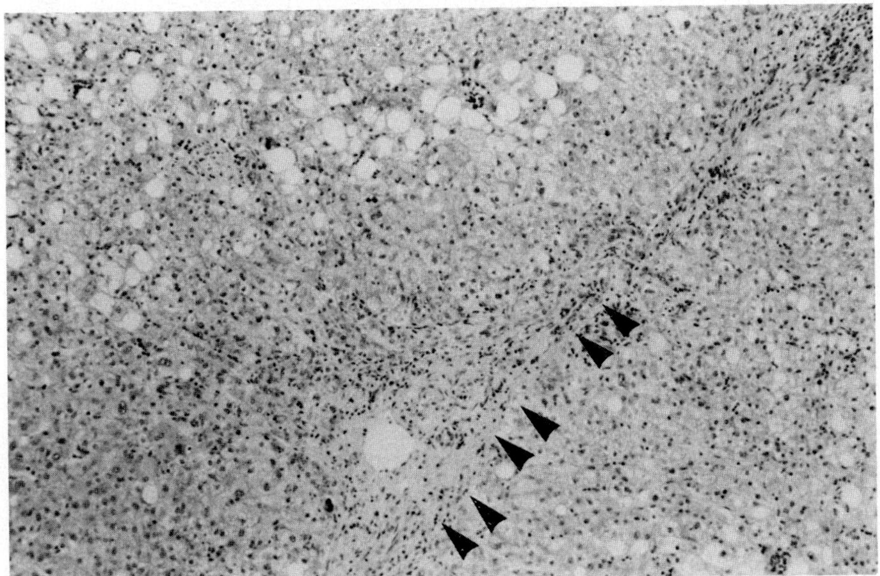

Figure 2. Moderate large-droplet fatty change, predominantly in a centrilobular location, in an adult patient who had been on parenteral nutrition for several months. In the portal triads and extending into the lobule there is chronic inflammation, fibrosis, and bile duct proliferation (arrowheads) with cholestasis. A focal chronic inflammatory reaction is also seen among the centrilobular hepatocytes. (Hematoxylin and eosin, ×85.)

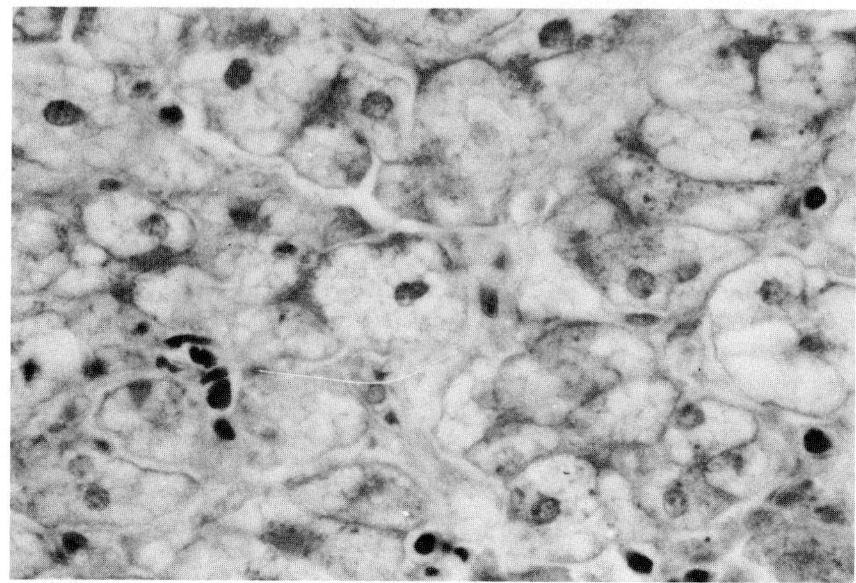

Figure 3. Fatty liver of pregnancy. Small, uniform fat droplets are seen in all hepatocytes. However, the hepatocyte nuclei are still central. (Hematoxylin and eosin, ×545.)

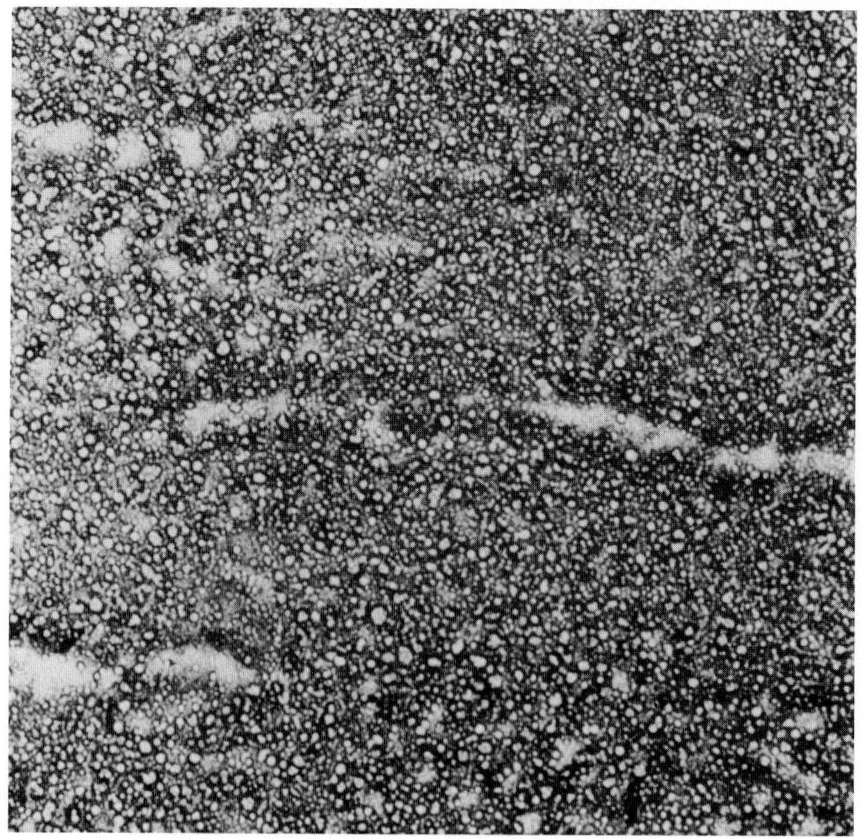

liver associated with minimal disability, while others, such as small-droplet fatty liver are generally associated with hepatic failure and death. These differences in clinical presentation most likely are related to biochemical differences (6). In some cases, fatty change may be associated with reversible portal hypertension. Abnormal liver enzyme tests suggest hepatocellular necrosis and inflammation. However, correlation between morphologic changes and liver function tests is often poor, particularly in the fatty liver of obesity and alcoholic liver disease (7). Apparently uncomplicated fatty liver may be associated with sudden death, particularly in alcoholics (8). Hyperbilirubinemia may be seen even with uncomplicated fatty change, particularly in alcoholics and as a result of parenteral hyperalimentation. Viral-like illnesses should suggest Q fever or, in children, Reye's syndrome in particular. Careful physical examination of the patient and a thorough history of drug and alcohol intake are clearly important.

PROGRESSION TO FIBROSIS AND CIRRHOSIS

Large-droplet fatty livers, complicated by hepatocellular necrosis as in alcoholics, may progress to fibrosis or cirrhosis (Chapter 13), even if the necrosis is rather inconspicuous. On the other hand, uncomplicated large-droplet fatty liver produced by obesity, diabetes mellitus, corticosteroids, or kwashiorkor, and small-droplet fatty liver generally do not tend to progress to fibrosis or cirrhosis (9). Fatty liver and any associated functional abnormalities usually are quickly reversible if the underlying cause is corrected. This is probably still true, even if there is mild or moderate fibrosis. Established cirrhosis, however, is not reversible, and this is probably also true for severe fibrosis.

LARGE-DROPLET STEATOSIS

Large-droplet steatosis, unassociated with inflammation or necrosis in Western society, is most frequently related to alcoholism (Chapter 5) or obesity, with or without intestinal bypass (Fig. 1). Severe fatty liver without inflammation or necrosis is also seen in protein deficiency states (kwashiorkor). Initially, small droplets are seen in periportal hepatocytes. As the disease progresses, vacuoles come to involve the liver in panlobular fashion. Mallory-like bodies have been seen in this condition (10). Noninflammatory steatosis is also seen in diabetes mellitus. It tends to be more pronounced in a centrilobular distribution; an additional clue is the presence of many glycogen nuclei most prominent in periportal hepatocytes. Although morphologically similar, the mechanism of fatty liver appears to differ in juvenile and maturity-onset diabetics (2). Cortisone therapy may produce a similar histologic picture (11). There are a number of neutral lipid-storage diseases in which vacuoles of cholesterol esters or triglycerides, or both may be found not only in liver cells, but in other organ

Figure 4. Fatty liver in Reye's syndrome. Fat droplets are distributed uniformly through the hepatocytes. (Giemsa stain, fresh-frozen section, ×80.) (Contributed by M. M. Thaler, M.D., ref. 27.)

Table 1. Principal Etiologic Factors Responsible for Fatty Liver

Etiology	*Principal Histologic Features*	*References*
Alcoholism	Large-droplet fat, alcoholic hepatitis	(Chapter 5)
Obesity	Large-droplet fat, "alcoholic hepatitis"	(7,12–14)
Intestinal bypass	Large-droplet fat, "alcoholic hepatitis," cirrhosis	(15,36–41)
Intestinal resection	Large-droplet fat, "alcoholic hepatitis"	(42,43)
Ulcerative colitis	Large-droplet fat, pericholangitis	(Chapter 7)
Psoriasis ± methotrexate	Large-droplet fat, portal fibrosis	(16,17)
Kwashiorkor	Large-droplet fat, mostly periportal	(10)
Diabetes mellitus	Large-droplet fat, glycogen nuclei	(2,10a)
Parenteral nutrition	Large-droplet fat, cholestasis	(18)
Corticosteroids	Usually large-droplet fat	(11)
Wilson's Disease	Focal large-droplet fat, chronic active hepatitis	(44)
Viral infections	Focal large-droplet fat, viral inclusions	(Chapter 3)
Q fever	Focal large-droplet fat, lipogranulomas	(45)
Malaria	Large-droplet fat portal fibrosis	(45a)
Galactosemia	Large droplet fat, portal fibrosis	(46)
Tyrosinemia	Large-droplet fat, portal fibrosis	(47)
Fructose intolerance	Large-droplet fat, portal fibrosis	(47)
Glycogenoses	Large-droplet fat	(48)
Hyperlipidemia	Large-droplet fat	(49)
Abetalipoproteinemia	Large-droplet fat	(50)
Weber-Christian's disease	Large-droplet fat	(51)
Wolman's disease	Large-droplet fat	(52)
Cholesterol ester storage	Mostly small-droplet fat	(24)
Tangier disease	Focal foamy macrophages	(53)
Total lipodystrophy	Large-droplet fat	(53a)
Reye's syndrome	Small-droplet fat, occasional periportal necrosis	(21,28,29,31)
Fatty liver of pregnancy	Small-droplet fat	(6)
Tetracycline fatty liver	Small-droplet fat	(22,23)
Carbon tetrachloride	Large-droplet fat, central necrosis	
Amanita phalloides	Large-droplet fat, central necrosis	(54,55)
Phosphorus poisoning	Large-droplet fat, portal necrosis	(20)
Hypervitaminosis A	Focal fat in Ito cells	(33–35)

systems as well. These include some hyperlipidemias, abetalipoproteinemia, Wollman's disease, cholesterol ester storage disease, and cerebrotendinous xathomatosis (Chapter 10). The glycogenoses, particularly type 1, also may be complicated by fatty change and hyperlipidemia (Chapter 10). These diseases are certainly rare and should only be considered once the more usual causes of fatty change have been ruled out.

Large-Droplet Steatosis with Inflammation

When large-droplet fatty liver is associated with an inflammatory infiltrate the cellular composition of the infiltrate may provide some clues as to the etiology of the fatty liver. Multiple small intralobular nests of polymorphonuclear leukocytes are strongly suspicious of alcoholic hepatitis. This diagnosis is supported by either Mallory bodies, enlarged mitochondria, or pericentral fibrosis. Similar changes have been reported in jejunoileal bypass patients and rarely in obese nonalcoholic patients as well (12–14a). However, in our experience, as in that of Piepkorn et al. (15), the full spectrum of alcoholic hepatitis is rare in these cases. Markers that will predict progression to fibrosis and cirrhosis have been difficult to find in jejunoileal bypass patients. Sclerosis surrounding the central vein may perhaps be such a marker (15a,15b). Groups of polymorphs in surgical wedge biopsy specimens, unassociated with Mallory bodies, must be suspected to be the result of operative trauma (Chapter 1, Fig. 9). Similar lesions may be seen in other types of hepatic trauma and in bacterial infections. Distinction of these reactions from alcoholic hepatitis is discussed in Chapter 5. Focal chronic inflammation, neutrophilic or lymphocytic, in conjunction with fatty change should also suggest psoriasis as a possible diagnosis. Whether these patients have received methotrexate or not, they tend to have fatty metamorphosis with lymphocytes in both lobular and portal areas. Marked variations in parenchymal nuclear size and density are often striking, and portal fibrosis is not uncommon. Cirrhosis may supervene (16,17).

Wilson's disease should be considered, particularly in children and young adults, in the presence of mild to moderate fatty change (Chapter 9, Fig. 5), striking glycogen nuclei, and a primarily lymphocytic portal inflammatory reaction, which may produce piecemeal necrosis at the limiting plate. Mallory bodies may be found in this disease as well. However, they tend to be fewer in number than in alcoholics and are generally limited to periportal hepatocytes.

In patients who have been on total parenteral nutrition, fatty change with severe cholestasis often develops that can be complicated by portal inflammation, fibrosis, and even cirrhosis (Fig. 2) (18,18a).

Acute infectious hepatitis is rarely associated with fatty change, except possibly non-A non-B hepatitis (Chapter 2). Fatty change is not unusual in chronic hepatitis, drug-related hepatitis, and other types of viral hepatitis (Chapter 2). Cytomegalovirus hepatitis, for instance, may cause moderate fatty change with focal polymorphonuclear leukocytes. The large distinctive eosinophilic intranuclear inclusions and amphophilic granular cytoplasm of infected cells can generally be found, if looked for carefully in hepatocytes or biliary epithelial cells. Q fever also may be associated with focal fatty change. Particularly suggestive of this diagnosis are lipogranulomas, consisting of a fairly large central lipid vacuole surrounded by eosinophils, neutrophilic leukocytes, and aggregates of Kupffer cells. Fragmentation of sinusoidal reticulin takes place in these areas of necrosis (Chapter 4). In acute pancreatitis, focal hepatic fat necrosis has been reported resembling that often seen in peripancreatic fat (19).

During the neonatal period, severe fatty change with ductal proliferation, which may progress to fibrosis or cirrhosis, should suggest galactosemia, tyrosinemia, or fructose intolerance (Chapter 9) (3). Focal nonspecific hepatic necrosis or nonspecific reactive hepatitis (Chapter 2) may be the only diagnosis one can render in the presence of mild fatty change and spotty areas of acute lobular inflammation. The patient's history, clinical presentation, and laboratory data may be required to narrow the search for an etiologic agent. Cultures of liver biopsy specimens for bacteria and viruses and electron microscopy must be considered in such patients.

Zonal hepatocellular swelling and necrosis associated with fatty change are characteristic of carbon tetrachloride administration, mushroom poisoning, or phosphorus ingestion. The lesions are most pronounced around central veins in the case of carbon tetrachloride and mushroom ingestion, and around portal areas with phosphorus (20). Inflammation is minor compared with the severity of the necrosis. The relatively few cases of Reye's syndrome with periportal hepatic necrosis (21) have to be distinguished from phosphorus poisoning (20). This is usually easy because of the characteristic small-droplet fat in Reye's syndrome.

SMALL-DROPLET STEATOSIS

Microvesicular fatty change is seen in idiopathic fatty liver of pregnancy (Fig. 3). In this condition, lipids have been reported to be free fatty acids rather than triglycerides (6). Small-droplet fatty change is also seen in patients treated with high dose, often intravenously administered, tetracycline (22,23) and with cholesterol ester storage disease (24).

The most common cause of microvesicular fatty liver is Reye's syndrome (acute encephalopathy with fatty degeneration of the viscera) (Fig. 4), which is generally, but not always, a disease of the pediatric age group (25–27a). Although the term "microvesicular" implies small droplets, in truth one can have difficulty perceiving the rather extensive fatty change present, for there are often no distinctly outlined vacuoles in hematoxylin and eosin-stained paraffin sections. The parenchymal cell cytoplasm has instead a rather swollen, occasionally pale, but more often reticulated appearance. This type of fatty change may mimic hydropic swelling and may even be overlooked when no history is given, particularly because the nuclei are not displaced toward the periphery of the cell. Severe (clinical stage IV) cases of Reye's syndrome are characterized by glycogen depletion (28) and may be associated with periportal ballooning degeneration or actual hemorrhagic liver cell necrosis (21,29) and portal inflammation. However, earlier or less severe stages of the disease may appear deceptively bland in routine paraffin sections stained with hematoxylin and eosin. It is best to use at least part of these patients' biopsy specimens for frozen sections for fat and glycogen. Oil-red-0 (28) is the standard stain for fat. However, we prefer to use a

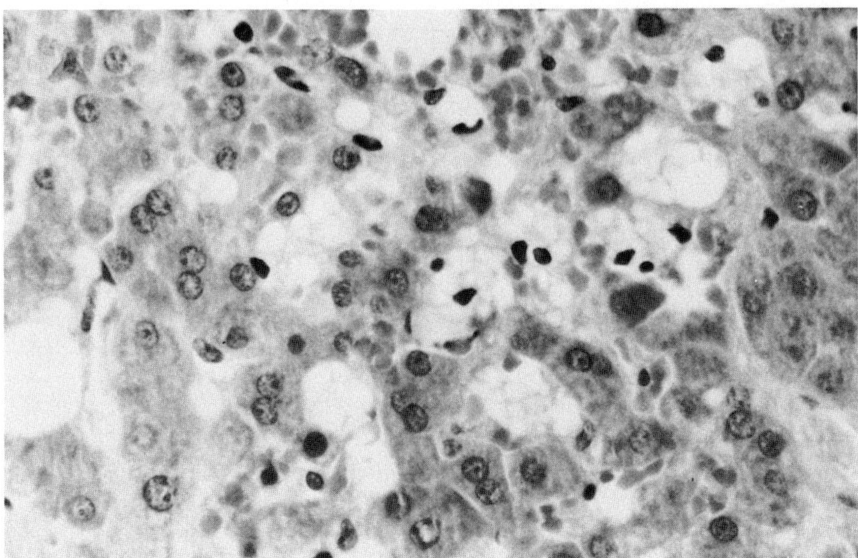

Figure 5. Hypervitaminosis A. Fat droplets are seen in the perisinusoidal (Ito) cells. (Hematoxylin and eosin, ×545.)

rapid Giemsa stain (Fig. 4) (30). One-μm-thick sections of blocks prepared for electron microscopy and viewed by light microscopy are very useful. By electron microscopy characteristic mitochondrial changes have been reported (31). A recent viral infection is usually thought to be most commonly responsible for this syndrome. However, aflatoxin ingestion and salicylate use have been suspected in some cases (Chapter 15). Jamaican vomiting sickness also produces a somewhat similar clinicopathologic picture to that of Reye's syndrome (3). Ornithine transcarbamylase deficiency should be suspected when the clinical picture of Reye's syndrome recurs and a liver biopsy specimen shows no fatty change (32).

HYPERVITAMINOSIS A

In this condition, a different type of fatty liver is seen. The fat can be called neither macro- nor microvesicular, since it is present not in parenchymal, but in sinusoidal Ito cells (Fig. 5) (33). In addition to the lipid, perisinusoidal fibrosis and central vein sclerosis with portal hypertension may develop (34). Even cirrhosis has been reported (35). Serum or liver vitamin A levels can be measured to verify the diagnosis. Carotinemic skin discoloration is a good clinical clue.

REFERENCES

1. Hilden M, Christoffersen P, Juhl E, et al: Liver histology in a "normal" population: Examinations of 503 consecutive fatal traffic casualties. *Scand J Gastroenterol* 12(5):593, 1977.
2. Hoyumpa AM, Greene HL, Dunn D, et al: Fatty liver: Biochemical and clinical considerations. *Dig Dis* 20:1142, 1975.
3. Colon A: Hepatic steatosis in children. *Am J Gastroenterol* 68:260, 1977.

4. Edmondson HA, Peters RL, Frankel HH, et al: The early stage of liver injury in the alcoholic. *Medicine* 41:119, 1967.
5. Hartroft WS: The liver—Nutritional guardian of the body, in Gall EA, Mostofi FK (eds): *The Liver.* Baltimore, Williams & Wilkins, 1973, p 131.
6. Eisele JW, Barker EA, Smuckler EA: Lipid content in the liver of fatty metamorphosis of pregnancy. *Am J Pathol* 81:545, 1975.
7. Galambos JT, Wills CE: Relationship between 505 paired liver tests and biopsies of 242 obese patients. *Gastroenterology* 74:1191, 1978.
8. Randall B: Fatty liver and sudden death. *Hum Pathol* 11:147, 1980.
9. Massarrat S, Jordan G, Sahrhage G, et al: Follow-up study on patients with non-alcoholic and non-diabetic fatty liver. *Acta Hepatogastroenterol (Stuttg)* 26:296, 1979.
10. Webber BL, Freiman H: The liver in kwashiorkor. A clinical and electron microscopical study. *Arch Pathol Lab Med* 98:400, 1974.
10a. Lorenz G: Bioptical changes in Mauriac syndrome. *Zbl allg Pathol u Pathol Anat* 125:303, 1981.
11. Hill RB: Fatal fat embolism from steroid-induced fatty liver. *N Engl J Med* 265(7):319, 1961.
12. Adler M, Schaffner F: Fatty liver hepatitis and cirrhosis in obese patients. *Am J Med* 67:811, 1979.
13. Miller DJ, Isimaru H, Klatskin G: Non-alcoholic liver disease mimicking alcoholic hepatitis and cirrhosis. *Gastroenterology* 77:A27, 1979.
14. Ludwig J, Viggiano TR, McGill DB, et al: Non-alcoholic steatohepatitis. Mayo Clinic experiences with a hitherto unnamed disease. *Mayo Clin Proc* 55:434, 1980.
14a. Nasrallah SM, Wills CE, Galambos JT: Hepatic morphology in obesity. *Dig Dis* 26:325, 1981.
15. Piepkorn MW, Mottet NK, Smuckler EA: Fatty metamorphosis of the liver associated with jejunoileal bypass. *Arch Pathol Lab Med* 101:411, 1977.
15a. Nasrallah SM, Wills CE, Galambos JT: Liver injury following jejunoileal bypass. Are there markers? *Ann Surg* 192:726, 1980.
15b. Haines NW, Baker AL, Boyer JL, et al: Prognostic indicators of hepatic injury following jejunoileal bypass performed for refractory obesity. A prospective study. *Hepatology* 1:161, 1981.
16. Podurgiel BJ, McGill DB, Ludwig J, et al: Liver injury associated with methotrexate therapy for psoriasis. *Mayo Clin Proc* 48:787, 1973.
17. Nyfors A, Poulsen H: Morphogenesis of fibrosis and cirrhosis in methotrexate-treated patients with psoriasis. *Am J Surg Pathol* I:235, 1977.
18. Sheldon G, Petersen S, Sanders R: Hepatic dysfunction during hyperalimentation. *Arch Surg* 113:504, 1978.
18a. Cohen C, Olsen MM: Pediatric total parenteral nutrition. *Arch Pathol Lab Med* 105:152, 1981.
19. Scully RE, Galdabini JJ, McNeely BU: Pancreatitis and hepatic fat necrosis. Case records of the Massachusetts General Hospital. *N Engl J Med* 293:764, 1975.
20. Fletcher GF, Galambos JT: Phosphorus poisoning in humans. *Arch Intern Med* 112:846, 1963.
21. Brown RE, Ishak KG: Hepatic zonal degeneration and necrosis in Reye's syndrome. *Arch Pathol Lab Med* 100:123, 1976.
22. Peters RL, Edmondson HA, Mikkelson WP, et al: Tetracycline induced fatty liver in nonpregnant patients. *Am J Surg* 113:622, 1967.
23. Lloyd-Still JD, Grand RJ, Vawter GF: Tetracycline toxicity in the differential diagnosis of postoperative jaundice. *Pediatrics* 84:366, 1974.
24. Slavin G, Wills EJ, Richmond JE, et al: Morphological features in a neutral lipid storage disease. *J Clin Pathol* 28(9):701, 1975.
25. Varma RR, Riedel CR, Komorowski RA, et al: Reye's syndrome in nonpediatric age groups. *JAMA* 242:1173, 1979.
26. Atkins JN, Haponik EF: Reye's syndrome in the adult patient. *Am J Med* 67:672, 1979.
27. Morse RS, Holmes AW, Levin S: Reye's syndrome in an adult. *Dig Dis* 20:1184, 1975.

27a. Thaler MM: Clinical and Enzymatic Indices of hepatic dysfunction in Reye's syndrome, in JFS Crocker (ed): *Reye's Syndrome. II.* 1979, p 115.

28. Bove KE, McAdams AJ, Partin JC, et al: The hepatic lesion in Reye's syndrome. *Gastroenterology* 69:685, 1975.

29. Bentz MS, Cohen C: Periportal hepatic necrosis in Reye's syndrome. One case in a review of eight patients. *Am J Gastroenterol* 73:49, 1980.

30. Wigger HJ: Frozen section of liver in the diagnosis of Reye's syndrome. *Am J Surg Pathol* 101:271, 1977.

31. Iancu TC, Mason WH, Neustein HB: Ultrastructural abnormalities of liver cells in Reye's syndrome. *Hum Pathol* 8:421, 1977.

32. Cox KL, Cannon RA: Recurrent Reye's syndrome without liver lipid deposition. *Hosp Pract* 16:45, 1981.

33. Hruban Z, Russell RM, Boyer JL, et al: Ultrastructural changes in livers of 2 patients with hypervitaminosis A. *Am J Pathol* 76:451, 1974.

34. Russell RM, Boyer JL, Bagheri SA, et al: Hepatic injury from chronic hypervitaminosis A resulting in portal hypertension and ascites. *N Engl J Med* 291:435, 1974.

35. Babb R, Kieraldo J: Cirrhosis due to hypervitaminosis A. *West J Med* 128:244, 1978.

36. Galambos JT: Jejunoileal bypass and nutritional liver injury. *Arch Pathol Lab Med* 100:229, 1976.

37. Marubbio AT Jr, Buchwald H, Schwartz MZ, et al: Hepatic lesions of central pericellular fibrosis in morbid obesity, and after jejunoileal bypass. *Am J Clin Pathol* 66:684, 1976.

38. Maxwell JG, Richards RC, Albo D: Fatty degeneration of the liver after intestinal bypass for obesity. *Am J Surg* 116:648, 1968.

39. Solhaug JH, Gluck E: Morphological and functional changes of the liver following small intestinal bypass for obesity. *Scand J Gastroenterol* 11:793, 1976.

40. Kroyer JM, Talbert WM: Morphologic liver changes in intestinal bypass patients. *Am J Surg* 139:855, 1980.

41. Gay TR, Peters RL: Death from hepatic failure as a late complication of jejunoileal bypass. *Am J Gastroenterol* 73:150, 1980.

41a. Hocking MP, Duerson MC, Alexander RW: Late hepatic histopathology after jejunoileal bypass for morbid obesity. Relation of abnormalities on biopsy and clinical course. *Am J Surg* 141:159, 1981.

42. Peura DA, Strohmeyer FW, Johnson LF: Liver injury with alcoholic hyalin after intestinal resection. *Gastroenterology* 79:128, 1980.

43. Craig RM, Neumann T, Jeejeebhoy KN, et al: Severe hepatocellular reaction resembling alcoholic hepatitis with cirrhosis after massive small bowel resection and prolonged total parenteral nutrition. *Gastroenterology* 79:131, 1980.

44. Sternlieb I: The development of cirrhosis in Wilson's disease. *Clin Gastroenterol* 4:367, 1975.

45. Bernstein M, Edmondson HA, Barbour BH: The liver lesion in Q fever. *Arch Intern Med* 116:491, 1965.

45a. Ghishan FK, Myers MG, Younszaik: Hepatic fatty metamorphosis in latent exoerythrocytic malaria. *Am J Gastroenterol* 74:532, 1980.

46. Applebaum MN, Thaler MM: Reversibility of extensive liver damage in galactosemia. *Gastroenterology* 69:496, 1975.

47. Hardwick DF, Dimmick JE: Metabolic cirrhosis of infancy and early childhood, in Rosenberg HS, Bolande RP (eds): *Perspectives in Pediatric Pathology*. Chicago, Year Book Medical Publishers, 1976, vol 3, p 103.

48. McAdams AJ, Hug G, Bove K: Glycogen storage disease types I–X. *Hum Pathol* 5:463, 1974.

49. Renger F, Hanefeld M, Jaross W, et al: Liver findings in primary hyperlipoproteinemia. *Dtsch Z Verdau Stoffwechselkr* 33:199, 1973.

50. Partin JS, Partin JC, Schubert WK, et al: Liver ultrastructure in abetalipoproteinemia: Evolution of micronodular cirrhosis. *Gastroenterology* 67:107, 1974.

51. Kimura H, Kako M, Yo K, et al: Alcoholic hyalin (Mallory bodies) in a case of Weber Christian disease: Electron microscopic observations of liver involvement. *Gastroenterology* 78:807, 1980.

52. Kane WJ, Sharp H: Metabolic liver diseases of childhood. *Pediatr Ann* 6:61, 1977.

53. Ferrans VJ, Frederickson DS: The pathology of Tangier disease. A light and microscopic study. *Am J Pathol* 78:101, 1975.

53a. Harbour JR, Rosenthal P, Smuckler EA: Ultrastructural abnormalities of the liver in total lipodystrophy. *Human Pathol* 12:856, 1981.

54. Panner BJ, Hanss RJ: Hepatic injury in mushroom poisoning. *Arch Pathol Lab Med* 87:35, 1969.

55. Wepler W, Opitz K: Histologic changes in the liver biopsy in amanita phalloides intoxication. *Hum Pathol* 3:249, 1972.

7
Hyperbilirubinemia and Cholestasis

UNCONJUGATED HYPERBILIRUBINEMIA

Hemolysis

In hemolytic anemia, there is generally only mild unconjugated hyperbilirubinemia unless there is hepatocellular dysfunction as well. The overall hepatic architecture is normal. Increased hemosiderin deposition is seen in Kupffer cells, portal macrophages, and to a lesser extent, in parenchymal cells. In sickle cell disease there may also be some elevation of conjugated bilirubin. Aggregates of sickled red blood cells can be seen most prominently in the centers of the lobules. Only mild scattered hepatocellular necrosis may be seen (Chapter 12) (1).

Gilbert's Syndrome

Familial, unconjugated, nonhemolytic hyperbilirubinemia (Gilbert's syndrome) is a mild and harmless condition. It is disputed whether patients with this syndrome suffer from a specific disease or whether they actually represent the extreme of normal variation (2). The etiology of this common condition may be a partial defect in bilirubin conjugation (3). By light microscopy, the liver appears normal except for excessive lipofuscinosis reported by some observers (4). Electron microscopically, an increase in the smooth endoplasmic reticulum has been shown in a proportion of cases (5,5a). This variability supports the suggestion that this syndrome may not be a single entity.

Crigler-Najjar Syndrome

Crigler-Najjar syndrome is associated with very high values of unconjugated serum bilirubin. Deficiency of the hepatic conjugating enzyme, uridine diphophoglucose (UDPG) transferase, can be demonstrated. Affected infants usually die during the first year of life from kernicterus, but some patients survive at least until adolescence (6,7). Histologically, bile pigment may be seen in Kupffer cells and in some canaliculi.

CONJUGATED HYPERBILIRUBINEMIA

Dubin-Johnson Syndrome

Dubin-Johnson syndrome, a rare inborn error of metabolism, is one of a great many hepatic disorders characterized by conjugated hyperbilirubinemia, but it differs from most of these in the absence of cholestasis (see below). The Dubin-Johnson syndrome was originally described as "chronic idiopathic jaundice with unidentified pigment in liver cells" (8). The jaundice becomes manifest at birth or puberty. Biochemically, there is an excretory defect with the accumulation of direct-reacting serum bilirubin, nonvisualization of the gallbladder on cholecystography, and retention of bromsulphalein. Grossly, the liver is deeply pigmented. The biopsy specimen appears black or greenish; histologically there are coarse brown pigment granules, predominantly in the central part of hepatic lobules (Chapter 11). The pigment granules are located principally in hepatocytes in the vicinity of the bile canaliculi. In size, location, and color they resemble lipofuscin. However, they are darker and larger. It is still disputed whether this pigment is related to lipofuscin or to melanin. Certainly the granules are not composed of bilirubin, nor are there bile plugs in the canaliculi. It seems likely that this pigment accumulation in hepatocytes is another result of the hepatic excretory defect responsible for the jaundice from which these patients suffer (9,10).

Rotor's Syndrome

Rotor's syndrome is another rare familiar disorder that resembles the Dubin-Johnson syndrome clinically. It is dissimilar in that there is no abnormal hepatic pigmentation, and oral cholecystography is frequently normal. With respect to porphyrin metabolism, Dubin-Johnson's and Rotor's syndromes are also separate and distinct clinical entities (11).

CHOLESTASIS

Cholestasis may be defined functionally as excretory failure of the liver cells with accumulation in the blood of all constituents normally excreted in the bile (12). This definition excludes unconjugated hyperbilirubinemia, as well as Dubin-Johnson's, and Rotor's syndromes, which are characterized by only partial impairment of hepatocytic excretion. Clinically, patients with cholestasis may complain of itching. Conjugated hyperbilirubinemia is usually present, and the serum alkaline phosphatase is generally elevated. There may also be an elevation of the serum cholesterol. Transaminase elevations are usually slight.

Morphology of Pure Cholestasis

The morphologic changes of cholestasis, irrespective of etiology ("pure cholestasis"), include grossly green discoloration of the liver. Microscopically, bile pigment in the liver confirms this observation, except for severe Crigler-Najjar disease (see p. 117). The most obvious histologic indication of cholestasis is the finding of brownish bile plugs in dilated canaliculi (Fig. 1). Occasionally the hepatocytes surrounding a bile plug are arranged in a pseudoacinar or pseudoglandular pattern (Fig. 2). Bile pigment is seen less frequently in the lumens of bile ducts. Bile pigment in granular form in the hepatocytes and Kupffer cells may be difficult to distinguish from other brownish pigments, such as hemosiderin or lipofuscin (Chapter 11). Hemosiderin is localized preferentially in periportal hepatocytes and lipofuscin in pericentral hepatocytes. Bile pigment, in most types of cholestasis, is predominantly localized in pericentral areas (13) (Fig. 3). However, in some conditions, particularly primary biliary cirrhosis, it may be predominantly periportal. If bile plugs cannot be found, it is generally wise to confirm that a brown pigment is not hemosiderin. The Prussian blue reaction is useful, since it stains hemosiderin blue and generally tends to give the bile pigment a greenish cast, the result of oxidation of bilirubin to biliverdin. This reaction is more likely to occur if the reagents for the Prussian blue stain are freshly made up. Lipofuscin is unaltered by the Prussian blue reaction. A more specific reaction for bilirubin is Glenner's stain (14). It should be noted that bile pigment observed in frozen sections may be washed out by fixation and tissue processing so that permanent paraffin sections prepared from the same specimen may show less or no cholestasis.

Electron microscopists have defined cholestasis as canalicular dilatation, a decrease of canalicular microvilli, thickening of the pericanalicular ectoplasm, and hypertrophy of the Golgi complexes. Bile pigment accumulation is not necessarily visible in cholestasis as defined electron microscopically (12,15).

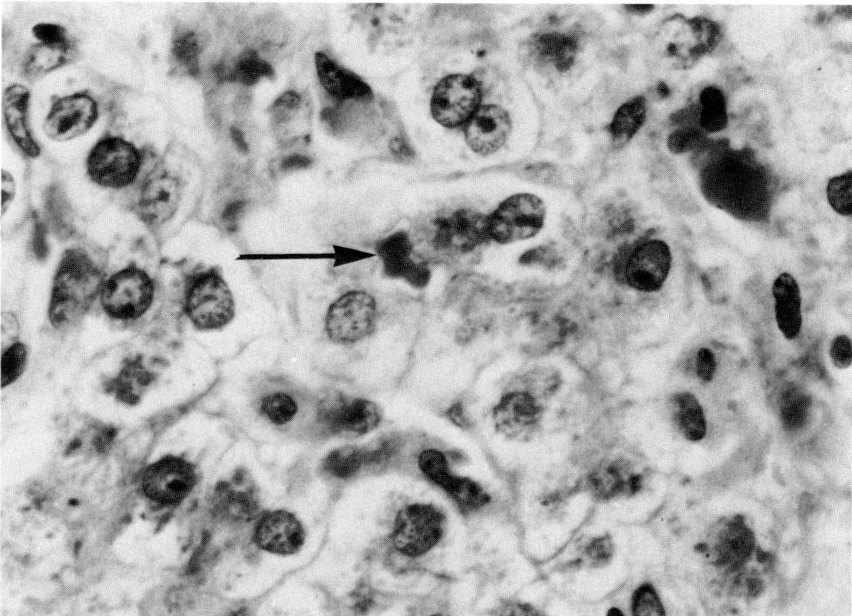

Figure 1. Bile plug (arrow) in a canaliculus in a patient with cholestasis associated with methandrostenolone (Dianabol) administration. (Hematoxylin and eosin, ×1,000.)

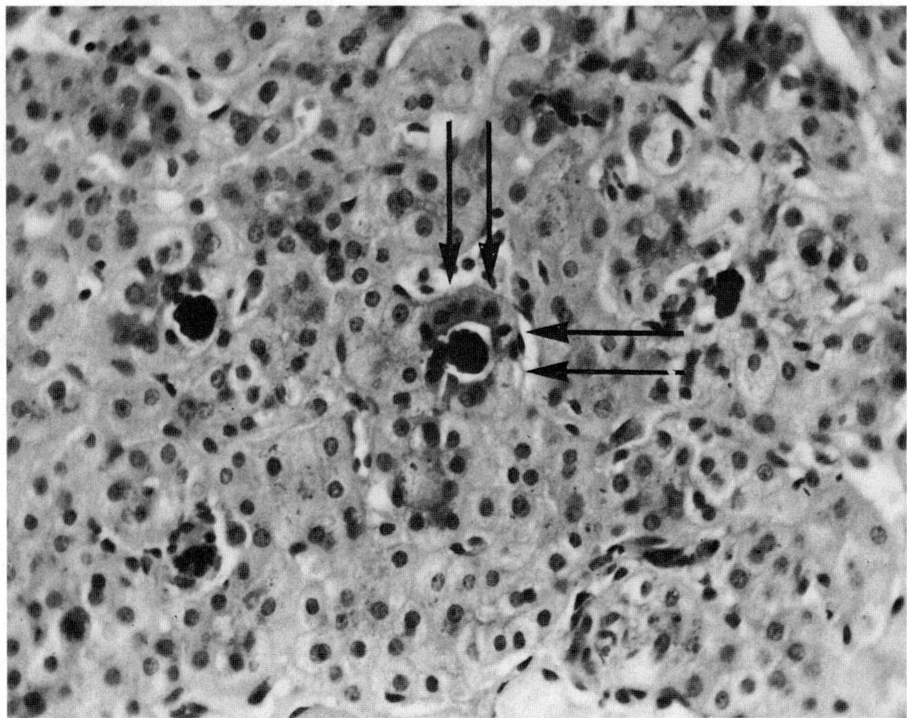

Figure 2. Pseudoglandular transformation of hepatocytes (arrows) with bile plug in central lumen. Several other bile plugs are shown as well in this field. Case of "neonatal hepatitis." (Hematoxylin and eosin, ×270.)

There are also striking alterations in hepatic histochemistry, particularly adenosine triphosphatase (ATPase) and alkaline phosphatase (12). Unfortunately, both electron microscopy and histochemistry are of little value in identifying the etiologic factor responsible for a patient's cholestasis.

The light microscopic changes found in pure cholestasis are not limited to the accumulation of bile pigment. Mallory's hyalin (Chapter 5) may be found in periportal hepatocytes and even in bile duct cells in some patients who have had cholestasis for several years. This is seen particularly in patients with primary biliary cirrhosis (PBC) (p. 127). Hepatic copper may also be elevated and copper stains may be positive in these patients, who must be distinguished from those with Wilson's disease (Chapter 9). Multiple orcein-staining brown granules, which probably represent a copper-binding protein, are often seen in the periportal hepatocytes of patients with long standing cholestatic liver diseases, particularly PBC (Fig. 4), but rarely in Wilson's disease (15a). These granules do not stain immunohistochemically for hepatitis B surface antigen (16–19). Hepatitis B surface antigen is also orcein positive (Chapter 2, Fig. 21) but is neither granular, pigmented, nor usually multiple, and it does not stain for copper.

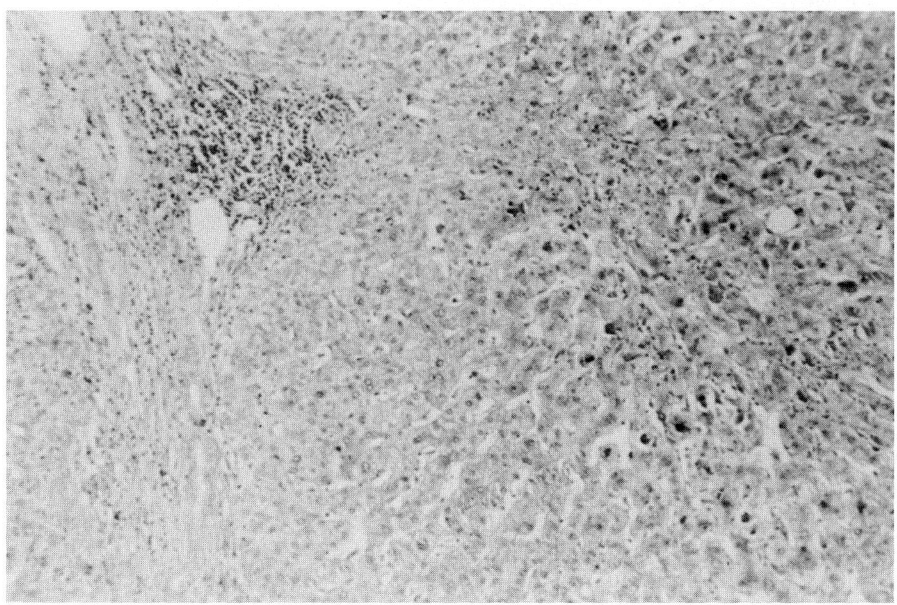

Figure 3. In a patient with extrahepatic obstruction, many dense bile plugs are seen in the right half of the field in canaliculi of the central part of a lobule. The portal triad in the left upper part of the field shows a moderate round cell infiltration. (Hematoxylin and eosin, ×85.)

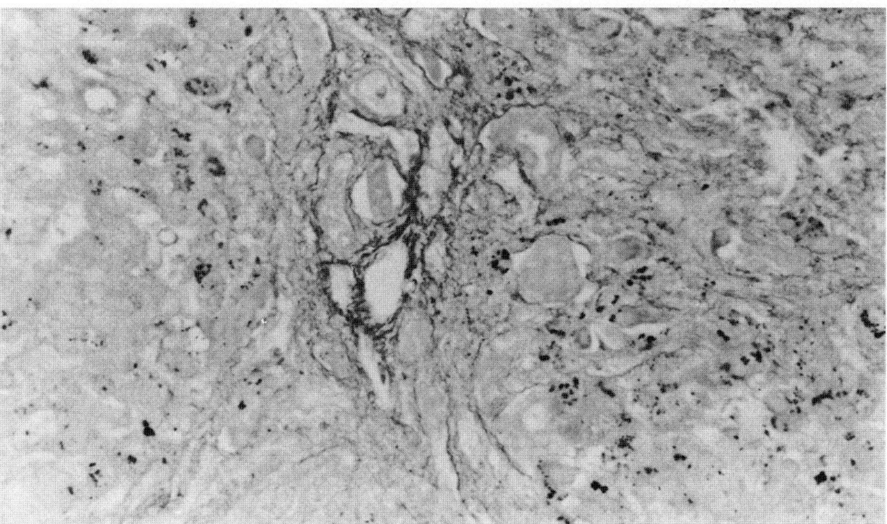

Figure 4. Small, dense granules associated with copper-binding protein are seen in many periportal hepatocytes in a case of Indian childhood cirrhosis. Note that elastic fibers in the portal triad are stained as well. (Orcein stain, ×214.)

Extra- and Intrahepatic Cholestasis

Cholestatic jaundice with conjugated hyperbilirubinemia is a prominent manifestation of a wide spectrum of hepatocellular, as well as biliary tract diseases. The management of patients with cholestasis, therefore, requires accurate etiologic diagnosis. A systematic approach to such patients has recently been outlined (20). Clinical, biochemical, and radiologic approaches are sometimes adequate to identify the lesion responsible for the cholestasis. However, in many cases a liver biopsy is required to establish a definitive diagnosis. A percutaneous needle biopsy should usually be the first step in reaching a morphologic diagnosis. Such a specimen may be obtained blindly or under direct vision with a laparoscope. If the needle biopsy is suggestive of extrahepatic obstruction, the needle biopsy is followed by a laparotomy and wedge biopsy, usually combined with exploration of the biliary system and operative cholangiography. Some investigators believe needle biopsy should be omitted if extrahepatic obstruction is strongly suspected on clinical grounds, but this opinon is not shared by all (21).

Since surgery is generally indicated in extrahepatic obstruction, it is particularly important to distinguish between biopsy specimens of patients with cholestasis due to hepatocellular disease and specimens with lesions of the biliary tract. This morphologic distinction involves two steps: (*1*) to attempt to identify any hepatocellular disease present (e.g., viral, drug-induced, alcoholic) by its characteristic morphologic picture, and (*2*) to look for morphologic evidence of extrahepatic biliary obstruction or biliary disease before making a definitive diagnosis. It is important always to take into account the clinical data. However, particularly in this area, it is best to evaluate the morphology first without knowledge of the clinical findings. Apparently, both extra- and intrahepatic cholestasis may be complications of hepatic transplantation (22–23a).

Morphology of Extrahepatic Cholestasis

The etiology of extrahepatic obstruction is discussed in Chapter 17. During the first 2 weeks of extrahepatic cholestasis, the histologic features are usually those of pure cholestasis, and morphologic changes suggestive of extrahepatic obstruction are often not found (24–24b). In any case, biopsy specimens are rarely obtained so soon after the onset of obstructive jaundice. Histologic features suggestive of extrahepatic obstruction may then develop (24–26), some of which have a higher degree of specificity than do others. Unfortunately, the most specific features, such as bile lakes (Fig. 8) and bile infarcts (Fig. 11), are seen relatively rarely. The differential diagnosis of obstructive jaundice, thus, continues to require a synthesis of all the data obtainable, including not only histopathology, but clinical history, biochemistry, and radiologic investigations as well (12). The morphology of the bile pigment in the liver in extrahepatic obstruction is that of pure cholestasis (p. 118). However, pigment deposition is generally relatively severe in extrahepatic obstruction, and Kupffer cells contain more pigment than is usually seen in cholestasis without mechanical obstruction.

Most useful in the diagnosis of extrahepatic obstruction are the alterations in the portal triads, particularly the main portal bile ducts and the connective tissue immediately surrounding them. Bile thrombi in the lumens of these bile ducts are certainly a suggestive finding, but there is no doubt that they can occasionally be seen when there is no mechanical obstruction. Periductal fibrous lamination ("onion skinning") is probably somewhat more specific. Often there is associated edema of the bile ducts and some infiltration with inflammatory cells (Fig. 5). Dilatation of portal bile ducts is seen rather rarely, but when present suggests mechanical obstruction. Proliferation of the interlobular bile ducts with periductal fibrosis is less prominent in adults than in children (Chapter 8), but when seen is highly suggestive of extrahepatic obstruction (Fig. 6). Polymorphs in the lining of interlobular ducts and particularly in their lumens are indicative of cholangitis. Since extrahepatic obstruction predisposes to cholangitis, the finding of polymorphs in bile ducts must always raise the suspicion that extrahepatic obstruction is also present. Marked portal fibrosis develops in extrahepatic obstruction of long standing, which may be partial (Fig. 7). A lesion rarely seen in patients without extrahepatic obstruction is the bile lake (Fig. 8), an accumulation of coarse aggregates of bile pigment that has totally replaced a group of cells. This lesion is often periportal. In long-standing obstruction, foamy histiocytes may accumulate in the vicinity of portal triads (Fig. 9). This may represent a late stage of a bile lake.

The cells in the lobules may undergo alterations that are more specific for extrahepatic obstruction than are most of the alterations in the portal triads. However, these lobular changes are also less common. Foci of hepatocytes and sometimes the adjacent Kupffer cells may undergo a series of changes that can be viewed as sequential steps, but that are probably a continuum. The earliest

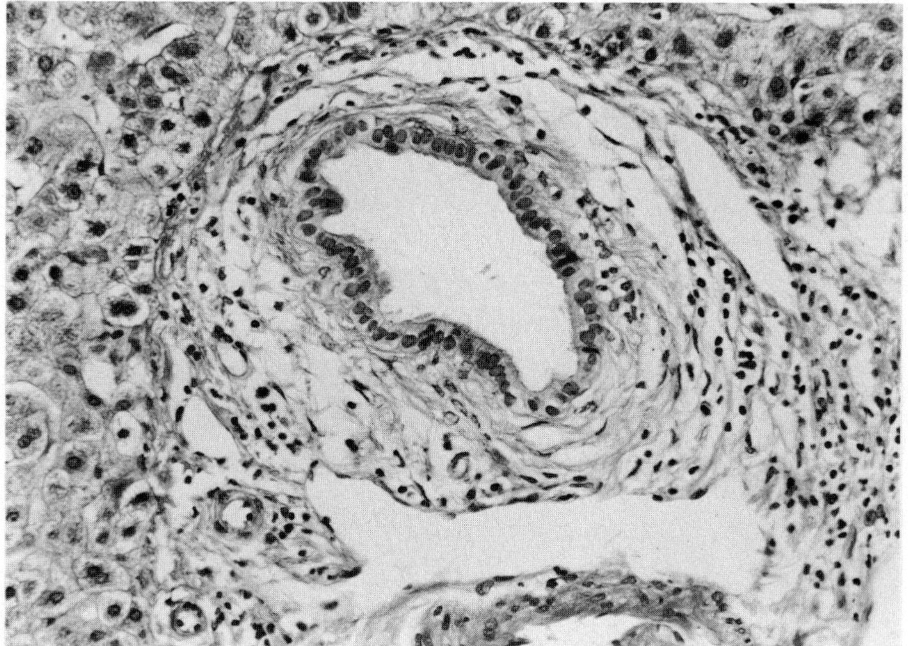

Figure 5. Extrahepatic obstruction in a patient in whom bile duct shows periductal edema and fibrous lamination ('onion skinning'). (Hematoxylin and eosin, ×250.)

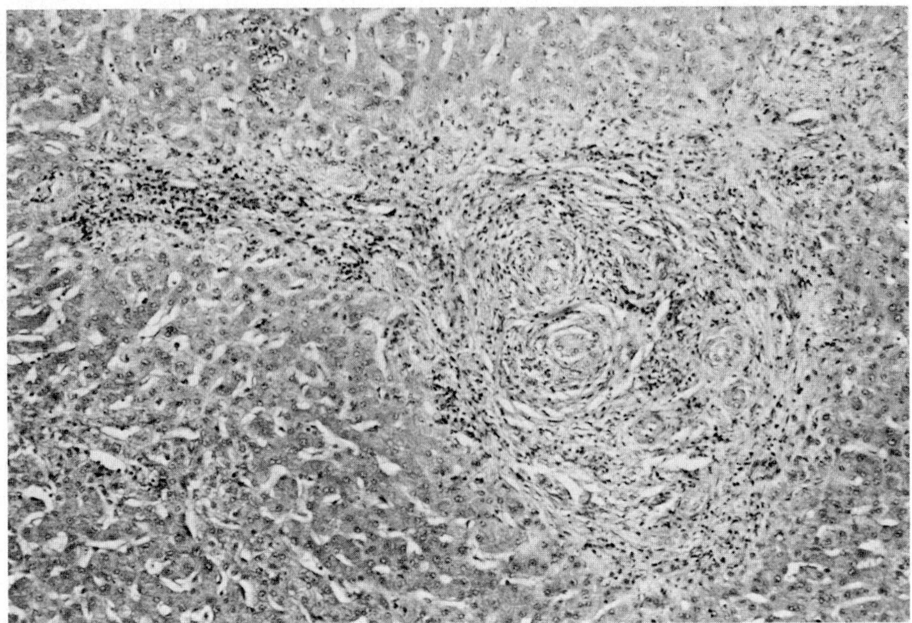

Figure 6. Recurrent cholangitis in a patient with extrahepatic obstruction associated with bile duct proliferation and periductal fibrosis. The bile ducts are surrounded by neutrophils, a few of which are within the bile ducts. There is also focal destruction of bile duct epithelium. (Hematoxylin and eosin, ×85.)

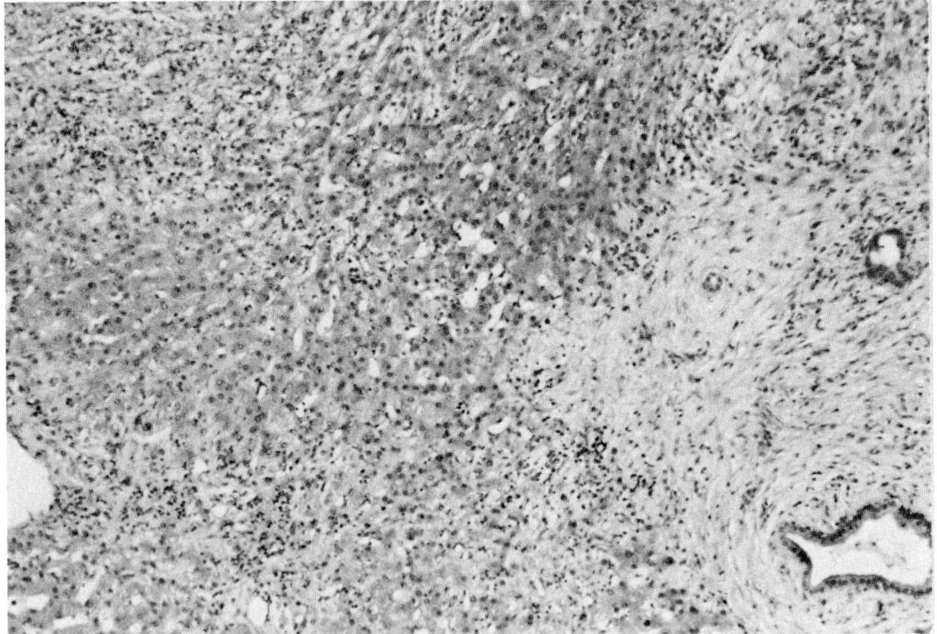

Figure 7. Severe portal fibrosis with relatively mild residual portal inflammation in a patient with long-standing cholangitis and extrahepatic obstruction. (Hematoxylin and eosin, ×85.)

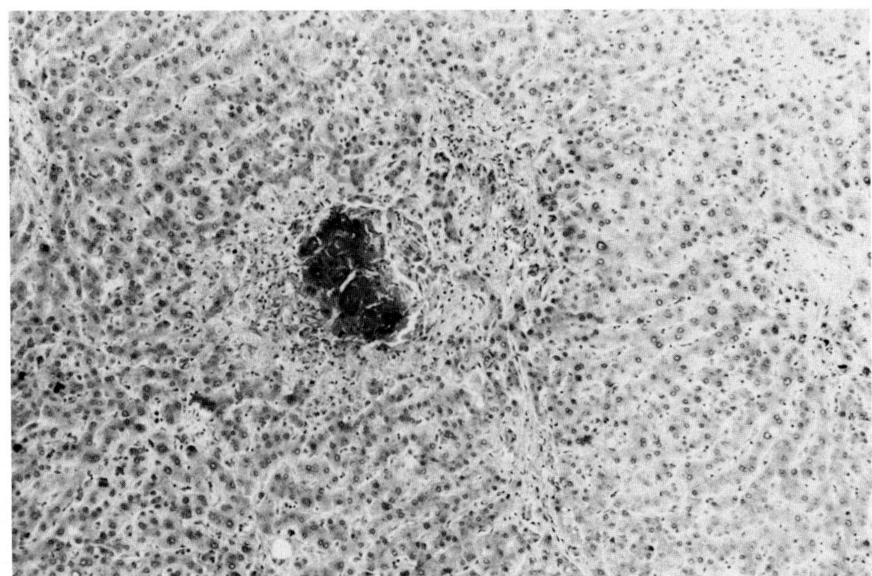

Figure 8. Extrahepatic obstruction, showing bile lake in the vicinity of a portal triad. (Hematoxylin and eosin, ×85.)

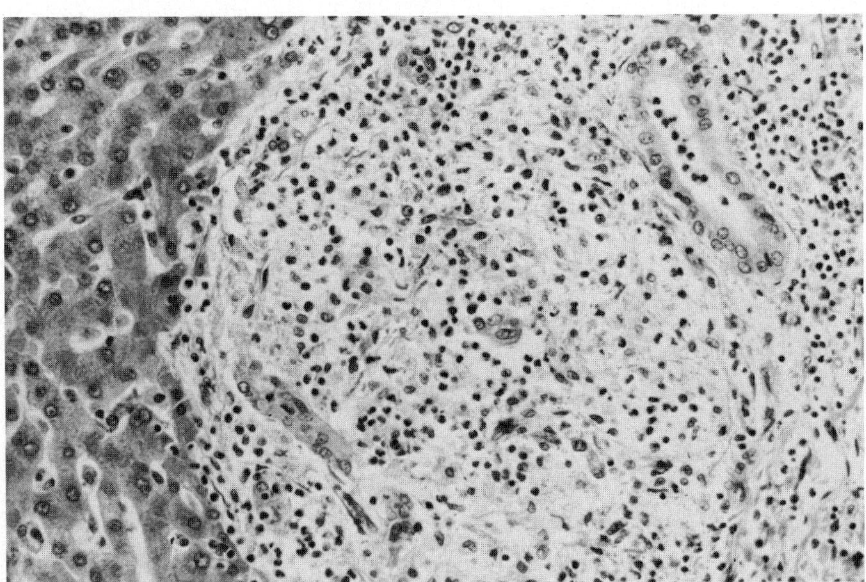

Figure 9. Extrahepatic obstruction, displaying mass of foam cells and neutrophils (old bile lake) in the vicinity of a large bile duct that contains a few neutrophils. (Hematoxylin and eosin, ×214.)

lobular change appears to be the accumulation of groups of foamy or xanthomatous cells (Fig. 10). Feathery degeneration is a term often used synonymously with xanthomatous change. Microscopically, there is reticular vacuolization affecting groups of cells that may be large enough to occupy a quarter of a hepatic lobule. It is often difficult to decide whether these swollen cells were originally hepatocytes or Kupffer cells. This lesion may superficially resemble some of the hepatocellular changes in alcoholic hepatitis, but in extrahepatic obstruction, cholestasis is usually more severe, and other evidence of alcoholic hepatitis is generally missing. The next step in the sequence is necrosis and diffuse staining with bilirubin, a bile infarct (Fig. 11).

In summary, although they have varying degrees of specificity, no single morphologic criterion, taken by itself, can be considered pathognomonic for extrahepatic obstruction. This includes even such time-honored criteria as bile thrombi in the interlobular bile ducts, feathery degeneration, or xanthomas, which are also seen in primary biliary cirrhosis, as well as bile lakes (12).

Suppurative Inflammatory Lesions of the Intrahepatic Biliary Tract

Cholecystitis and cholelithiasis may be associated with alterations in liver biopsies. However, there is some disagreement about the frequency and severity of such alterations (27,28). According to some authors about 20% of biopsy speci-

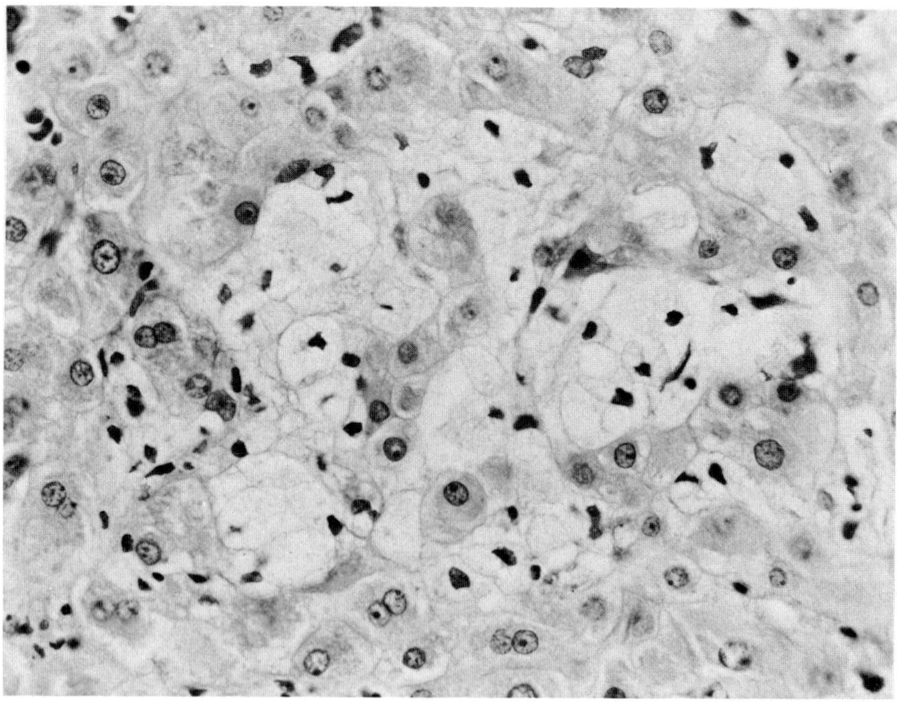

Figure 10. Extrahepatic obstruction, showing swelling ("feathery degeneration") of many hepatocytes. (Hematoxylin and eosin, ×400.)

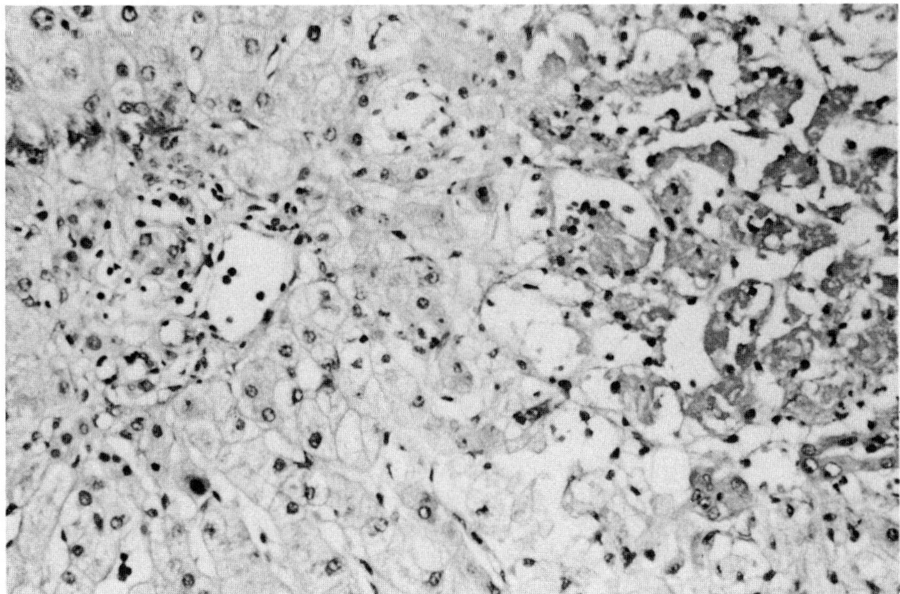

Figure 11. Extrahepatic obstruction, showing a bile infarct in the right half of the field. A portal triad with edema and inflammation is seen on the left. (Hematoxylin and eosin, ×214.)

mens showed histologic changes of extrahepatic biliary obstruction, while in another series only nonspecific reactive hepatitis was detected. In our experience, patients with uncomplicated cholecystitis and cholelithiasis rarely have significant hepatic histopathology.

Acute suppurative cholangitis is quite rare (29). Such patients are generally jaundiced and have a spiking temperature. Acute cholangitis is usually associated with an extrahepatic duct lesion (Chapter 17). Less frequently it may be seen in patients with acute cholecystitis, enteritis pancreatitis, or the toxic shock syndrome (29a). The histologic changes of extrahepatic obstruction are therefore usually present in addition to those of acute cholangitis. In the liver, the histologic hallmark of acute suppurative cholangitis is the presence of neutrophils in the lumens and lining cells of interlobular bile ducts. It is sometimes difficult to be sure whether the inflammatory cells are related more closely to the bile ducts or to the portal veins (pylephlebitis). Occasionally both lesions coexist. Necrosis of biliary epithelium is usually also present in cholangitis and may resemble that seen in primary biliary cirrhosis. However, neutrophils within bile ducts are not characteristic of primary biliary cirrhosis. The clinical picture of primary biliary cirrhosis is also quite different from that of acute suppurative cholangitis.

Primary Biliary Cirrhosis

Primary biliary cirrhosis (PBC) (chronic nonsuppurative destructive cholangitis) affects principally middle-aged women and is presently always fatal. The patients suffer from jaundice and itching. In addition to an elevation of bilirubin, the alkaline phosphatase is usually elevated, and antimitochondrial antibodies are positive in more than 90% of cases. Primary biliary cirrhosis may be an immune-complex disease (30) and is sometimes associated with other clinical conditions that may have an immune etiology, such as scleroderma (31). More patients have recently been diagnosed in the asymptomatic stage on the basis of the biochemical and biopsy findings (32,33). Although the term PBC is well established, it is not really appropriate, because cirrhosis develops only late in the disease. The term chronic destructive nonsuppurative cholangitis is more appropriate than PBC, but it is rather cumbersome (34,35). Extrahepatic obstruction, which may be associated with suppurative cholangitis by histologic, clinical, biochemical, and radiologic data must always be considered in the differential diagnosis. Occasionally, this may require laparotomy with wedge biopsy and operative cholangiography. Four pathologic stages of PBC are generally recognized. However, the criteria employed by different authors differ somewhat (18,34). The different stages appear to change gradually into one another and may coexist in the same biopsy specimen. "Early" lesions are still found occasionally when the disease is advanced clinically and pathologically (12,18,34,36).

The hallmark of stage I is the "florid duct lesion" (Figs. 12,13,15). It affects the larger and medium-sized interlobular bile ducts. The epithelium of the affected ducts is irregular, sloughed, necrotic, or shows evidence of focal regeneration. This is the most specific morphologic lesion in PBC. Mononuclear inflammatory

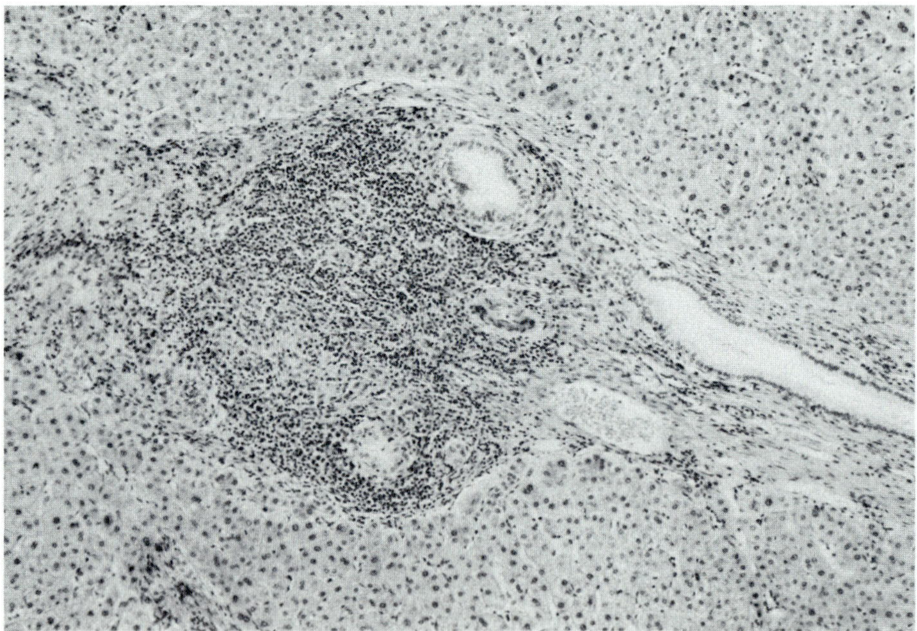

Figure 12. Primary biliary cirrhosis, low-power view, showing a marked portal inflammatory infiltrate without any significant penetration of the limiting plate (piecemeal necrosis). Note irregular arrangement of biliary epithelium in the bile ducts ("florid bile duct lesion"). (Hematoxylin and eosin, ×85.)

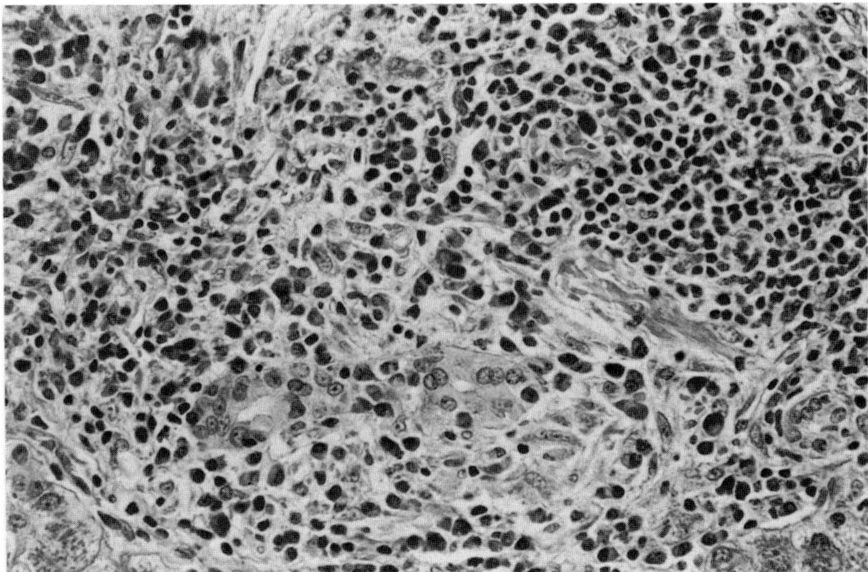

Figure 13. Primary biliary cirrhosis, higher-power view, showing the inflammatory cells in a portal triad. Note the irregular, jumbled arrangement of the biliary epithelium. ("florid bile duct lesion"). (Hematoxylin and eosin, ×300.)

cells, mostly lymphocytes, surround the bile ducts and can actually be seen within the lumens. Unfortunately, this classic duct lesion is relatively rarely seen in needle biopsy specimens and is usually better represented in wedge biopsy specimens. Nakanuma and Ohta (35) recently studied these bile duct lesions histometrically. Fibrinoid necrosis (Fig. 14) and granulomas in the vicinity of the portal triads and bile ducts are not uncommon at this stage. Some granulomas are classic, noncaseating tubercles with Langhans' giant and epithelioid cells (Figs. 15,16). Others consist simply of histiocytes or may resemble foreign body granulomas (Fig. 17). The presence of hepatic granulomas raises the possibility of a wide variety of disease states (Chapter 4). Stains for acid-fast bacilli and fungi should always be done, foreign material should be looked for, and if possible, the biopsy specimen should be cultured for tuberculosis and fungi. Hepatic sarcoidosis may also occasionally resemble PBC (37). Still, in the presence of the characteristic morphologic, biochemical, serologic, and clinical features of PBC, the correct diagnosis can generally be made. The granulomas are usually located within lymphocytic aggregates which sometimes have germinal centers. The specific duct lesions and the granulomas are usually accompanied, and may be overshadowed, by nonspecific histologic changes. These include portal inflammation and infiltration of these inflammatory cells through the limiting plate into the lobule (piecemeal necrosis). Occasionally, the portal infiltrates are severe enough to suggest lymphoma or leukemia. Lymphomatous infiltration, however, is generally composed of cells which are more uniform and generally immature. Moreover, the bile duct lesions of PBC are absent in lymphomas. In PBC a focal increase of lymphocytes and other mononuclear cells is also frequently seen in the sinusoids. Bile thrombi may be seen, but are relatively rare at this stage. At this point the principal differential diagnosis is chronic active

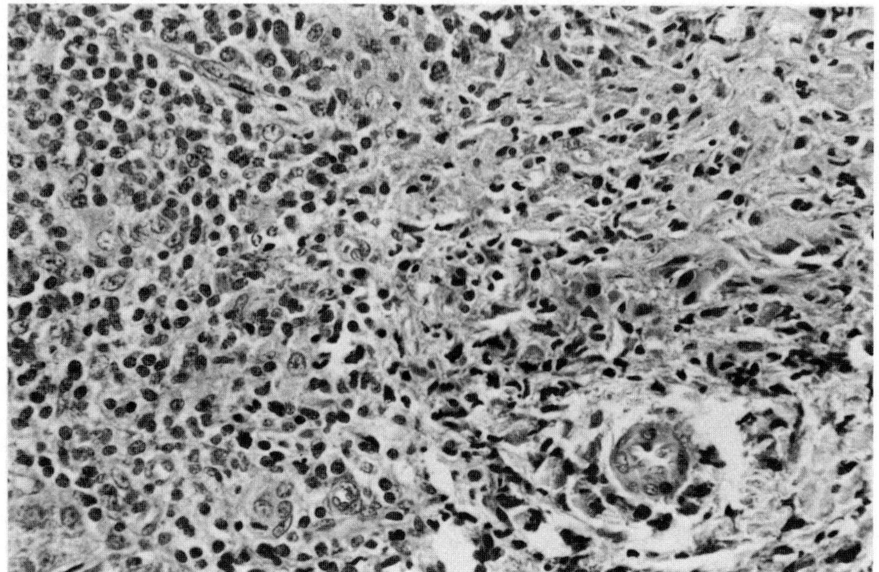

Figure 14. Primary biliary cirrhosis, showing inflammatory cells in a portal triad, in which only a hepatic artery in the lower right can be identified. The upper right of the field shows an area of fibrinoid necrosis. (Hematoxylin and eosin, ×300.)

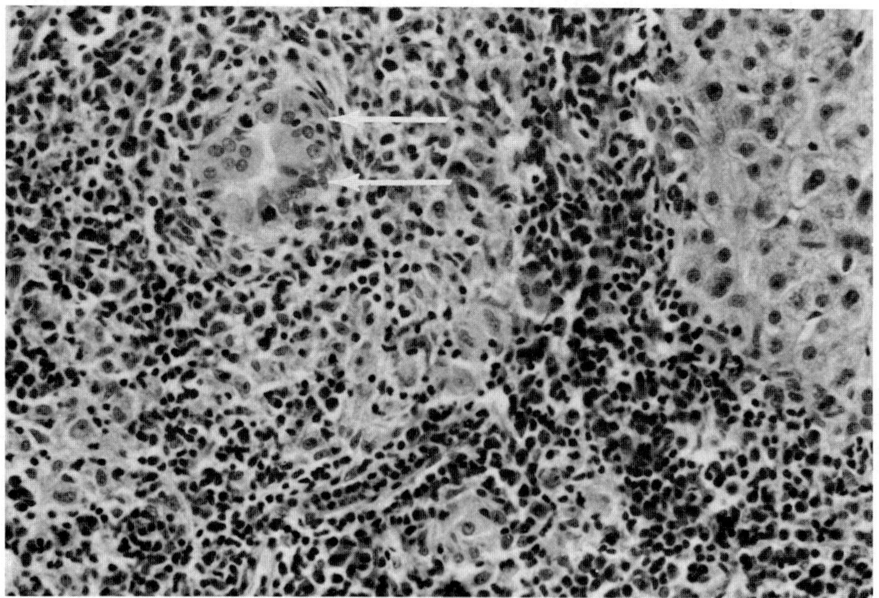

Figure 15. Primary biliary cirrhosis, higher power view, showing a portal triad infiltrated by chronic inflammatory cells. Note the irregular arrangement and some pyknosis (arrows) of bile duct lining cells (florid bile duct lesion) in the left upper part of the field. A small group of epithelioid cells is seen in the inflammatory cells both to the right of the duct and below. (Hematoxylin and eosin, ×250.)

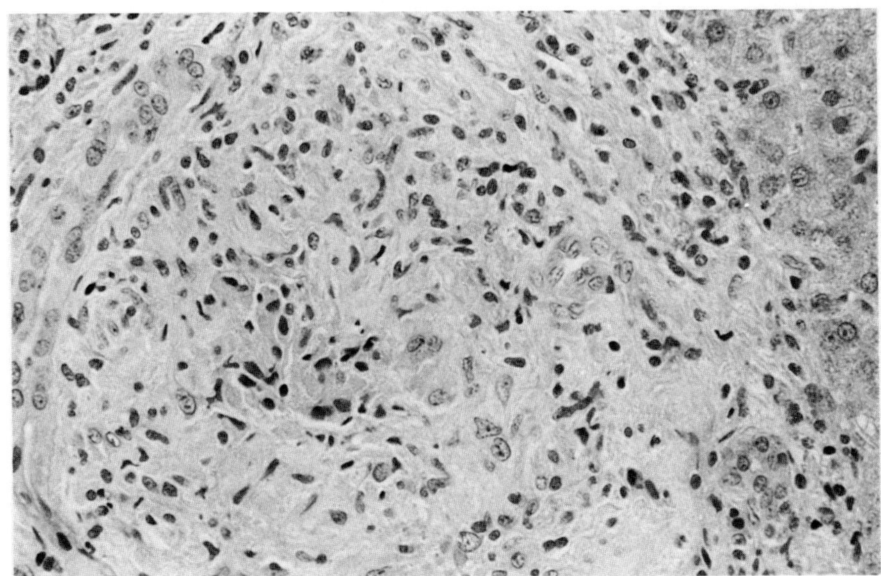

Figure 16. Primary biliary cirrhosis, showing a well-formed epithelioid cell granuloma in a portal triad. The adjacent bile ducts show some distortion. (Hematoxylin and eosin, ×300.)

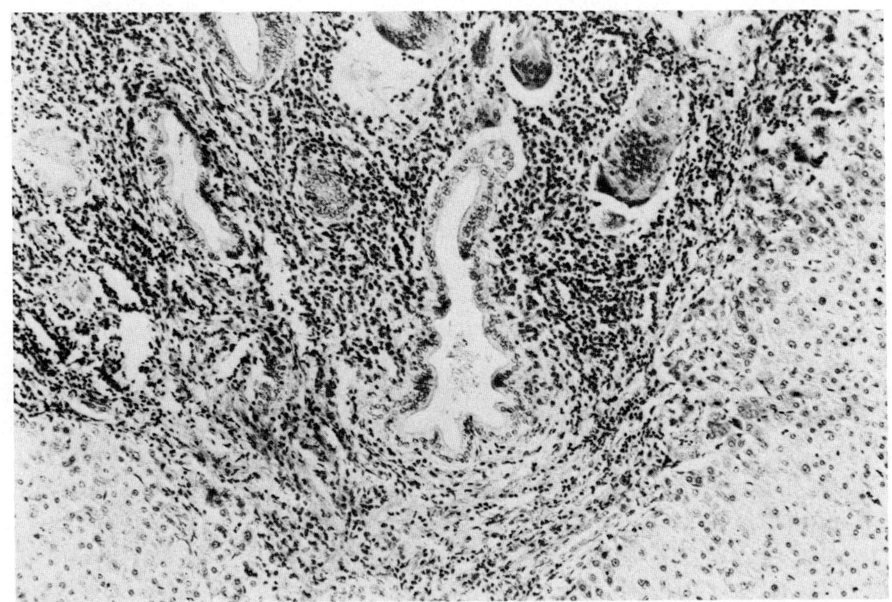

Figure 17. Primary biliary cirrhosis, exhibiting an increased number of portal bile ducts, some of which show epithelial irregularities. The ducts are surrounded by chronic inflammatory cells and by some foreign-body type giant cells. (Hematoxylin and eosin, ×100.)

hepatitis, because piecemeal necrosis may be present in both entities. The florid bile duct lesion of PBC resembles the abnormal bile ducts reported in acute and chronic active hepatitis (Chapter 2) (38) and similar lesions may be seen in pericholangitis (see below).

During the second stage, florid bile duct lesions may still be present. More striking is a paucity or decrease of portal bile ducts as a result of the initial destructive lesions. In adults an absence of ducts in 60% of portal tracts is considered significant, if 20 portal tracts are counted (39). It is rarely possible to find enough portal triads in needle biopsy specimens to make such a count significant. Wedge biopsies, however, are generally adequate for this purpose. Coupled with the decrease in portal bile ducts, there is proliferation of the small ductules, a characteristic lesion at this stage. The ductular proliferation originates in the portal triads but may extend somewhat into the periportal parenchyma. Although proliferating ductules are characteristic of this stage, they are not specific for PBC. Ductular proliferation occurs in viral hepatitis, alcoholic hepatitis, and even in extrahepatic obstruction, to mention only a few entities. The proliferating ductules are surrounded by inflammatory cells, fibroblasts, and scanty collagen fibers. Inflammatory aggregates still infiltrate the portal triads. These are mostly mononuclears with a few neutrophils and eosinophils. Mild piecemeal necrosis may still be present. Lymphoid follicles and granulomas are still seen occasionally but are less distinct. Groups of xanthomatous cells in the lobules are seen quite commonly.

Fibrosis is the predominant change in the third, or "precirrhotic," stage. Dense fibrous septa with a few ductules and inflammatory cells extend from portal triads. Adjacent triads are frequently joined, but regenerative nodules are absent. Cholestasis is often quite striking in the periphery of the lobules. Hepatocytes in the lobular periphery and even bile duct epithelial cells may contain Mallory's hyalin (Chapter 5). The diagnostic florid duct lesions are rarely seen and even the ductular proliferation of the previous stage is much less striking. However, the reduced number of large bile ducts, occasional portal lymphoid follicles, and foam cell aggregates within the lobules may permit suspicion of the diagnosis. Such a suspicion is strengthened if periportal cholestasis is present.

Cirrhosis ultimately develops. This is the fourth, last, and least specific stage of the disease. The pattern of the cirrhosis may be micronodular or macronodular (Chapter 13). The changes described in the previous stage may persist but often have to be diligently searched for. Hepatocarcinoma is a rare complication (40).

In the differential diagnosis of PBC chronic active hepatitis (Chapter 2), pericholangitis, sclerosing cholangitis, and destruction of portal bile ducts by fungal infection (41,42); by the cytomegalovirus (CMV) or the graft versus host reaction (43) have to be considered in particular. Morphologically the florid bile duct lesion is the only diagnostic feature of PBC. Fungi and intranuclear inclusions should always be looked for carefully in patients with destructive bile duct lesions, particularly in immunosuppressed patients. Serologic studies for CMV are also indicated in this group. Degenerative changes and actual destruction of portal bile ducts and periportal cholestasis may also be features of a graft-versus-host reaction (Figs. 18,19) (43–48) and possibly of chronic rejection in transplanted livers (22). Paraquat may produce a similar lesion (Chapter 15). However, granulomas appear to be seen only in PBC (45).

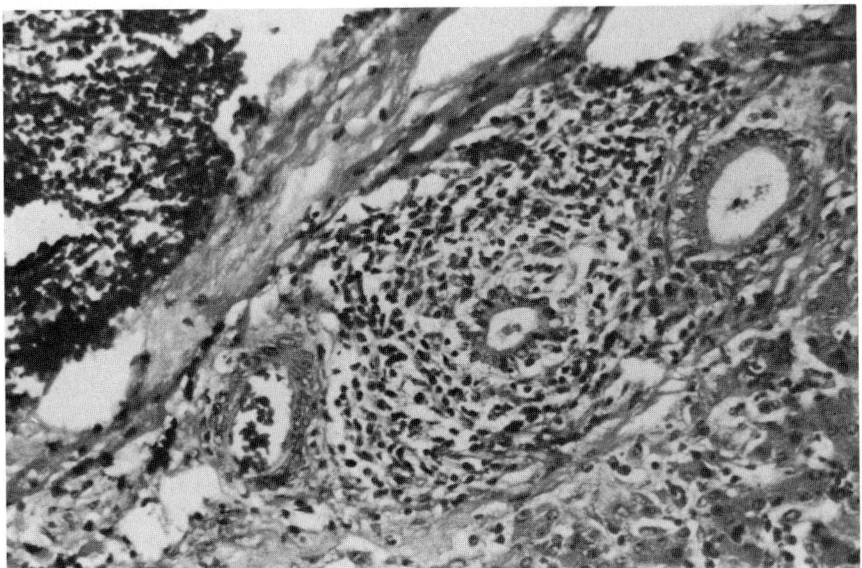

Figure 18. Graft-versus-host reaction in a premature infant treated by transfusions. Note acute inflammatory cells surrounding a portal bile duct, the lining cells of which show edema and early necrosis. (Hematoxylin and eosin, ×24.)

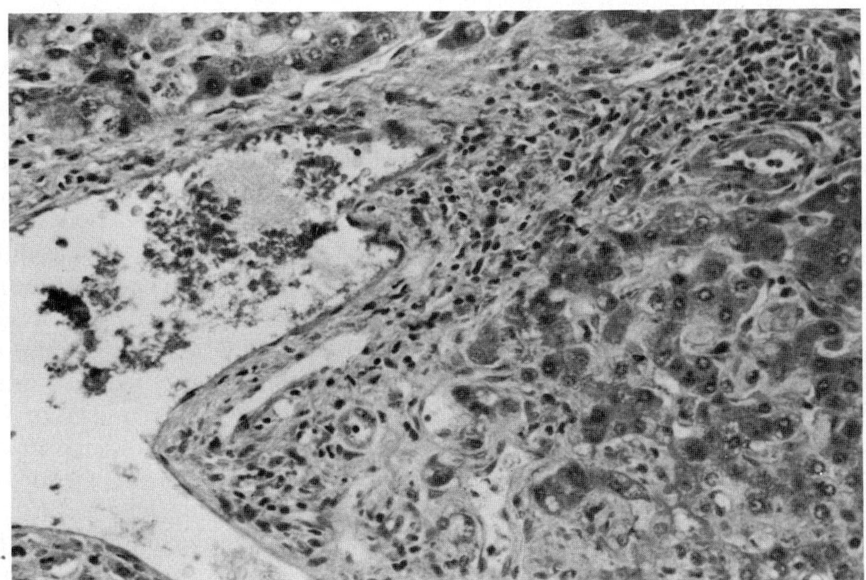

Figure 19. Graft-versus-host reaction after bone marrow transplantation, showing moderate round cell infiltration of a portal triad. No bile duct can be seen in this triad, which is typical of the great majority of triads in this liver. (Hematoxylin and eosin, ×214.)

Pericholangitis

Pericholangitis is the name usually given to an inflammatory lesion of varying severity seen in about 70% of patients with ulcerative colitis and Crohn's disease (49,50a). The lesion consists of portal inflammation, often associated with degenerative changes in the bile ducts and ductular proliferation. Mild to moderate periductal fibrosis is common, and the fibrosis occasionally extends into the lobules. Focal hepatocellular necrosis may also be present. These changes are not specific and may be seen in patients without inflammatory bowel disease, particularly in primary biliary cirrhosis and extrahepatic obstruction. Hepatic granulomas are said to be present in a few cases of ulcerative colitis (50). However, granulomas are more common in Crohn's disease; it is difficult not to suspect the possibility that these "ulcerative colitis" patients may really have had Crohn's disease.

Cholestasis tends to be centrilobular rather than peripheral, as in PBC. Antimitochondrial antibodies are present in 90% of cases of PBC, but are rare in pericholangitis. The pericholangitis may regress if colectomy is performed in patients with ulcerative colitis (50,51). Fatty change of the liver is seen in one-half of the patients with ulcerative colitis. It is related to the severity of the colitis but unrelated to other histologic changes (50). Piecemeal necrosis (Chapter 2) is seen in some patients with pericholangitis in the absence of markers for hepatitis B or "lupoid hepatitis." It is debatable whether these patients should be diagnosed as pericholangitis or chronic active hepatitis. Cirrhosis is seen in 3–5% of patients with inflammatory bowel disease and may well be the end result of pericholangitis with or without piecemeal necrosis.

Primary Sclerosing Cholangitis

Primary sclerosing cholangitis is diagnosed in patients with progressive obstructive jaundice who have had no previous surgery and no evidence of biliary calculi or congenital biliary anomalies. There is generalized thickening and stenosis of the extra- and sometimes the intrahepatic biliary system as well. Endoscopic retrograde cholangiography is very helpful. Primary sclerosing cholangitis is frequently associated with other diseases, such as chronic inflammatory bowel disease and retroperitoneal fibrosis. This condition is more common in men than in women, and antimitochondrial antibodies are generally absent. Eosinophilia is found in some cases (52). Hepatic needle biopsy is essential in these patients. It may show the histologic features of extrahepatic obstruction or a rather characteristic massive periductal fibrosis of the intrahepatic bile ducts, principally affecting the lamina propria. Whereas such a biopsy specimen alone may not be able to differentiate primary sclerosing cholangitis from pericholangitis or PBC, it is generally helpful in excluding fungal infection (41,42,50a,52a). In association with the characteristic clinical and cholangiographic findings, the diagnosis of sclerosing cholangitis can generally be made with considerable confidence. Laparotomy with biopsy of the thickened bile duct and wedge biopsy of the liver are generally desirable in confirming the diagnosis. Very rarely, it is virtually impossible to be sure whether a patient has primary biliary cirrhosis or sclerosing cholangitis, or possibly a combination of both (53,54). Involvement of the extrahepatic biliary system is more suggestive of sclerosing cholangitis, but even this may not be an absolute criterion.

The histologic distinction between cholangiocarcinoma and sclerosing cholangitis in bile duct biopsies may be difficult and is discussed in Chapter 17. Granulomatous infections (41) and parasitic infections (55) of the ducts can generally be excluded fairly easily. Wedge biopsy of the liver is desirable, because the characteristic lesions of PBC are more easily found in wedge specimens than in needle biopsy specimens. Biopsy of enlarged lymph nodes in the porta hepatis of patients suspected of sclerosing cholangitis is also helpful, since deposits of cholangiocarcinoma or of epithelioid tubercles in such nodes would, of course, exclude the diagnosis.

Parasitic Infections of the Biliary Tract

Infection of the biliary tract by *Clonorchis sinensis* is quite common in China and Japan, where raw fish is a common item in the diet. Grossly, the liver shows considerable periductal fibrosis in the portal triads (56). Histologically, many of the larger portal bile ducts contain adult *C. sinensis*. The bile ducts themselves show mucinous metaplasia and adenomatous hyperplasia of the duct epithelium and periductal fibrosis (Fig. 20). Cholangiocarcinoma is quite a common complication of this infection (57). *Fasciola hepatica* has a life cycle similar to that of clonorchis. The gross and microscopic changes are similar, except that ulcerative lesions of the bile ducts are more characteristic of *Fasciola* (58,59).

Morphology of Intrahepatic Cholestasis

A great variety of hepatocellular diseases may, at times, produce unusually severe cholestasis mimicking clinically the picture of extrahepatic obstruction (60). This includes viral and drug-induced hepatitis (Chapters 2 and 3) (61,62),

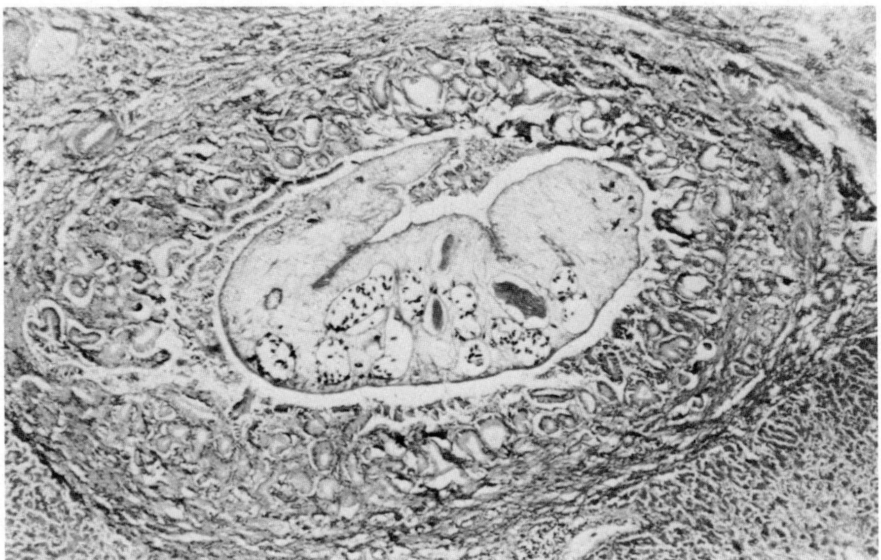

Figure 20. *Clonorchis sinensis* in a portal bile duct. Note proliferation of surrounding bile duct epithelium. (Hematoxylin and eosin, ×34.)

granulomatous hepatitis (Chapter 4), alcoholic liver disease (Chapter 5), and fatty liver (Chapter 6) (63). Congestive heart failure (Chapter 12) (64) and preeclampsia (Chapter 3) (65) also may occasionally be associated with cholestasis. In such patients, the clinical and morphologic features of the primary disorder can generally be detected. Postoperative cholestasis should be suspected when jaundice appears within 48 hours of major surgery (66,67). Often, little is seen on the biopsy specimen, except for a few small centrilobular bile plugs. Shock and sepsis are generally also present and may, in addition, cause central necrosis or focal necrosis and inflammation. Cholestasis may be an important feature of the hepatic complications of total parenteral nutrition (68,69). Occasionally, cholestasis may be the only symptom of hepatic amyloidosis (70). It may also be the presenting sign of bacterial infections, particularly Gram-negative septicemia and pneumonia (71,72), of Hodgkin's disease (73), and of space-occupying lesions including cysts, neoplasms, and abscesses (74,75). These conditions should, therefore, be searched for carefully both clinically and pathologically in patients with cholestasis of obscure etiology.

The differential diagnosis of patients with pure cholestasis (see above) is particulary difficult. The great majority suffer from drug-induced cholestasis (Chapter 15), recurrent jaundice of pregnancy, benign recurrent cholestasis, or extrahepatic obstruction too early to be diagnosable morphologically (see above). Some drugs, particularly contraceptive and anabolic steroid, are typically associated with pure cholestasis. The pathologist should also suspect a drug etiology, particularly a phenothiazine, when a biopsy specimen shows cholestasis with mild focal necrosis and intense periportal edema and inflammation, particularly if eosinophils are prominent in the periportal infiltrate. Of course a drug etiology should also be considered in every case of hepatitis, whether associated with cholestasis or not. Cholestatic viral hepatitis (Chapter 2) may mimic pure cholestasis but some histologic evidence of hepatitis can usually be found.

Recurrent cholestasis of pregnancy usually occurs during the last trimester of pregnancy and is particularly common in Scandinavia and Chile. Intense pruritus is usually present. Histologically, the picture is identical with that produced by contraceptive steroids (76,77).

Benign recurrent intrahepatic cholestasis is a disorder of unknown etiology, which frequently occurs in siblings. It usually starts in childhood and is characterized by multiple transient episodes of cholestasis. These are separated by intervals of months to years during which there is complete clinical, biochemical, and morphologic normality (78–80). Histologically, there is centrilobular bile stasis with canalicular bile thrombi, minimal hepatocellular necrosis, and Kupffer cell activation in the vicinity of the bile thrombi.

REFERENCES

1. Rosenblate HJ, Eisenstein R, Holmes AW: The liver in sickle cell anemia. *Arch Pathol Lab Med* 90:235, 1970.
2. Bailey A, Robinson D, Dawson AM: Does Gilbert's disease exist? *Lancet* 1:931, 1977.
3. Berthelot P, Dhumeaux D: New insights into the classification and mechanisms of hereditary, chronic, non-haemolytic hyperbilirubinaemias. *Gut* 19:474, 1978.

4. Berk PD, Javitt NB: Hyperbilirubinemia and cholestasis. *Am J Med* 64:311, 1978.
5. McGee JOD, Allan JG, Russell I, et al: Liver ultrastructure in Gilbert's syndrome. *Gut* 16:220, 1975.

5a. Dawson J, Carr-Locke DL, Talbot IC, et al: Gilbert's syndrome: Evidence of morphological heterogeneity. *Gut* 20:848, 1979.

6. Gardner WA, Konigsmark BW: Familial non-hemolytic jaundice: Bilirubinosis and encephalopathy. *Pediatrics* 43:365, 1969.
7. Huang PWH, Rozdilsky B, Gerrard JW, et al: Crigler-Najjar syndrome in four of five siblings with postmortem findings in one. *Arch Pathol Lab Med* 90:536, 1970.
8. Dubin IN: Chronic idiopathic jaundice. A review of fifty cases. *Am J Med* 24:268, 1958.
9. Ware AJ, Eigenbrodt EH, Shorey J, et al: Viral hepatitis complicating the Dubin-Johnson syndrome. *Gastroenterology* 63:331, 1972.
10. Lo NS, Chan CW, Hutchison JH: Dubin-Johnson syndrome with some unusual features in a Chinese family. *Arch Child* 54:529, 1979.
11. Evans J, Lefkowitch J, Lim CK: Fecal porphyrin abnormalities in a patient with features of Rotor's syndrome. *Gastroenterol* 81, 1125, 1981.
12. Desmet VJ: Morphologic and histochemical aspects of cholestasis, in Popper H, Schaffner F (eds): *Progress in Liver Disease.* New York, Grune & Stratton, 1972, vol IV, p 97.
13. Dubin IN, Peterson L: An explanation for the centrolobular localization of intrahepatic bile stasis in acute liver diseases. *Am J Med Sci* 336(1):45, 1958.
14. Glenner G: Simultaneous demonstration of bilirubin, hemosiderin and lipofuscin in tissue sections. *Am J Clin Pathol* 27:1, 1957.
15. Jones AL, Schmucker DL, Renston RH, et al: The architecture of bile secretion. A morphological perspective of physiology. *Dig Dis Sci* 25:609, 1980.

15a. Evans J, Newman SP, Sherlock S: Observations on copper associated protein in childhood liver disease. *Gut* 21:970, 1980.

16. Sipponen P: Orcein positive hepatocellular material in long-standing biliary diseases. I Histochemical characteristics. *Scand J Gastroenterol* 11:545, 1976.

16a. Sipponen P: Orcein positive hepatocellular material in long-standing biliary diseases. II. Ultrastructural studies. *Scand J Gastroenterol* 11:553, 1976.

17. Salaspuro MP, Sipponen P, Ikkala E, et al: Clinical correlations and significance of orcein positivity in chronic active hepatitis and primary biliary cirrhosis. *Ann Clin Res* 8:206, 1976.
18. Ludwig J, Dickson ER, McDonald GSA: Staging of chronic nonsuppurative destructive cholangitis (syndrome of primary biliary cirrhosis). *Virchows Arch* [*Pathol Anat*]379:103, 1978.
19. Nakanuma Y, Karino T, Ohta G: Orcein positive granules in the hepatocytes in chronic intrahepatic cholestasis. Morphological, histochemical and electron X-ray microanalytical examination. *Virchows Arch* [*Pathol Anat*] 382:21, 1979.
20. Fischer MG, Gelb AM, Weingarten, LA: Cholestatic jaundice in adults. Algorithms for diagnosis. *JAMA* 245:1945, 1981.
21. Morris JS, Gallo GA, Scheuer PJ, et al: Percutaneous liver biopsy in patients with large bile duct obstruction. *Gastroenterology* 68:750, 1975.
22. Roddy H, Putnam CW, Fennel RH Jr: Pathology of liver transplantation. *Transplantation* 22(6):625, 1976.
23. Starzl TE, Putnam CW, Hansbrough JF, et al: Biliary complications after liver transplantation: With special reference to the biliary cast syndrome and techniques of secondary duct repair. *Surgery* 81(2):212, 1977.

23a. Fennel RH Jr, Vierling JM: Non-suppurative cholangitis in chronic rejection of transplanted livers. *Gastroenterology* 79:1016, 1980.

24. Shorter R, Baggenstoss A: Extrahepatic cholestasis: I. Histologic changes in hepatic interlobular bile ducts and ductules in extra-hepatic cholestasis. *Am J Clin Pathol* 32(1):1, 1959.

24a. Shorter R, Baggenstoss A: Extrahepatic cholestasis: II. Histologic features of diagnostic importance. *Am J Clin Pathol* 32(1):5, 1959.

24b. Shorter R, Baggenstoss A: Extrahepatic cholestasis: III. Chronology of histologic changes in the liver. *Am J Clin Pathol* 32(1):10, 1959.

25. Gall EA, Dobrogorski O: Hepatic alterations in obstructive jaundice. *Am J Clin Pathol* 41:126, 1964.

26. Desmet VJ: Morphologic features of intrahepatic cholestasis, in Gentilini P, Popper H, Sherlock S, et al (eds): *Problems in Intrahepatic Cholestasis*. Basel, Karger, 1979, p 11.

27. Triger DR, MacIver AG, Gamlen TR, et al: Liver abnormalities and gallstones: A prospective combined clinical, histological and surgical study. *Br J Surg* 63:272, 1976.

28. Falkmer S, Sjöstrom B: Histological changes in the liver in diseases of the biliary tract. *Gastroenterology* 91:223, 1959.

29. Welch JP, Donaldson GA: The urgency of diagnosis and surgical treatment of acute suppurative cholangitis. *Am J Surg* 131:527, 1976.

29a. Ishak KG, Rogers WA: Cryptogenic acute cholangitis—Association with toxic shock syndrome. *Am J Clin Path* 76:619, 1981.

30. Thomas JC, Potter BJ, Sherlock S: Is primary biliary cirrhosis an immune complex disease? *Lancet* 2:1261, 1977.

31. Miller F, Lane B, Soterakis J, et al: Primary biliary cirrhosis and scleroderma. *Arch Pathol Lab Med* 103:505, 1979.

32. Long RG, Scheuer PJ, Sherlock S: Presentation and course of asymptomatic primary biliary cirrhosis. *Gastroenterology* 72:1204, 1977.

33. Fleming CR, Ludwig J, Dickson ER: Asymptomatic primary biliary cirrhosis. Presentation, histology, and results with D-penicillamine. *Mayo Clin Proc* 53:587, 1978.

34. Rubin E, Schaffner F, Popper H: Primary biliary cirrhosis. Chronic nonsuppurative destructive cholangitis. *Am J Pathol* 46:387, 1965.

35. Nakanuma Y, Ohta G: Histometric and serial section observations of the intrahepatic bile ducts in primary biliary cirrhosis. *Gastroenterology* 76:1326, 1979.

36. Popper H: The problem of histologic evaluation of primary biliary cirrhosis. *Virchows Arch [Pathol Anat]* 379:99, 1978.

37. Rudzki C, Ishak KG, Zimmerman HJ: Chronic intrahepatic cholestasis of sarcoidosis. *Am J Med* 59:373, 1975.

38. Poulsen H, Christoffersen P: Abnormal bile duct epithelium in chronic aggressive hepatitis and cirrhosis. *Hum Pathol* 3:217, 1972.

39. Baggenstoss AH, Foulk W, Butt HL, et al: The pathology of primary biliary cirrhosis with emphasis on histogenesis. *J Clin Pathol* 42:259, 1964.

40. Mallet L, Petite JP, Amat D, et al: Carcinome hepatocellulaire au cours de la cirrhose primitive. *Gastroent Clin Biol* 5:379, 1981.

41. Lefton HB, Farmer RG, Buchwald R, et al: Cryptococcal hepatitis mimicking primary sclerosing cholangitis. *Gastroenterology* 67:511, 1974.

42. Teixera F, Gayotto LC, DeBrito T: Morphological patterns of the liver in South American blastomycosis. *Histopathology* 2:231, 1978.

43. Beschorner WE, Pino J, Boitnott JK, et al: Pathology of the liver with bone marrow transplantation, effects of busulfan, carmastine, acute graft versus host disease and cytomegalovirus infection. *Am J Pathol* 99:369, 1980.

44. Beschorner WE, Pino JL, Boitnott JK, et al: Liver pathology following bone marrow transplantation. *Lab Invest* 40:241, 1979.

45. Jones EA: Primary biliary cirrhosis and liver transplantation. *N Engl J Med* 306:41, 1982.

46. Sloane JP, Farthing MJG, Powles RL: Histopathological changes in the liver after allogeneic bone marrow transplantation. *J Clin Pathol* 33:344, 1980.

47. Rothko K, Moore GW, Hutchins GM: Analysis of cause of death following bone marrow transplantation. A clinicopathologic study of forty-three patients. *Lab Invest* 42:146, 1980.

48. Woodruff JM, Hansen JA, Good RA, et al: The pathology of the graft versus host reaction (GVHR) in adults receiving bone marrow transplants *Transplant Proc* 8:675, 1976.

49. Dew MJ, Thompson H, Allan RN: The spectrum of hepatic dysfunction in inflammatory bowel disease. *Q J Med* 189:113, 1979.

50. Eade MN, Cooke WT, Brooke BN: Liver disease in ulcerative colitis. II. Long term effect of colectomy. *Ann Intern Med* 72:475, 1970.

50a. Ludwig J, Barham SS, La Russo NF: Morphologic features of chronic hepatitis associated with primary sclerosing cholangitis and ulcerative cholangitis. *Hepatology* 1:632, 1981.

51. Toghill PJ, Benton KPE, Smith PG: Chronic liver disease associated with childhood ulcerative colitis. *Postgrad Med J* 50:9, 1974.

52. An unusual cholangitis, editorial. *Br Med J* 2:1090, 1976.

52a. Chapman RWG, Arborgh BA, Rhodes JM, et al: Primary sclerosing cholangitis. A review of its clinical features, cholangiography and hepatic histology. *Gut* 21:870, 1980.

53. Fee HJ, Gewirtz H, Schiller J, et al: Sclerosing cholangitis and primary biliary cirrhosis—A disease spectrum? *Am Surg* 186(5):589, 1977.

54. Galambos JT, Brooks WS: Atypical biliary cirrhosis—or sclerosing cholangitis. *J Clin Gastroenterology* 2:43, 1980.

55. Danzi J, Makipour H, Farmer R: Primary sclerosing cholangitis. A report of nine cases and clinical review. *Am J Gastroenterology* 65:109, 1976.

56. Hou PC: The pathology of *clonorchis sinensis* infestation of the liver. *J Pathol* 70:53, 1955.

57. Hou PC: The relationship between primary carcinoma of the liver and infestation with clonorchis sinensis. *J Pathol* 72:239, 1956.

58. Acosta FW, Vercelli-Retta J, Falconi LM: Fasciola hepatica human infection. *Virchows Arch [Pathol Anat]* 383:319, 1979.

59. Ash JE, Spitz S: Pathology of tropical diseases. An atlas. *Am Registry Pathol.* Washington, D.C., 279, 1945.

60. Gentilini P, Popper H, Sherlock S, (eds): *Problems in intrahepatic cholestasis,* Second International Symposium on Cholestasis. Basel, New York, Karger, 1979.

61. Cooksley WG, Powell LW, Kerr JF, et al: Cholestasis in active chronic hepatitis. *Dig Dis* 17:495, 1972.

62. Ishak KG: Light microscopic morphology of viral hepatitis. *Am J Clin Pathol* 65:787, 1976.

63. Perillo RP, Griffin R, De Schryber-Kecskemeti K, et al: Alcoholic liver disease presenting with marked elevation of serum alkaline phosphatase. A combined clinical and pathologic study. *Dig Dis* 23:1061, 1978.

64. Buhac I, Agrawal AB, Park SK, et al: Jaundice and bridging centrilobular necrosis of liver in circulatory failure. *NY State J Med* 76:678, 1976.

65. Long RG, Scheuer PJ, Sherlock S: Pre-eclampsia presenting with deep jaundice. *J Clin Pathol* 30:212, 1977.

66. Kantrowitz PA, Jones WA, Greenberger NJ, et al: Severe postoperative hyperbilirubinemia simulating obstructive jaundice. *N Engl J Med* 276:591, 1967.

67. Hampel N, Lichtig C, Gersh I, et al: Postoperative intrahepatic cholestasis. *Int Surg* 62(1):51, 1977.

68. Sheldon G, Petersen S, Sanders R: Hepatic dysfunction during hyperalimentation. *Arch Surg* 113:504, 1978.

69. Cohen CC, Olsen MM: Pediatric total parenteral nutrition. *Arch Pathol Lab Med* 105:152, 1981.

70. Rollinghoff W, Braun HJ, Schad FJ: Intrahepatische Cholestase als Leitsymptom einer primaren Amyloidose. *Dtsch Med Wochenschr* 101:1838, 1976.

71. Tugwell P, Williams AO: Jaundice associated with lobar pneumonia. *Q J Med* (New ser) XLVI, 181:97, 1977.

72. Zimmerman HJ, Fang M, Utili R, et al: Jaundice due to bacterial infection. *Gastroenterology* 77:362, 1979.

73. Perera DR, Greene ML, Fenster LF: Cholestasis associated with extrabiliary Hodgkin's Disease. *Gastroenterology* 67:680, 1974.

74. Ramachandran S, Pakianathan V, Aiyathural JEJ: Severe obstructive jaundice due to amoebic liver abscess. *Med J Aust* 1:925, 1976.

75. Santman FW, Thijs LG, Vander Veen EA, et al: Intermittent jaundice: A rare complication of a solitary nonparasitic liver cyst. *Gastroenterology* 72:325, 1977.

76. Misra PS, Evanov FA, Wessely Z, et al: Idiopathic intrahepatic cholestasis of pregnancy. Report of an unusual case and a review of the recent literature. *Am J Gastroenterol* 73:54, 1980.

77. Medline A, Ptak T, Gryfe A, et al: Pruritus of pregnancy and jaundice induced by oral contraceptives. *Am J Gastroenterol* 65:156, 1976.

78. Summerskill WHJ, Walshe JM: Benign recurrent intrahepatic "obstructive" jaundice. *Lancet* 2:686, 1959.

79. Tygstrup N, Petersen P, Bremmelgaard A: Idiopathic intermittent intrahepatic cholestasis, in Javitt NB (ed): *Neonatal Hepatitis and Atresia,* Washington, D.C. U.S. Department of Health, Education, and Welfare 79-1296. 1977, p 195.

80. La Russo N, Dickson ER, Pineda AP: Plasma perfusion and studies of copper metabolism in benign recurrent cholestasis. Novel procedures in a rare syndrome. *Mayo Clin Proc* 55:450, 1980.

8
Hyperbilirubinemia and Cholestasis in Infancy

Jaundice in infancy and childhood differs considerably from jaundice in adults, not only with respect to etiologic factors, but in its microscopic manifestations as well. Several recent monographs deal with this subject (1–4). Thaler (5) outlined a systematic approach to the problem of jaundice in infancy.

UNCONJUGATED HYPERBILIRUBINEMIA

Elevation of unconjugated bilirubin up to 10 mg/100 ml is physiologic during the neonatal period. Unconjugated hyperbilirubinemia is present when the bilirubin is above this level; less than 15% of the total bilirubin is of the direct-reacting type. Excessive unconjugated hyperbilirubinemia of 20 mg/100 ml or more may give rise to kernicterus. Apart from severe Crigler-Najjar disease (Chapter 7, p 117), neonatal unconjugated hyperbilirubinemia is generally not associated with hepatic pathology.

CHOLESTASIS

Cholestatic jaundice with conjugated hyperbilirubinemia (Chapter 7) is the most prominent manifestation of hepatocellular disease during the neonatal period. Other evidence of liver disease, including hepatomegaly and abnormal biochemical tests such as elevation of the transaminase enzymes is usually present, but not consistently. Mechanical biliary obstruction in the neonate is generally accompanied by clinical and biochemical findings closely resembling those of hepatocellular disease at this age period. The differential diagnosis of conjugated hyperbilirubinemia during infancy thus covers a broad spectrum of hepatic disorders and biliary tract lesions. The distinction between these two broad groups is of clinical importance because some abnormalities of the extrahepatic system are amenable to surgery. On the other hand, surgery is not indicated in infants with intrahepatic cholestasis, for whom a thorough clinical workup is required. The serum alpha-1-antitrypsin should always be measured, as there is a deficiency of this enzyme (Chapter 9) in a significant proportion of neonates with conjugated hyperbilirubinemia. If the enzyme is decreased, the infant should be phenotyped by serum electrophoresis. Unfortunately, standard liver function tests are not helpful in distinguishing mechanical obstruction from hepatocellular disease at this age. A rapidly rising serum alkaline phosphatase and cholesterol may represent an exception to this statement suggesting a paucity of the intrahepatic bile ducts (intrahepatic atresia) (5). A substantial proportion of infants who present in this manner possess a characteristic facies, congenital heart defects, and vertebral malformations (6,7). The "Bronze Baby" syndrome also is seen in this age group (7a). It is particularly important in infants with cholestasis to eliminate treatable conditions. Congenital syphilis and bacterial infections may cause hepatocellular jaundice and should be tested for. Galactosemia, fructose intolerance, and tyrosinemia (Chapter 9) should also be excluded, because they represent treatable causes of hepatocellular jaundice.

Role of Liver Biopsy

Liver biopsy in infants with cholestasis is part of a multidisciplinary approach aimed at distinguishing between extrahepatic biliary tract lesions and hepatocellular diseases unaccompanied by extrahepatic biliary obstruction, "neonatal hepatitis." According to Danks et al. (8), conjugated hyperbilirubinemia occurs approximately once in 5,000 births. In his series, approximately one-half of these patients had an abnormality of the extrahepatic biliary tree, while the other had "neonatal hepatitis." Liver biopsy may be performed by a percutaneous approach with a biopsy needle or by open surgical wedge biopsy, usually combined with exploration of the biliary system and operative cholangiography, if feasible. Percutaneous liver needle biopsy should, in general, be the first step in reaching a morphologic diagnosis. There has been much controversy as to the correct timing of this approach. If performed too early (i.e., before the age of 2 months), the diagnostic histologic changes of extrahepatic obstruction may not be apparent. If performed later, the biliary cirrhosis produced by extrahepatic obstruction may have become irreversible. Recently the trend has been toward earlier surgery. Performance of a percutaneous liver biopsy at 2 months or even earlier is, therefore, recommended, even though the histologic evidence of extrahepatic obstruction may not yet be fully developed.

Normal Infant Liver

The histology of the normal infant liver during the neonatal period differs in certain respects from that of the adult. At birth, even in the mature fetus, a few islands of erythropoietic tissue are still present, scattered throughout the lobular parenchyma. They are even more striking in premature infants (Chapter 1). During the first few days after birth, these erythropoietic islands disappear, except in infants suffering from anoxia, most often caused by the pulmonary distress syndrome. Scanty hemosiderin may also be present in the periportal zones of normal neonates. Hepatocellular disease, particularly "neonatal hepatitis" (see below) may be associated with persistent extramedullary hemopoiesis (Fig. 6) and excessive hemosiderin deposition (9,9a). Excessive hepatic hemosiderosis in infancy is also a feature of Zellweger's (p. 165) and Donohue's (p. 165) syndromes and is discussed further in Chapter 11. Hemopoiesis surrounding the portal triads, consisting of both red and white cell precursors, is seen relatively rarely in the mature neonate. In this location, both leukopoiesis and erythropoiesis occur. Hemopoiesis in this location is seen in prematures and particularly in infants with erythroblastosis fetalis. Copper levels and levels of orcein-positive copper-associated protein are relatively high in normal newborn infants (10,10a). Parenchymal cell nuclei appear more uniform in normal neonates than in adults. This is presumably because almost all hepatocytes are tetraploid and there is a smaller number of octaploids than in adults. The organization of the hepatic lobules in premature infants differs little from that of adults, with the exception that the liver cell plates consist of a double layer of cells, rather than a single layer. This persists up to the age of 5 years (11). It is important to note from which lobe a biopsy specimen is taken, because the left lobe is more vulnerable to shock in the postnatal period. Hemopoiesis, iron concentration, and fatty change also are often more marked in this lobe (12).

Differentiation of "Neonatal Hepatitis" and Biliary Atresia

After identifying the relatively few infants with cholestasis due to bacterial and treatable metabolic causes or drugs, such as erythromycin estolate (13), it is found that the great majority suffer from either extrahepatic biliary atresia (14), or cholestasis with a normal biliary tree, the "neonatal hepatitis" group. In a few cases of "neonatal hepatitis," etiologic agents, including antitrypsin deficiency, a virus (rubella, herpes, or cytomegalovirus), or toxoplasma, can be demonstrated serologically or by culture.

If extrahepatic biliary atresia and "neonatal hepatitis" are pathogenetically distinct, it is clearly important to identify those patients who have extrahepatic obstruction, because they may be surgically curable. However, if "infantile obstructive cholangiopathy," a concept including both groups of conditions, has a common pathogenetic mechanism (2,15,16), the distinction between them may become less important. Evidence in favor of a common pathogenesis includes the finding that some of the diseases that usually injure hepatocytes primarily, such as rubella (17), cytomegalovirus (18), and 17-18 trisomy (19), appear to be also associated occasionally with extrahepatic atresia. However, extrahepatic atresia, unlike "neonatal hepatitis," is rarely familial and has a different sex incidence. How much overlap there is between these two groups remains uncertain. Treatment at present has to be based on the morphologic diagnosis in order to benefit those patients who may have a chance of being cured surgically.

The histologic criteria for differential diagnosis between biliary obstruction and "neonatal hepatitis" are quite well established (9,20,21) and are listed in Table 1.

The most important criteria favoring mechanical obstruction of the extrahepatic biliary tract are proliferation of large interlobular bile ducts and portal fibrosis (Figs. 1–3). Proliferation of small ductules is not as helpful in this differentiation, because it is also seen in the "neonatal hepatitis" group. However,

Table 1. Differentiation of Extrahepatic Obstructive Lesions and "Neonatal Hepatitis"

Finding	*Extrahepatic Atresia*	*"Neonatal Hepatitis"*
Bile duct proliferation	+++	±
Ductular proliferation	++	+
Portal fibrosis	+++	+
Diffuse fibrosis	−	±
Portal bile thrombi	+	±
Bile lakes	+	−
Hepatocellular lesions including giant cell transformation	±	++
Persistent extramedullary hemopoiesis	±	++

the distinction between ductules and ducts can be difficult. We find it convenient to characterize as ducts those structures having lumens adjacent to portal vascular structures, and as ductules those smaller structures lacking lumens in the vicinity of the limiting plate. We have not found the presence of bile thrombi in portal bile ducts helpful in making this differential diagnosis. Bile lakes or bile infarcts are strongly suggestive of extrahepatic atresia but, unfortunately, are rare and therefore not often useful.

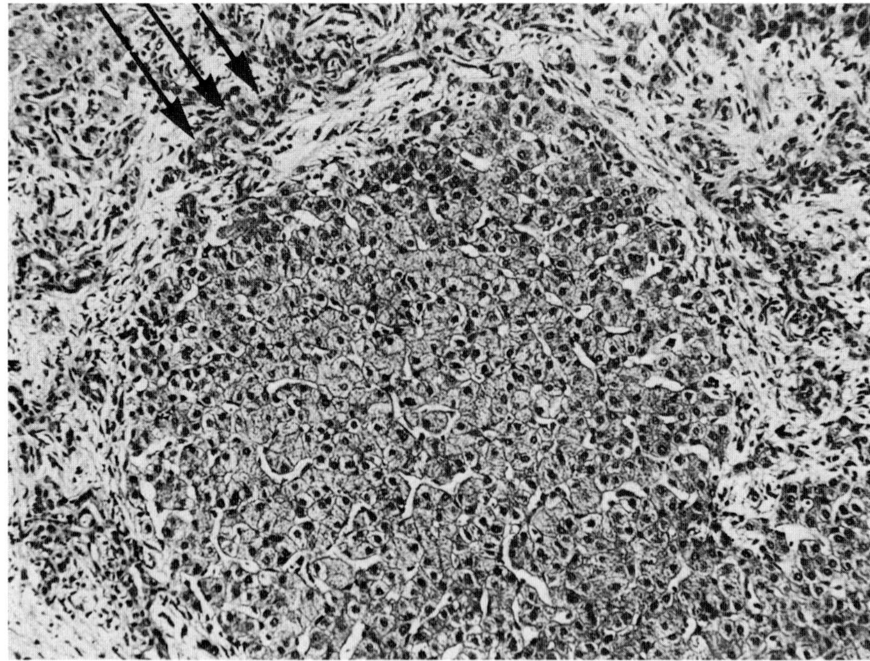

Figure 1. Extrahepatic biliary atresia in an infant age 3 months, showing marked proliferation of the portal bile ducts (arrows), as well as portal fibrosis. (Hematoxylin and eosin, ×110.)

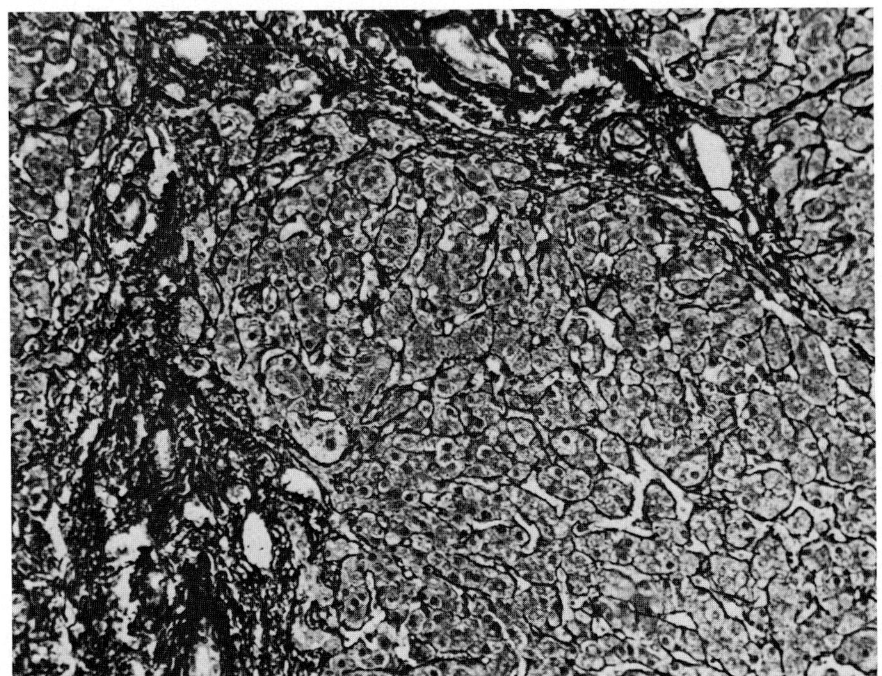

Figure 2. Extrahepatic biliary atresia in the same patient described in Figure 1. Note marked increase in periportal reticulin. The proliferated bile ducts stand out as empty spaces among the reticulin fibers. (Reticulin stain, ×110.)

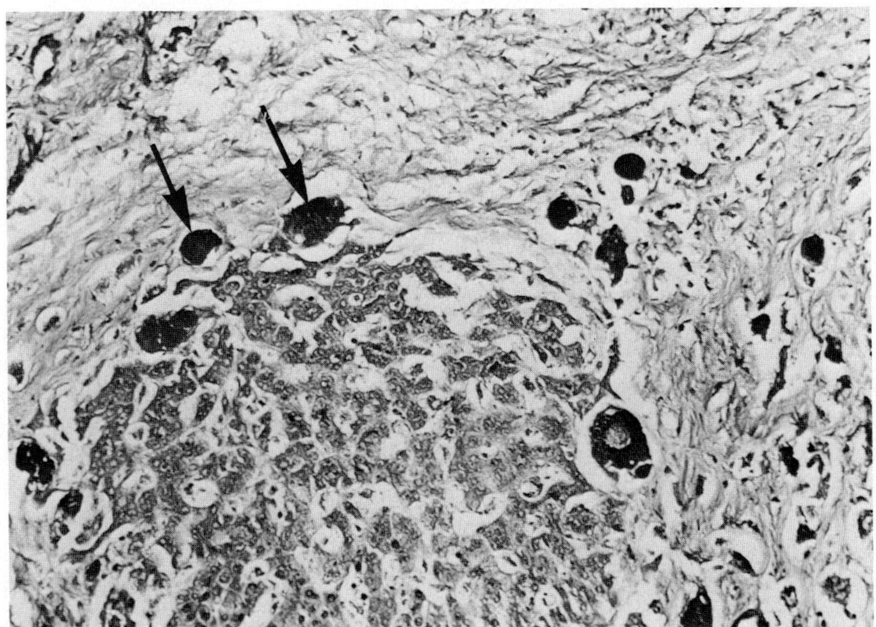

Figure 3. Extrahepatic biliary atresia, showing a more advanced lesion than that shown in Figures 1 and 2. Note marked increase in portal fibrosis and relatively small number of bile ducts. Large bile plugs are seen in several portal bile ducts (arrows). (Hematoxylin and eosin, ×140.)

Included under hepatocellular lesions in Table 1 are hydropic swelling and hyalinization of hepatocytes, acidophilic bodies, proliferation and prominence of Kupffer cells, and round cells in the lobules and portal triads. These "hepatitic" alterations are less severe, on the average, in extrahepatic obstruction than in hepatocellular disease. However, in individual cases they are not helpful in differential diagnosis. This also applies to giant cell transformation (GCT) of hepatocytes, which is more striking in "neonatal hepatitis," but is also quite common in extrahepatic obstruction (Figs. 4,5). Although GCT is generally seen in infants with severe "hepatitis," GCT unaccompanied by the other changes of "hepatitis" is occasionally observed. Unfortunately, the term giant cell hepatitis has been used not only for GCT with hepatitis, but also as a synonym for pure GCT. The significance and histogenesis of the hepatocellular giant cells in GCT remains obscure. They appear to represent a nonspecific response of the neonatal liver to a variety of injurious agents. Rarely giant cell hepatitis is seen in adults with viral or drug-induced liver injury (22,23). Extramedullary hemopoiesis (Fig. 6) and hemosiderin deposition are also generally more pronounced in infants with "neonatal hepatitis" (9). The diagnostic significance of neonatal iron storage, particularly whether neonatal hemochromatosis is a diagnostic entity, remains uncertain (Chapter 11) (9,9a). Fibrosis in neonatal hepatitis tends to develop gradually during the first year of life; it involves the portal triads relatively mildly, but extends into the lobules (Fig. 7). Nodular regeneration and well-developed cirrhosis may develop subsequently.

Neonatal Cholestasis Associated with Extrahepatic Obstruction

When clinical workup and needle biopsy specimen suggest extrahepatic obstruction (see above), the infant's extrahepatic biliary system should be explored surgically. A hepatic wedge biopsy specimen is taken, and if a bile-containing duct or gallbladder can be found, an intraoperative cholangiogram is done. Because the extrahepatic biliary system is often minute, surgical exploration is often very difficult. The more thorough the preoperative workup, the more likely the correct surgery will be performed (24). Lack of an extrahepatic biliary system (atresia), or presence of abnormally minute extrahepatic ducts (hypoplasia), used to be considered static congenital malformations that do not change after birth. This may be true in some cases. However, there is now good evidence that mechanical extrahepatic obstruction of the newborn may be progressive (25), and also that hypoplasia of the extrahepatic biliary system may be functional and reversible (24), the result of a primary hepatocellular disorder such as alpha-1-antitrypsin deficiency or "neonatal hepatitis." There are many different anatomic types of atresia of the biliary tract which may be classified surgically according to Kasai (Chapter 17, Figs. 4–6) (26). If a localized obstruction of the extrahepatic system is found, the proximal bile-containing segment is anastomosed to the duodenum (choledochojejunostomy or cholecystjejunostomy). Correctable lesions of this type are unfortunately rare in most series (26,27). Dilated bile ducts containing inspissated bile have been found in the hilum of the liver (28); anastomosis of these structures to the gut has been advocated. However, these ducts may not communicate with the rest of the biliary system (29).

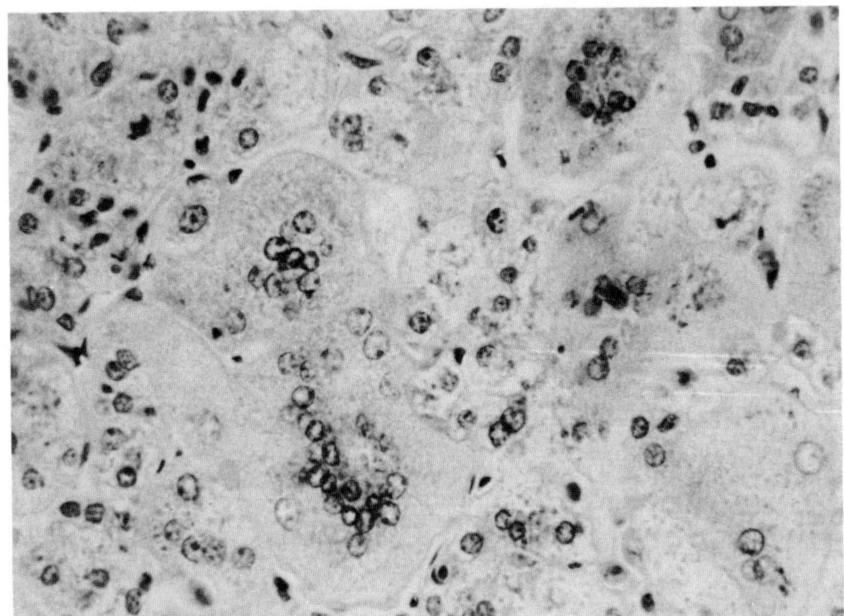

Figure 4. Multinucleated hepatocytic giant cell from a patient with "neonatal hepatitis." (Hematoxylin and eosin, ×400.)

If choledochojejunostomy or cholecystjejunostomy proves to be impossible because no obvious site of blockage of the extrahepatic system is found at laparotomy, then a distinction has to be made between progressive mechanical extrahepatic obstruction (25) and functional hypoplasia (24) as a result of hepatocellular disease. If hepatic biopsy and other available evidence, such as serum alpha-1-antitrypsin levels, suggest hepatocellular disease or intrahepatic atresia, then no biliary surgery is indicated. If, however, the biopsy suggests extrahepatic obstruction, and if the extrahepatic biliary system is hypoplastic, atretic or absent, then a hepatic portoenterostomy (26) may be indicated (for details, see Chapter 17).

A small proportion of cases of extrahepatic obstruction will, at laparotomy, prove to be due to a choledochal cyst. A mass is often palpable in these patients, who may also complain of pain. Although congenital, this lesion may not become symptomatic until adulthood (30–33). Five types of choledochal cyst are recognized (Chapter 17).

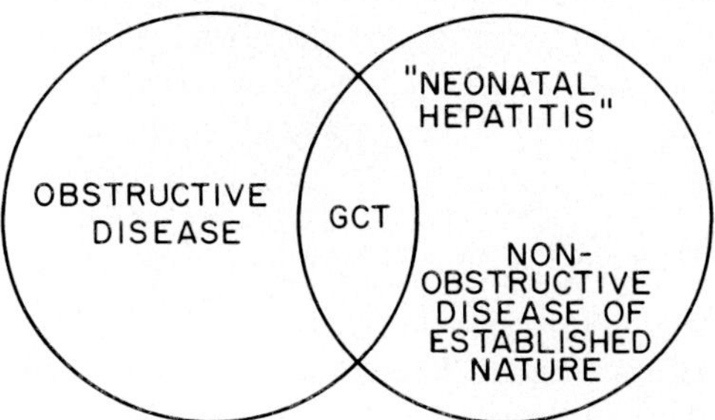

Figure 5. Possible etiologies for giant cell transformation (GCT).

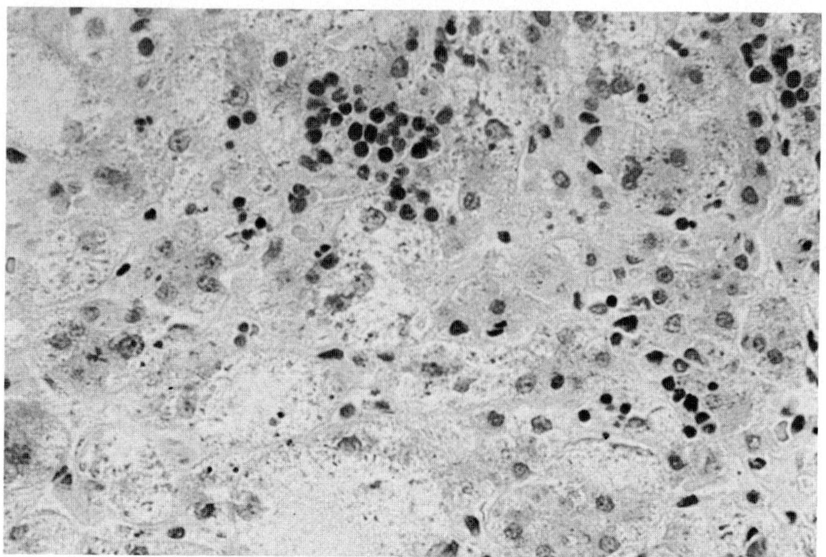

Figure 6. "Neonatal hepatitis" in a 2-month-old infant showing a group of hemopoietic cells. Some of the hepatocytes are enlarged and appear to be undergoing degenerative changes. (Hematoxylin and eosin, ×250.)

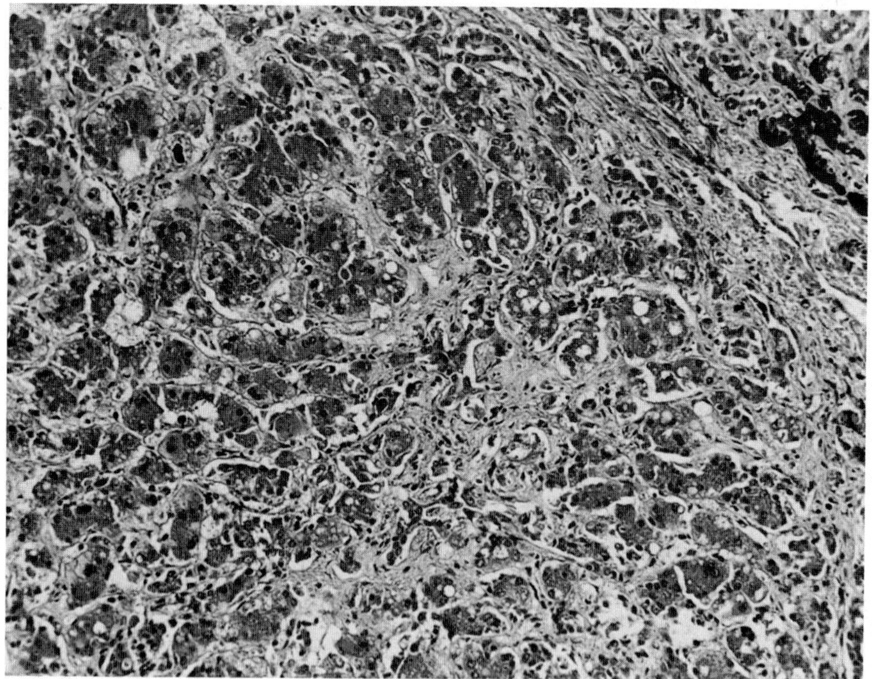

Figure 7. Infant with "neonatal hepatitis." The extrahepatic biliary system was injected with India ink to prove its patency, as shown at upper right. There is some portal fibrosis which also extends into the lobule. (Hematoxylin and eosin, ×110.)

The prognosis of extrahepatic atresia has usually been considered poor, since choledochoduodenostomy or cholecystjejunostomy are rarely feasible. The results of the Kasai operation are still controversial. In the absence of a successful operation, biliary cirrhosis develops in patients with extrahepatic atresia. For those who survive more than a year, the proliferated bile ducts in the fibrous septa tend to disappear, and the cirrhosis comes to resemble portal cirrhosis closely. Hepatocellular carcinoma is an occasional complication of biliary atresia (34,35).

Neonatal Cholestasis Without Mechanical Obstruction of the Extrahepatic Biliary System ("Neonatal Hepatitis")

The term "neonatal hepatitis" is often used as a synonym for hyperbilirubinemia without organic biliary obstruction (36). In recent years it has become clear that a great variety of etiologic factors can produce the hepatic morphologic pattern described above (Table 2), as it can be seen in diseases of established nature, of infectious, metabolic, chromosomal, or congenital origin, or it may be the result of blood group incompatibility (Table 2).

Generally, however, only a minority of cases of "neonatal hepatitis" can be associated with the known etiologic factors enumerated in Table 2. In most recent series homozygous alpha-1-antitrypsin deficiency (PiZZ) (Chapter 9) has been responsible for most of these. Morphologically, different patterns may be observed in antitrypsin deficiency. Typical "neonatal hepatitis," rarely with giant cells, is seen in one group; dense periportal fibrosis with ductular proliferation in another and paucity of intrahepatic bile ducts (see below) in a third. The PAS-positive diastase resistant droplets in periportal hepatocytes characteristic of this disease should be looked for in all pediatric patients with liver disease. The diagnosis is confirmed by demonstrating antitrypsin immunohistochemically in these droplets and by showing serum levels of antitrypsin to be low. Patients with antitrypsin deficiency should be phenotyped by serum electrophoresis. It should be noted that the highly characteristic PAS-positive droplets are rarely present before the age of 3 months (57). Immunohistochemistry, however, is more sensitive, becomes positive earlier, and is virtually specific (58) in cases of "neonatal hepatitis" in infants less than 3 months of age. Alpha-1-antitrypsin deficiency should therefore be excluded by examination of the serum. The prognosis of infants with antitrypsin deficiency is not necessarily as grave as might be expected, particularly in those infants who have the clinical and morphologic features of neonatal hepatitis (39,59). However, severe fibrosis in infancy and early childhood appears to carry a poor prognosis (60). During an epidemic, rubella can also account for a substantial proportion of infants with "neonatal hepatitis." In all cases of "neonatal hepatitis," careful clinical, serologic, and histopathologic studies are required to investigate the possible presence of the etiologic agents enumerated in Table 1. Viral inclusions of herpes and cytomegalovirus (Chapter 3) should be looked for in particular.

"Neonatal hepatitis," unassociated with any of the above etiologic factors, is usually sporadic but may be familial (61). The familial type appears to have a higher morbidity and mortality. Aagenaes et al. (62) described a hereditary

Table 2. Etiologic Factors that May Be Associated with "Neonatal Hepatitis"

Alpha-1-antitrypsin deficiency (37–40)	Gaucher's disease (22)
Rubella (41,19)	Down's syndrome (42)
Cytomegalovirus (43)	17-18 trisomy (19)
Herpes simplex (44)	Mucolipidosis (22)
Coxsackie virus (22)	Turner's syndrome (22)
Hepatitis B (45)	Indian childhood cirrhosis (47)
Toxoplasmosis (46)	ABO and Rh incompatibility (49)
Congenital syphilis (48)	Spherocytosis (51)
Escherichia *coli* pyelonephritis (50)	Anomalous pulmonary venous return to portal vein (22)
Cystic fibrosis (22)	Endocardial cushion defect (22)
Galactosemia (52)	Arnold-Chiari malformation (22)
Myeloproliferative disorder (22)	Zellweger's syndrome (55)
Niemann-Pick disease (53,54)	
Total parenteral nutrition (56)	

recurrent type of "neonatal hepatitis," associated with edema of the legs. Hepatocellular giant cells persist until adulthood (63). The long-term prognosis of "neonatal hepatitis" is uncertain and may depend on etiology. Some patients recover completely, some develop cholestasis and the morphologic picture of paucity of intrahepatic bile ducts, and a few die of cirrhosis. Some patients had persistent cholestasis with gradual improvement (64). Cases with complete giant cell transformation appear to have a relatively good chance of clinical recovery, while cases with persistent inflammation and intralobular fibrosis, as well as familial cases, tend to have a high mortality and a considerable risk of developing cirrhosis. Hepatocellular carcinoma has been described as a complication of "neonatal hepatitis" (65).

Hepatitis A and B in Infancy

There is no evidence that hepatitis A plays a role in neonatal hepatitis or extrahepatic atresia (66). Clinically evident "neonatal hepatitis" as described above is rarely associated with hepatitis B (45,66). Many infants born to asymptomatic Hb_sAg carrier mothers develop serologic evidence of infection and some develop mild, usually subclinical, chronic persistent hepatitis (67,68). Characteristically, HB_cAg can be demonstrated in the nuclei of their hepatocytes but HB_sAg is absent. In spite of this nonaggressive histologic appearance, the long-term prognosis of these infants must remain guarded, since some may develop cirrhosis and even hepatocellular carcinoma after many years. Chronic active hepatitis has rarely been reported in these infants. (68a). There is no evidence linking hepatitis B to extrahepatic atresia (66).

Neonatal Cholestasis Associated with Intrahepatic Atresia (Paucity of Intrahepatic Bile Ducts)

Neonatal cholestasis associated with intrahepatic atresia is a mysterious condition of uncertain, probably multiple, etiologies which, in most series, is quite rare in comparison with both extrahepatic atresia and "neonatal hepatitis." Arteriohepatic dysplasia or Alagille's syndrome (6) is the most clearly established entity included under this heading (Fig. 8). Rubella, 17-18 trisomy, and alpha-

1 antitrypsin deficiency are among the other reported etiologic factors (17,19,69). The graft-versus-host reaction in children with bone marrow transplants can produce this picture (Chapter 7), as can Byler's disease and an inherited anomaly of trihydroxycoprostanic acid metabolism (see p. 152). Clinically and pathologically, intrahepatic atresia progresses more slowly to hepatic fibrosis than extrahepatic atresia (70). Ultimately however, the picture of biliary cirrhosis may develop with xanthomas, elevated serum cholesterol (71), and a striking elevation of alkaline phosphatase. Some of these patients may never progress to cirrhosis (72).

The distinction of intrahepatic atresia from extrahepatic atresia is usually possible even in needle biopsy specimens, because in intrahepatic atresia there is a paucity of interlobular bile ducts with only slight fibrosis, rather than the ductal proliferation and marked fibrosis found in the early stages of extrahepatic atresia. The distinction of intrahepatic atresia from "neonatal hepatitis" is difficult and may be impossible, particularly in needle specimens (64). Intrahepatic atresia is suspected if there is a paucity of interlobular bile ducts (less than 0.4 per portal triad). Wedge biopsy and a count of 10–20 portal triads are generally required to make a definitive morphologic diagnosis (6). However, liver histology in Alagille's syndrome appears to be more variable than previously realized (64a).

Other Cholestatic Disorders

Cholestasis in infancy and childhood in the absence of mechanical extrahepatic obstruction is the predominant feature of several syndromes. A diagnosis of one

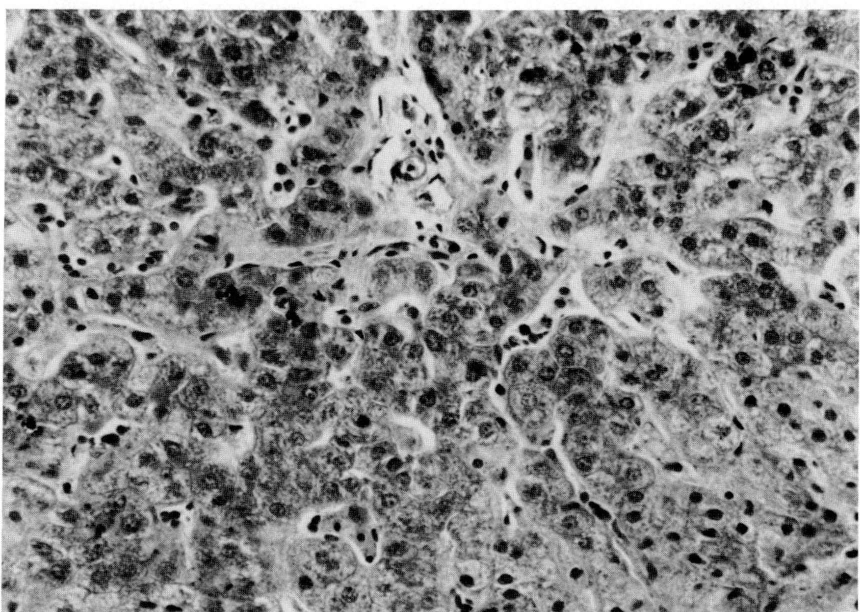

Figure 8. Infant with intrahepatic atresia. Upper middle portion shows small portal triad without a bile duct. There is no portal fibrosis. Liver cell plates are two cells thick. Parenchyma, however, appears essentially normal. (Hematoxylin and eosin, ×250.)

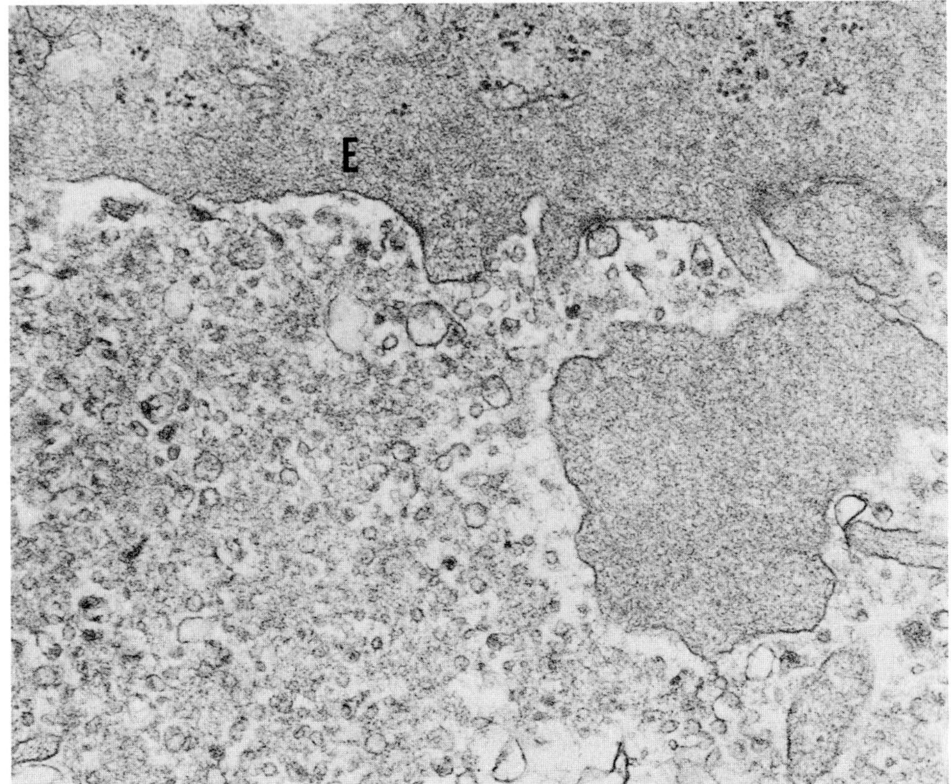

Figure 9. Byler's disease, showing marked ectoplasmic thickening (E). The microvilli are widened and blunted. The lumen of the bile duct contains coarse particulate material characteristic of this disease. (×60,000). (Contributed by B. Dahms, M.D.)

of these syndromes should be made only after a thorough search has ruled out viral hepatitis, drug toxicity, intra- and extrahepatic atresia, and the numerous etiologies associated with "neonatal hepatitis." One of these syndromes is benign recurrent cholestasis (Chapter 7) (73). However, this condition rarely commences during the neonatal period. There are symptom-free intervals of months to years. Histologically, centrilobular cholestasis, occasional single cell necrosis, and minimal portal inflammation occur.

Fatal familial progressive cholestasis (Byler's disease) usually has an onset after the age of 6 months. The hepatic histopathology is not specific. Portal fibrosis with ductular proliferation and mild portal inflammation is found. In the later stages there may be paucity of intrahepatic bile ducts. Canalicular bile plugs and pseudoglandular transformation of hepatocytes are seen, and death from cirrhosis usually occurs before the age of 10 years (74,75). Electron microscopically, a peculiar appearance of the canalicular bile plugs has been found (Fig. 9) (76). Whether this finding is specific remains unclear. Hepatocellular carcinoma has developed in these patients (p. 243).

A syndrome has been described in which infants with severe cholestatic liver disease have large amounts of trihydroxycoprostanic acid, a bile acid precursor in their serum, bile, and urine, which appears to be inherited as an autosomal recessive trait (77,78).

Total parenteral nutrition may be associated with severe cholestasis in infants and children (56). Hepatocellular giant cell transformation has been reported in these patients. Fatty change and extramedullary hemopoiesis are also seen (79). Portal fibrosis may develop (80).

REFERENCES

1. Bill AH, Kasai M, (eds): Biliary atresia and choledochal cyst. New concepts of cause and treatment, in *Progress in Pediatric Surgery*. Baltimore, University Park Press, 1974, vol 6.
2. Perez-Soler A: The inflammatory and atresia-inducing disease of the liver and bile ducts. *Monographs in Pediatrics*. Basel, New York, Karger, 1976, vol 8.
3. Rosenberg HS, Bolande RP, (eds): Perspectives in pediatric pathology, in *Year Book*. Chicago, Year Book Medical Publishers, 1976, Vol. 3, pp 1–135.
4. Javitt NB: *Neonatal Hepatitis and Biliary Atresia*, NIH 79-1296. Washington, D.C., U.S. Department of Health, Education, and Welfare, 1977.
5. Thaler MM: Jaundice in the newborn. Algorithmic diagnosis of conjugated and unconjugated hyperbilirubinemia. *JAMA* 237:58, 1977.
6. Alagille D, Odievre M, Gautier M, et al: Hepatic ductular hypoplasia associated with characteristic facies, vertebral malformations, retarded physical, mental and sexual development and cardiac murmur. *J Pediatr* 86:63, 1975.
7. Henriksen MT, Langmark F, Sorland SJ, et al: Hereditary cholestasis combined with peripheral pulmonary stenosis and other anomalies. *Acta Paediatr Scand* 66:7, 1977.

7a. Balazs M, Mark ZS, Lukazs VF: Light- and electron microscopic studies of the liver in Bronze Baby Syndrome. *Path Res Pract* 172:196, 1981.

8. Danks DM, Campbell PE, Jack D, et al: Studies of the aetiology of neonatal hepatitis and biliary atresia. *Arch Dis Child* 52:360, 1977.
9. Ruebner BH, Miyai K: The pathology of neonatal hepatitis and biliary atresia with particular reference to hemopoiesis and hemosiderin deposition. *Ann NY Acad Sci* 111:375, 1963.

9a. Goldfischer S, Grotsky HW, Change CH, et al: Idiopathic neonatal iron storage involving the liver, pancreas, heart, and endocrine and exocrine glands. *Hepatology* 1:58, 1981.

10. Irons R, Schenk E, Lee J: Cytochemical methods for copper. *Arch Pathol Lab Med* 101:298, 1977.

10a. Goldfischer S, Popper H, Sternlieb I: The significance of variations in the distribution of copper in liver disease. *Am J Pathol* 99:715, 1980.

11. Morgan JD, Hartroft W: Juvenile liver. *Arch Pathol Lab Med* 71:86, 1961.
12. Emery JL: Functional asymmetry of the liver. *Ann NY Aca Sci* 111:37, 1963.
13. Krowchuk D, Seashor JH: Complete biliary obstruction due to erythromycin estolate administration in an infant. *Pediatrics* 64:956, 1979.
14. Witzleben CL: Extrahepatic biliary atresia. Concepts of cause, diagnosis and management, in Rosenberg HJ, Bolande RP (ed): *Perspectives in Pediatric Pathology*. New York, Masson Publishing, 1979, vol 5, p 41.
15. Landing BH, Mahnovski V, Dahms B: Considerations of certain aspects of the pathogenesis of neonatal hepatitis and biliary atresia, in Javitt NB (ed): *Neonatal Hepatitis and Biliary Atresia*, NIH 79-1296. Washington, D.C., US Department of Health, Education, and Welfare, 1979, p 315.
16. Grishan FK, LaBreque DR, Mitros FA, et al: The evolving nature of infantile obstructive cholangiopathy. *J Pediatr* 97:27, 1980.
17. Strauss L, Bernstein J: Neonatal hepatitis in congenital rubella. *Arch Pathol Lab Med* 86:317, 1968.
18. Oppenheimer EH, Esterley JR: Congenital cytomegalovirus infection and bile duct obstruction in newborn infant with cystic fibrosis of pancreas. *Lancet* 2:1031, 1973.
19. Alpert LI, Strauss L, Hirschhorn K: Neonatal hepatitis and biliary atresia associated with trisomy 17-18 syndrome. *N Engl J Med* 280:16, 1969.

20. Bennett DE: Problems in neonatal obstructive jaundice. *Pediatrics* 33:735, 1964.
21. Brough AJ, Bernstein J: Morphological approach to the evaluation of infantile conjugated hyperbilirubinemia, in Javitt NB (ed): *Neonatal Hepatitis and Atresia,* NIH 79-1296. Washington, D.C., US Department of Health, Education, and Welfare, 1977, p 381.
22. Montgomery CK, Ruebner BH: Neonatal hepatocellular giant cell transformation, a review, in Rosenberg HS, Bolande RP (eds): *Perspectives in Pediatric Pathology.* Chicago, Year Book Medical Publishers, 1976, p. 85.
23. Richey J, Rogers S, Van Thiel DH, et al: Giant multinucleated hepatocytes in an adult with chronic active hepatitis. *Gastroenterology* 73:570, 1977.
24. Lilly JR: Surgical jaundice in infancy. *Ann Surg* 186(5):549, 1977.
25. Koop CE: Biliary obstruction in the newborn. *Surg Clin North Am* 56:373, 1976.
26. Kasai M: Treatment of biliary atresia with special reference to hepatic portoenterostomy and its modifications. *Prog Pediatr Surg* 6:5, 1974.
27. Bunton GL, Cameron R: Regeneration of liver after biliary cirrhosis. *Ann NY Acad Sci* 111:412, 1963.
28. Danks DM, Campbell PE: Extrahepatic biliary atresia. Comments on the frequency of potentially operable cases. *J Pediatr* 69:21, 1966.
29. Fonkalsrud EW, Arima E: Bile lakes in congenital biliary atresia. *Surgery* 77:384, 1975.
30. Barlow B, Tabor E, Blanc WA, et al: Choledochal cyst: A review of 19 cases. *J Pediatr* 89(6):934, 1976.
31. Kimura K, Tsugawa C, Ogawa K, et al: Choledochal cyst. *Arch Surg* 113:159, 1978.
32. Loubeau J-M, Steichen FM: Dilation of intrahepatic bile ducts in choledochal cyst. *Arch Surg* 111:1384, 1976.
33. Muakkasah K, Obeid S, Slim M: Congenital choledochal cysts. *Arch Surg* 111(10):1112, 1976.
34. Deoras M, Dicus W: Hepatocarcinoma associated with biliary cirrhosis. *Arch Pathol Lab Med* 86:338, 1968.
35. Kulkarni PB, Beatty EC: Cholangiocarcinoma associated with biliary atresia. *Am J Dis Child* 131:442, 1977.
36. Craig JM, Landing BH: A form of hepatitis in the neonatal period simulating biliary atresia. *Arch Pathol Lab Med* 54:321, 1952.
37. Glasgow JF, Lynch MJ, Hercz A, et al: Alpha-1-antitrypsin deficiency in association with both cirrhosis and chronic obstructive lung disease in two sibs. *Am J Med* 54:181, 1973.
38. Brunt PW: Antitrypsin and the liver. *Gut* 15:573, 1974.
39. Hirschberger M, Stickler GB: Neonatal hepatitis and alpha-1-antitrypsin deficiency. The prognosis in five patients. *Mayo Clin Proc* 52:214, 1977.
40. Hadchouel M, Gautier M: Histopathologic study of the liver in the early cholestatic phase of alpha-1-antitrypsin deficiency. *J Pediatr* 89:211, 1976.
41. Esterly JR, Slusser RJ, Ruebner BH: Hepatic lesions in the congenital rubella syndrome. *J Pediatr* 71:676, 1967.
42. Mori W: Liver changes in Down's syndrome. *Acta Hepatogastroenterol* 18:363, 1971.
43. Medearis DN Jr: Observations concerning human cytomegalovirus infection and disease. *Johns Hopkins Med J* 114:181, 1964.
44. Nahamias AJ, Alford CA, Korones SB: Infection of the newborn with herpesvirus hominis. *Adv Pediatr* 17:185, 1970.
45. Kattamis C, Demetrios D, Karambula K, et al: Neonatal hepatitis associated with Australia antigen (Au-1). *Arch Dis Child* 48:133, 1973.
46. Sumegi I: Riesenzellenhepatitis bei Neugeborenen. *Acta Pathol Microbiol Scand* [*A*] 47:259, 1959.
47. Smetana HF, Hadley GG, Sirsat SM: Infantile cirrhosis. An analytical review of the literature and a review of 50 cases. *Pediatrics* 28:107, 1961.
48. Peace R: Fatal hepatitis and cirrhosis in infancy. *Arch Pathol Lab Med* 61:107, 1956.
49. Dunn PM: Obstructive jaundice and hemolytic disease of the newborn. *Arch Dis Child* 38:54, 1963.

50. Bernstein J, Brown AK: Sepsis and jaundice in early infancy. *Pediatrics* 29:873, 1962.
51. Bain GO, Wang GC, Misanik LF: Giant cell hepatitis associated with hereditary spherocytosis. *J. Pediatr* 51:549, 1957.
52. Suzuki H, Gilbert EF, Anido V, et al: Galactosemia. A report of 200 fatal cases. *Arch Pathol Lab Med* 82:602, 1966.
53. Ivemark BI, Svennerholm L, Thoren C, et al: Niemann-Pick disease in infancy. Report of two siblings with clinical, histological and chemical studies. *Acta Paediatr Scand* 52:391, 1963.
54. Ashkenazi A, Yarom R, Gutman A, et al: Niemann-Pick disease and giant cell transformation of the liver. *Acta Paediatr Scand* 60:285, 1971.
55. Gilchrist KW, Gilbert EF, Goldfarb S, et al: Studies of malformation syndromes of man XIB: The cerebro-hepatorenal syndrome of Zellweger: Comparative pathology. *Eur J Pediatr* 121:99, 1976.
56. Bernstein J, Chang CH, Brough AJ, et al: Conjugated hyperbilirubinemia in infancy associated with parenteral alimentation. *J Pediatr* 90(3):361, 1977.
57. Talbot IC, Mowat AP: Liver disease in infancy: Histological features and relationship to alpha-1-antitrypsin phenotype. *J Clin Pathol* 28:559, 1975.
58. Bradfield JWB, Blenkinsopp WK: Alpha-1-antitrypsin globules in the liver and PiM phenotype. *J Clin Pathol* 30:464, 1977.
59. Odievre M, Valayer J, Razemon-Pinta M, et al: Hepatic port-enterostomy or cholecystostomy in the treatment of extrahepatic biliary atresia. *J Pediatr* 88:774, 1976.
60. Strobel S, Bender JW, Posselt HG, et al: Alpha-1-antitrypsin deficiency: Fulminant course in early infancy. *Helv Paediatr Acta* 35:75, 1980.
61. Lawson EE, Boggs JD: Long term follow-up of neonatal hepatitis. Safety and value of surgical exploration. *Pediatrics* 53:650, 1974.
62. Aagenaes O, Van Der Hagen CB, Refsum S: Hereditary recurrent intrahepatic cholestasis from birth. *Arch Dis Child* 43:646, 1968.
63. Sándor T, Surinya M, Mónus Z: Familial occurrence of giant cell hepatitis in infancy. *Acta Hepatogastroenterol (Stuttg)* 23:101, 1976.
64. Heathcote J, Deodhar KP, Scheuer PJ, et al: Intrahepatic cholestasis in childhood. *N Engl J Med* 295:801, 1976.
64a. Dahms BB, Petrelli M, Wyllie R: Arteriohepatic dysplasia: A longitudinal study of liver biopsy in infants and children. *Lab Invest* 46:4, 1981.
65. Fajers CM, Falkmer S, Frisell E, et al: Primary carcinoma of the liver and giant-cell hepatitis in infancy. *Acta Paediatr Scand* 49:96, 1960.
66. Ballistreri WF, Tabor E, Gerety RJ: Negative serology for hepatitis A and B viruses in 18 cases of neonatal cholestasis. *Pediatrics* 66:269, 1980.
67. Shiraki K, Yoshihara N, Kawana T, et al: Hepatitis B surface antigen and chronic hepatitis in infants born to asymptomatic carrier mothers. *Am J Dis Child* 131:644, 1977.
68. Schweitzer IL, Dunn AEG, Peters RL, et al: Viral hepatitis B in neonates and infants. *Am J Med* 55:762, 1973.
68a. Shinozaki T, Saito K, Shiraki K: HBsAg positive giant cell hepatitis with cirrhosis in a 10 month old infant. *Arch Dis Child* 56:64, 1981.
69. Perrault J: Paucity of interlobular bile ducts. Getting to know it better. *Dig Dis Sci* 26:485, 1981.
70. Branski D, Lebenthal E, Hatch TF, et al: Intrahepatic cholestasis for 15 years without cirrhosis. *J Clin Gastroenterol* 2:251, 1980.
71. Haas L, Dobbs RH: Congenital absence of the intrahepatic bile ducts. *Arch Dis Child* 33:396, 1959.
72. Berman MD, Ishak KG, Schaefer LJ: Syndromatic hepatic ductular hypoplasia (arteriohepatic dysplasia. *Dig Dis Sci* 26:485, 1981.
73. Summerskill WHJ, Walshe JM: Benign recurrent intrahepatic obstructive jaundice. *Lancet* 2:686, 1959.
74. Clayton RJ, Iber FL, Ruebner BH, et al: Byler Disease. Fatal familial intrahepatic cholestasis in an Amish kindred. *Am J Dis Child* 117:112, 1969.

75. Odievre M, Gautier M, Hadchouel M, et al: Severe familial intrahepatic cholestasis. *Arch Dis Child* 48:806, 1973.

76. Linarelli LG, Williams CN, Phillips MJ: Byler's Disease: Fatal intrahepatic cholestasis. *J Pediatr* 81:484, 1972.

77. Eyssen H, Parmentier G, Compernolle F, et al: Trihydroxycoprostanic acid in the duodenal fluid of two children with intrahepatic bile duct anomalies. *Biochim Biophys Acta* 273:212, 1972.

78. Hansen RF, Isenberg JN, Williams GC, et al: The metabolism of 3α 7α 12α trihydroxy 5β cholestan 26 oic acid in two siblings with cholestasis due to intrahepatic bile duct anomalies. *J Clin Invest* 56:577, 1975.

79. Cohen L, Olsen M: Liver histopathology associated with pediatric total parenteral nutrition. *Lab Invest* 42:107, 1980.

80. Dahms BB, Helpin TC: Serial liver biopsies in parenteral nutrition associated cholestasis of early infancy. *Lab Invest* 42:170, 1980.

9
Metabolic Diseases Associated with Hepatocellular Necrosis

The possibility of a metabolic disease should be considered in infants with jaundice and liver enzyme abnormalities, after all possible infectious causes for the clinical picture of "neonatal hepatitis" by appropriate cultures and titers have been excluded and after the diagnosis of extrahepatic atresia has been ruled out. Morphologically, hepatocellular pathology of variable severity is observed, which in some of the conditions described in this chapter cannot be distinguished from "neonatal hepatitis" (Chapter 8). Abnormal storage products are not conspicuous in this group of diseases. A considerable proportion of patients progress to fibrosis, and eventually to cirrhosis. In some metabolic diseases, the early stages of hepatocellular injury may be clinically inconspicuous, and the patients may have no complaints until they present with cirrhosis in childhood or even as adults. Cirrhosis may also develop in some diseases in which an abnormal storage product is the predominant lesion. These are dealt with in Chapter 10 and include glycogenosis types III and IV, Wolman's disease, Niemann-Pick's disease, Gaucher's disease, and the mucopolysaccharidoses. Iron overload, which may be associated with cirrhosis, is described in Chapter 11. Reye's syndrome, which may be associated with hepatocellular necrosis, has been described in Chapter 6.

ALPHA-1-ANTITRYPSIN DEFICIENCY

Deficiency of this protease inhibitor (alpha-1-antitrypsin) is associated with liver disease in a considerable proportion of homozygous children of genotype PiZZ (1,2). Antitrypsin deficiency is one of the most frequently responsible etiologic factors in infantile cholestasis, surpassed in frequency only by extrahepatic biliary atresia. Hepatosplenomegaly and a bleeding diathesis are common in these infants. The trypsin inhibitory capacity of the serum should be measured in all cases of infantile obstructive jaundice. Phenotyping by immunoelectrophoresis should be done in all patients with low serum antitypsin. A variable spectrum of histologic abnormalities has been described. The changes may be those of "neonatal hepatitis", paucity of intrahepatic bile ducts, or cirrhosis

(Chapter 8) (3,4). Whereas emphysema develops in most PiZZ homozygous adults, in only about 10% does hepatic pathology develop. The most striking histologic feature found in virtually all homozygotes after the age of 3 months (5) is roughly spherical droplets within hepatocytes, predominantly in periportal zones. These droplets are faintly eosinophilic and may be inconspicuous in hematoxylin and eosin-stained sections. In sections stained by the PAS method, the droplets are brilliantly purplish red, even after diastase digestion (Figs. 1–3) (6). The finding of such droplets is strongly suspicious, but not diagnostic (7). A virtually conclusive diagnosis is reached by immunohistochemistry, which has shown the droplets to consist of alpha-1-antitrypsin. We prefer the horseradish immunoperoxidase method over immunofluorescence (8). This reaction is more sensitive than is PAS staining and is positive in very young infants when PAS-positive droplets are absent. Immunohistochemistry should always be confirmed by serum electrophoresis, since apparently typical droplets reacting with specific antisera have been found in patients with normal phenotype (9,9a). Electron microscopically the droplets consist of amorphous material located within the dilated cisternae of the endoplasmic reticulum (Fig. 4) (10,11).

The characteristic PAS-positive droplets can be demonstrated not only in those who have hepatic pathology, but also in those who do not (12). Chronic active hepatitis and cirrhosis have been claimed to be associated with heterozygous antitrypsin deficiency (PiMZ, PiFZ, PiSZ) (13–16c). PAS staining after diastase digestion has therefore been recommended in cases of cryptogenic cirrhosis (13). If this is positive, the diagnosis should be confirmed by immunohistochemistry. Hepatocarcinoma develops in some adult patients with cirrhosis

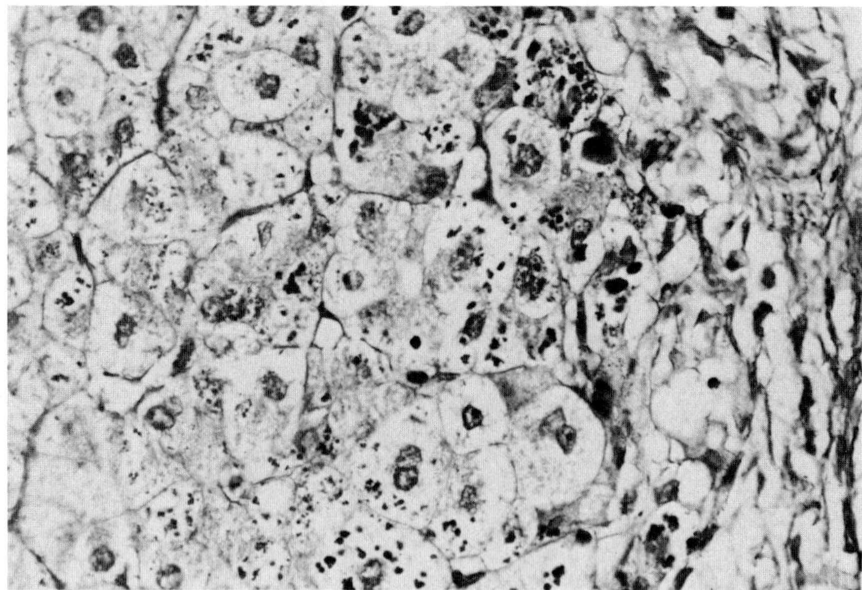

Figure 1. Alpha-1-antitrypsin deficiency. Biopsy from a 1-year-old child with moderate portal fibrosis (right). Many small droplets containing alpha-1-antitrypsin are seen in periportal hepatocytes. (PAS reaction with diastase digestion, ×520.)

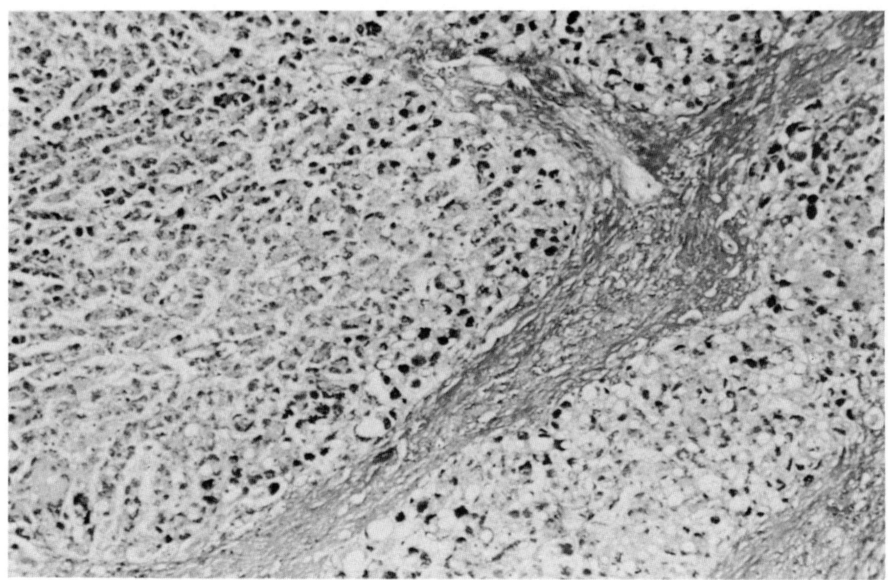

Figure 2. Alpha-1-antitrypsin deficiency. Autopsy of a 3-year-old child with severe cirrhosis. Masses of droplets containing alpha-1-antitrypsin are seen in periportal hepatocytes. (PAS with diastase, ×85.)

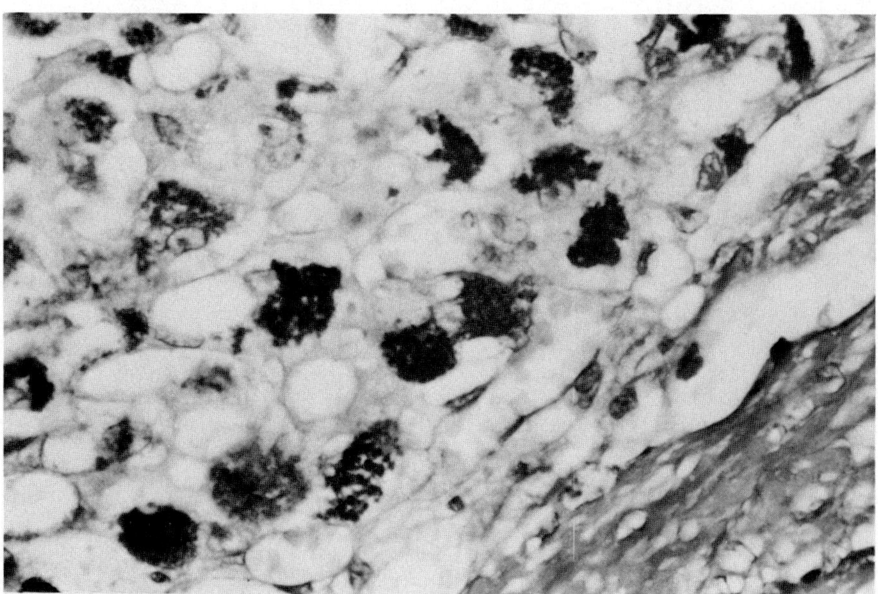

Figure 3. High-power of same specimen shown in Figure 2. Note striking number of PAS-positive granules in hepatocytes. (PAS with diastase, ×545.)

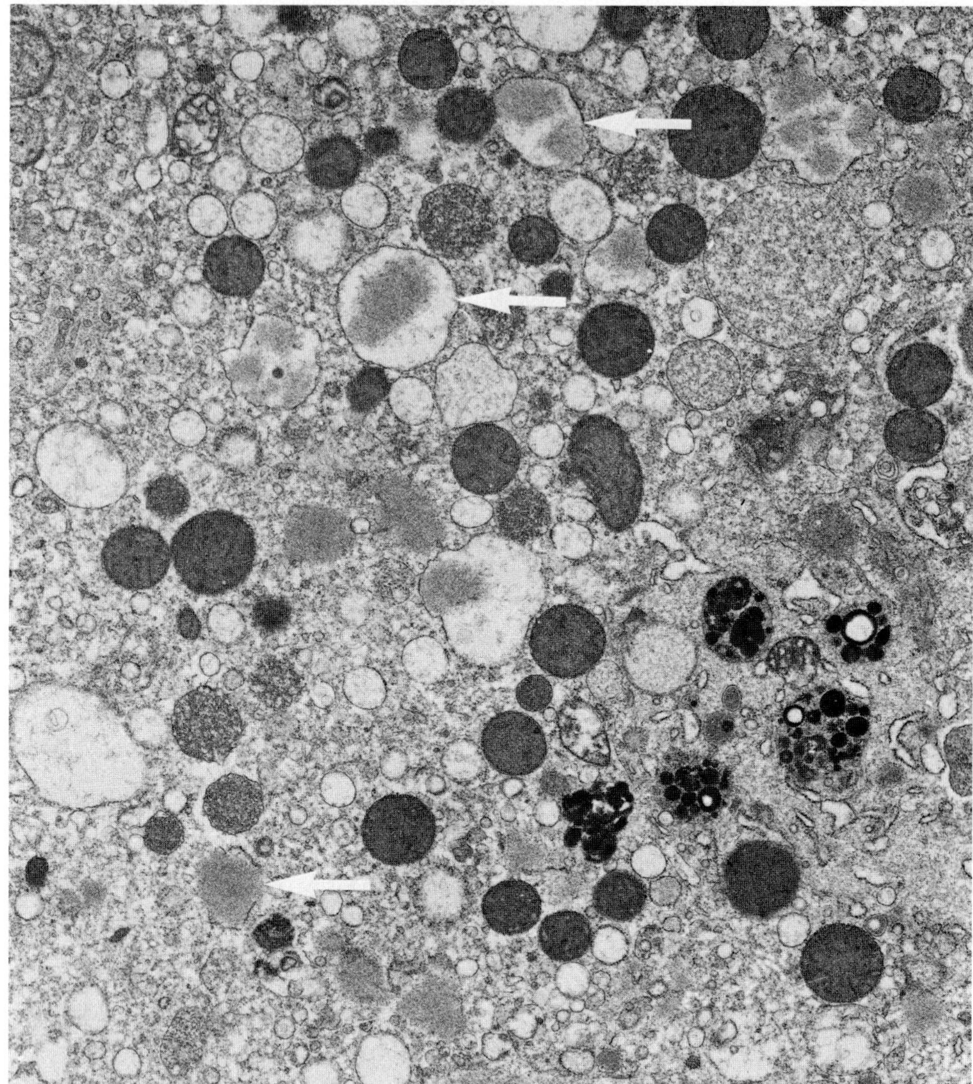

Figure 4. Alpha-1-antitrypsin deficiency, showing moderately dense amorphous material in cisternae of dilated endoplasmic reticulum of a hepatocyte. (×10,000.) (Contributed by J. Lawrie, M.D.)

associated with alpha-1-antitrypsin deficiency (17). Most frequently these patients have PiZZ deficiency, but hepatocarcinoma has been reported in heterozygous patients (14,17a,18).

FAMILIAL HYPOFIBRINOGENEMIA

Weakly PAS-positive droplets may be demonstrated in this disease. These have been proven to consist of fibrinogen. Like alpha-1-antitrypsin deficiency familial hypofibrinogenemia appears to be due to a failure of hepatic secretion (18a).

WILSON'S DISEASE

Wilson's disease (hepatolenticular degeneration) is a disturbance of copper metabolism inherited as an autosomal recessive (19). The disease is expressed only in homozygotes. It is apparently caused by deficient excretion of copper in bile canaliculi. In Wilson's disease, hepatic copper increases in concentration from a normal value of less than 100 μg/g hepatic dry weight to a value generally higher than 500 μg. Patients most commonly present during the second decade. However, the diagnosis has been made at 4 years (20). The earliest sign of the disease is asymptomatic hepatosplenomegaly, followed by jaundice, edema, and ascites. Kayser-Fleischer rings and neurologic dysfunction are common. The characteristic biochemical changes in the serum consist of low ceruloplasmin and copper with excessive urinary copper excretion.

Liver biopsy is helpful in early diagnosis. The tissue obtained at needle biopsy should be subdivided into three parts. Unfixed dried tissue that can be kept at room temperature is employed to estimate copper concentration. More than 250 μg/g dry weight is considered diagnostic, except in patients with long-standing cholestasis caused by extrahepatic obstruction, hepatocellular disease or primary biliary cirrhosis (21–23).

The second portion of the biopsy specimen is fixed for light microscopy. The finding in hepatocytes of granules staining with rubeanic acid or rhodamine (24) provides a reasonable screening method in the diagnosis of excessive hepatic tissue copper levels. A complementary, somewhat more sensitive and probably less specific, stain is orcein. This stain was found (25) to stain granules of a copper associated protein in the hepatocytes of patients with elevated hepatic copper. However, it must be recognized that in the early stages of Wilson's disease copper stains are negative, despite high hepatic copper levels. On the other hand, copper stains may be positive in a variety of hepatic diseases, particularly those with prolonged cholestasis (Chapter 7), including primary biliary cirrhosis, alcoholic cirrhosis, and Indian childhood cirrhosis (see p. 165), as well as normal neonates (26,27).

The earliest histologic changes in Wilson's disease consist of small- or large-droplet fatty change (Fig. 5), glycogen nuclei (Chapter 1), and lipofuscin deposition (Chapter 11). The histologic picture of chronic active hepatitis (Chapter 2) follows these early changes (26,27). The severity of the parenchymal necrosis seems to determine the rapidity with which cirrhosis develops. Degeneration and necrosis of parenchymal cells may continue even in the cirrhotic stage of Wilson's disease. The periportal hepatocytes of such patients often contain Mallory's "alcoholic" hyalin (Chapter 5). Cholestasis, including bile thrombi in ductules, may be seen. Cirrhosis may be macronodular or mixed micro–macronodular (30). End-stage cirrhosis may be seen even in childhood (31). However, the development of hepatocarcinoma is rare (19).

The third portion of the biopsy specimen is fixed for ultrastructural studies. Electron microscopically the mitochondria show the most striking changes (Fig. 6). They are enlarged and vacuolated and contain crystalline inclusions. Their matrix shows increased electron density and is retracted from the surrounding membranes (28,32).

Unfortunately, neither the early stage of fatty change nor the later stages of chronic active hepatitis, cholestasis, and cirrhosis are specific for Wilson's disease.

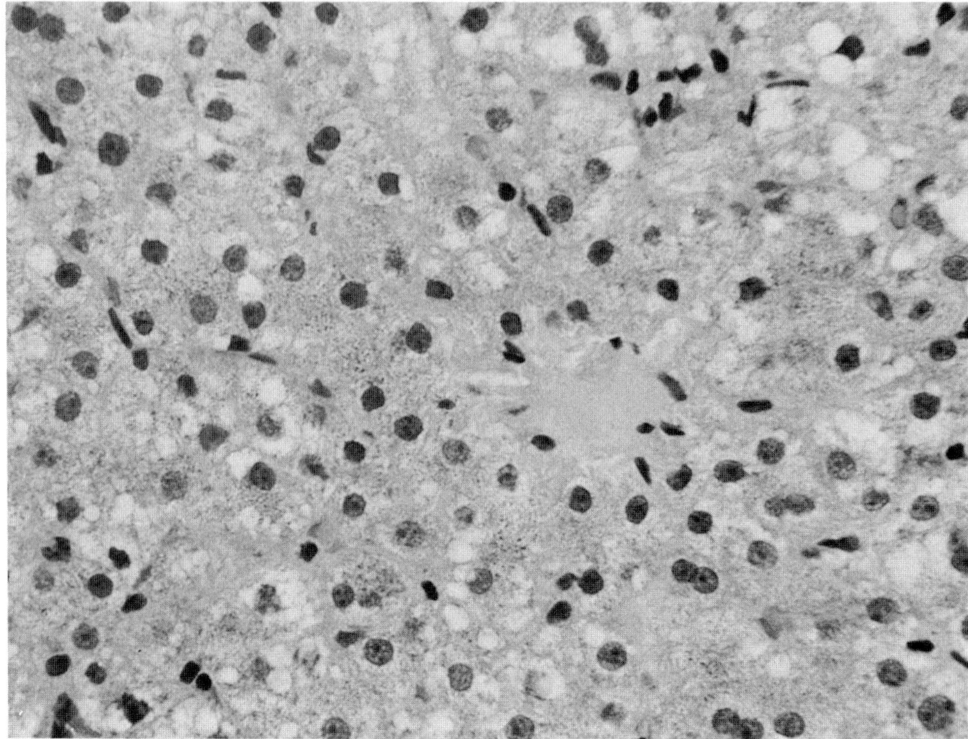

Figure 5. Early stage of Wilson's disease in a child. There is mild fatty change and minimal inflammation. (Hematoxylin and eosin, ×160.)

Timely treatment can prevent the serious cerebral and hepatic changes. Therefore, a high index of suspicion should be maintained for children or adults under 30 presenting with the clinicopathologic manifestations described above. As screening procedures, rhodamine and orcein stains should be done on such specimens. For a definitive diagnosis, however, measurement of the hepatic copper level is usually required.

GALACTOSEMIA

Galactosemia is an autosomal recessive hereditary metabolic disease due to deficiency of galactose-1-phosphate uridyl transferase. Apart from classic galactosemia, there are several variants of this disease (20,33). Symptoms appear in infants within a few days of milk ingestion. Vomiting, jaundice, hypoglycemia, and hepatosplenomegaly are conspicuous. The diagnosis is confirmed by absence of the enzyme in red blood cells.

Histologically, fatty change occurs involving parenchymal cells throughout the lobules (Fig. 7). Pseudoglandular transformation of the liver cell plates is at first minimal. Later this becomes much more striking. The dilated canaliculi

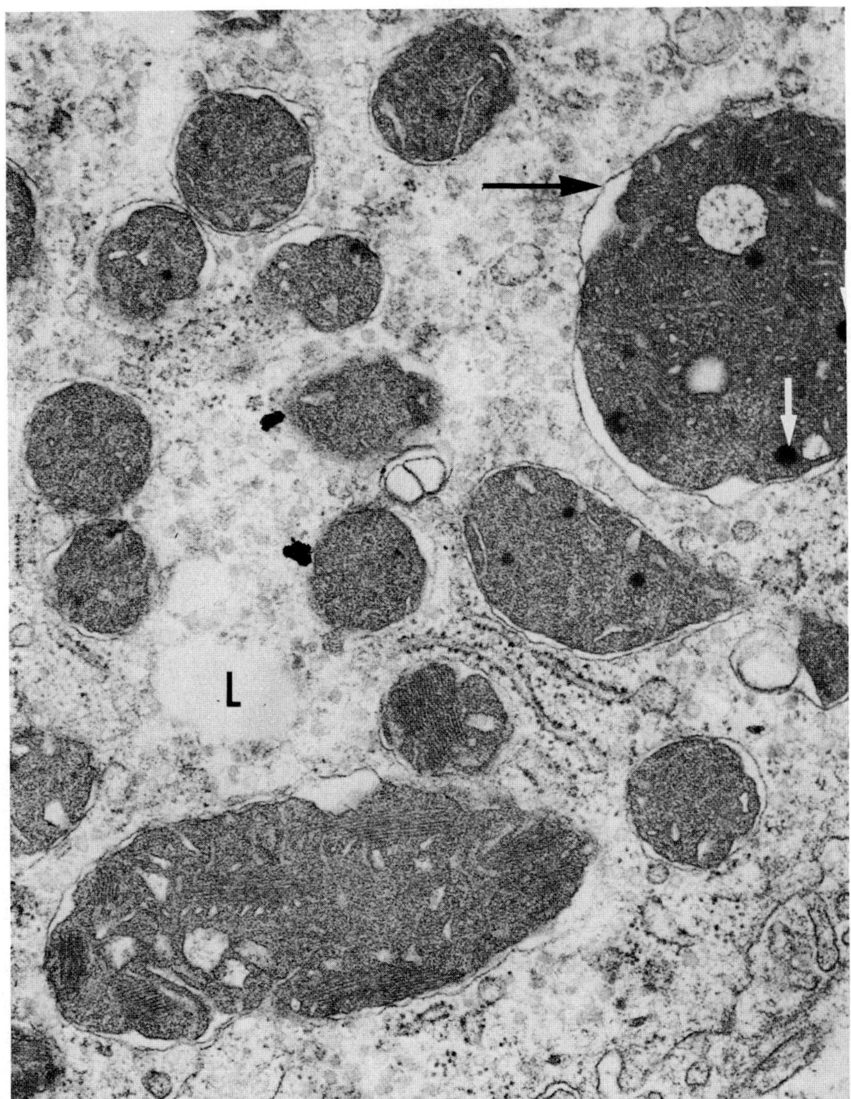

Figure 6. Wilson's disease in a 24-year-old woman. Characteristic mitochondrial lesion in a fragment of a hepatocyte. Note enlarged mitochondrial granules (white arrows), separation of outer and inner membranes (black arrows), and dilated cristae. Lipid droplets (L) are also seen. (Uranyl acetate, and lead citrate, ×23,000.) (Contributed by I. Sternlieb, M.D.)

composing the lumens of the pseudoglandular spaces often contain bile thrombi. Hepatocellular giant cells have been reported in this condition. As ductular proliferation and portal fibrosis develop, the fatty change becomes less conspicuous. If milk products are withdrawn, these changes, including the fibrosis, appear to be reversible (34). If the disease is not adequately treated, cirrhosis supervenes. The pseudo-glandular pattern fades as cirrhosis develops.

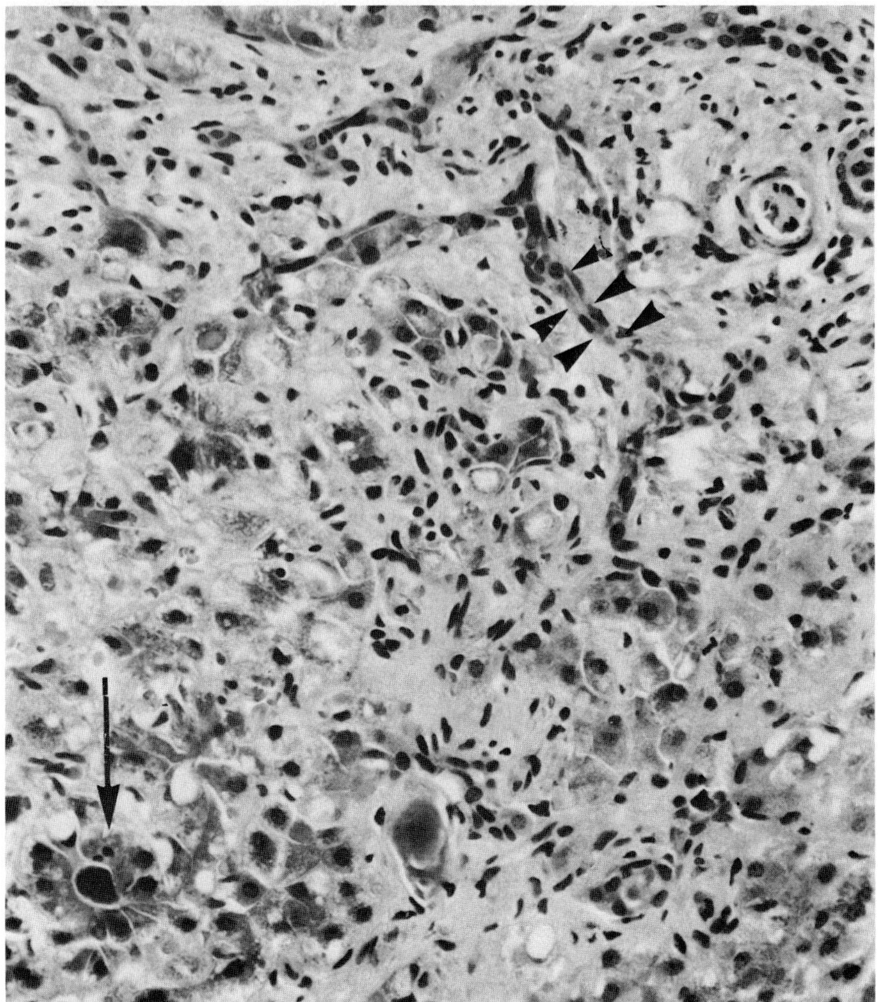

Figure 7. Galactosemia in a 28-day-old infant. Hepatocytes show moderate fatty change and focal glandular transformation with bile plugs (arrow). Note marked proliferation of portal bile ducts (arrowheads) and portal fibrosis. (Masson's trichrome, ×250.) (Contributed by M. Thaler, M.D., ref. 34).

HEREDITARY TYROSINEMIA AND HEREDITARY FRUCTOSE INTOLERANCE

The clinical presentation and hepatic pathology of these conditions resemble those of galactosemia. Hereditary tyrosinemia is poorly understood. It is supposedly due to lack of parahydroxyphenylpyruvic acid oxidase and plasma tyrosine levels are elevated. In the acute form symptoms appear within the first 6 months and death occurs in infancy. Patients with the chronic form present later in childhood with cirrhosis (20,33) and have a high risk of developing hepatocarcinoma. Hereditary fructose intolerance is best diagnosed by a fructose tolerance test (33a).

ZELLWEGER'S CEREBROHEPATORENAL SYNDROME

Zellweger's cerebrohepatorenal syndrome is an autosomal recessive condition leading to early death (35). The underlying metabolic defect is not understood. There are cerebral lesions and renal cysts. Hepatic hemosiderosis is a feature in some patients. Lobular disarray, hepatocellular necrosis, bile duct proliferation, fibrosis, and even cirrhosis may be seen. Giant cell transformation has been reported (36). Electron microscopy shows mitochondrial abnormalities and absence of peroxisomes (20,37,38). A slight variant of this condition was recently described (39).

DONOHUE'S LEPRECHAUNISM

Donohue's Syndrome is another obscure, rare, lethal, autosomal recessive condition characterized by multiple endocrine abnormalities. The liver shows excessive hemosiderosis and nodular transformation (37).

DISORDERS OF THE UREA CYCLE

Ornithine transcarbamylase (OTC) and carbamyl phosphate synthetase deficiency are among the enzymopathies of the urea cycle associated with elevated blood ammonia levels (40). Citrullinemia may also be present. The clinical symptoms consist of vomiting, lethargy, seizures, and ataxia. Light microscopically, the liver shows only non-specific changes. The diagnosis is made chemically on a liver biopsy. OTC deficiency can be diagnosed histochemically (40a). Electron microscopy shows alterations of the mitochondria and endoplasmic reticulum.

INDIAN CHILDHOOD CIRRHOSIS

Indian childhood cirrhosis is a mysterious, generally fatal disease seen only in children born in India. It affects infants between the ages of 1 and 3 years and is more common in males. Histologically, there is hepatocellular ballooning and focal necrosis with diffuse fibrosis. Abundant Mallory's hyalin (Chapter 5) is a common finding in hepatocytes (41), which also contain a copper binding protein, as demonstrated by orcein positive deposits (Chapter 7) (42,43). Hepatic copper levels of these patients are elevated. The inflammatory cells in the lobules include lymphocytes, histiocytes, and neutrophils. Canalicular and hepatocellular cholestasis vary in amount. Typically there is little fat and giant cell transformation is rare. Bile ductular proliferation occurs, but regenerative nodules are poorly developed (44). The microscopic picture thus resembles fairly closely certain types of alcoholic hepatic injury, most particularly central hyaline sclerosis of alcoholics. However, fatty change is much more striking in alcoholics, and of course, the age incidence of alcoholic hepatitis is very different. Only a few cases have been studied by electron microscopy (44a).

HEPATIC PORPHYRIAS

The porphyrias are associated with overproduction of heme precursors. In the hepatic porphyrias, porphyria cutanea tarda, protoporphyria, acute intermittent porphyria, porphyria variegata, and hereditary coproprophyria, the liver is the major site of biochemical abnormality (45).

Porphyria Cutanea Tarda

Porphyria cutanea tarda (PCT) is the commonest hepatic porphyria in western countries. Males are affected predominantly. Most patients suffer from photosensitivity, which may be severe. Large amounts of uroporphyrin are excreted in the urine. Most patients are alcoholics and many have cirrhosis of the liver. Uropor-

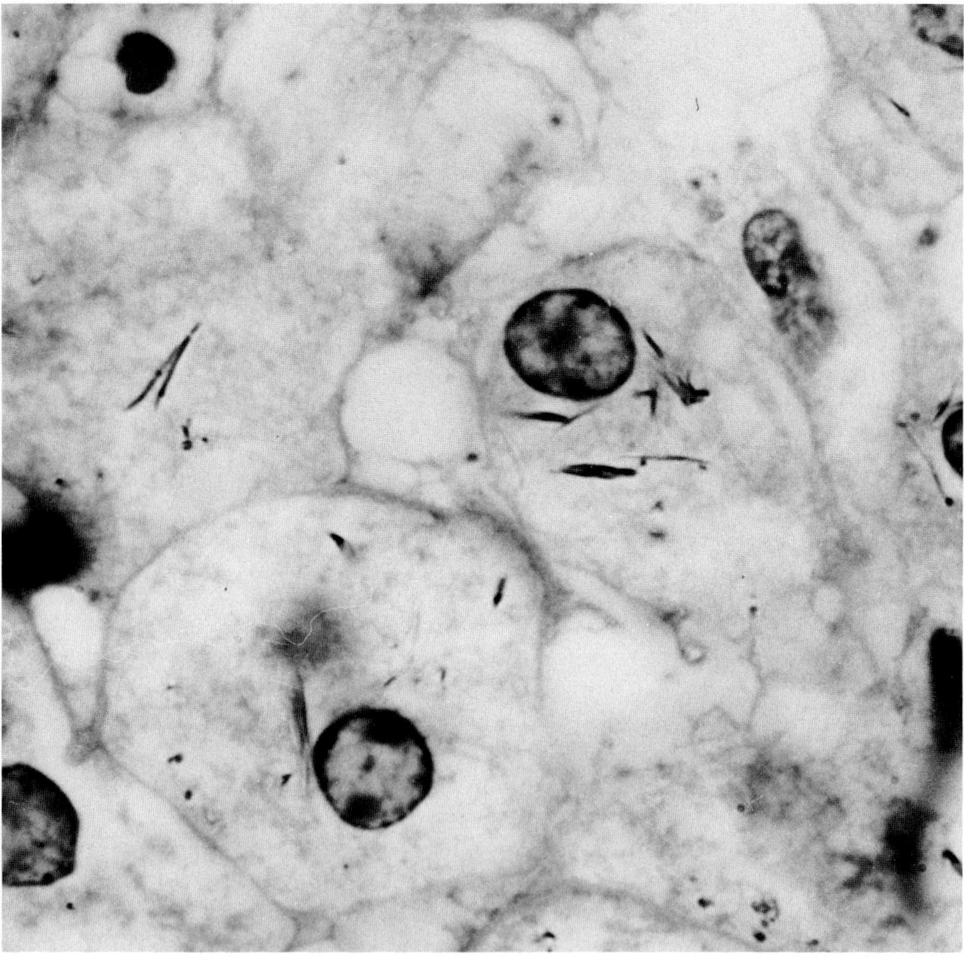

Figure 8. Porphyria cutanea tarda, showing needle-shaped inclusions in the cytoplasm of hepatocytes. These are of variable length and may be pigmented. (Hematoxylin and eosin, ×1,000.) (Contributed by J. M. Cortes, M.D., ref. 47.)

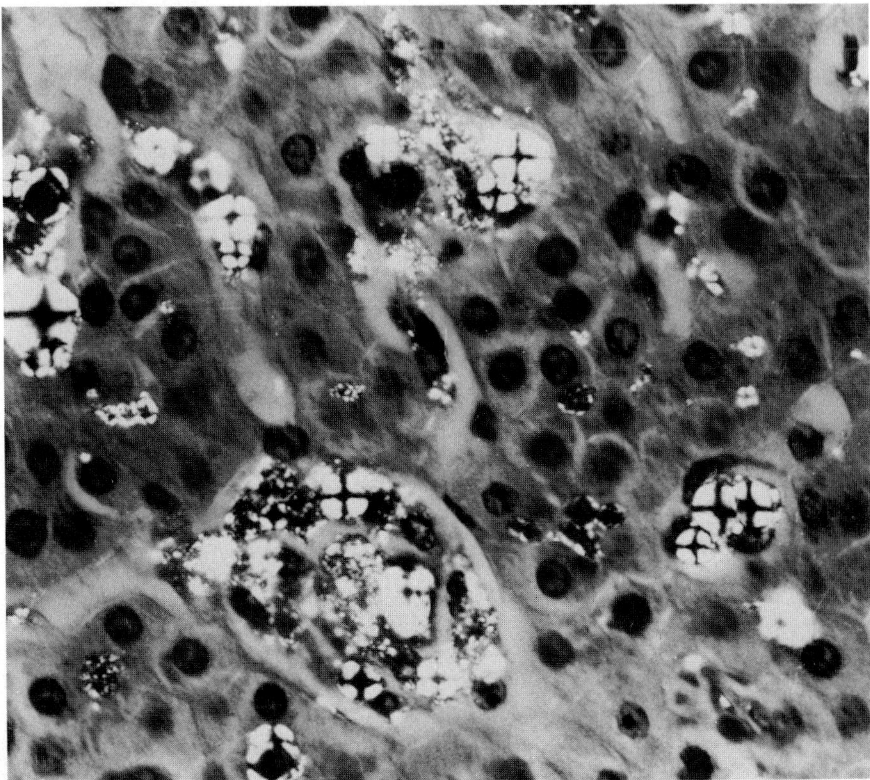

Figure 9. Polarization microscopy of a specimen from a patient with protoporphyria shows that some of the brown pigment of protoporphyrin is birefringent with the appearance of a central dark Maltese cross. (Contributed by R. Bloomer, M.D., ref. 54.)

phyrin has a highly characteristic flamingo to orange-red autofluorescence that is easily demonstrated in ultraviolet light. This makes it possible to detect uroporphyrin in liver biopsies of patients with porphyria cutanea tarda. Since there are many subclinical cases who have no symptoms referable to the skin, we suggest that every liver biopsy specimen be looked at, unfixed, under ultraviolet light for autofluorescence, as soon as it has been transferred from the syringe into a small dish. Porphyrins are light sensitive and are quickly destroyed by the ordinary methods of fixation. They can therefore be demonstrated by fluorescence when viewed with ultraviolet light only in unfixed air-dried frozen sections or touch preparations. Hepatic fluorescence, which fades much faster in daylight than the fluorescence found in PCT, has also been noted in protoporphyria, and in some cases of porphyria variegata, but not in acute intermittent porphyria, since porphobilinogen does not fluoresce.

Liver disease is common in PCT. However, the degree of hepatic damage is quite variable. In the United States fewer than 10% of patients have cirrhosis (45). Histologically, the liver shows a characteristic combination of lesions consisting of focal large-droplet fatty change, moderate siderosis and nonspecific reactive hepatitis (46), with focal aggregates of lipofuscin containing mac-

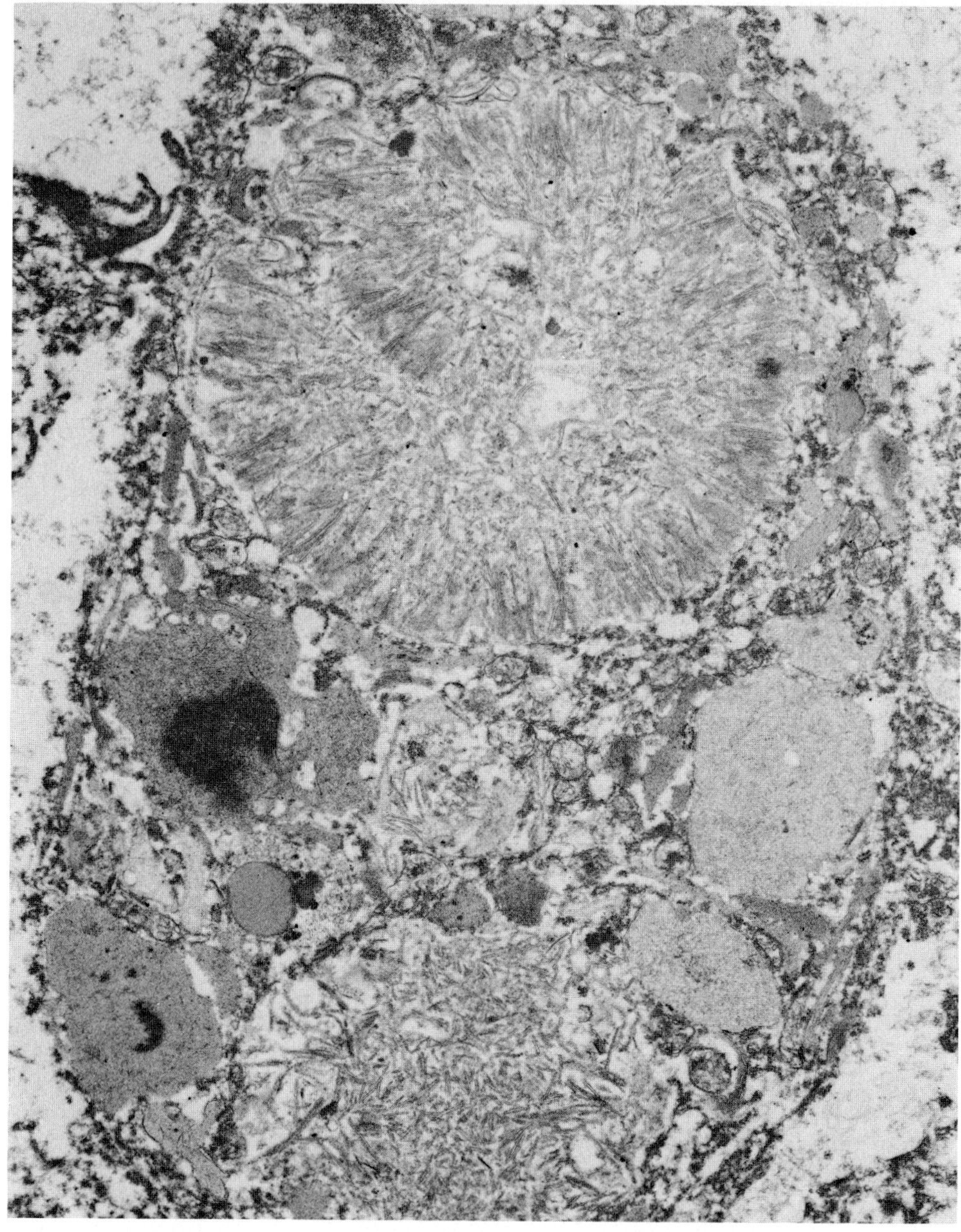

Figure 10. Erythropoietic protoporphyria. Characteristic "star-burst" crystal. (×13,400.) (Contributed by L. Russell, M.D.)

rophages (47). Accumulation of lymphocytes is often seen in the portal triads. Portal bile ducts, however, show no lesions (47). Fibrosis may also be present. While some of these features suggest alcoholic liver disease, the entire constellation is not typical of alcoholic hepatitis and Mallroy's hyalin is unusual (47). Cirrhosis and hepatocellular carcinoma appear to be common complications of this disease (48). Apparently specific birefringent needlelike cytoplasmic inclusions in hepatocytes visible by light microscopy in unstained frozen or paraffin sections, or in rapidly stained hematoxylin and eosin-stained sections have recently been described in PCT (Fig. 8) (47,49). These crystals enable the pathologist to suspect the diagnosis, even if liver biopsy specimens are submitted in fixative. However, gross observation of fresh liver specimens under ultraviolet light continues to be desirable to make the diagnosis.

Erythropoietic Protoporphyria

Erythropoietic protoporphyria, in which there is lifelong photosensitivity, is the only hepatic porphyria which manifests itself before puberty. The incidence of hepatic involvement in this disease is unknown, but probably is small (33). Cholelithiasis occurs in some patients (45). However, protoporphyria itself may simulate biliary obstruction (50). Portal fibrosis with bile duct proliferation and round cell infiltration and even cirrhosis may occur (50–53a). Granules of dark brown pigment resembling bile are seen within hepatocytes and Kupffer cells, as well as intracanalicular plugs. This pigment has a rapidly fading red autofluorescence under ultraviolet light. With polarized light, the pigment is generally strikingly birefringent and can have a punctate or diagnostic Maltese-cross appearance (Fig. 9) (54,55). Electron microscopically, this material has a characteristic crystalline appearance (Fig. 10) (56,57).

Acute Intermittent Porphyria

Acute intermittent porphyria is characterized by mild hepatic involvement consisting principally of fatty change and iron overload (46).

REFERENCES

1. Böhm N: Antitrypsin and its deficiency states. *Pathol Res Pract* 168:1, 1980.
2. Cutz E, Cox DW: Alpha-1-antitrypsin deficiency. The spectrum of pathology and pathophysiology, in Rosenberg HJ, Bolande RP (eds): *Perspectives in Pediatric Pathology.* New York, Masson Publishing, 1979, vol 5, p 1.
3. Triger DR, Millward-Sadler GH, Czaykowsky AA, et al: Alpha-1-antitrypsin deficiency and liver disease in adults. *Q J Med* NS 45:351, 1976.
4. Palmer PE, Wolfe HJ, Dayal Y, et al: Immunocytochemical diagnosis of alpha-1-antitrypsin deficiency. *Am J Surg Pathol* 2:275, 1978.
5. Talbot IC, Mowat AP: Liver disease in infancy. Histological features and relationship to alpha-1-antitrypsin phenotype. *J Clin Pathol* 28:559, 1975.
6. DeLellis RA, Balogh K, Merk FB, et al: Distinctive hepatic cell globules in adult alpha-1-antitrypsin deficiency. *Arch Pathol Lab Med* 94:308, 1972.

7. Popper H, Paronetto F, Barka T: PAS-positive structures of nonglycogenic character in normal and abnormal liver. *Arch Pathol Lab Med* 70:300, 1960.

8. Palmer PE: Three-layer immunoenzyme bridge method for alpha-1-antitrypsin tissue localization. *Am J Surg Pathol* 2:327, 1978.

9. Bradfield JWB, Blenkinsopp WK: Alpha-1-antitrypsin globules in the liver and PiM phenotype. *J Clin Pathol* 30:464, 1977.

9. Carlson J, Eriksson S, Hagerstrand I: Intra- and extracellular $alpha_1$-antitrypsin in liver disease with special reference to Pi phenotype. *J Clin Pathol* 34:1020, 1981.

9a. Pariente EA, DeGott C, Martin JP: Hepatocytic PAS positive diastase-resistant inclusions in the absence of alpha-1-antitrypsin deficiency—High prevalence in alcoholic cirrhosis. *Am J Clin Pathol* 76:299, 1981.

10. Feldman G, Bignon J, Chahinian P, et al: Hepatocyte ultrastructural changes in alpha-1-antitrypsin deficiency. *Gastroenterology* 67:1214, 1974.

11. Yunis EJ, Agostini RM Jr, Glew RH: Fine structural observations of the liver in alpha-1-antitrypsin deficiency. *Am J Pathol* 82(2):265, 1976.

12. Reintoft I: Alpha-1-antitrypsin globules in livers from a medicolegal autopsy material. *Acta Pathol Microbiol Scand* [*A*] 87:447, 1979.

13. Brand B, Bezahler GH, Gould R: Cirrhosis and hetorozygous FZ alpha-1-antitrypsin deficiency in an adult. *Gastroenterology* 66:264, 1974.

14. Theodoropoulos G, Fertakis A, Archimandritis A, et al: Alpha-1-antitrypsin phenotypes in cirrhosis and hepatoma. *Acta Hepatogastroenterol* 23:114, 1976.

15. Chan CH, Steer CJ, Vergalla J, et al: Alpha-1-antitrypsin deficiency with cirrhosis associated with the protease inhibitor phenotype SZ. *Am J Med* 65:978, 1978.

16. Kelly JK, Taylor TV, Milford-Ward A: Alpha-1-antitrypsin Pi S phenotype and liver cell inclusion bodies in alcoholic hepatitis. *J Clin Pathol* 32:706, 1979.

16a. Palmer P, Gherardi G, Baldwin J, et al: Adult liver disease in SZ phenotype alpha-1-antitrypsin deficiency. *Ann Intern Med* 88:59, 1978.

16b. Hodges JR, Millward-Sadler GH, Balbatis C, et al: Heterozygous MZ alpha-1-antitrypsin deficiency in adults with chronic active hepatitis and cryptogenic cirrhosis. *N Engl J Med* 304:557, 1981.

16c. Roggli VL, Hausner RI, Askew JB: Alpha-1-antitrypsin globules in hepatocytes of elderly persons with liver disease. *Am J Clin Pathol* 75:538, 1981.

17. Reintoft I, Hagerstrand I: Demonstration of alpha-1-antitrypsin in hepatomas. *Arch Pathol Lab Med* 103:495, 1979.

17a. Reintoft I, Hagerstrand IE: Does the Z gene variant of alpha-1-antitrypsin predispose to hepatic carcinoma? *Hum Pathol* 10(4):419, 1979.

18. Rawlings W, Moss J, Copper HS et al: Hepatocellular carcinoma and partial deficiency of alpha-1-antitrypsin (MZ). *Ann Intern Med* 81:771, 1974.

18a. Pfeiffer U, Ormanns W, Klinge O: Hepatocellular fibrinogen storage in familial hypofibrinogenemia. *Virch Arch Pathol Anat B* 36:247, 1981.

19. Sternlieb I: Copper and the liver. *Gastroenterology* 78:1615, 1980.

20. Hardwick DR, Dimmick JE: Metabolic cirrhoses of infancy and early childhood, in Rosenberg HS, Bolande RP (eds): *Perspectives in Pediatric Pathology*. Chicago, Year Book Medical Publishers, 1976, vol 3, p 103.

21. Evans J, Newman S, Sherlock S: Liver copper levels in intrahepatic cholestasis of childhood (IHCC). *Gastroenterology* 75:875, 1978.

22. Fleming CR, Dickson ER, Baggenstoss AH, et al: Copper and primary biliary cirrhosis. *Gastroenterology* 67:1182, 1974.

23. Owen CA, Dickson ER, Goldstein NP, et al: Hepatic subcellular distribution of copper in primary biliary cirrhosis. Comparison with other hyperhepatocupric states and review of the literature. *Mayo Clin Proc* 52:73, 1977.

24. Irons R, Schenk E, Lee J: Cytochemical methods for copper. *Arch Pathol Lab Med* 101:298, 1977.

25. Sipponen P, Salaspuro MP, Makkonene H: Histologic characteristics of chronic hepatitides and primary biliary cirrhosis with special reference to orcein positive hepatocellular accumulations. *Ann Clin Res* 8:200, 1976.

26. Berresford PA, Sunger JP, Harrison V, et al: Histologic demonstration and frequency of intrahepatocytic copper in patients suffering from alcoholic liver disease. *Histopathology* 4:637, 1980.

27. Goldfischer S, Popper H, Sternlieb I: The significance of variations in the distribution of hepatic copper in liver disease. *Am J Pathol* 99:715, 1980.

28. Sternlieb I: The development of cirrhosis in Wilson's disease. *Clin Gastroenterol* 4(2):367, 1975.

29. Scott J, Gollan J, Samourian S, et al: Liver physiology and disease. Wilson's disease, presenting as chronic active hepatitis. *Gastroenterology* 74(4):645, 1978.

30. Stromeyer FW, Ishak KG: Histology of the liver in Wilson's disease. A study of 34 cases. *Am J Clin Pathol* 73:12, 1980.

31. Adler R, Mahnovski V, Heuser ET et al: Fulminant hepatitis. A presentation of Wilson's disease. *Am J Dis Child* 131:870, 1977.

32. Lough J, Wiglesworth FW: Wilson disease. Comparative ultrastructure in a sibship of nine. *Arch Pathol Lab Med* 100(12):659, 1976.

33. Kane WJ, Sharp HL: Metabolic liver disease of childhood. *Pediatr Ann* 6:318, 1977.

33a. Steinmann B, Gitzelmann R: The diagnosis of hereditary fructose intolerance. *Helv Paed Acta* 36:297, 1981.

34. Applebaum MN, Thaler MM: Reversibility of extensive liver damage in galactosemia. *Gastroenterology* 69(2):496, 1975.

35. Gilchrist KW, Gilbert EF, Shahidi NT, et al: The evaluation of infants with the Zellweger (cerebro-hepato-renal) syndrome. *Clin Genet* 7:413, 1975.

36. Carlson BR, Weinberg AG: Giant cell transformation cerebrohepatorenal syndrome. *Arch Pathol Lab Med* 102:596, 1978.

37. Finegold MJ: Cholestatic syndromes in infancy, in Rosenberg HS, Bolande RP (eds): *Perspectives in Pediatric Pathology.* Chicago, Year Book Medical Publishers, 1976, vol 3, p 41.

38. Pfeiffer U, Sandhage K: Licht-und Elektronenmikroskopische Leberbefunde beim Cerebro-hepato-renalen Syndrom nach Zellweger (Peroxisome-defizienz). *Virchows Arch* [*Pathol Anat*]384:269, 1979.

39. Müller Hocker J, Bise K, Endres W, et al: Morphology and diagnosis of Zellweger syndrome. *Virchows Arch A* 393:103, 1981.

40. Zimmermann A, Bachmann C, Colombo JP: Ultrastructural pathology in congenital defects of the urea cycle: Ornithine transcarbamylase and carbamyl phosphate synthetase deficiency. *Virchows Arch A* 393:321, 1981.

40a. Snodgrass PJ: Biochemical aspects of urea cycle disorders. *Pediatrics* 68:273, 1981.

41. Nayak NC, Roy S: Morphological types of hepatocellular hyalin in Indian childhood cirrhosis: An ultrastructural study. *Gut* 17:791, 1976.

42. Portmann B, Tanner MS, Mowat AP, et al: Orcein-positive liver deposits in Indian childhood cirrhosis. *Lancet* 1:1338, Jun 1978.

43. Popper H, Goldfischer S, Sternlieb I et al: Cytoplasmic copper and its toxic effects. Studies in Indian childhood cirrhosis. *Lancet* 1:1205, Jun 1979.

44. Nayak NC, Sachdeva R, Dhar A, et al: Demonstration of hepatitis B virus surface component in human hepatocellular cancer cells. *Indian J Med Res* 69:161, 1979.

44a. Bhagwat AG, Vashishta KK, Valia BNS, et al: Ultrastructure of liver in the siblings of Indian childhood cirrhosis. *Bull Postgrad Inst Med Ed and Res, Chandigarh* 14:140, 1980.

45. Bloomer J: The hepatic porphyrias. *Gastroenterology* 71(4):689, 1976.

46. Biempica L, Kosower N, Ma M, et al: Hepatic porphyrias. *Arch Pathol Lab Med* 98:336, 1974.

47. Cortes JM, Oliva H, Paradinas FJ, et al: The pathology of the liver in porphyria cutanea tarda. *Histopathology* 4:471, 1980.

48. Kordac V: Frequency of occurrence of hepatocellular carcinoma in patients with porphyria cutanea tarda during long-term observation. *J Clin Chem Clin Biochem* 16(1):67, 1978.

49. Waldo ED, Tobias H: Needle-like cytoplasmic inclusions in the liver in porphyria cutanea tarda. *Arch Pathol Lab Med* 96:368, 1973.

50. Singer J, Plaut A, Kaplan M: Hepatic failure and death from erythropoietic protoporphyria. *Gastroenterology* 74:588,1978.

51. Bloomer JR, Phillips MJ, Davidson DL, et al: Hepatic disease in erythropoietic protoporphyria. *Am J Med* 58:869, 1975.

52. Thompson RPH, Molland EA, Nicholson DC, et al: "Erythropoietic" protoporphyria and cirrhosis in sisters. *Gut* 14:934, 1973.

53. Cripps DJ, Goldfarb SJ: Erythropoietic protoporphyria: Hepatic cirrhosis. *Br J Dermatol* 98(3):349, 1978.

53a. Eales L: Erythopoietic protoporphyria (EP). *Int J Biochem* 12:915, 1980.

54. Katskin G, Bloomer JR: Birefringence of hepatic pigment deposits in erythropoietic protoporphyria. *Gastroenterology* 67:294, 1974.

55. Matilla A, Molland EA: A light and electron microscopic study of the liver in the case of erythrohepatic protoporphyria and in griseofulvin-induced porphyria in mice. *J Clin Pathol* 27:698, 1974.

56. Wolff K, Wolff-Schreiner E, Gschnait F: Liver inclusions in erythropoietic protoporphyria. *Eur J Clin Invest* 5:21, 1975.

57. Nakanuma Y, Wada M, Kono N: An autopsy case of erythropoietic protoporphyria with cholestatic jaundice and hepatic failure, and a review of the literature. *Virchows Arch A* 393:123, 1981.

58. Klinge O and Alexandrakis E: Hepatic reactions in erythropoietic protoporphyria. *Virchows Arch B* 37:369, 1981.

10 Diseases with Abnormal Hepatic Storage Products

The group of diseases associated with abnormal hepatic storage products is characterized by excessive deposition of material normally found in the liver or formation of a substance normally not present in the liver. Most of these diseases are the result of enzyme deficiencies (1). Hepatocellular injury and cirrhosis are unusual in this group of disorders but may be seen in glycogenosis types III and IV, Wolman's disease, Niemann-Pick disease, Gaucher's disease, and the mucopolysaccharidoses. Clinically, hepatomegaly may be the only sign of these disorders. However, cholestasis and liver failure may also be present.

In hematoxylin and eosin-stained, formalin-fixed paraffin sections, most of the compounds discussed in this section are colorless. They are usually intracellular and can be deposited in hepatocytes or Kupffer cells, or both. Affected cells usually appear swollen and pale and may have distinct vacuoles. The PAS reaction, with and without diastase digestion, is always indicated. It will show whether glycogen is present and also whether a neutral mucopolysaccharide may be involved. Stains for acid mucopolysaccharides, such as the Alcian blue reaction, are also desirable in most cases. Additional stains may be indicated in certain cases. Alcohol fixed sections are desirable for highly water-soluble compounds such as cystine. Frozen sections of fresh tissue are desirable for the demonstration of lipid-soluble compounds by fat stains such as Oil red O.

Light-microscopic examination of 1-μm-thick plastic sections of tissue embedded for electron microscopy is most useful in this group of disorders. Such sections allow clear visualization of small droplets. Distinction of greenish lipid droplets from empty-appearing droplets containing water soluble substances is usually easy. The same blocks can then be studied under the electron microscope, often showing characteristic stored materials that, in some cases, are crystalline. Abnormal lysosomes are also seen. Lipid-containing inclusions often have a characteristic lamellated structure (Fig. 5) that gives some indication of the chemical identity of the stored material (2). Polysaccharide- or mucopolysaccharide-containing inclusions, on the other hand, tend to have an electron lucent, flaky, or reticulated appearance that permits no further morphologic differentiation (Fig. 8) (2,2a).

In most cases chemical analysis of the stored product and often of the enzymes involved in its metabolism is essential for diagnosis. Needle biopsies may supply sufficient material for such studies but surgical biopsies may be required. In many of these conditions, the enzyme defect responsible for the storage disease has been identified. Assay of the enzyme in question is desirable in such cases. Definitive diagnosis must take into account clinical and biochemical features, as well as morphology.

GLYCOGEN STORAGE DISEASES (GLYCOGENOSES)

Glycogen storage diseases are genetically determined conditions in which the glycogen content of a tissue is increased (3,4). Clinically, the various types of glycogenosis may present as hepatomegaly, cardiomegaly, weakness, or a central nervous sytem disorder. In patients suspected of having glycogenosis, a thorough history (including family history), physical examination, and serum biochemical studies, including a glucose tolerance test, and, if possible, analysis of leukocyte glycogen, are indicated. Liver biopsy is often an important step in diagnosis. The biopsy specimen must be subdivided. One part is not fixed and is used to estimate glycogen concentration chemically (normal = 6% of hepatic wet weight or less) and enzymes, such as glucose-6-phosphatase. The rest of the specimen is fixed for light and electron microscopy. Fixation of glycogen in formalin is capricious, fixation in alcohol more reliable. However, alcohol is a poor fixative for morphology. Gendre's fluid may be a better fixative than alcohol for morphology and better than formalin for glycogen preservation. To prevent loss of glycogen during fixation, tissues should be fixed as briefly as possible, consistent with good morphology. Frozen sections are generally superior to paraffin sections for the demonstration of glycogen. Since quantitative assessment of glycogen by microscopy is difficult, if not impossible, chemical estimation is virtually essential and qualitative identification of the type of carbohydrate is often desirable.

Type I Glycogenosis

Type I glycogenosis (von Gierke's disease) is clinically associated particularly with hypoglycemia in infants. Hyperlipidemia may also be present. The light microscopic changes may be suggestive of the disease but are not diagnostic. The hepatocytes are large and pale in hematoxylin and eosin-stained sections. This enlargement of the hepatocytes may obscure their normal plate arrangement. PAS stains generally show a large amount of positive cytoplasmic material that is diastase labile and is thus identified as glycogen. Nuclear glycogen deposition (Chapter 1, Fig. 9) may occasionally be seen in liver biopsy specimens from normal children. However, in type I glycogenosis, glycogen nuclei tend to be strikingly prominent. Fatty change may be present, varying from mild to severe (Fig. 1). Fat droplets are probably best demonstrated in 1-μm-thick sections prepared as for electron microscopy. The ultrastructure of this type has been described (5). Benign hepatic tumors and hepatocarcinomas have developed in a few of these patients (6).

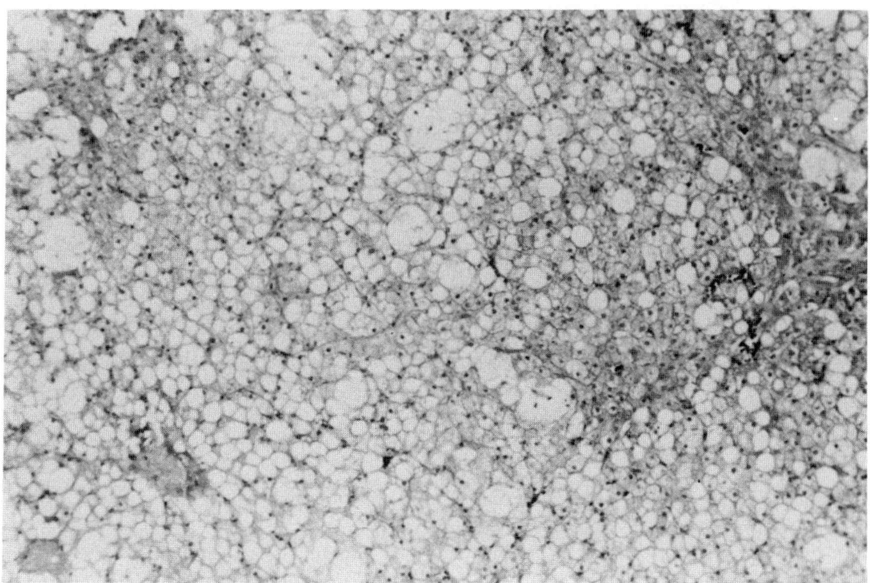

Figure 1. Infant with glycogen storage disease type 1. Note marked fatty change. (Hematoxylin and eosin, ×85.)

Type II Glycogenosis

Type II glycogenosis (Pompe's disease) has hypotonia, cardiomegaly, and mild hepatomegaly in infancy as its principal manifestations (7). Light microscopically, the hepatocytes are only mildly distended by uniformly distributed cytoplasmic glycogen. Glycogen nuclei are not seen. The hepatocytes contain small spherical clear areas that are somewhat indistinct in hematoxylin and eosin-stained sections. Electron microscopically, these clear areas are shown to consist of glycogen-containing, membrane-bounded, vacuoles (8). Histochemically, these vacuoles are found to have acid phosphatase activity and are, therefore, presumed to be lysosomes. Hepatic lysosomal alpha-1-4-glycosidase is deficient biochemically (7,9).

Type III Glycogenosis

Patients with type III glycogenosis (Cori's disease; limit dextrinosis) accumulate an abnormal glycogen with excessive branching because of a deficiency of debrancher enzyme (amino-1, 6-glucosidase). These children present with marked hepatomegaly and fasting hypoglycemia. The liver morphologically resembles that of type I, particularly in the presence of excessive cytoplasmic glycogen and in the presence of glycogen nuclei limited to glycogenosis types I and III. Patients of type III, unlike those of type I, may show delicate fibrous septa and may even develop cirrhosis. However, lipid vacuoles that may be prominent in type I are not a prominent feature of type III.

Type IV Glycogenosis

In type IV glycogenosis (amylopectinosis), there is a deficiency of brancher enzyme. An abnormal glycogen with decreased branch points and increased chain length is therefore formed. These patients present with hepatomegaly. Microscopically, the hepatocytes are enlarged, and a large deposit of slightly basophilic, sharply outlined material is seen in virtually every hepatocyte (10,11). These deposits are PAS positive but are only slowly and partially digested by diastase (Fig. 2). The inclusions are positive when stained with colloidal iron and weakly positive with alcian blue stains. They resemble Lafora bodies seen in myoclonic epilepsy. Similar bodies have been seen by light microscopy in alcoholics treated with disulfuram (antabuse) or cyanamide. However, they differed electron microscopically (12,13). Micronodular cirrhosis usually develops by the second year of life in type IV glycogenosis (Fig. 3).

Other Types of Glycogenosis

Types V and VII do not involve the liver. Glycogen storage diseases type VI and VIII, IX, and X have low hepatic phosphorylase in common (14). Hepatomegaly is generally the only clinical manifestation. Microscopically, the hepatocytes are irregularly enlarged, particularly at the lobular periphery. Diffuse fibrosis may develop. Glycogen storage disease type VIII is fatal in childhood. The exact biochemical defect remains obscure. Groups of hepatocytes are spectacularly enlarged.

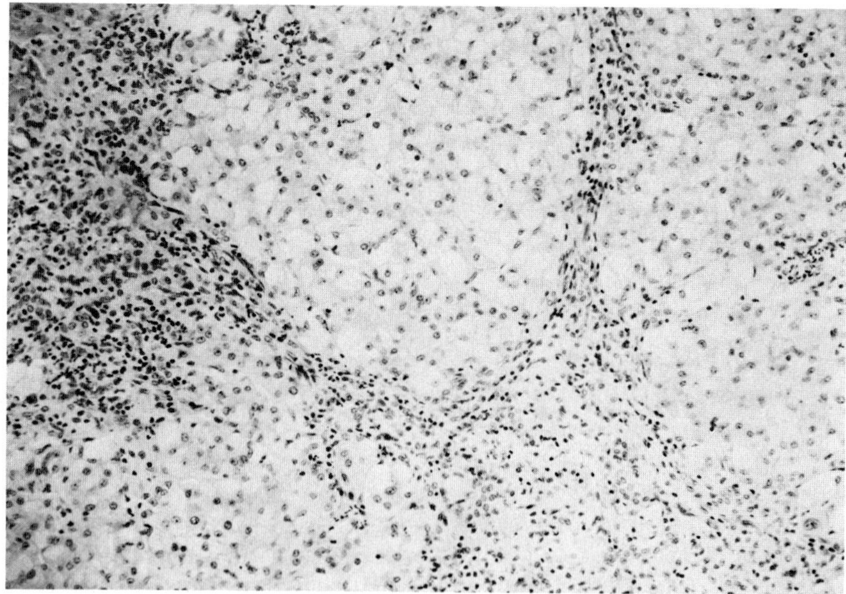

Figure 2. Biopsy from a child with type IV glycogen storage disease. Note clear vacuoles in hepatocytes, as well as portal fibrosis and inflammation. (Hematoxylin and eosin, ×124.)

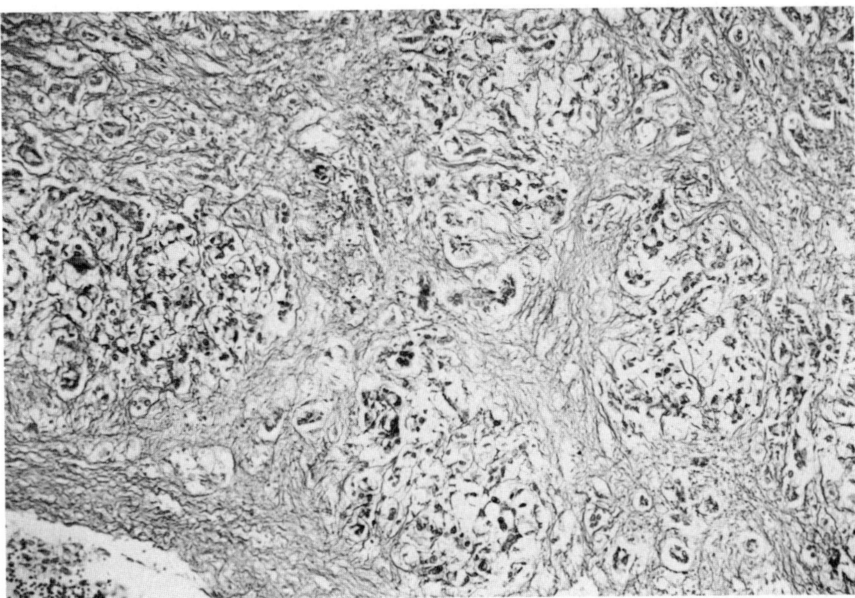

Figure 3. Autopsy specimen from child with type IV glycogen storage disease in same patient described in Figure 3. Note micronodular cirrhosis. (Reticulin stain, ×124.)

CHOLESTEROL ESTER STORAGE DISEASE

Cholesterol ester storage disease is a rare, usually relatively benign familial disorder of lipid metabolism. It generally presents in normal-growing children as asymptomatic hepatosplenomegaly. Chemically, it is characterized by accumulation of cholesterol esters and neutral fat in the liver, as well as in the intestine and bone marrow. The disease appears to be due to a deficiency of lysosomal acid lipase (3,15). Serum cholesterol esters, phospholipids, and triglycerides are usually elevated. Type II hyperlipoproteinemia may be found (15). Serum bile salts may also be increased. A fatal outcome with childhood cirrhosis has occasionally been reported in this condition (16). Wolman's disease is similar biochemically but progresses to cirrhosis in infancy (3).

Grossly the liver in these patients is enlarged and orange yellow. Biopsy specimens float in formalin. Frozen sections demonstrate Sudan IV positive lipid droplets in hepatocytes and Kupffer cells (15–17). Polarized light shows these droplets to be doubly refractile and also demonstrates needle-shaped cholesterol crystals in the droplets. The PAS reaction on paraffin-embedded material is negative (18).

CEREBROTENDINOUS XANTHOMATOSIS

This is a rare disease characterized by xanthomas, cataracts, progressive cerebellar ataxia, and dementia. Chemically, there is excessive deposition of cholesterol and cholestanol. Light microscopically, the liver appears essentially normal apart from the presence of lipofuscin-like granules, as well as mild fatty change and fibrosis. Electron microscopy shows large numbers of small lipid droplets, thick bands of collagen in the space of Disse, bizarre, giant mitochondria, and rather striking cytoplasmic crystals of unknown composition (19).

HYPERLIPOPROTEINEMIA

Liver biopsy specimens from patients with type II hyperlipoproteinemia generally show neither significant fatty change nor any other distinct morphologic lesions. Fatty change is, however, found in the vast majority of patients with types I, III, IV, and V (20). Few other light microscopic changes are present in hepatic biopsy specimens. However, by electron microscopy, mitochondrial enlargement, and paracrystalline inclusions are frequently seen.

ABETALIPOPROTEINEMIA

Abetalipoproteinemia is a genetic disorder with malabsorption of lipid, steatorrhea, inability to produce chylomicra, and absence of serum betalipoprotein. There is hepatomegaly and the transaminases may be elevated. The hepatocytes show severe large droplet fatty change, mostly triglycerides (21).

TANGIER DISEASE

Tangier is a rare disease in which there is severe deficiency or absence of alpha-(high-density) lipoproteins. Foamy macrophages containing cholesterol esters are seen in the portal triads and in the lobules (22). The hepatocytes are involved only minimally, if at all.

NIEMANN-PICK DISEASE

Niemann-Pick disease is characterized by accumulation of sphingomyelin. The disease is caused by a deficiency of sphingomyelinase. Clinically, this condition has been subdivided into several types (3). The great majority of patients, however, present in infancy with hepatosplenomegaly, anemia, and neurologic involvement.

Light microscopically, the lipid is stored in large foamy macrophages found in the sinusoids (Fig. 4) and portal triads of the liver, as well as in other reticuloendothelial organs (23). These "Pick cells" are filled with large lipid granules which stain positively with fat stains, such as Oil red O in frozen sections. The lipid is extracted by alcohol, giving the Pick cells a foamy appearance in paraffin sections. In hematoxylin and eosin-stained sections, the foamy Pick cells may be mistaken for parenchymal cells. In PAS-stained preparations, however, the negative staining of the Pick cells usually contrasts strongly with the PAS-positive hepatocytes. Electron microscopically, the hepatocytes are stuffed with typical,

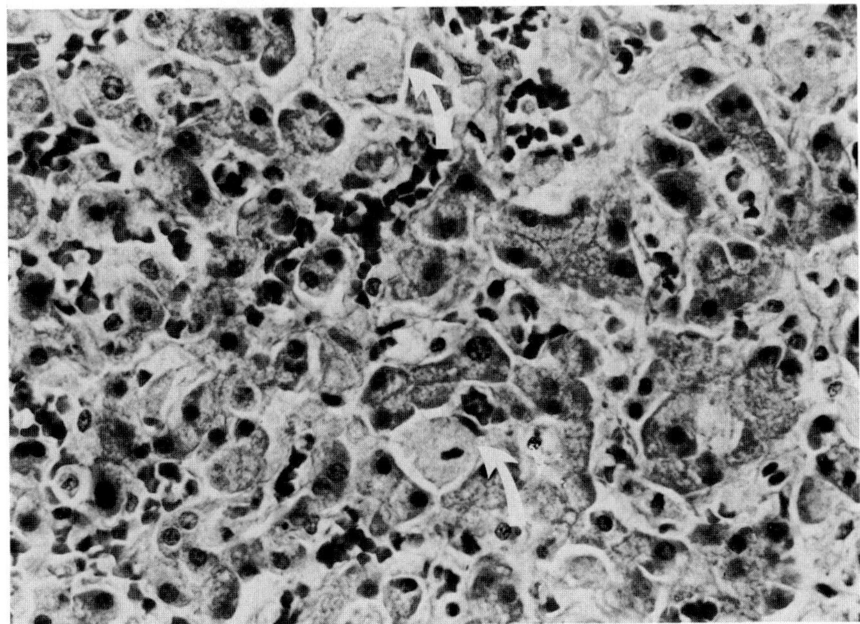

Figure 4. Niemann-Pick disease, showing swollen macrophages (Pick cells) in sinusoids (arrows). (Hematoxylin and eosin, ×425.)

polyglobular inclusions containing whorls of lamellated material (Fig. 5) (1). Niemann-Pick disease has been found to be associated with the "syndrome of the sea blue histiocyte" (24,25) and "ceroid storage disease" (Chapter 11) (26).

GAUCHER'S DISEASE

Gaucher's disease is a storage disease in which glucocerebroside, a glycolipid, accumulates (27) because of glucocerebrosidase deficiency. Gaucher's is an autosomal recessive disorder that clinically appears in several forms (3). Hepatosplenomegaly is a feature of all types. In the commonest type, the adult form, progression is slow and patients have a normal life span. In the infantile form, the disease is usually fatal by the second year of life.

Microscopically large, lipid-laden histiocytes with striated or "wrinkled tissue paper" cytoplasm are found in the sinusoids, and to a lesser extent around central veins and in portal triads (Fig. 6). The striations are often better seen in Masson's trichrome stain than in hematoxylin and eosin. In paraffin sections stained with PAS, the cytoplasm, even after distase digestion, is positive. Lipid can be demonstrated by fat stains such as Oil red O in frozen sections, but usually not in paraffin sections. Electron microscopically, the cerebroside forms characteristic tubules of varying diameter, sometimes with a helical substructure (1). In the infantile form, hepatocellular giant cells may be seen. Hepatic abnormalities including fibrosis and cirrhosis have occasionally been reported in all types of this disease (3,28a).

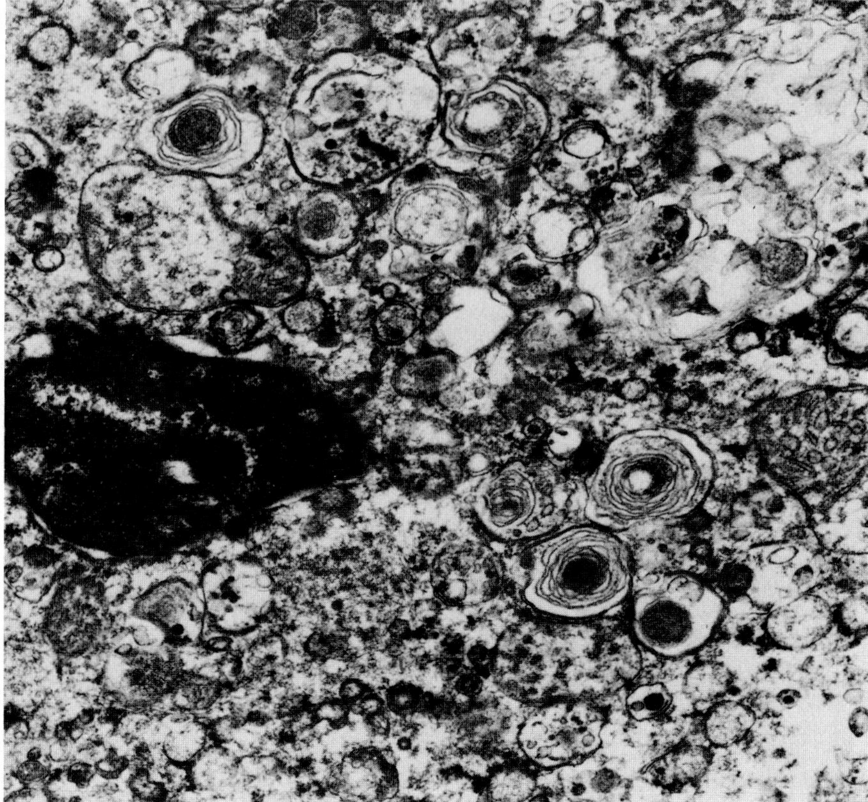

Figure 5. Niemann-Pick disease, showing whorls of lamellated material in a Pick cell. (×20,000.) (Contributed by J. E. Dimmick, M.D.)

GANGLIOSIDOSES

GM1 Gangliosidosis

GM1 gangliosidosis is caused by a deficiency of beta-galactosidase. It was first described as "Tay Sachs disease with visceral involvement." Two clinical variants are recognized which also show some morphologic differences (29). This condition becomes manifest in early infancy or childhood. The most prominent clinical features are retardation of locomotion and mental development, skeletal deformities, and hepatosplenomegaly. The affected children generally die between the first and second year of life. The clinical features, thus, are similar to those of the mucopolysacchridoses. Microscopically, the hepatocytes contain fine vacuoles that are PAS negative after diastase digestion. The Kupffer cells contain small vacuoles and fine fibrils which are weakly PAS positive, even after diastase digestion. These vacuoles are also positive for acid mucopolysaccharides (29). Distinctive vacuoles are seen in hepatocytes and characteristic tubular inclusions in most Kupffer cells by electron microscopy (1).

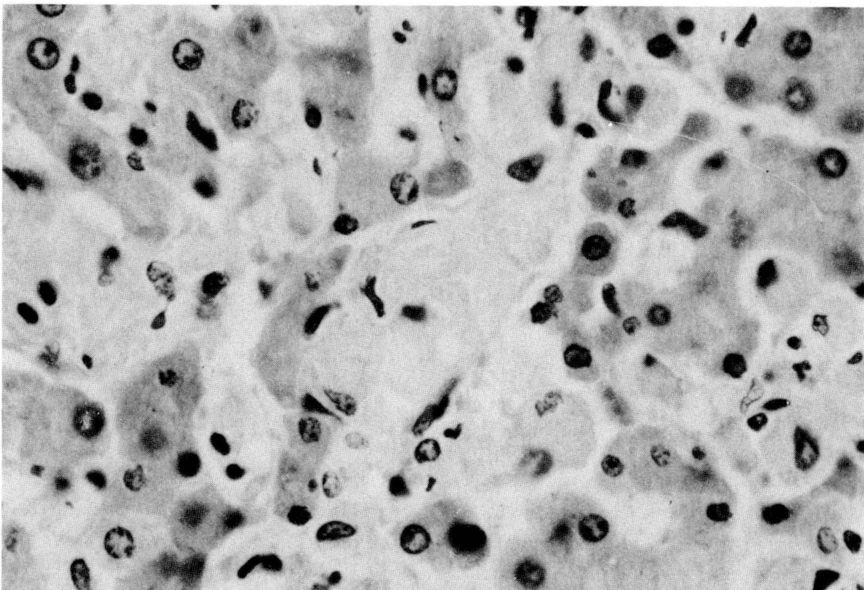

Figure 6. Gaucher's disease. Note large cells in the sinusoids with "wrinkled tissue paper" cytoplasm. (Hematoxylin and eosin, ×545.)

Tay-Sachs Disease

Tay-Sachs disease (GM_2 gangliosidosis), an early infantile form of familial amaurotic idiocy, is caused by a lack of hexosaminidase A. Clinically and light microscopically, hepatic involvement cannot be demonstrated. However, small amounts of GM_2 ganglioside have been isolated from the liver (30). Electron microscopically, concentric membranous whorls are seen in hepatocytes (1).

Sandhoff's Disease

Sandhoff's disease, which resembles Tay-Sachs disease clinically, is caused by a deficiency of hexosaminidase A and B. This metabolic disturbance results in storage of GM_2 ganglioside and of a neutral glycosphingolipid, globoside, in the viscera. The Kupffer cells contain positive granules by the PAS and Luxol fast blue stains. The hepatocytes, however, appear virtually normal in routine sections. By electron microscopy tightly laminated, osmophilic structures can easily be identified in Kupffer cells and hepatocytes (3,31,31a).

An Unusual Rare Glycosphingolipidosis

An unusual rare glycosphingolipidosis has been reported in which ceramide and globoside accumulate in both hepatocytes and Kupffer cells that appear foamy. These cells are PAS negative, but Sudan black positive (32). Cirrhosis may develop. Foam cells with similar staining characteristics have been found in the "sea-blue histiocyte" syndrome (32) and in drug-induced phospholipidosis (33,34).

MUCOPOLYSACCHARIDOSES

The mucopolysaccharidoses constitute a group of disorders, six of which (Hurler's, Hunter's, Sanfilippo's, Maroteaux's, type VII and aspartylglucosaminuria) are associated with hepatosplenomegaly (35–41). During the last few years, hereditary defects of lysosomal enzymes have been identified in nearly all mucopolysaccharidoses (42). The morphologic findings in these diseases are essentially similar. Hurler's syndrome will be described in detail as a typical example. Distinction between the different mucopolysaccharidoses must be on a biochemical basis.

Hurler's Syndrome

Hurler's syndrome (lipochondrodystrophy, dysostosis multiplex, gargoylism) is generally associated with hepatosplenomegaly. The syndrome is caused by a deficiency of alpha-1-iduronidase. In the liver, spleen, and other organs two heparin-like mucopolysaccharides, heparitin sulfate, and chondroitin sulfate B, accumulate. Light microscopically, the hepatocytes are enlarged about two or three times and appear empty or faintly vacuolated; the nuclei remain centrally placed (Fig. 7). The Kupffer cells also are swollen. Small droplets composed of water-soluble complex mucopolysaccharide can be demonstrated with difficulty in formalin-fixed material (36,39). Special fixation methods, such as Bouin's, Zenker's, Lindsay's, or Susa's, have therefore been advocated (35). The material is probably best demonstrated by the alcian blue or colloidal iron methods. Electron microscopically, finely granular material of low-electron density is seen in paren-

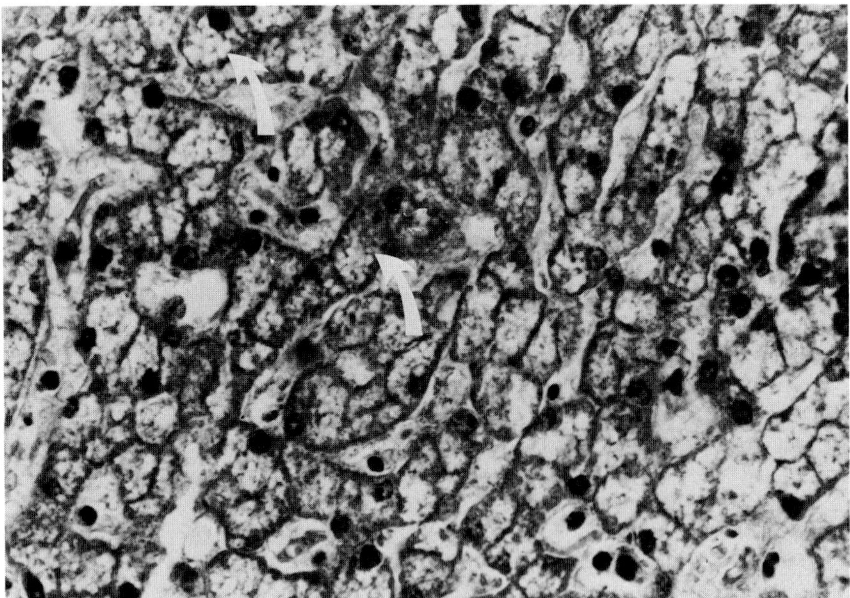

Figure 7. Mucopolysaccharidosis, in which the cytoplasm of the hepatocytes is strikingly vacuolated (arrows). (Hematoxylin and eosin, ×425.)

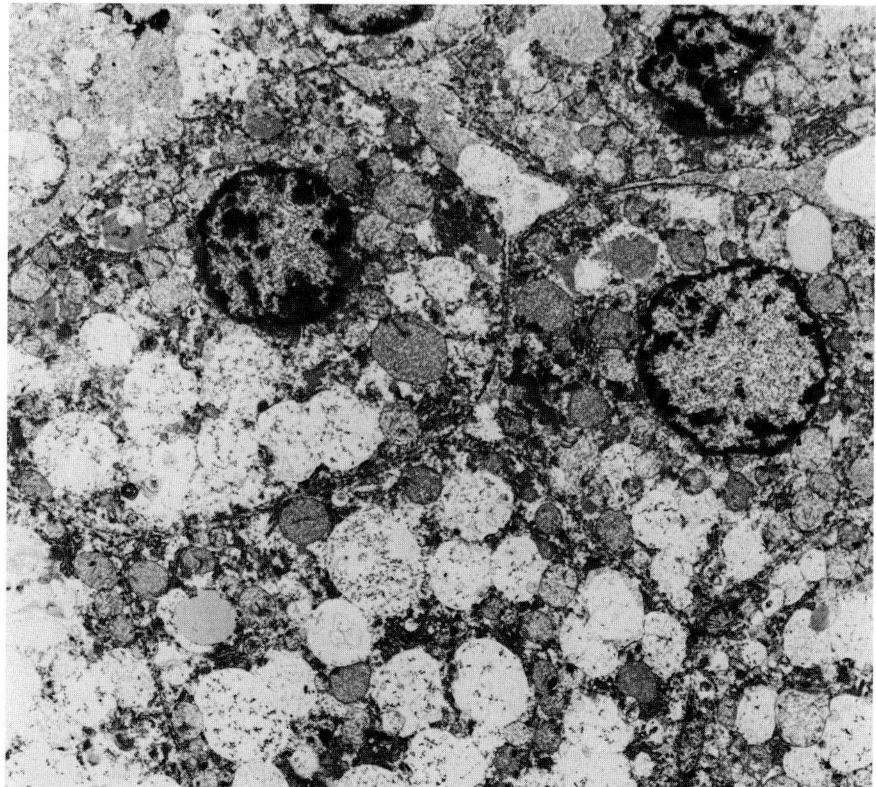

Figure 8. Mucopolysaccharidosis, showing cytoplasmic vacuoles containing uniform finely granular material. (×3,300.) (Contributed by J. E. Dimmick, M.D.)

chymal cells, Kupffer cells, and lipocytes, where it is stored in multiple single membrane-bound cytoplasmic vacuoles, which are generally considered to be lysosomes (Fig. 8). In the portal triads, this stored material is contained in macrophages, which are frequently aggregated into groups.

MANNOSIDOSIS

Mannosidosis is a recessive disease with accumulation of mannose-rich oligosacharides in many organs. The hepatocytes contain cytoplasmic vacuoles resembling those seen in the mucopolysaccharidoses (43).

MUCOLIPIDOSES

Mucolipidoses are rare conditions that share features of both the mucopolysaccharidioses and the lipidoses (44–47). Mental retardation is seen in all types and hepatosplenomegaly in some. Kupffer cells and parenchymal cells contain cytoplasmic vacuoles. Electron microscopically, abnormal cytoplasmic bodies are seen which, most likely, indicate defective degradation of both lipids and carbohydrates (44).

CYSTINOSIS

Cystinosis is a recessive metabolic disorder characterized by renal tubular abnormalities (the Fanconi syndrome), rickets, and ocular problems. Liver biopsy specimens may show mild fatty change and minimal necrosis (48). Fibrosis and cirrhosis have been reported but are inadequately documented. Cystine crystals may be demonstrated in Kupffer cells in frozen sections or in alcohol fixed paraffin sections. By electron microscopy the Kupffer cells appear unusually dark and many of them contain rectangular or hexagonal crystals. Changes in the hepatocytes are nonspecific (49). Definitive identification of the crystals requires x-ray diffraction.

AMYLOIDOSIS

Amyloidosis, of course, is not a metabolic disease, but may be an immunologic disorder with extracellular deposition of an abnormal protein. Hepatic involvement is seen in about one-half of all patients with amyloidosis. Hepatomegaly, splenomegaly, and ascites are commonly found (50). Occasionally, severe cholestatic jaundice and portal hypertension may occur (51,52,52a). Liver failure, however, is rare in patients with amyloidosis.

Grossly, livers involved by amyloidosis are often enlarged; the hepatic surface is generally smooth. Pallor and a firm consistency are often present in biopsy specimens and at autopsy. However, even if these features are present, they are easy to overlook, and amyloidosis is generally diagnosed only histologically.

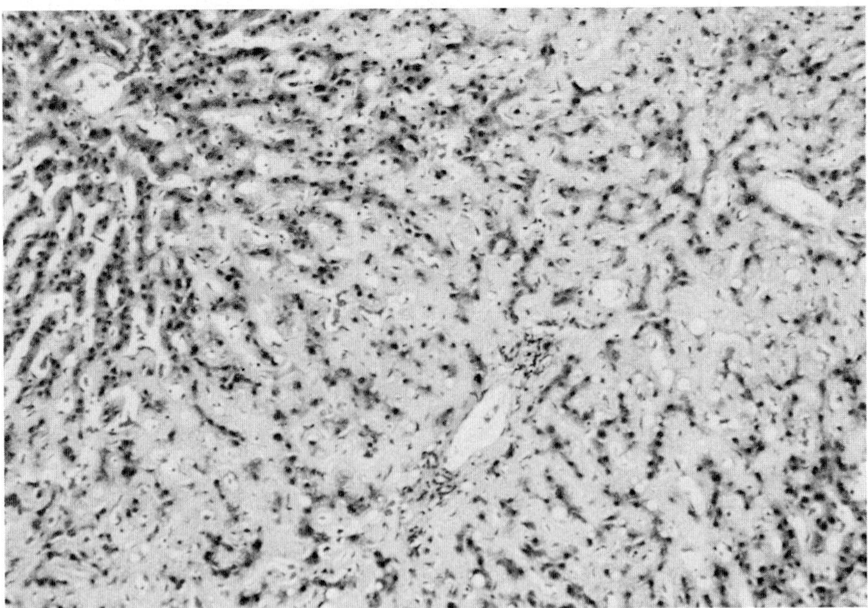

Figure 9. Amyloidosis with a myloid deposition most marked in the peripheral part of the lobule. Where the hepatocytes are not totally obliterated, the amyloid can be seen to be located principally in the spaces of Disse. (Hematoxylin and eosin, ×545.)

Histologically, if stained with hematoxylin and eosin, amyloid is a pink hyaline extracellular material (Fig. 9). There are many histologic methods whereby amyloid can be stained selectively. These include metachromasia after staining with methyl violet. Sirius R and thioflavin T are also popular stains. However, most of these methods are rather capricious and nonspecific. The best light microscopic method makes use of the strong affinity of amyloid for Congo red. This results in an orange appearance of the amyloid. The amyloid containing section, stained by Congo red, is then viewed under polarized light. If looked at in this way, amyloid lights up as pale apple green material in one direction and red at 90 degrees to the green axis.

Amyloid in the liver is localized at one or both of two sites. In the intralobular type, most characteristically seen in secondary amyloidosis, amyloid is deposited in the spaces of Disse (53). If the deposition is severe, there is compression atrophy of the adjacent hepatocytes and considerable narrowing, or even apparent occlusion of the adjacent sinusoidal spaces. Massive deposition of amyloid occasionally leads to focal disappearance of heptocytes and Kupffer cells. At first glance, the pink amorphous hyaline resembles collagen. Congo red stains should always be used if amyloid is considered a possibility. In the portal type, amyloid is deposited in the walls of the hepatic arteries and their branches. This arrangement is most typical of primary amyloidosis. Portal periarterial amyloidosis is easily overlooked in liver biopsies because it is often patchy, or if the arterial hyalinization is observed, it is attributed to hyaline arteriosclerosis of the portal branches of the hepatic artery. Confirmation of the diagnosis of amyloidosis by Congo red staining is particularly indicated in such cases. It should be noted that the differential localization of hepatic amyloid in primary and secondary amyloidosis is disputed (50). Rarely, amyloid may be deposited in the form of globular amyloid bodies (54,55). Light microscopically, these faintly eosinophilic hyaline bodies appear to be within hepatocytes and may be confused with megamitochondria or Mallory's hyalin.

REFERENCES

1. O'Brien JF: The lysosomal storage diseases. *Mayo Clin Proc* 57,192, 1982.
2. Spycher MA: Electron microscopy. A method for the diagnosis of inherited metabolic storage diseases. *Pathol Res Pract* 167:118, 1980.
2a. Allison AC: Lysosomes in pathology, in Anthony PP, Woolf N (eds): *Recent Advances in Histopathology*, ed 3. Edinburgh, Churchill Livingston, 1978, p 69.
3. Kane WJ, Sharp HL: Metabolic liver disease of childhood. *Pediatr Ann* 6:318, 1977.
4. McAdams A, Hug G, Bove K: Glycogen storage disease types 1 to X. *Hum Pathol* 5:463, 1974.
5. Riede UN, Spycher MA, Gitzelmann R: Glycogenosis type I (glucose-6-phosphatase deficiency). I. Ultrastructural morphometric analysis of juvenile liver cells. *Pathol Res Pract* 167:136, 1980.
6. Pizzo CJ: Type I glycogen storage disease with focal nodular hyperplasia of the liver and vasoconstrictive pulmonary hypertension. *Pediatrics* 65:341, 1980.
7. Hug G, Schubert W: Glycogenosis Type II glycogen distribution in tissues. *Arch Pathol Lab Med* 84:141, 1967.
8. McAdams AJ, Wilson HE: The liver in generalized glycogen storage disease. *Am J Pathol* 49(1):99, 1966.

9. Peters TJ, Jenkins W, Dubowitz V: Subcellular fractionation studies on hepatic tissue from a patient with Pompe's disease (Type II glycogen storage disease). *Clin Sci* 59:7, 1980.

10. Sidbury JB, Mason J, Burns WB Jr, et al: Type IV glycogenosis. Report of a case proven by characterization of glycogen and studied at necropsy. *John Hopkins Med J* 111:157, 1962.

11. Bannayan GA, Dean WJ, Howell RR: Type IV glycogen-storage disease. Light-microscopic, electronmicroscopic and enzymatic study. *Am J Clin Pathol* 66(4):102, 1976.

12. Vazquez JJ, Pardo-Mindan J: Liver cell injury bodies similar to Lafora's in alcoholics treated with disulfiram (antabuse). *Histopathology* 3:377, 1979.

13. Vazquez JJ, Cervera S: Cyanamide-induced liver injury in alcoholics. *Lancet* 1:361, Feb 1980.

14. Hug G, Chuck G, Walling L, et al: Liver phosphorylase deficiency in glycogenosis Type VI: Documentation by biochemical analysis of hepatic biopsy specimens. *J Lab Clin Med* 84:26, 1974.

15. Wolf H, Hug G, Michaelis R, et al: A rare hereditary disease with cholesterol ester storage in the liver. *Helv Paediatr Acta* 29(2):105, 1974.

16. Beaudet A, Ferry G, Nichols B, et al: Cholesterol ester storage disease: Clinical, biochemical, and pathological studies. *Pediatrics* 90:910, 1977.

17. Carter AR, France NE, Lewis BW, et al: Cholesterol ester storage disease. Radiological features. *Pediatr Radiol* 2:1315, 1974.

18. Pfeiffer U, Jeschke R: Cholesterol ester storage disease. *Virchows Arch* [*Cell Pathol*] 33:17, 1980.

19. Boehme DH, Sobel HJ, Marquet E: Liver in cerebrotendinous xanthomatosis (CTX). A histochemical and EM study of four cases. *Pathol Res Pract* 170:192, 1980.

20. Renger F, Hanefeld M, Jaross W, et al: Liver findings in primary hyperlipoproteinemia (HLP). *Dtsch Z Verdau Stoffwechselkr* 33(4/5):199, 1973.

21. Partin JS, Partin JC, Schubert WK, et al: Liver ultrastructure in abetalipoproteinemia: Evolution of micronodular cirrhosis. *Gastroenterology* 67:107, 1974.

22. Ferrans VJ, Fredrickson DS: The pathology of Tangier disease. A light and electron microscopic study. *Am J Pathol* 78:101, 1975.

23. Elleder M, Smid F, Harzer K, et al: Niemann-Pick disease. Analysis of liver tissue in sphingomyelinase deficient patients. *Virch Arch* [*Pathol Anat*] 385:215, 1980.

24. Long RG, Lake BD, Pettit JE, et al: Adult Niemann-Pick disease. Its relationship to the syndrome of the sea-blue histiocyte. *Am J Med* 62:627, 1977.

25. Wenger DA, Barth G, Githens JH: Nine cases of sphingomyelin lipidosis, a new variant in Spanish-American children. *Am J Dis Child* 131:955, 1977.

26. Jonas O: Ceroid storage in a child with a Niemann-Pick type syndrome. *Med J Aust* 2:441, 1966.

27. Brady RO: The lipid storage diseases: New concepts and control. *Ann Intern Med* 82:257, 1975.

28. Fellows KE, Grand RJ, Colodny AH, et al: Combined portal and vena caval hypertension in Gaucher disease: The value of preoperative venography. *J Pediatr* 87(5):739, 1975.

28a. James SP, Stromeyer FW, Chang C, et al: Liver abnormalities in patients with Gaucher's disease. *Gastroenterology* 80:126, 1981.

29. Petrelli M, Blair JD: The liver in GM_1 gangliosidosis types 1 and 2. *Arch Pathol Lab Med* 99:111, 1975.

30. Eeg-Olofsson L, Kristensson K, Sourander P, et al: Tay-Sachs disease. A generalized metabolic disorder. *Acta Paediatr Scand* 55:546, 1966.

31. Hadfield MG, Mamunes P, David RB: The pathology of Sandhoff's disease. *J Pathol* 123:137, 1977.

31a. Tatematsu M, Imaida K, Ito N, et al: Sandhoff disease. *Acta Path Jap* 31:503, 1981.

32. Miyasaki K, Saito K: Glycosphingolipidosis. Accumulation of ceramide trihexoside and globoside. *Arch Pathol Lab Med* 96:362, 1973.

33. Lagerson A: Cellules de Kupffer et dyslipoidoses. *Med Chir Dig* 6:453, 1977.

34. De La Iglesia F, Feuer G, Takada A, et al: Morphological studies on secondary phospholipidosis in human liver. *Lab Invest* 30(4):539, 1974.

35. Haust MD: The genetic mucopolysaccharidoses, in Richter GW, Epstein MA (eds): *International Review of Experimental Pathology*. New York, Academic Press, 1973, 12:251.

36. Haust MD, Orizaga M, Bryans AM, et al: The fine structure of liver in children with Hurler's syndrome. *Ex Mol Pathol* 10:141, 1969.

37. Konyar E, Tondeur M, Resibois A: Histochemical demonstration of acid mucopolysaccharides in Sanfilippo's disease: An ultrastructural study of the liver. *Virch Arch [Cell Pathol]* 11:224, 1972.

38. Cain H, Egner E, Kresse H: Mucopolysaccharidosis IIIA (Sanfilippo disease type A). Histochemical, electron microscopical and biochemical findings. *Beitr Pathol* 160:58, 1977.

39. Callahan WP, Lorincz AE: Hepatic ultrastructure in the Hurler syndrome. *Am J Pathol* 48:277, 1966.

40. Isenberg JN, Sharp H: Aspartylglucosaminuria: Unique biochemical and ultrastructural characteristics. *Hum Pathol* 7:469, 1976.

41. Witting CHR, Mullker KM, Kresse H, et al: Morphological and biochemical findings in a case of mucopolysaccharidosis type III A (Sanfilippo's disease type A). *Beitr Pathol* 154:324, 1975.

42. Neufeld EF: Mucopolysaccharidoses: The biochemical approach. *Hosp Pract* 7:107, 1972.

43. Dickersin GR, Lott IT, Kolodny EH, et al: A light and electron microscopic study of Mannosidosis. *Hum Pathol* 11:245, 1980.

44. Livni N, Merin S: Mucolipidosis IV. Ultrastructural diagnosis of a recently defined genetic disorder. *Arch Pathol Lab Med* 102:600, 1978.

45. Freitag F, Blümcke S, Spranger J: Hepatic ultrastructure in mucolipidosis I (lipomucopolysaccharidosis). *Virchows Arch [Cell Pathol]* 7:189, 1971.

46. Kenyon KR, Sensenbrenner JA, Wyllie RG: Hepatic ultrastructure and histochemistry in mucolipidosis II (I-cell disease). *Pediatr Res* 7(6):560, 1973.

47. Blank E, Linder D: I-cell disease (mucolipidosis 11): A lysosomopathy. *Pediatrics* 54:797, 1974.

48. Hardwick DF, Dimmick JE: Metabolic cirrhoses of infancy and early childhood, in Rosenberg HS, Bolande RP (eds): *Perspectives in Pediatric Pathology*. Chicago, Year Book Medical Publishers, 1976, vol 3, p 103.

49. Scotto J, Stralin H: Ultrastructure of the liver in a case of childhood cystinosis. *Virchow's Arch [Pathol Histol]* 377:43, 1977.

50. Levy M, Polliack A, Lender M, et al: The liver in amyloidosis. *Digestion* 10:40, 1974.

51. Rubinow A, Koff RS, Cohen AS: Severe intrahepatic cholestasis in primary amyloidosis. *Am J Med* 64:937, 1978.

52. Melkebeke P, Vandepitte J, Hannon R et al: Huge hepatomegaly, jaundice and portal hypertension due to amyloidosis of the liver. *Digestion* 20:351, 1980.

52a. Finkelstein SD, Fonasier VL, Prudzanski W: Intrahepatic cholestasis with predominant pericentral deposition in systemic amyloidosis. *Human Pathol* 12:470, 1981.

53. Eguchi T, Fukuda K, Okugawa N, et al: Ultrastructure of the liver in human amyloidosis. *Kurume Med J* 24(4):229, 1977.

54. French SW, Schloss GT, Stillwan AE: Unusual Amyloid bodies in human liver. *Am J Clin Pathol* 75:400, 1981.

55. Kanel CG, Uchida T, Peters RL: Globular hepatic amyloid—an unusual hepatic presentation. *Hepatology* 1:647, 1981.

11
Hepatic Pigments

It is not uncommon to find pigment granules on microscopic examination of hepatocytes or Kupffer cells. Most of these pigments are brownish, and the Prussian blue reaction is a good first step in distinguishing among the three principal ones: lipofuscin, hemosiderin, and bilirubin. By this reaction, hemosiderin is stained blue, bilirubin often becomes slightly greenish, and lipofuscin is unchanged. Excessive deposition of hemosiderin and lipofuscin is discussed in this chapter, bilirubin in the chapters on cholestasis (Chapter 7 and 8).

IRON OVERLOAD

Hemosiderosis

Hemosiderin is a refractile brown pigment containing ferric iron, which, unlike the tissue iron in ferritin, can be demonstrated histochemically by the Prussian blue reaction. Hemosiderosis, therefore, can be defined as the deposition of stainable iron in tissues. Hemosiderin granules within the hepatocytes, at least during the earlier stages of this condition, are seen predominantly in a pericanalicular location (Fig. 1). In the hepatic lobule, they are localized preferentially in the lobular periphery. The degree of hemosiderosis is a good quantitative indication of iron content. Hepatic iron measurements can be made on biopsy specimens of 10 mg (1). While it is desirable to estimate iron content on fresh tissues, prolonged storage in formol saline seems to produce no significant alterations (1). The normal hepatic iron content varies in different parts of the world and normal standards should probably be established for each population. Published standards for normal hepatic iron, therefore, are somewhat arbitrary. Normal hepatic iron is said to be less than 40 μg/100 mg wet liver (2) or 230 μg/100 mg dry liver (1). Such normal livers contain either no stainable iron (grade 0) (3) or contain hemosiderin in only 5–10 hepatocytes per biopsy specimen (grade 1) (3). In hemosiderosis grade 2 (3), which is considered marginally elevated (1), 5–10% of hepatocytes contain easily visible hemosiderin. These iron-laden cells are located in the periphery of the lobules. In grade 3, about 40% of parenchymal cells are hemosiderin laden. Hepatocytes in the pericentral zone are generally free of iron. In grade 4, most parenchymal cells are heavily laden with hemosiderin. The presence of hemosiderin in Kupffer cells is noted but is not taken into account in this classification. Hemosiderosis, thus, may be normal (grade 1), may indicate marginal hepatic iron elevation (grade 2), or may

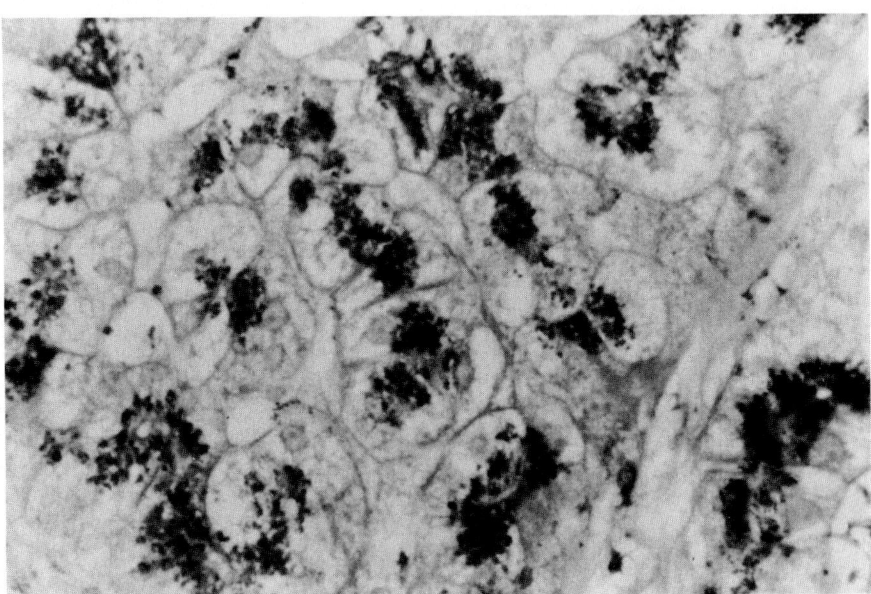

Figure 1. Hemosiderosis. Note hemosiderin granules located principally in the center of the liver plates, an indication of their location in pericanalicular lysosomes of hepatocytes. (Prussian blue reaction for hemosiderin, ×545.)

indicate excessive hepatic iron (grades 3 and 4). Moderate or severe Kupffer cell hemosiderosis is also abnormal and is seen particularly in transfusion hemosiderosis.

Hemochromatosis

Hemochromatosis is often familial, commoner in males, and may be defined as a pathologic entity with the following characteristics: markedly increased iron stores in the liver, generally grade 4 siderosis, and more than 1000 μg/100 g dry weight with hepatic fibrosis or cirrhosis and increased iron stores in other parenchymal organs, such as pancreas, heart, pituitary, and adrenals (2,4). Repeated phlebotomy, the treatment for hemochromatosis, appears to be capable of decreasing iron stores and fibrosis, but not necessarily of preventing the development of hepatocarcinoma, a relatively common complication of hemochromatosis. The definition of hemochromatosis given above does not include patients with greatly increased stainable iron (grades 3 or 4) without hepatic fibrosis. Such patients may quite possibly suffer from latent hemochromatosis (2); treatment should be seriously considered in such cases if they are thought to be at risk of developing overt hemochromatosis. Patients with grade 2 siderosis usually have only slight elevations of iron stores and are often patients with alcoholic cirrhosis or shunts (5). Phlebotomy is not indicated in these patients.

Hemochromatosis, as defined above, may be caused by (4,6) (*1*) idiopathic (familial) hemochromatosis; (*2*) chronic refractory anemias (thalassemia, sideroblastic anemia, pyridoxine-responsive anemia, hereditary spherocytosis); (*3*) dietary overload, e.g., in Bantus and health fadists (7); (*4*) congenital transferrin deficiency; and (5) porphyria cutanea tarda (Chapter 9). Cases of idiopathic neonatal hemochromatosis have been reported (8).

Iron overload may also occur in other conditions, such as pancreatic insufficiency, folic acid deficiency, vitamin B_{12} deficiency in hemodialysis patients (9,10), and in Zellweger's and Donohue's syndromes and hypermethionemia (tyrosinemia) (8) in the neonatal period (Chapter 9). However, the causal relationship between iron overloading and these conditions remains disputed (4).

Hemochromatosis has been shown to develop in some patients with refractory anemia (e.g., thalassemia), even in the absence of transfusions (11). Such patients may be clinically and pathologically distinguishable from cases of idiopathic hemochromatosis. In some anemias, on the other hand (e.g., aplastic anemia), iron absorption is not increased, and iron accumulation is entirely transfusional in origin. In such patients, Kupffer cell hemosiderosis is generally more marked than parenchymal cell hemosiderosis. Only in relatively few of these patients does cirrhosis seem to develop (4,12). This may be because few of these patients survive long enough to accumulate sufficient iron stores. It is also possible that the development of cirrhosis in this group of patients may be related more directly to posttransfusion hepatitis than to increased iron stores.

Grossly, hepatic tissue from patients with iron overload is rusty brown. Portal fibrosis may be visible as a diffuse whitish mottling. In the earlier stages of hemochromatosis the cirrhosis is micronodular, while later it becomes macronodular (13).

Microscopically, as described above, most parenchymal cells are laden with hemosiderin (grade 4 hemosiderosis). Generally, the pigment is diffusely distributed through the hepatocytes and no longer limited to a pericanalicular location (Fig. 2). In classic hemochromatosis, hemosiderin is found in Kupffer cells, but this is usually relatively mild, In addition, hemosiderin is frequently found in ductal and ductular cells and in fibrous septa. Ferrocalcinosis (Gamna-Gandi-like bodies) is occasionally seen (11).

If a fibrotic or cirrhotic liver has the gross and microscopic appearance described above, then in the absence of clinical data, the only diagnosis that can be made is pigmentary cirrhosis, compatible with hemochromatosis. The differential diagnosis includes all the causes of iron overload described above, and the final diagnosis has to be made on the basis of a combination of clinical and pathologic data.

Cirrhosis with Secondary Iron Overload

Patients with cirrhosis, particularly those who have had a portacaval shunt, may develop increased hepatic stores of iron. In a few cases, the intensity of iron deposition approaches that found in hemochromatosis. This is seen particularly in alcoholics who ingest drinks containing excessive iron and in cirrhotics with portacaval shunts, which can predispose to hepatic iron accumulation. Biopsy specimens from this relatively small group of cirrhotics who have severe hepatic iron deposition may have virtually all the microscopic features of primary hemochromatosis (see above). However, cirrhotics with secondary iron overload usually have relatively scanty hemosiderin deposition in the fibrous septa and generally show some continuing activity of their alcoholic hepatitis.

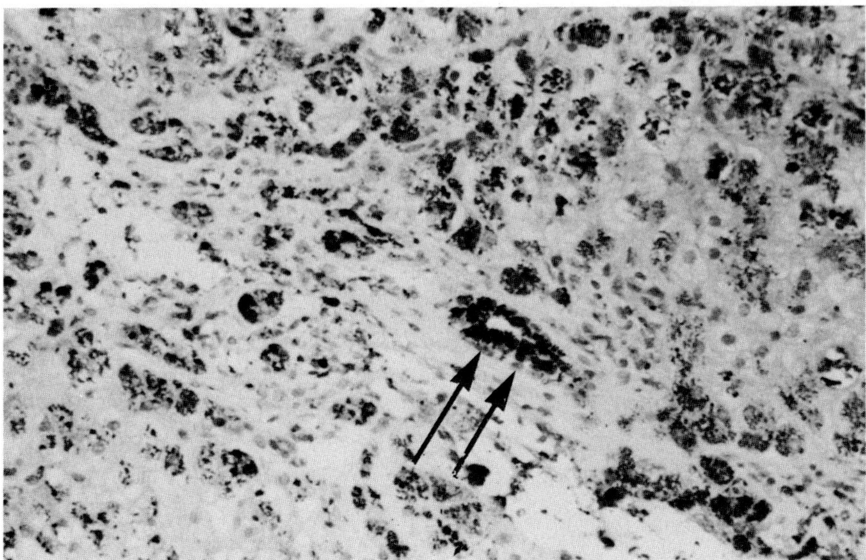

Figure 2. Hemochromatosis. Note massive deposition of hemosiderin pigment in hepatocytes and bile duct cells (arrows). Granules in hepatocytes are dispersed throughout the cells and are no longer localized to the pericanalicular region. There is considerable fibrosis, possibly early cirrhosis. (Prussian blue reaction for hemosiderin, ×214.)

EXCESSIVE LIPOFUSCIN DEPOSITION

Lipofuscin consists of small, pale, yellowish brown pigment granules. These granules are a normal constituent of hepatocytes, certainly in adults, but may be found even in newborns (14). Like hemosiderin, lipofuscin is found in the pericanalicular lysosomes of hepatocytes. This results in a characteristic pattern of localization resembling that of hemosiderin (Fig. 1). Unlike hemosiderin granules, lipofuscin granules are distinctly more prominent in the central parts of the lobules than in periportal zones. The pigment granules, if present in normal amounts, may be easily overlooked in routine hematoxylin and eosin-stained sections, particularly if these are heavily stained. The granules are better seen in sections stained by pale stains, such as the nuclear fast red employed as a counterstain in the Prussian blue reaction for hemosiderin. The lipofuscins, traditionally classified as "wear-and-tear pigment," are similar to, if not identical with, the ceroids (15). Chemically, they consist of complex lipids. Histochemically, these pigments are generally PAS positive, even after diastase digestion. They may also be acid fast, have a yellow-brown autofluorescence, and may be stained with fat stains, even after paraffin embedding (15). Ultrastructurally, the granules are shown to consist of multilobular bodies of varying density, generally in a pericanalicular location.

Lipofuscin, unlike Dubin-Johnson pigment (see below), cannot be detected grossly. Quantitative microscopic or biochemical measurements of the normal amount of lipofuscin in parenchymal cells at various ages do not appear to have been made, and excessive lipofuscin deposition has not been defined quantitatively. One should, therefore, speak preferably of unusual prominence of this pigment rather than of an absolute increase. Lipofuscin excess in hepatocytes is not associated with any functional impairment and must be distinguished principally from Dubin-Johnson pigment (see below). Lipofuscin tends to be more prominent in the elderly, as well as in starvation and cachexia. Lipofuscin-like pigment has also been reported to be prominent in some cases of Gilbert's syndrome (16), porphyria (17), cerebrotendinous xanthomatosis (17a), and after chronic phenacetin ingestion or drugs, such as chlorpromazine (18).

Lipofuscin may be found focally in groups of macrophages (often mixed with hemosiderin) within the lobules and in portal triads. This lesion represents "gravestones of hepatocytes" and indicates focal necrosis in the recent past (Chapter 2). A pigment resembling lipofuscin, but not acid fast, and birefringent under polarized light, may develop in the parenchymal and Kupffer cells after prolonged parenteral nutrition with lipid emulsions (19,20).

Ceroid Storage Disease

Accumulation of this material in hepatocytes and Kupffer cells has been described in a small number of young children (21). Clinically, these patients have hepatosplenomegaly, anemia, and thrombocytopenia. As pointed out, ceroid is similar to, if not identical with, lipofuscin. The etiology of ceroid storage disease is uncertain. Certainly, a metabolic lesion has not been defined so far.

Microscopically, the portal triads are infiltrated by macrophages loaded with granules of brown pigment with the characteristics of lipofuscin. The Kupffer cells contain similar material. Cirrhosis may develop in these patients. Ceroid accumulation resembling that in ceroid disease has also been reported in the "syndrome of the sea-blue histiocyte," which may be primary or secondary to a great variety of metabolic and hematologic disorders (22–24).

DUBIN-JOHNSON SYNDROME

In this syndrome (see chapter on jaundice) the liver biopsy specimen is grossly dark or even black. Pigment granules with many of the characteristics of lipofuscin are found in hepatocytes (Fig. 3). Compared with the lipofuscins found in normal subjects, the granules are darker, larger, and more coarse. The Dubin-Johnson pigment is not typical of most lipofuscins in its reactions with special stains and electron microscopically. It is still disputed whether the Dubin-Johnson pigment is a lipofuscin or whether it is related to the melanins.

PROTOPORPHYRIA

In protoporphyria a brownish iron negative pigment is found in hepatocytes, Kupffer cells, and bile canaliculi. This pigment is described in greater detail in Chapter 9 (Fig. 10).

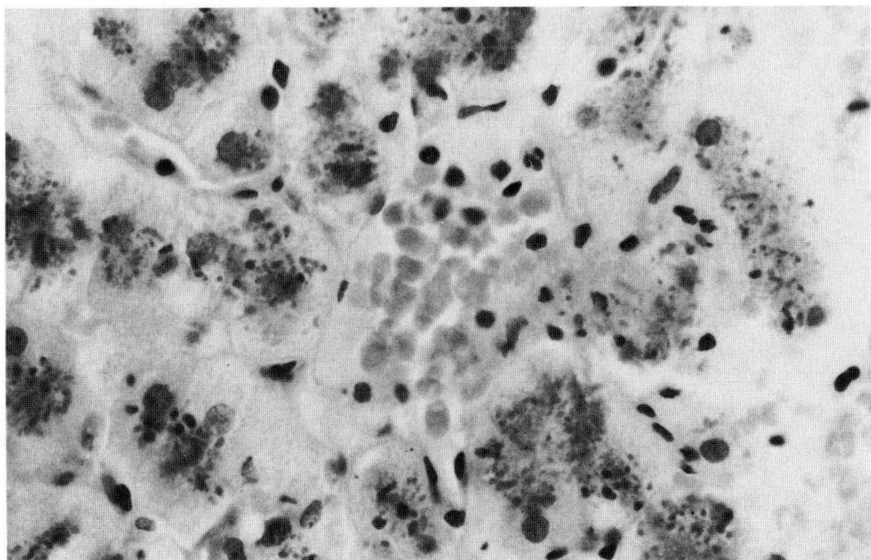

Figure 3. Dubin-Johnson syndrome. Note pigment granules with characteristic pericanalicular localization. (Hematoxylin and eosin, ×545.)

OTHER HEPATIC PIGMENTS

Most of the other pigments found in the liver are not products of abnormal metabolism, but are exogenous in origin. A practical method for the identification of particulate and crystalline material has recently been described (25).

Formalin Pigment

Formalin pigment is dark brown, microcrystalline, iron negative, and doubly refractile. It has no particular cellular localization and is formed from hemoglobin when tissues rich in blood are fixed in formalin at an acid pH. The pigment is readily bleached by hydrogen peroxide and may be extracted with saturated picric acid (5 minutes) or a mixture of 50 ml acetone and 50 ml 3% hydrogen peroxide with 1 ml 25% ammonia water (1–5 minutes) (26).

Malaria

Malarial pigment is seen in malarial parasites and in Kupffer cells of some patients who lived for a long time in an endemic area. The pigment consists of coarse black-brown granules and is believed to be a hematin. Its appearance and staining reactions are similar to those of formalin pigment (26).

Anthracosilicosis

Anthracosis is an occasional finding in liver biopsy specimens that has no clinical significance. The pigment consists of coarse black granules that are deposited in portal macrophages. It resembles malarial pigment and formalin pigment, but is not dissolved in any of the common solvents. It is undoubtedly carried to the liver from thoracic lymph nodes. In anthracosilicosis (27), the granules are located in Kupffer cells and portal macrophages. Silica may be identified by viewing the specimen under polarized light. Aggregates of such pigment-containing macrophages may be seen in the walls of central veins. Antracosilicosis does not seem to be associated with significant hepatic pathology, but it does suggest pulmonary involvement.

Thorotrast

Thorotrast is a radioactive contrast agent that is no longer used. Microscopically, it appears as yellowish gray granules in Kupffer cells and portal macrophages that can be shown to be radioactive by autoradiography. Identification of thorotrast may be made by electron microscopic x-ray microanalysis (28). Thorotrast deposition leads to hepatic fibrosis and malignant tumors, particularly hemangiosarcoma (Chapters 14 and 15).

Silver

Argyria is produced by chronic ingestion of silver-containing drugs. It results not only in silvery skin pigmentation, but also in the deposition of fine black granules in portal macrophages and, to a lesser extent, in Kupffer cells (28a).

Polyvinylpyrrolidine

Polyvinylpyrrolidine is a plasma expander that is stored in Kupffer cells. In hematoxylin and eosin-stained, sections it appears gray-blue. It stains positively with Congo red, but does not have the characteristic birefringence of amyloid. Staining reactions and electron microscopy of this material have been discussed by Reske-Nielson et al. (29), who recommend spectrophotometric analysis to confirm the diagnosis.

REFERENCES

1. Barry M: Liver iron concentration, stainable iron, and total body storage iron. *Gut* 15:411, 1974.
2. Edwards CQ, Carroll M, Bray P, et al: Hereditary hemochromatosis: Diagnosis in siblings and children. *N Engl J Med* 297:7, 1977.
3. Scheuer PJ, Williams R, Muir AR: Hepatic pathology in relatives of patients with hemochromatosis. *J Pathol* 84:53, 1962.
4. Grace ND, Powell LW: Iron storage disorders of the liver. *Gastroenterology* 64:1257, 1974.
5. Barry M: Progress report. Iron and the liver. *Gut* 15:324, 1974.
6. Powell LW, Bassett ML, Halliday JW: Hemochromatosis: 1980 update. *Gastroenterology* 78:374, 1980.
7. Hennigar GR, Greene WB, Walker EM, et al: Hemochromatosis caused by excessive vitamin iron intake. *Am J Pathol* 96:611, 1979.
8. Goldfischer S, Grotsky HW, Chang CC, et al: Idiopathic neonatal iron storage involving the liver, pancreas, heart and endocrine and exocrine glands. *Hepatology* 1:58, 1981.

9. Ali M, Fayemi O, Rigolosi R, et al: Hemosiderosis in hemodialysis patients. An autopsy study of 50 cases. *JAMA* 244:323, 1980.
10. Kothari T, Swami AP, Lee JCK, et al: Hepatic hemosiderosis in maintenance hemodialysis (MHD) patients. *Dig Dis Sci* 25:363, 1980.
11. Iancu TC, Landing BH, Neustein HB: Pathogenetic mechanisms in hepatic cirrhosis of thalassemia major: Light and electron microscopic studies. *Pathol Annu* 12:171, 1977.
12. Abe A, Goto S, Aizawa Y, et al: A female case of secondary hemochromatosis. Long term observations on the clinical course. *Acta Hepatol Jpn* 21:890, 1980.
13. Kent G, Popper H: Liver biopsy in diagnosis of hemochromatosis. *Am J Med* 44(6):837, 1968.
14. Goldfischer S, Bernstein J: Lipofuscin (aging) pigment granules of the newborn human liver. *J Cell Biol* 42:253, 1969.
15. Pearse AGE: *Histochemistry, Theoretical and Applied*, ed 3. Baltimore, Williams & Wilkins, 1972, vol 2, p 1077.
16. Berk PD, Bloomer SR, Howe RB, et al: Constitutional hepatic dysfunction (Gilbert's syndrome). A new definition based on kinetic studies with unconjugated radio-bilirubin. *Am J Med* 49:296, 1970.
17. Bruguera M, Esquerda JE, Mascaro JM, et al: Erythropoietic protoporphyria. A light, electron, and polarization microscopical study of the liver in three patients. *Arch Pathol Lab Med* 100:587, 1976.
17a. Boehme DH, Sobel HJ, Marquet E: Liver in cerebrotendinous Xanthomatosis (CTX). A histochemical and EM study of four cases. *Pathol Res Pract* 170:192, 1980.
18. Scheuer PJ: Long-term effects on the liver. *J Clin Pathol* 28(9):71, 1975.
19. Thompson SW: *The Pathology of Parenteral Nutrition with Lipids.* Springfield, Ill, Charles C. Thomas, 1974.
20. Koga Y, Swanson VL, Hays DM: Hepatic "intravenous fat pigment" in infants and children receiving lipid emulsion. *J Pediatr Surg* 10:641, 1975.
21. Björkerud S, Schelin U: Liver changes in ceroid storage disease in childhood. *Acta Pathol Microbiol Scand* [*A*] 60:512, 1964.
22. Jonas O: Ceroid storage in a child with a Niemann-Pick type syndrome. *Med J Aust* 2:551, 1966.
23. Varela-Duran J, Roholt PC, Ratliff NB: Sea blue histiocyte syndrome. A secondary degenerative process of macrophages. *Arch Pathol Lab Med* 104:30, 1980.
24. Long RG, Lake BD, Pettit JE, et al: Adult Niemann-Pick disease. Its relationship to the syndrome of the sea-blue histiocyte. *Am J Med* 62:627, 1977.
25. Crocker PR, Doyle DV, Levison DA: A practical method for the identification of particulate and crystalline material in paraffin embedded tissue specimens. *J Pathol* 131:165, 1980.
26. Barka T, Anderson PJ: *Histochemistry, Theory, Practice and Bibliography.* New York, Hoeber–Harper & Row, 1963, p 189.
27. Dirschmd K, Kiesler J: Morphology of the liver in anthracosilicosis. *Leber Magen Darm* 10:115, 1980.
28. Odegaard A, Ophus EM, Larsen AM: Identification of thorium dioxide in human liver cells by electron microscopic X-ray microanalysis. *J Clin Pathol* 31:893, 1978.
28a. Rauber G, Duprez A, Bibas H: Argyrism avec localisation hépatique. A propos d'un cas. *Med Chir Dig* 10:319, 1981.
29. Reske-Nielsen E, Bojsen-Moller M, Vetner M, et al: Polyvinylpyrrolidone-storage disease. *Acta Pathol Microbiol Scand* [*A*] 84:397, 1976.

12
Vascular Lesions of the Liver

HEPATIC CONGESTION

Centrilobular sinusoidal congestion is probably the most frequent hepatic vascular lesion. Microscopically, the congestion is shown to be accompanied by dilatation of the central sinusoids. Often it is difficult to be certain whether this lesion is truly present in biopsy material. One reason is that the blood easily drains out of a needle biopsy and even out of the periphery of a wedge biopsy. To mention other variables, hepatic tissue is compressed and traumatized during the process of obtaining it, and paraffin sections are teased and traumatized in hot water baths before ever reaching a slide. Clearly, the number of red blood cells within sinusoids, as well as the degree of sinusoidal dilatation, will vary from biopsy to biopsy and area to area. It is best, therefore, to accept considerable variation as normal. However, a definite recurrent microscopic pattern of pericentral sinusoidal engorgement or a gross "nutmeg" appearance has to be considered significant, particularly if associated with canalicular centrilobular bile plugs (1).

Chronic Passive Congestion

Heart failure is the principal entity that may be responsible for this morphologic lesion. Clinically, these patients have hepatomegaly that can be associated with ascites, upper abdominal pain, and even portal encephalopathy (2). Hyperbilirubinemia and transaminase elevations may also be present. This can lead to a clinical diagnosis of acute or chronic hepatitis (3), or even of extrahepatic obstruction. In addition to centrilobular congestion, central atrophy is characteristic of congestive failure (Fig. 1) (4), but central hepatic necrosis may also be seen, not only in right-sided heart failure, but in left-sided heart failure as well (4a). The hepatocytes in the central parts of the liver plates may be replaced by red blood cells (Fig. 2) (3,5). In prolonged hepatic congestion, central fibrosis develops that can become associated with a nodular appearance of the liver. However, the overall hepatic architecture tends to remain intact, and true cirrhosis hardly ever develops. The term "cardiac cirrhosis" is frequently, if rather loosely, applied to this condition (Chapter 13).

Hepatic space-occupying lesions may also cause central congestion (6) and occasionally no explanation can be found for this observation (7).

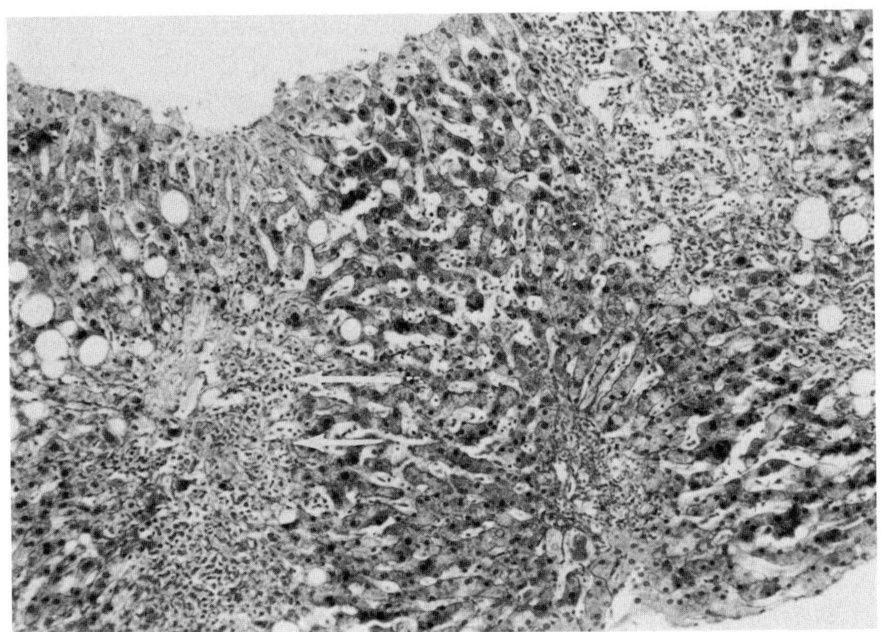

Figure 1. Cardiac failure. Chronic passive congestion. Note marked centrilobular accumulation of red blood cells with central atrophy of hepatic plates. (Reticulin stain, ×85.)

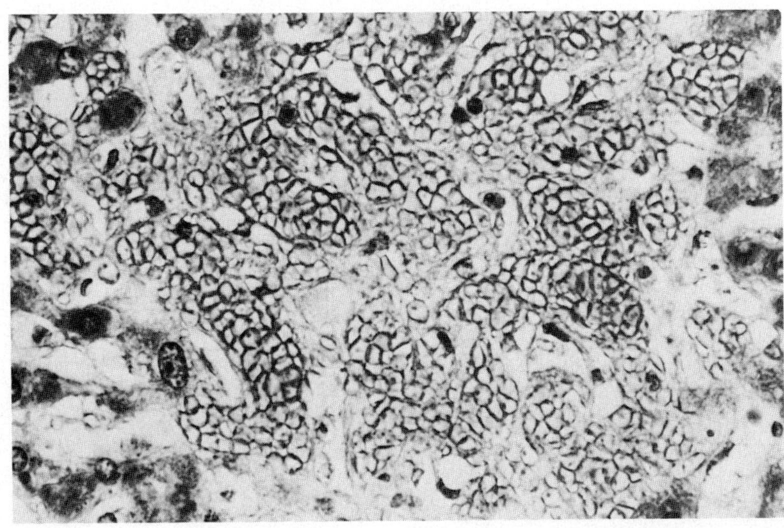

Figure 2. Cardiac failure, high-power view. The hepatic plates in the vicinity of a central vein have been replaced by red blood cells. (Trichrome, ×174.) (Contributed by G. Kanel, M.D., ref. 5.)

Zahn's infarcts are well-demarcated hyperemic areas in patients with extensive centrilobular congestion. These lesions are not true infarcts, although centrilobular atrophy and necrosis may be seen. Classically seen at autopsy and associated with portal vein occlusion, their etiology remains debatable (8).

Budd-Chiari Syndrome

The Budd-Chiari syndrome, due to hepatic venous outflow obstruction, resembles chronic passive congestion produced by heart failure quite closely in its hepatic manifestations, both clinically and morphologically (Fig. 3). However, these two conditions are usually easily distinguished by clinical examination of the patient's cardiovascular system. Central necrosis tends to be more pronounced in the Budd-Chiari syndrome, which is usually associated with thrombi in varying stages of organization in the larger hepatic veins or the vena cava, or both. Thrombi are therefore seen only occasionally in needle biopsy specimens, or even in wedge biopsy specimens. The commonest etiologic factors responsible for the thrombosis in the Budd-Chiari syndrome are polycythemia vera and oral contraceptives (9–11). Other possible factors include congenital bands (12), neoplasms, pregnancy (13,14), and even alveolar hydatid disease (15) and paroxysmal nocturnal hemoglobinuria (14a). Pericentral fibrosis and a nodularity resembling that seen in chronic passive congestion may develop in the Budd-Chiari syndrome. These nodules must not be confused with hepatocellular neoplasms (9,16).

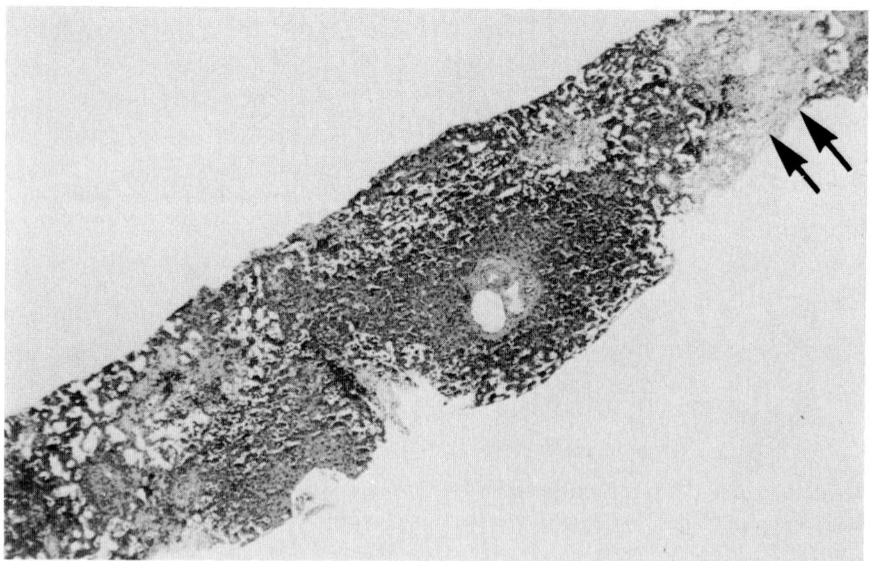

Figure 3. Budd-Chiari syndrome. Low power view of needle biopsy specimen from a young woman who had been on contraceptives. Note centrilobular dilatation of the sinusoids and centrilobular necrosis (arrows). (Hematoxylin and eosin, ×34.)

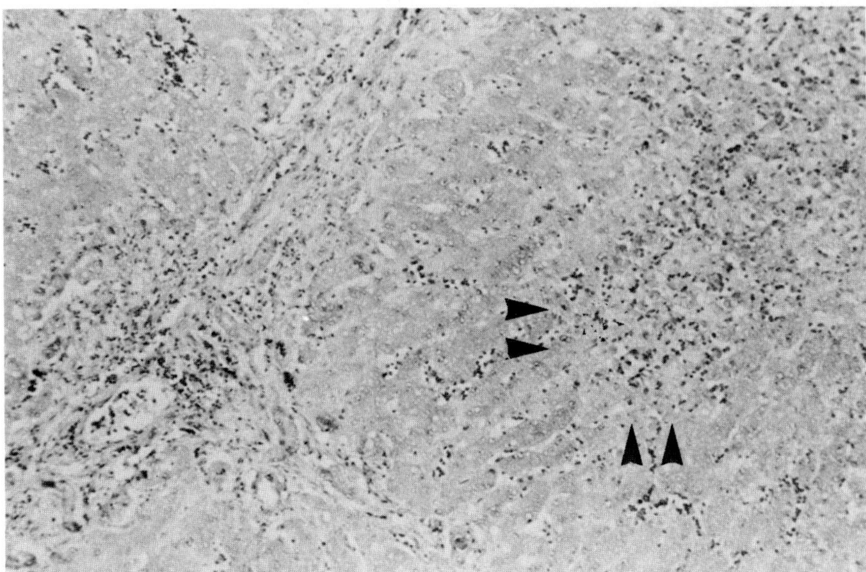

Figure 4. "Shock liver." Centrilobular necrosis (arrowheads) with relatively mild congestion. (Hematoxylin and eosin, ×85.)

Shock Liver

"Shock liver," like chronic passive congestion, is characterized by centrilobular sinusoidal congestion, often associated with cholestasis. However, there is generally more striking centrilobular liver cell degeneration, usually hydropic. Overt hyaline necrosis and cell dropout may also occur (Fig. 4) (17). Both inflammation and phagocytic activation of Kupffer cells are generally mild or absent. However, the inflammatory reaction may be quite striking and consist predominantly of neutrophils (18). In the recovery phase, when the degenerative changes have disappeared, this lesion may resemble chronic passive congestion quite closely. With the help of clinical data, this distinction usually presents no great difficulty. In cirrhotics who have suffered from shock most frequently due to bleeding varices, the necrosis is located in the centers of cirrhotic nodules.

Sickle Cell Anemia

In sickle cell anemia, there is predominantly centrilobular, but sometimes panlobular, sinusoidal congestion, particularly during crises (Fig. 5). Clumps of sickled erythrocytes are always present (Fig. 6). The periportal sinusoids tend to be greatly dilated, presumably because of vascular obstruction by centrilobular agglutinates. Sickled red blood cells are easily seen in formalin-fixed material, but not after Zenker fixation. Although the clinical picture resembles that of acute viral hepatitis, there is virtual absence of the lobular disarray and of the inflammatory response characteristic of acute viral hepatitis. However, there may be mild hepatocellular necrosis, including scattered acidophilic bodies and cholestasis. Focally, there may be some increase in reticulin. Electron microscopy

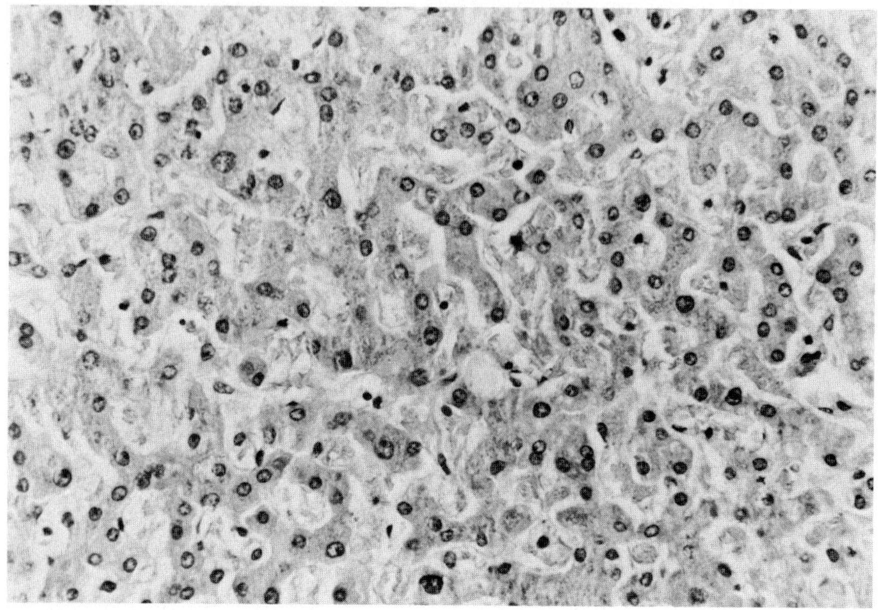

Figure 5. Sickle cell disease. Hepatic sinusoids are markedly congested. (Hematoxylin and eosin, ×250.)

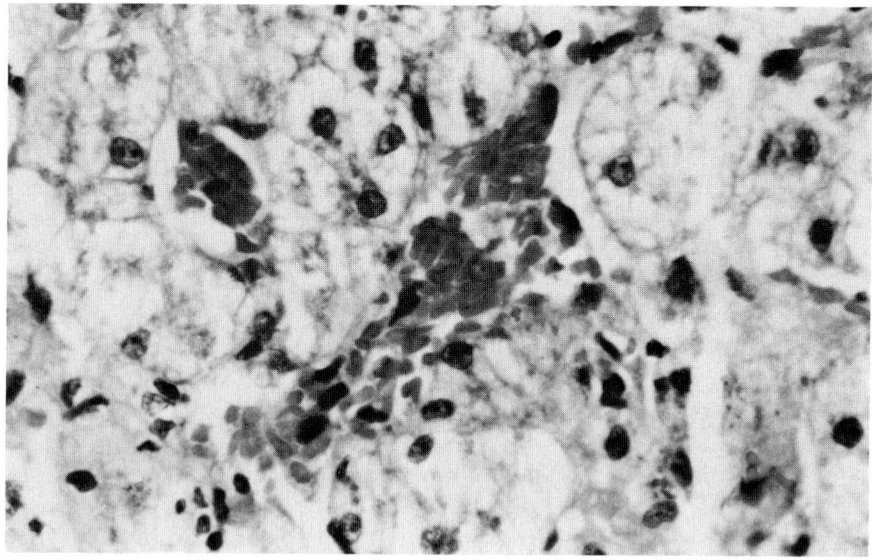

Figure 6. Sickle cell disease, higher power view. Red blood cells clumped in a sinusoid can now be seen to be sickled. (Hematoxylin and eosin, ×545.)

shows the aggregates of sickled red cells to be within Kupffer cells. It is well to recall that patients with sickle cell anemia are at high risk of contracting viral hepatitis and features of both entities may be seen in the same biopsy specimen. Serologic studies may be helpful in verifying concurrent viral infection (19). Hepatic fibrosis is not uncommon in these patients, but there is doubt whether it is directly attributable to sickle cell disease or to chronic hepatitis (20,20a).

Veno-Occlusive Disease

Veno-occlusive disease is a relatively rare cause of striking central congestion. To verify this diagnosis, one should look for loose connective tissue occupying part or all of the lumens of centrilobular and sublobular veins (Figs. 7,8). During the later stages of the disease the connective tissue may become quite dense. The relationship of this lesion to thrombosis remains in dispute. Endothelial injury of central veins may trigger fibrin deposition followed by fibrous occlusion (21–27). As the disease progresses, bridging fibrosis links central veins (24,25). Ultimately, severe sinusoidal and even portal fibrosis with cirrhosis and portal hypertension may supervene. The disease was reported originally in Jamaican children as secondary to ingestion of the pyrrolizidine group of alkaloids in "bush-tea poisoning." Veno-occlusive disease, however, is certainly not confined to children in Jamaica, but may be seen in India, Afghanistan, South America, South Africa, Britain, and the United States (22,27–28). Antimetabolites, immunosuppressive drugs, such as urethane and azathioprine (Chapter 15), and irradiation (26,29,30) can produce the same picture in adults. Allogeneic bone marrow transplantation associated with graft-versus-host disease may also be an etiologic factor (31). A few cases in infants with presumed immunodeficiency states have also been reported (24).

Periportal Sinusoidal Congestion

Periportal sinusoidal congestion has been seen in patients on contraceptives (32). No vascular obstructing lesion could be found to explain this phenomenon.

VASCULAR LESIONS AFFECTING PREDOMINANTLY THE PORTAL TRIADS

Osler-Weber-Rendu Disease

Large, dilated, thin-walled portal vascular structures are observed in a significant proportion of patients with Osler-Weber-Rendu disease (33,34). These vessels may be surrounded by bands of fibrous tissue and may also be found in the periportal parts of the lobules. As these lesions grow larger, entire lobules and even multiple lobules may be replaced by the telangiectases. The telangiectatic vessels are lined by benign appearing endothelial cells and embedded in a fibrous stroma that can be delicate or quite dense. The lesions involving adjacent triads may coalesce and may also extend to central veins. Fibrosis, possibly secondary to thrombosis, may occur in the vicinity of the telangiectatic vessels.

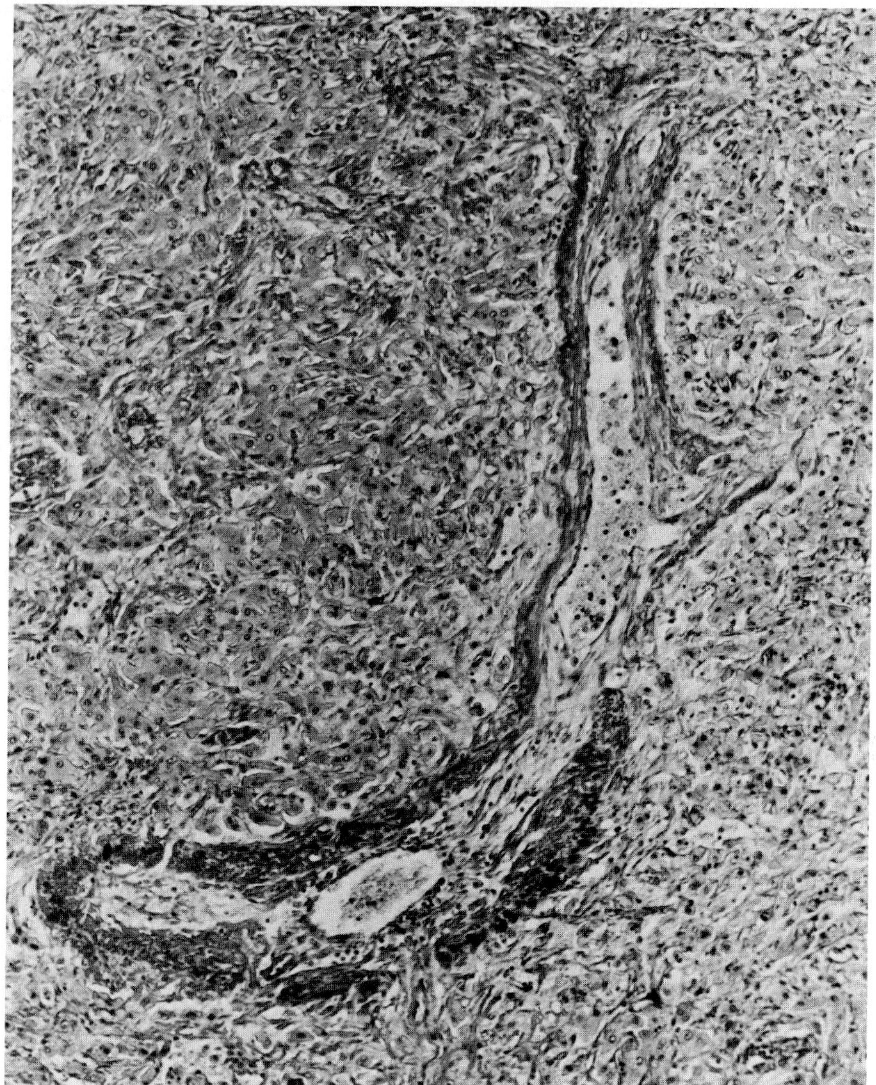

Figure 7. Veno-occlusive disease in a Jamaican patient. The central vein is almost completely occluded by fibrous tissue. (Mallory trichrome, ×140.) (Contributed by G. Bras, M.D.)

Nodules may develop, resulting in a lesion which has been termed atypical cirrhosis (35) or pseudocirrhosis (36). Clinically, these patients have hepatomegaly, occasionally portal hypertension, and rarely, hepatic coma.

Hairy Cell Leukemia

Peculiar hepatic angiomatous lesions have been reported in conjunction with hairy cell leukemia (37). Cystic spaces resembling blood vessels are seen in numerous portal areas. Filled with erythrocytes, the spaces are lined by leukemic

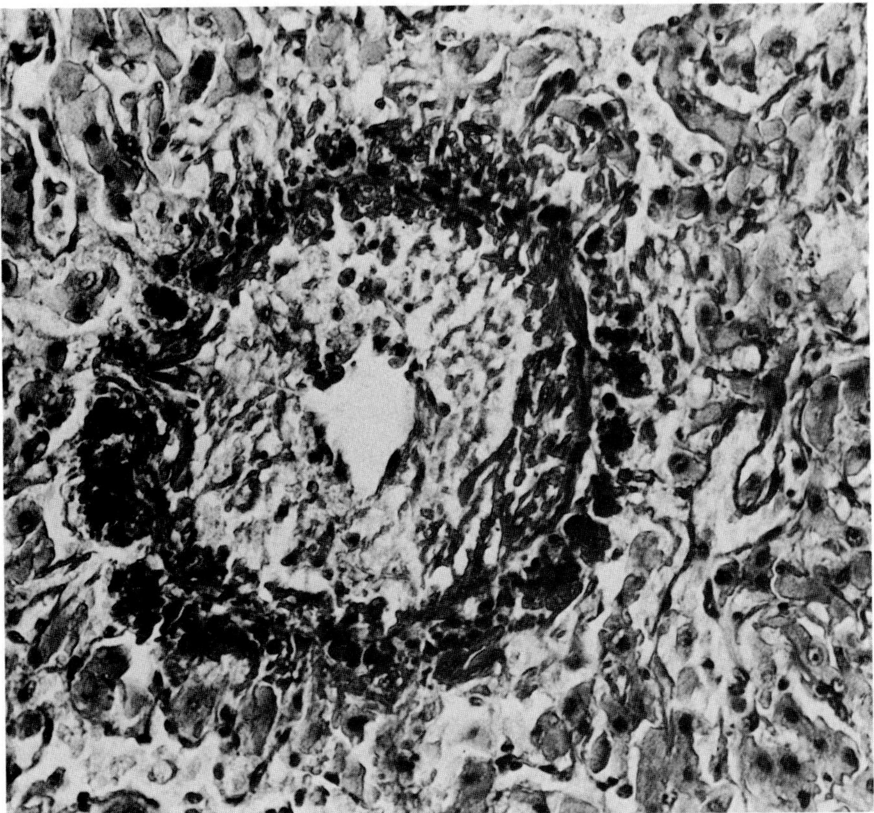

Figure 8. Veno-occlusive disease in a Jamaican patient. Higher-power view of lesion is similar to that in Figure 7. (Mallory trichrome, ×290.) (Contributed by G. Bras, M.D.)

cells that can be shown to have a tartrate-resistant acid phosphatase (Chapter 14). Isolated lesions of a similar type may be found in some lobules. When the lesions extend from portal to portal areas, the gross appearance resembles that of a "nutmeg liver" (see p. 196). Similar lesions may be seen in the spleen.

Arteritis

Necrotizing arteritis of the main hepatic artery or of its intrahepatic branches may be seen in patients with polyarteritis nodosa, systemic lupus erythematosis, or rheumatoid arthritis. The vascular lesion consists of fibrinoid necrosis and acute inflammation, which is usually followed by organization (Fig. 9). Secondary aneurysms and/or hemorrhage may also develop. Since hepatic involvement in polyarteritis is said to be found in 65% of patients, one would expect biopsy specimens, especially wedge biopsy specimens, to show these characteristic lesions fairly frequently (38). However, the authors have personally only seen two cases, one from a needle and another from a wedge biopsy. Spontaneous rupture of the liver in polyarteritis nodosa has been reported (39). The hepatitis B virus is now recognized to be causative in a significant number of patients with polyarteritis nodosa. These are usually either asymptomatic carriers of hepatitis

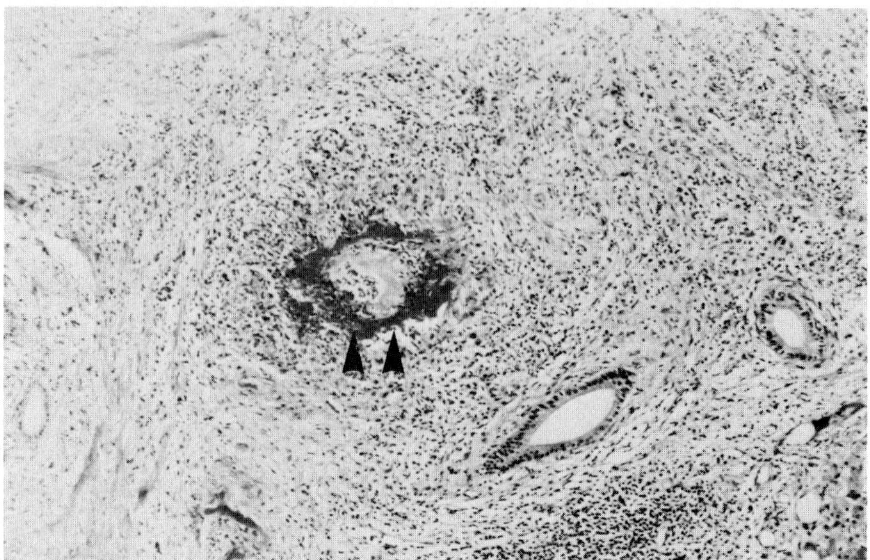

Figure 9. Polyarteritis nodosa. Fibrinoid necrosis (arrowheads) in hepatic artery branch in a portal triad. The artery is surrounded by acute inflammatory cells. Two bile ducts are also seen. (Hematoxylin and eosin, ×85.)

B or suffer from chronic persistent hepatitis (Chapter 2). Chronic active hepatitis is rare in this group of patients (40,41).

Arteriosclerosis and Amyloidosis

Hyaline arteriosclerosis of the arteries in the portal triads may be commoner in systemic hypertension. Fibroproliferative arteriolosclerosis definitely does suggest hypertension (41a). Amyloidosis of these arteries may resemble hyaline arteriosclerosis. Amyloidosis, however, is distinguished by its positive staining with Congo red and birefringence under polarized light (Chapter 11).

Arteriovenous Fistulae

Fistulae between the hepatic arterial and hepatic venous systems are difficult to demonstrate histologically and are best diagnosed radiologically. They occur most frequently in infantile hemangioendotheliomas (Chapter 14) (42), but may also be found in Osler-Weber-Rendu disease (see p. 201) (35). Symptoms tend to be cardiac in nature with tachycardia, increased cardiac output, widened pulse pressure, and possibly congestive heart failure. A hepatic bruit is usually present. There are generally no major changes in liver function tests. Diagnosis may be made by selective celiac arteriography.

Fistulae between the hepatic artery and portal vein resemble cavernous hemangiomas microscopically and may be congenital or traumatic. They may be located either intra- or extrahepatically. Portal hypertension, ascites, or esophageal varices may be produced (43–46a).

Pathology of the Extrahepatic Blood Supply to the Liver

Congenital absence of the extrahepatic portal vein is very rare but may be a harmless anomaly (47). Portal vein occlusion may occur in association with hepatic disease, carcinomatosis, sepsis, polycythemia, cryoglobulinemia, or abdominal trauma (48). It has also been reported after jejunoileal bypass (49). These patients develop portal hypertension, rarely associated with ascites. Results of liver biopsy are generally virtually normal.

Aneurysms of the hepatic artery are rare (50). They are frequently multiple and may be congenital or acquired. The usual mode of presentation is gastrointestinal bleeding, colicky pain, and jaundice. Only a few cases of dissecting aneurysm of the hepatic artery have been reported.

VASCULAR LESIONS WITHOUT LOBULAR LOCALIZATION

Peliosis Hepatis

Peliosis hepatis is characterized by blood-filled hepatic spaces that are usually multiple, have no particular lobular localization, and range from 0.2 to several cm in diameter (Figs. 10,11) (51–53). Clinically, this lesion may be associated with hepatomegaly and hepatic failure. However, it may also be an incidental autopsy finding. In a few patients intraperitoneal hemorrhage and shock have been reported. Two types of this lesion have been described. In one of these, the parenchymal type, cysts lack an endothelial or Kupffer cell lining and may be associated with liver cell necrosis and destruction of the reticulin framework (54). In the other, the phlebectatic type, the spaces are endothelially-lined, dilated sinuses. Liver cell necrosis is not seen in this type. Both morphologic types may coexist in the same patient (55), and distinction between them is probably not clinically significant (56). In the past, peliosis was most commonly reported with tuberculosis. It is currently seen most frequently in patients receiving androgenic-anabolic steroids and is frequently associated with hepatocellular neoplasms (Chapter 14). A case has been reported in a child with a steroid producing adrenal tumor (57). In most series a few cases are not associated with any recognized predisposing factors. One such case occurred in a newborn infant (58). In recent years peliosis has evolved from a puzzling autopsy finding into a clinically significant entity (56). St. George disease of cattle in Australia (59) is a naturally occurring model of the disease caused by a poisonous plant (59a). Experimental models have also been described (54,60–62). Nonetheless, the etiology and histogenesis of peliosis hepatis are not clearly established.

Infarction

Hepatic infarction is traditionally held to be a relatively uncommon event because of the liver's dual blood supply. Nonetheless, infarcts do occur with hepatic artery lesions, such as atherosclerosis, hypoplasia, thrombosis, embolism, dissecting aneurysm, polyarteritis, and combined arterial and venous lesions (63–65).

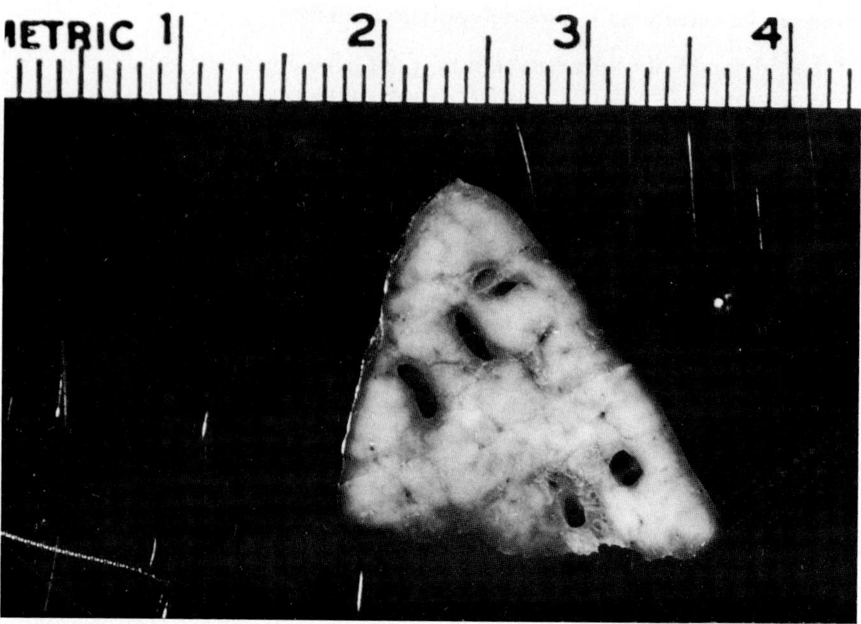

Figure 10. Peliosis hepatis. Roughly spherical dark vascular spaces can be seen in this gross specimen.

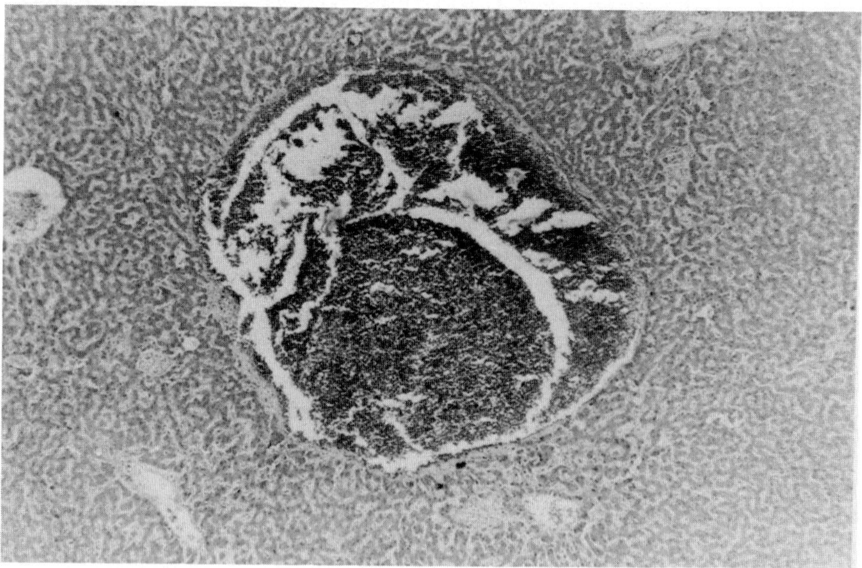

Figure 11. Peliosis hepatis showing a blood-filled space that has no particular lobular localization. The lesion illustrated has no definite endothelial lining. (Hematoxylin and eosin, ×34.)

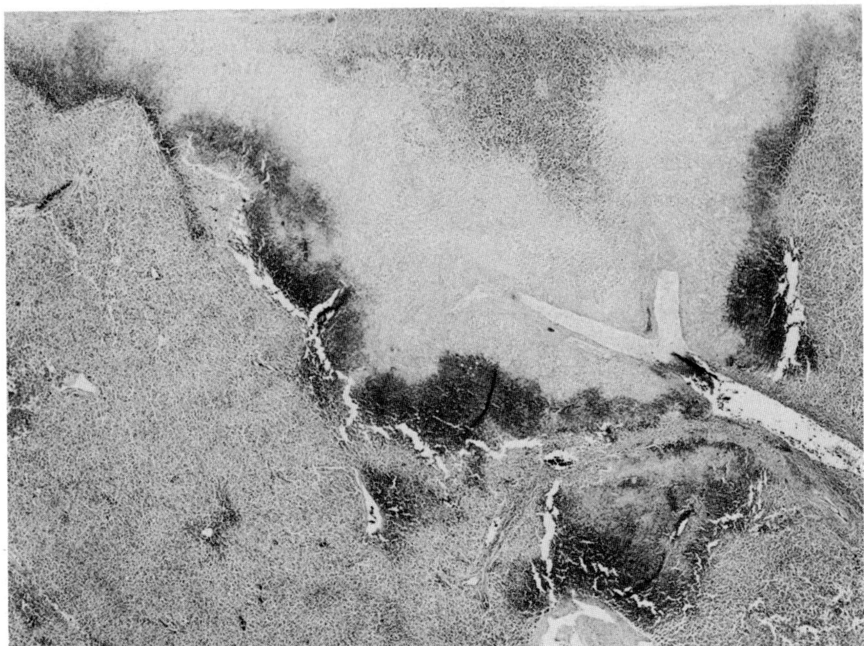

Figure 12. Hepatic infarct. Note wedge-shaped pale lesion with hemorrhagic border. (Hematoxylin and eosin, ×12.)

Less commonly, infarcts are associated with thromboemboli blocking the portal vein or its radicals (66,67). In a significant proportion of cases vascular obstruction appears to be absent (64,65). The clinical features of hepatic infarcts are difficult to define, because these lesions are usually associated with a primary disease such as congestive heart failure or shock. Clinically manifest hepatic infarcts are rare. Such patients develop epigastric pain or tenderness and may develop spontaneous hepatic rupture (67a). Elevations of SGOT and SGPT have also been reported. Hepatic scans show a space occupying cold lesion.

Infarcted areas are most frequently wedge shaped and may measure up to 15 cm in diameter. However, they do not necessarily abut Glisson's capsule. Initially hemorrhagic, the infarcted areas become pale with peripheral hyperemia within 24–72 hours. Ultimately, they become converted into retracted scars. Microscopically, there is coagulative hyaline necrosis involving several lobules, the necrotic area later becoming replaced by granulation tissue and then by scarring (Fig. 12) (68).

REFERENCES

1. Gadeholt H, Haugen J: Centrilobular hepatic necrosis in cardiac failure. *Acta Med Scand* 176:525, 1964.
2. Kisloff B, Schaffer G: Fulminant hepatic failure secondary to congestive heart failure. *Dig Dis* 21:895, 1976.
3. Cohen J, Kaplan M: Left-sided heart failure presenting as hepatitis. *Gastroenterology* 74:583, 1978.

4. Safran A, Schaffner F: Chronic passive congestion of the liver in man. *Am J Pathol* 50:447, 1967.

4a. Arcidi JM, Moore GW, Hutchins GM: Hepatic morphology in cardiac dysfunction. A clinicopathologic study of 1000 subjects at autopsy. *Am J Pathol* 104:159, 1981.

5. Kanel GC, Ucci AA, Kaplan MM, et al: Perivenular hepatic lesion associated with heart failure. *Am J Clin Pathol* 73:235, 1980.

6. Bruguera M, Aranguibel F, Ros E, et al: Incidence and clinical significance of sinusoidal dilatation in liver biopsies. *Gastroenterology* 75:474, 1978.

7. Poulsen H, Winkler K, Christoffersen P: The significance of centrilobular sinusoidal changes in liver biopsies. *Scand J Gastroenterol* 7:103, 1970.

8. Horrocks P, Tapp E: Zahn's "infarcts" of the liver. *J Clin Pathol* 19:475, 1966.

9. Tavill AS, Wood EJ, Kreel L, et al: The Budd-Chiari syndrome: Correlation between hepatic scintigraphy and the clinical, radiological, and pathological findings in nineteen cases of hepatic venous outflow obstruction. *Gastroenterology* 68:509, 1975.

10. Alpert LI: Veno-occlusive disease of the liver associated with oral contraceptives. Case report and review of literature. *Hum Pathol* 7(6):709, 1976.

11. Hoyumpa AM, Schiff L, Helfman EL: Budd-Chiari syndrome in women taking oral contraceptives. *Am J Med* 50:137, 1970.

12. Espana P, Figuera D, De Miguel JM, et al: Membranous obstruction of the inferior vena cava and hepatic veins. *Am J Gastroenterol* 1:28, 1980.

13. Cabrera J, Bruguera M, Navarro F, et al: Budd-Chiari syndrome due to a membranous obstruction of the inferior vena cava in a child. *J Pediatr* 96:435, 1980.

14. Khuroo MS, Datta DV: Budd-Chiari syndrome following pregnancy. Report of 16 cases with roentgenologic, hemodynamic and histologic studies of the hepatic outflow tract. *Am J Med* 68:113, 1980.

15. Khuroo MS, Datta DV, Khoshy A, et al: Alveolar hydatid disease of the liver with Budd-Chiari syndrome. *Postgrad Med J* 56:197, 1980.

16. Parker RGF: Occlusion of the hepatic veins in man. *Medicine* 38:369, 1959.

17. Shoemaker WC, Szanto PB, Anderson D: Hepatic hemodynamic and morphologic changes in shock. *Arch Pathol Lab Med* 80:76, 1965.

18. Coen R, McAdams J: Visceral manifestations of shock in congenital heart disease. *Am J Dis Child* 119:389, 1970.

19. Rosenblate HJ, Eisenstein R, Holmes AW: The liver in sickle cell anemia. *Arch Pathol Lab Med* 90:235, 1970.

20. Omata M, Johnson CS, Tong MJ: Pathological spectrum of sickle cell liver disease. *Gastroenterol* 79:118, 1980.

20a. Bauer TW, Moore GW, Hutchins GM: The liver in sickle cell disease. A clinicopathologic study of 70 patients. *Am J Med* 69:833, 1980.

21. Marubbio AT, Danielson B: Hepatic veno-occlusive disease in a renal transplant patient receiving azathioprine. *Gastroenterol* 69:739, 1975.

22. Lyford CL, Vergara GG, Moeller DD: Hepatic veno-occlusive disease originating in Ecuador. *Gastroenterol* 70:105, 1976.

23. Griner PF, Elbacawi A, Packman CH: Veno-occlusive disease of the liver after chemotherapy of acute leukemia. *Ann Intern Med* 85:578, 1976.

24. Mellis C, Bale PM: Familial hepatic veno-occlusive disease with probable immune deficiency. *J Pediatr* 88:236, 1976.

25. Bras G: Aspects of hepatic vascular diseases, in Gall EA, Mostofi FK (eds): *The Liver*. Baltimore, Williams & Wilkins, 1973, p 406.

26. Fajardo LF, Colby TV: Pathogenesis of veno-occlusive disease after radiation. *Arch Pathol Lab Med* 104:584, 1980.

27. McGee J O'D, Patrick RS, Wood CB: A case of veno-occlusive disease of the liver in Britain associated with herbal tea assumption. *J Clin Path* 29:788, 1976.

27a. Tandon BN, Tandon HD, Tandon RK, et al: An epidemic of veno-occlusive disease of liver in central India. *Lancet* 2:271, Aug 1976.
28. Mohabbat O, Shafiq Younos M. Merzad AA, et al: An outbreak of hepatic veno-occlusion disease in Northwestern Afghanistan. *Lancet* 2:269, Aug 1976.
29. Lewin K, Willis RR: Human radiation hepatitis: A morphologic study with emphasis on the late changes. *Arch Pathol Lab Med* 96:21, 1973.
30. Reed G, Cox A: The human liver after radiation injury. A form of veno-occlusive disease. *Am J Pathol* 48(4):597, 1966.
31. Berk PD, Popper H, Kruger GRF, et al: Veno-occlusive disease of the liver after allogeneic bone marrow transplantation. Possible association with graft versus host disease. *Ann Intern Med* 90:158, 1979.
32. Poulsen H, Winkler K: Liver disease with periportal sinusoidal dilatation. *Digestion* 8:441, 1973.
33. Feizi O: Hereditary hemorrhagic telangiectasia presenting with portal hypertension and cirrhosis of the liver. *Gastroenterology* 63:660, 1972.
34. Daly JJ, Schiller AL: The liver in hereditary hemorrhagic telangiectasia (Osler-Weber-Rendu disease). *Am J Med* 60:723, 1976.
35. Martini GA: The liver in hereditary haemorrhagic teleangiectasia: An unborn error of vascular structure with multiple manifestations: A reappraisal. *Gut* 19:531, 1978.
36. Cooney T, Sweeney E, Coll R: "Pseudocirrhosis" in hereditary haemorrhagic telangiectasis. *J Clin Pathol* 30:1134, 1977.
37. Nanba K, Soban EJ, Bowling MC, et al: Splenic pseudosinuses and hepatic angiomatous lesions. Distinctive features of hairy cell leukemia. *Am J Clin Pathol* 67:415, 1977.
38. Mowrey IH, Lundborg EA: Clinical manifestations of essential polyangitis (periarteritis nodosa) with emphasis on hepatic manifestations. *Ann Intern Med* 40:1145, 1954.
39. Li AKC, Rhodes JM, Valentine AR: Spontaneous liver rupture in polyarteritis nodosa. *Br J Surg* 66:177, 1979.
40. Strohmeyer G, Berger M, Jacobi E, et al: Periarteritis nodosa, liver disease, and persistent hepatitis B antigen. *Z Gastroenterol* 13(4):452, 1975.
41. Trepo C, Thivolet J, Lambert R: Four cases of periarteritis nodosa associated with persistent Australia antigen. *Digestion* 5:100, 1972.
41a. Tracy RE, Johnson WD, Lopez CR, et al: Hypertension and arteriolar sclerosis of the kidney, pancreas, adrenal gland and liver. *Vich Arch Pathol Anat* 391:91, 1981.
42. Mattioli L, Lee KR, Holder TM: Hepatic artery ligation for cardiac failure due to hepatic hemangioma in the newborn. *J Pediatr Surg* 9:859, 1974.
43. Fulton RL, Wolfel DA: Hepatic artery-portal vein arteriovenous fistula. *Arch Surg* 100:307, 1970.
44. Okuda K, Kotoda K, Igarashi M, et al: Intrahepatic arteriovenous fistula resulting from needle biopsy: A case report. *Acta Hepatogastroenterol* 21(6):422, 1974.
45. Baer, JW: Hepatic arterioportal fistula related to a liver biopsy. *Gastroenterol Radiol* 2(3):297, 1977.
46. Van Waes K, Demeulenaere L, Van Damme W, et al: Hepaticoportal fistula and portal hypertension. *Dig Dis* 24:565, 1979.
46a. Rogers WA, Suter PF, Breznock FM, et al: Intrahepatic arteriovenous fistulae in a dog resulting in portal hypertension, portocaval shunts and reversal of portal blood flow. *J Am Anim Hosp Assoc* 13:470, 1977.
47. Marois D, Heerden JA, Carpenter HA, et al: Congenital absence of the portal vein. *Mayo Clin Proc* 54:55, 1979.
48. Nayak NC, Ramalingaswami V: Obliterative portal venopathy of the liver. *Arch Pathol Lab Med* 87:359, 1969.
49. Metz R, Gray R, Goldstein L: Portal venous occlusion; an unusual cause of ascites in a patient with jejunoileal bypass. *Dig Dis* 23:59s, 1978.

50. Hubens A, De Schepper A: Hepatic artery aneurysm: A pitfall in biliary surgery. *Br J Surg* 66:259, 1979.
51. Nuernberger SP, Ramos CV: Peliosis hepatis in an infant. *J Pediatr* 87:424, 1975.
52. Nadell J, Kosek J: Peliosis hepatis. Twelve cases associated with oral androgen therapy. *Arch Pathol Lab Med* 101:405, 1977.
53. Chopra S, Edelstein A, Koff RS, et al: Peliosis hepatis in hematologic disease. *JAMA* 240:1153, 1978.
54. Bagheri SA, Boyer JL: Peliosis hepatis associated with androgenic-anabolic steroid therapy. *Ann Intern Med* 81:610, 1974.
55. Usatin MS, Wigger HJ: Peliosis hepatis in a child. *Arch Pathol Lab Med* 100:419, 1976.
56. Taxy JB: Peliosis: A morphologic curiosity becomes an iatrogenic problem. *Hum Pathol* 9:331, 1978.
57. Willen H, Willen R, Gad A, et al: Peliosis hepatis as a result of endogenous steroid hormone production. *Virchows Arch [Pathol Anat]* 383:233, 1979.
58. Kawamoto S, Wakabayashi T: Peliosis hepatis in a newborn infant. *Arch Pathol Lab Med* 104:444, 1980.
59. Seawright AA, Francis J: Peliosis hepatis—A special liver lesion in St. George disease of cattle. *Aust Vet J* 47:91, 1971.
59a. Kelly WR, Seawright AA, Pimelea SPP: Poisoning of cattle, in Keeler RF, Van Kampen KR, James LF (eds): *Effects of Poisonous Plants on Livestock.* New York, Academic Press, 1978, p 293.
60. Naeim F, Copper PH, Semion AA: Peliosis hepatis. Possible etiologic role of anabolic steroids. *Arch Pathol Lab Med* 95:284, 1973.
61. Ruebner BH, Watanabe K, Wand JS: Lytic necrosis resembling peliosis hepatis produced by lasiocarpine in the mouse liver. *Am J Pathol* 60:247, 1970.
62. Mendenhall CL, Chedid A: Peliosis hepatis. Its relationship to chronic alcoholism, aflatoxin B, and carcinogenesis in male Holtzman rats. *Dig Dis Sci* 25:587, 1980.
63. Trojanowski JQ, Harrist TJ, Athanasoulis CA, et al: Hepatic and splenic infarctions. Complications of the therapeutic transcatheter embolization. *Am J Surg* 139:272, 1980.
64. Seeley TT, Blumenfeld CM, Ikeda R, et al: Hepatic infarction. *Hum Pathol* 3(2):265, 1972.
65. Hartveit F, Maehle B, Borsting S: Post-natal infarction of the right lobe of the liver. *Acta Paediatr Scand* 63(3):453, 1974.
66. Henrich WL, Huehnergarth RJ, Rosch J, et al: Gallbladder and liver infarction occurring as a complication of acute bacterial endocarditis. *Gastroenterology* 68:1602, 1975.
67. Ghandur-Mnaymneh L: Anemic infarction of the liver resulting from hepatic and portal vein thrombosis. *Johns Hopkins Med J* 139:78, 1976.
67a. Hocking WG, Lasser K, Ungerer R, et al: Spontaneous hepatic rupture in rheumatoid arthritis. *Arch Int Med* 141:792, 1981.
68. Chen V, Hamilton J, Qizilbash A: Hepatic infarction. *Arch Pathol Lab Med* 100:32, 1976.

13
Fibrosis, Nodules, and Cirrhosis

DEFINITION OF FIBROSIS AND CIRRHOSIS

Hepatic fibrosis can be defined as an increase in the proportion of fibrous connective tissue to parenchyma. Chemically, the normal liver contains about 5–8 mg of collagen per gram wet liver (1). One type of fibrosis is caused by a dropout of parenchymal cells, lack of hepatocellular regeneration, and collapse of the preexisting reticulin framework of the liver. This results in the formation of passive septa that stain for reticulin rather than collagen and tend to be relatively slender and acellular. A second type of hepatic fibrosis is caused by accelerated collagen biosynthesis. This type of fibrosis also is usually associated with hepatic injury. Excessive collagen formation leads to the development of active septa that generally stain for collagen and elastic fibers (1a), as well as reticulin, and are usually broad and often infiltrated by inflammatory cells. In most cases of hepatic fibrosis, both collapse and increased collagen biosynthesis take place. Of these, increased biosynthesis is probably the more important. Fibrosis may be predominantly portal, central, or focal (i.e., patchy and without any lobular localization). Fibrous septa may join portal to portal areas, central to central areas, or portal to central areas. In the past few years there have been some exciting advances in our understanding of the biochemistry of collagen. Type I and Type III collagen have been demonstrated in the portal triads and in the reticulin fibers of the lobules. Fibrotic livers also show both types in a proportion roughly similar to that of normal liver. Basement membrane collagens (Types IV and V) are normally mostly found in vessel walls and bile ducts. Type IV may be demonstrable in the lobule in acute hepatic injury when fibrosis cannot yet be demonstrated histologically (1–5a).

The term *cirrhosis* is applied to a liver that, in addition to marked fibrosis, shows distinct nodular transformation of the hepatic architecture (6–9). Chemically, there is a four- to sevenfold increase in collagen. In cirrhosis all types of collagen found in the normal liver are increased. In cirrhotic livers containing more than 20 mg of collagen per gram of wet liver, type I collagen appears to predominate (1). The morphologic definition of cirrhosis given above is not universally adhered to. In fact, some pathologists still use the terms fibrosis and cirrhosis synonymously. An advantage of defining cirrhosis as fibrosis with nodular transformation is that patients with this type of liver disease usually have portal hypertension. Patients with fibrosis alone usually do not have portal hypertension. Gradually increasing fibrosis generally precedes cirrhosis. However, not all patients with fibrosis necessarily develop cirrhosis. In fact, when the stimulus for fibrosis is removed, the amount of collagen may decrease or even disappear (10). By contrast, cirrhosis is virtually irreversible because of the associated diffuse nodular transformation of the hepatic architecture. Histologically, the cirrhotic liver generally lacks portal triads and the nodules are composed of liver cell plates more than one cell thick. In cirrhosis, fibrosis and nodular transformation are diffuse and involve the entire organ, although not necessarily each and every one of its lobules. The gradual progression of fibrosis to cirrhosis explains why, especially in borderline cases, the histologic distinction between fibrosis and cirrhosis may be a subjective matter. This is particularly true in the case of small needle biopsy specimens, which may not necessarily be representative of the predominant histologic alterations in the rest of the liver. Fragmentation of a needle biopsy specimen is always an indication to search particularly carefully for clues pointing to cirrhosis, such as micronodules surrounded by reticulin or collagen. It has been suggested that cirrhosis should not be diagnosed in a biopsy, unless there is widespread fibrosis associated with at least two parenchymal nodules completely surrounded by connective tissue. Lesser changes may warrant a diagnosis of probable cirrhosis (8a).

NONPROGRESSIVE HEPATIC FIBROSIS

Most, but not all, etiologic factors that can cause hepatic fibrosis may eventually cause cirrhosis. However, some fibrous lesions generally do not progress to cirrhosis. This section describes congenital hepatic fibrosis, cystic disease of the liver, and hepatoportal sclerosis. Osler-Weber-Rendu disease was described in Chapter 12.

Congenital Hepatic Fibrosis

Congenital hepatic fibrosis is characterized by diffuse periportal fibrosis and septation, associated with hyperplasia and cystic dilatation of bile ducts within the fibrous tissue. The ductal structures often contain inspissated bile. The liver in congenital hepatic fibrosis may grossly appear nodular and resemble cirrhosis (11). However, it becomes apparent on histologic examination that true nodules and architectural disorganization do not develop (Figs. 1,2) (12). The hepatic ultrastructure of this condition has been described in a family with associated congenital heart disease (12a). Grossly obvious hepatic cystic structures are rare (13), but cysts of the extrahepatic biliary system may be associated with this condition (Chapter 17). The renal lesions associated with congenital hepatic fibrosis are relatively mild. Clinically, congenital hepatic fibrosis most frequently presents as variceal bleeding or ascites due to portal hypertension in adolescents or young adults (13a,b). It may be complicated by acute suppurative cholangitis (12,14,15). Cholangiocarcinoma is a rare complication (16,17). Congenital hepatic fibrosis is rarely seen for the first time in older patients (18,19). The hepatic abnormalities of the fetal alcohol syndrome may resemble congenital hepatic fibrosis (20).

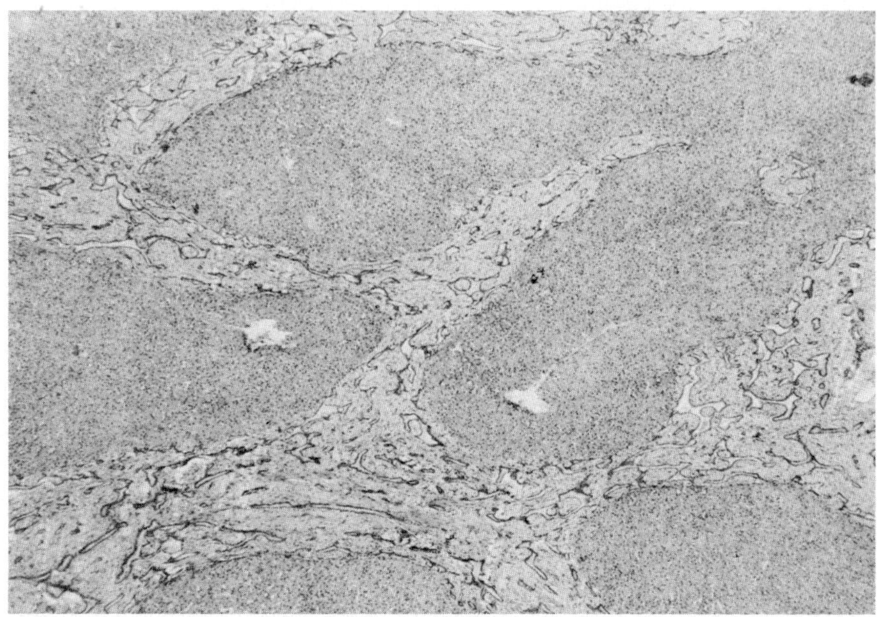

Figure 1. Congenital heptic fibrosis. Note regular arrangement of proliferated bile ducts in a fibrous stroma. Intact central veins are shown, with no cirrhosis. (Hematoxylin and eosin, ×34.)

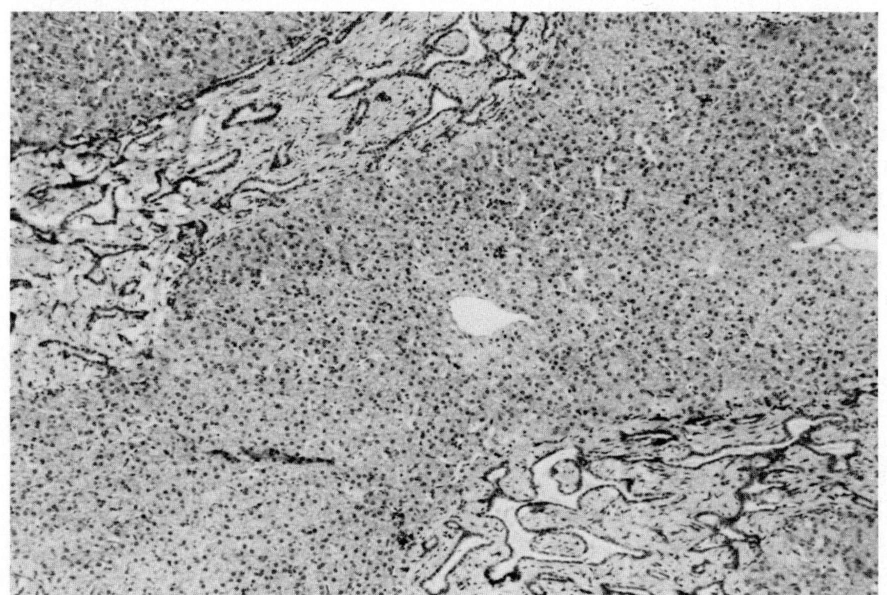

Figure 2. Congenital hepatic fibrosis. Note well-organized, regular pattern of proliferated bile ducts in a fibrous stroma and the normal central vein. (Hematoxylin and eosin, ×85.)

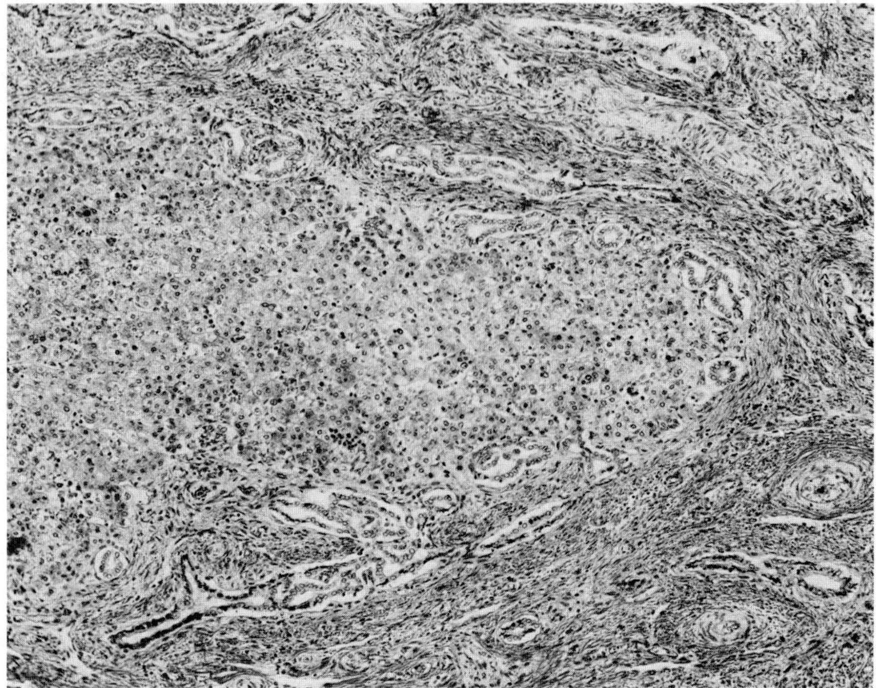

Figure 3. Congenital cystic disease in a stillborn infant. Note irregularly proliferated bile ducts embedded in fibrous tissue. Foci of hemopoiesis are scattered among the hepatocytes. The infant also had cystic kidneys. (Hematoxylin and eosin, ×100.)

Cystic Disease of the Liver

Congenital cystic disease of the liver is virtually indistinguishable, microscopically, from congenital hepatic fibrosis. However, the cystic dilatation may be more striking and the portal fibrosis less severe (Fig. 3). Polycystic disease of the liver usually presents with systemic hypertension and renal failure. The renal lesions of polycystic disease are much more severe than those of congenital hepatic fibrosis and can usually be distinguished from them (21,22). Because of the differences in clinical presentation, most workers consider congenital hepatic fibrosis and hepatic polycystic disease to be different entities. The various types of hepatic cystic disease have been reviewed recently (23).

Hepatoportal Sclerosis

Noncirrhotic portal hypertension has also been called idiopathic hepatoportal sclerosis, hepatosplenic fibrosis, noncirrhotic portal fibrosis, perisinusoidal fibrosis, intrahepatic obliterative portal venopathy, or since its first description in India, tropical splenomegaly (24,25,25a). It seems likely that many of these patients were previously diagnosed as Banti's syndrome. Thrombosis of the extrahepatic portal vein must be excluded before making a diagnosis of hepatoportal sclerosis. Cases have been reported not only from India, but also from Japan, Mexico, France, and the United States. Some cases have been associated with Felty's syndrome (26). The liver shows only mild to moderate portal

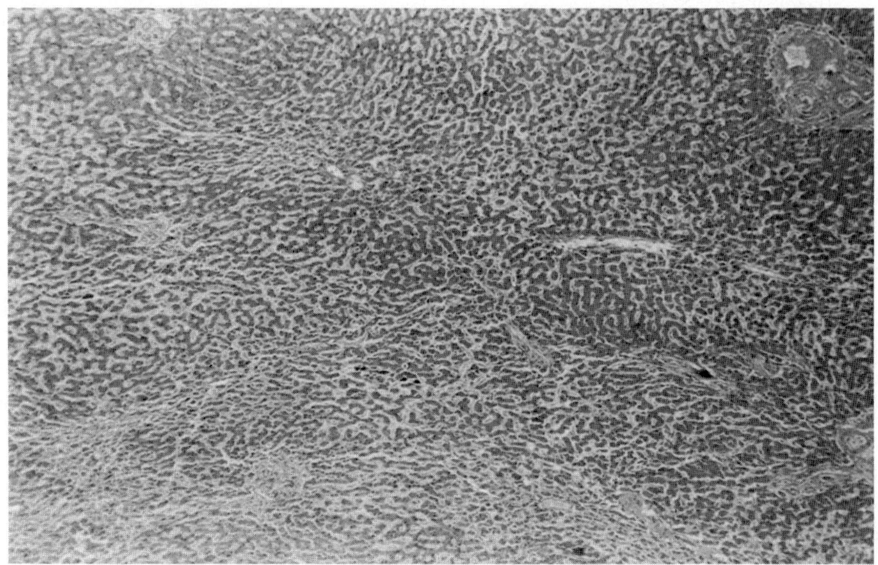

Figure 4. Hepatoportal sclerosis. Note relatively mild fibrosis of portal triad in right upper corner. The lobular arrangement of the hepatic plates seems somewhat jumbled. (Hematoxylin and eosin, ×34.)

fibrosis, and even septal fibrosis, with mild disturbance of the basic hepatic architecture (Fig. 4). Although there is no true cirrhosis, this condition is associated with portal hypertension. Hepatoportal sclerosis occurs predominantly in adults, mostly in males, and is more common in tropical than in temperate climates.

Grossly, the liver is smooth during the early stages of the disease. Later, its surface becomes wrinkled. Since the lesions tend to be irregular in distribution and involve the larger portal triads, needle biopsy yields few, if any clues. Wedge biopsy is more apt to be useful diagnostically, although it has been said that subcapsular fibrosis may become so extreme as to mimic cirrhosis (27). The portal vein branches may be small and narrow or widely patent. The larger portal vein branches may show some intimal thickening or thrombosis with recanalization. It is uncertain whether the changes in the portal vein branches are primary or secondary to the portal hypertension. If the portal vein changes were primary, then this condition would be an intrahepatic variant of portal vein thrombosis. Whenever feasible, the intrahepatic portal venous system must be studied carefully (28). Sinusoidal stenosis due to obliteration of the space of Disse by increased reticulin fibers has also been observed in noncirrhotic portal hypertension (29–31). Intrahepatic bile duct lesions have also been considered to be possibly responsible for this syndrome (32).

Clinically, hepatoportal sclerosis manifests itself by massive splenomegaly without hepatomegaly, hemorrhage from esophageal varices, or hypersplenism with anemia, leukopenia, and thrombocytopenia. In most cases, the etiology of this condition is unknown. Patients who have been exposed to inorganic arsenicals (33,34), vinyl chloride (35,36), thorotrast (37), or possibly antimetabolites (38) may develop periportal fibrosis with septa formation and the clinicopathologic picture may resemble quite closely that of idiopathic hepatoportal sclerosis. The etiology may be ascertainable only by a careful history. However, thorotrast can be demonstrated in the tissues as an amorphous pigmented radioactive material (Chapter 11), and arsenic concentrations have also been measured (39).

CLASSIFICATION OF CIRRHOSIS

The division of cirrhosis into subtypes has remained somewhat controversial for several reasons. The predominant pattern may vary in different parts of the same liver. Moreover, one morphologic type may transform into another over a period of time. For example, micronodular cirrhosis may develop into mixed and then macronodular cirrhosis (40). Primarily because of this, some etiologic agents are not too well correlated with a particular morphologic subtype of cirrhosis. Nevertheless, cirrhosis is usually subdivided morphologically because there is some relationship between morphologic subtypes and etiologic factors.

Micronodular Cirrhosis

Micronodular cirrhosis is grossly characterized by small nodules, almost uniform in size. Different investigators have considered the maximum diameter of the nodules in this type of cirrhosis to be anywhere from 0.1 to 1.0 cm. Probably the most useful compromise is 0.3 cm (6,7). Histologically, only occasional portal tracts and hepatic veins can be seen. Fibrous septa are fairly uniform in width (Figs. 5–8). This type of cirrhosis has also been called portal, nutritional, or Laennec's cirrhosis. It is characteristically seen in alcoholics, but may also be associated with a great variety of other etiologic factors, such as obesity, jejunolileal bypass, hemochromatosis, Wilson's disease, Indian childhood cirrhosis, and, rarely, with chronic active hepatitis.

Macronodular Cirrhosis

Macronodular cirrhosis is characterized by nodules varying greatly in size, measuring from 0.3 cm up to 5 cm in diameter or even more. Fibrous septa vary greatly in width, and broad septa are common (Figs. 9–11). Grossly, the liver may appear severely deformed, particularly in the left lobe. Histologically, the larger nodules may contain several central veins, a feature that suggests that the nodule originated from several adjacent lobules. This type of cirrhosis has also been called postnecrotic cirrhosis. It is the most common type of cirrhosis developing as a sequel to chronic active hepatitis. However, patients with chronic active hepatitis may also develop micronodular cirrhosis.

Incomplete Septal Cirrhosis

Incomplete septal cirrhosis has also been called mixed micro- and macronodular or posthepatitic cirrhosis (41). In this type of cirrhosis, which appears to be relatively uncommon, nodules vary considerably in size, but septa are relatively

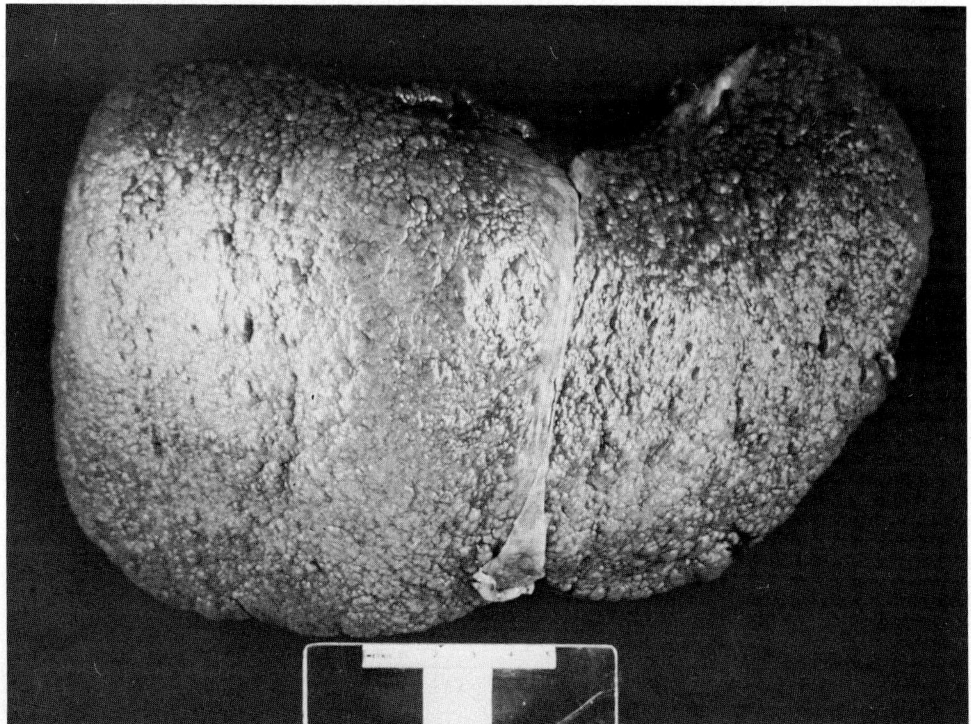

Figure 5. Micronodular cirrhosis. Gross photograph. Note fine uniform granularity. Nodules are less than 0.5 cm in diameter.

slender and may end blindly without linking portal tracts and central veins. This type of cirrhosis is usually of uncertain etiology but is often suspected to be the result of viral hepatitis.

Congestive Cirrhosis

Congestive cirrhosis or cardiac cirrhosis may rarely result from prolonged chronic passive congestion of the liver (Chapter 12). After some weeks or months, chronic passive congestion leads to central fibrosis, which can be followed by the formation of septa running from the central veins through the lobules towards the portal triads. Congestive fibrosis is not uncommon and is seen particularly in patients with mitral stenosis, tricuspid insufficiency, constrictive pericarditis, or hepatic vein occlusion (Budd-Chiari syndrome). In a very few patients who have had chronic passive congestion for months or years, the septa connect central veins to portal triads and become associated with nodular transformation of the parenchyma. True congestive cirrhosis, unlike congestive fibrosis, is, therefore, a very rare finding. Centrilobular fibrosis, similar to that seen in congestive heart failure, may be seen in alcoholics, particularly patients with central hyaline sclerosis (Chapter 5). Biopsy specimens from such patients

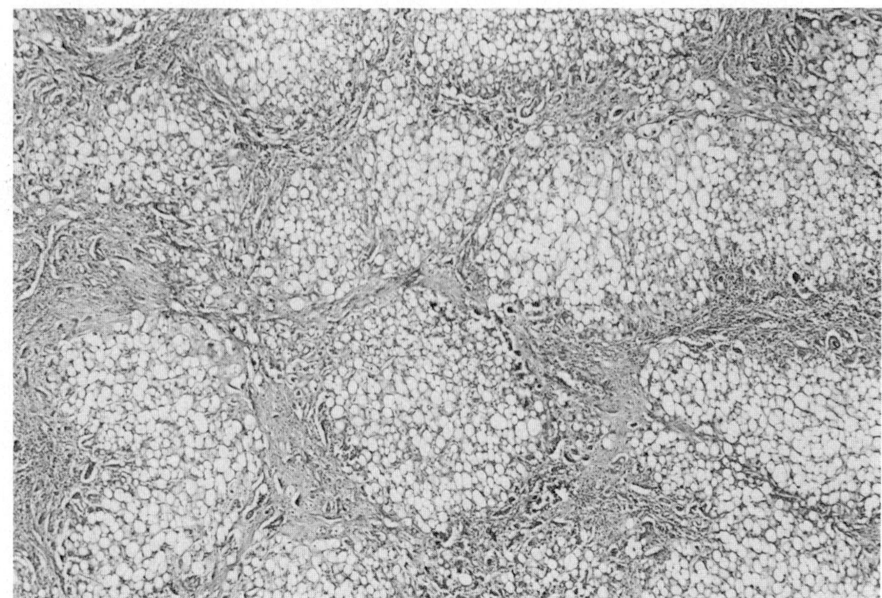

Figure 6. Micronodular cirrhosis with marked fatty change. Note small, relatively uniform nodules of hepatocytes separated by fibrous septa. (Hematoxylin and eosin, ×40.)

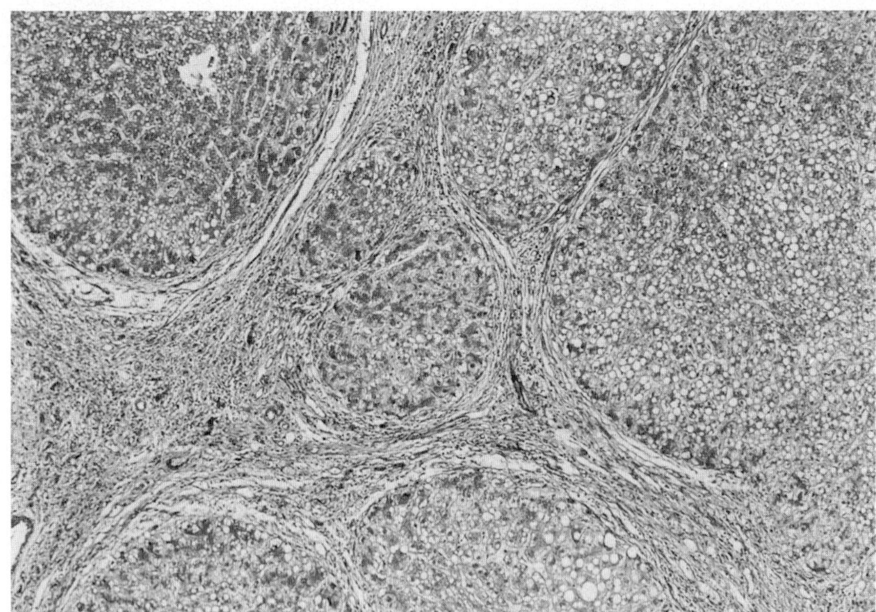

Figure 7. Micronodular cirrhosis with mild fatty change. Note hepatic nodules separated by fibrous septa. The nodules are somewhat larger and more variable than those shown in Figure 6, and the fibrous septa appear slightly wider. (Hematoxylin and eosin, ×60.)

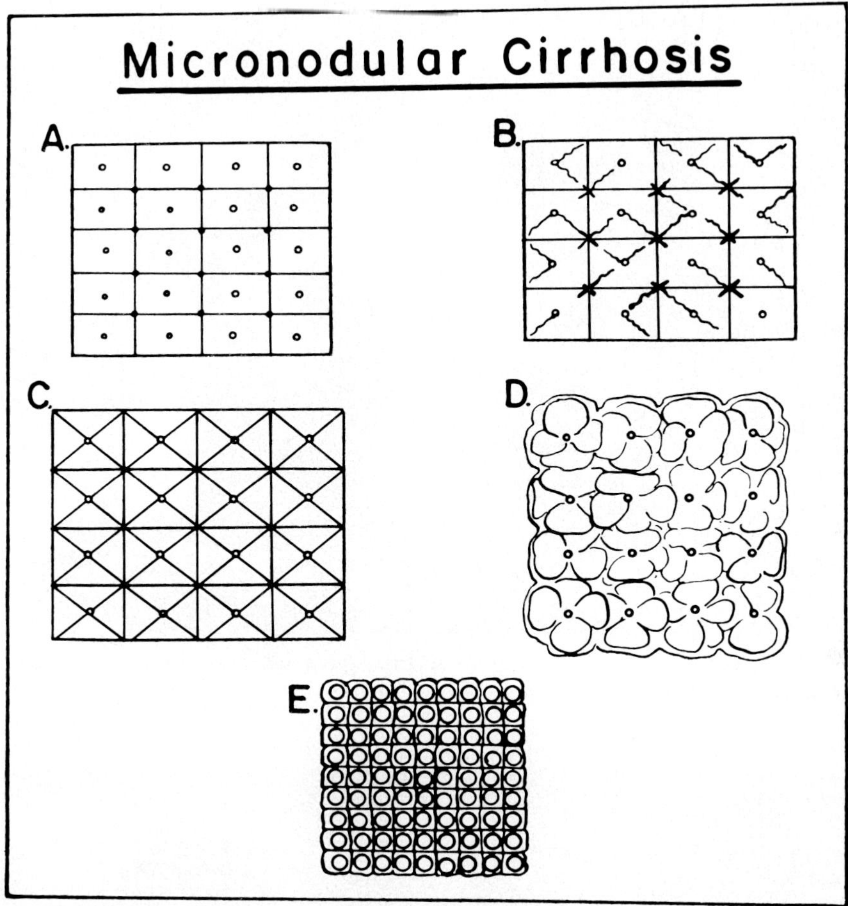

Figure 8. Schematic histogenesis of micronodular cirrhosis. (*a*) Normal liver. Lobules are shown as squares. Central circles represent central veins. (*b*) Portal and central fibrosis have developed. (*c*) Fibrosis bridges portal triads and central veins. (*d* and *e*) Fibrosis has increased and micronodules have developed. (Reproduced from Gall, ref. 41.)

generally also show fatty change and Mallory's hyalin. Such a picture has also been reported in diabetics who had no history of alcoholism (42).

Secondary Biliary Cirrhosis

Secondary biliary cirrhosis is the result of prolonged mechanical obstruction of large intrahepatic or of extrahepatic bile ducts. Initially such biliary obstruction causes portal fibrosis, then septa formation, and eventually fully developed cirrhosis with nodular transformation of the hepatic parenchyma. Extrahepatic biliary atresia is the most common cause of secondary biliary cirrhosis in children, but choledochal cyst or cystic dilatation of the bile ducts (Caroli's syndrome) also have to be considered. The rare case of congenital hepatic fibrosis with acute cholangitis (p. 212) can be difficult to distinguish from extrahepatic

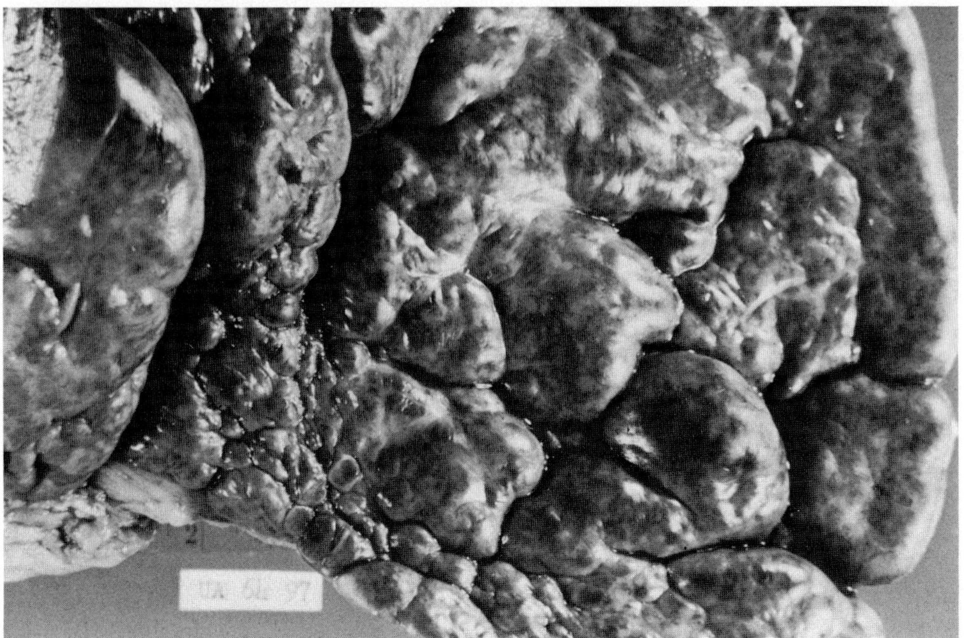

Figure 9. Macronodular cirrhosis, gross section. Note variation in size of nodules, the largest of which are several centimeters in diameter.

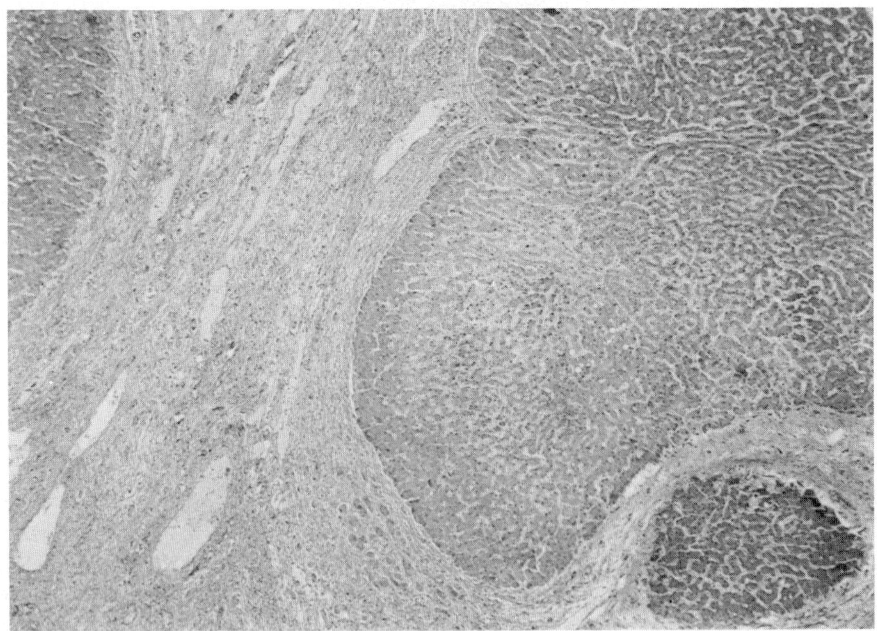

Figure 10. Macronodular cirrhosis. Note nodules varying greatly in size, separated by wide, fibrous septa. (Hematoxylin and eosin, ×40.)

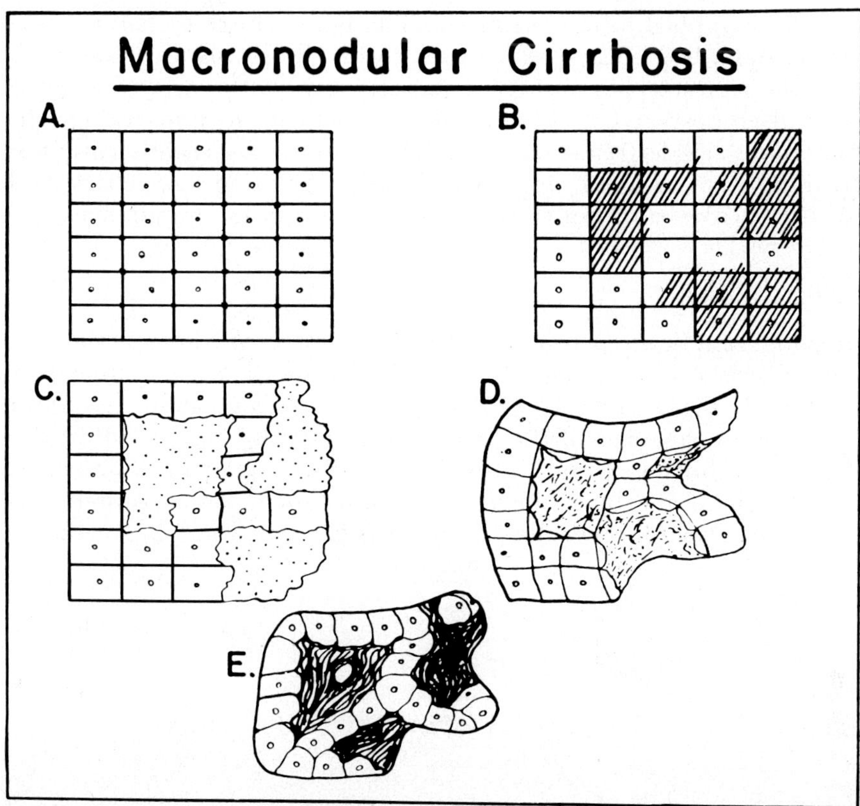

Figure 11. Schematic histogenesis of macronodular cirrhosis. (*a*) Normal liver; (*b*) Shaded areas represent massive necrosis; (*c*) dotted areas represent dropout of parenchyma; (*d*) areas of necrosis have undergone stromal collapse; (*e*) the stroma has undergone collagenization (darkened areas), and the surviving lobules have undergone some hypertrophy. (Reproduced from Gall, ref. 41.)

obstruction and cholangitis. In adults, secondary biliary cirrhosis may be the result of duct stricture following surgical injury of the extrahepatic bile ducts, or of obstruction by gallstones or neoplasms, Before the development of cirrhosis, the livers of these patients show the characteristic features of extrahepatic obstruction, including severe cholestasis and bile duct proliferation, usually with cholangitis (Chapters 7 and 8). As fibrosis increases and cirrhosis develops, the number of bile ducts in the septa decreases, and cholestasis becomes less conspicuous. Fully developed biliary cirrhosis ultimately becomes difficult to distinguish from micronodular cirrhosis.

Primary Biliary Cirrhosis

Primary biliary cirrhosis starts as a destructive lesion of the bile ducts, and cirrhosis is only a late feature. This is why the condition has also been called chronic, nonsuppurative, destructive cholangitis, a better, though cumbersome term. In the past such terms as Hanot's cirrhosis and xanthomatous biliary cirrhosis were applied to this condition. The noncirrhotic earlier stages of this disease are described in Chapter 7 dealing with cholestasis. In advanced biliary cirrhosis the characteristic histologic picture seen in the earlier stages of the disease is often obscured, and the cirrhosis may be difficult to distinguish from the micronodular type. However, even in late cases with cirrhosis, careful search will frequently reveal clues suggestive of the earlier stages of biliary cirrhosis, such as destructive lesions of the bile ducts or periportal granulomas.

Focal Biliary Cirrhosis

The hepatic complications of cystic fibrosis have recently been reviewed (42a). The characteristic morphologic hepatic change in 10–25% of cases has been termed "focal biliary cirrhosis" (43,44). This lesion is generally asymptomatic. However, almost one-half of the cases of cystic fibrosis have a nonfunctioning gallbladder on cholangiography (45). The microscopic hepatic lesion consists of focal dilatation of the interlobular portal bile ducts, which contain strongly acidophilic material (43). Periductal fibrosis is present (Fig. 12). In about 2% of

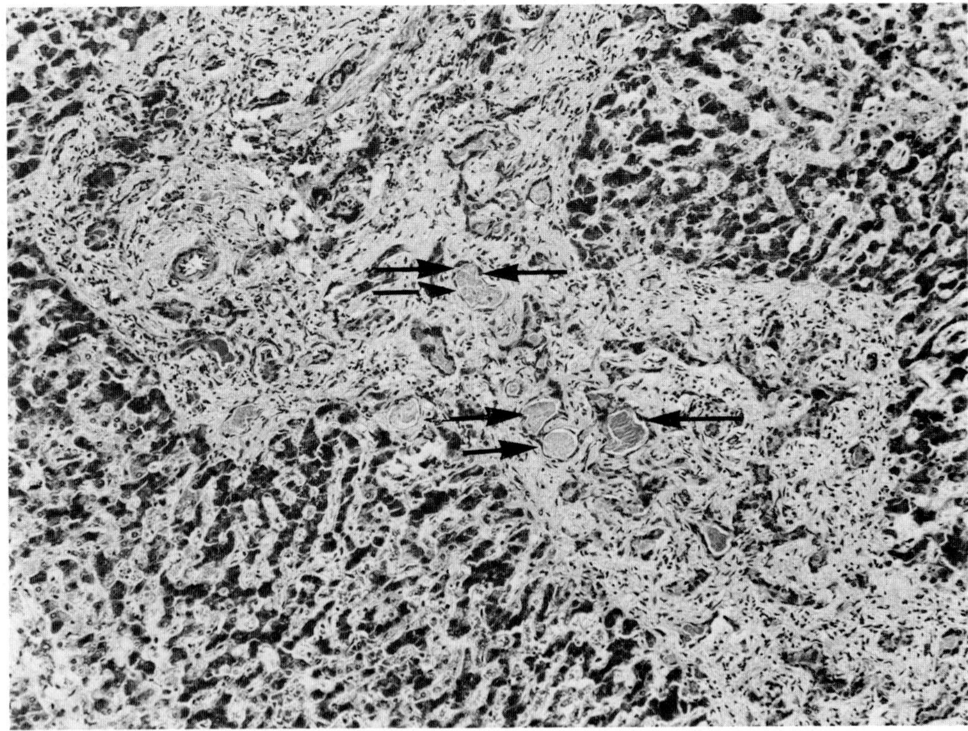

Figure 12. Focal biliary cirrhosis in fibrocystic disease. Note dilated bile ducts containing inspissated material (arrows) and embedded in fibrous tissue. (Hematoxylin and eosin, ×140.)

cases, this lesion progresses to micronodular (11) or even to macronodular (Fig. 9) cirrhosis. The characteristic inspissation of bile ducts with acidophilic material may persist into the cirrhotic stage. The presenting symptom in these patients is usually portal hypertension and, rarely, liver failure.

ETIOLOGY OF FIBROSIS AND CIRRHOSIS

Most cases of hepatic fibrosis that progress to cirrhosis belong to one of the following categories: (*1*) chronic hepatitis (Chapter 2), (*2*) alcoholic liver disease (Chapter 5), or (*3*) cryptogenic fibrosis or cirrhosis. This latter is seen most frequently in elderly patients, particularly women, and is most commonly of the macronodular or incomplete septal types. The liver is often scarred or decreased in size. It seems quite likely that most cases in the third category really belong to one of the first two. Evidence seems to be accumulating that cryptogenic cirrhosis is often the result of chronic hepatitis. Idiopathic familial cirrhosis has also been described (46). Morphologic clues to the etiology of hepatic fibrosis or cirrhosis may be obtained from the morphologic subtype, as pointed out above. In addition, viewing of fresh biopsy specimens under ultraviolet light is desirable, since fluorescence is produced in porphyria cutanea tarda and in erythropoietic protoporphyria. Certain microscopic features should be looked for in every case of cirrhosis. However, the more advanced the cirrhosis, the less likely one is to find such etiologic clues.

Fatty Change

Large-droplet hepatocellular fatty change is common in cirrhotic livers (Chapter 6). Apart from alcoholism, this may be seen in obesity, especially after intestinal bypass surgery, after parenteral nutrition, in psoriatics, particularly those on methotrexate, in Wilson's disease, and, to a lesser extent, in chronic active hepatitis, especially in patients on cortisone and in diabetics. In infancy, fatty change coupled with ductular proliferation, fibrosis and cirrhosis is seen in galactosemia, hereditary fructose intolerance, and tyrosinemia (Chapter 9).

Alcoholic Hepatitis

Mallory's hyalin (Chapter 5, Fig. 1), if prominent throughout the lobules, and particularly if associated with features of central hyaline sclerosis or alcoholic hepatitis, suggests alcoholism, morbid obesity, or jejunoileal bypass. In infants and children massive hyalin deposition suggests Indian childhood cirrhosis. Mallory's hyalin in lesser amounts in periportal hepatocytes, particularly in the presence of cholestasis, is less specific and suggests Wilson's disease, primary biliary cirrhosis, or chronic active hepatitis. Round or oval hyaline droplets, usually enlarged mitochondria, are also common in alcoholics (Chapter 5, Fig. 3).

Chronic Active Hepatitis

Piecemeal necrosis, particularly if associated with ground-glass cells positive for HB_sAg, suggests chronic active hepatitis (Chapter 2). Hepatocytes may also be positive for HB_sAg without having a ground-glass appearance. Apart from hepatitis non-A non-B, few if any other viruses are known to cause fibrosis or cirrhosis.

Antitrypsin Deficiency

PAS-positive, diastase-resistent droplets in the periphery of lobules or nodules suggest alpha-1-antitrypsin deficiency (Chapter 9). These patients may develop portal fibrosis, micronodular cirrhosis, or macronodular cirrhosis, sometimes with a rather characteristic hyaline circumferential scarring (Fig. 13).

Metabolic Disorders

Significant hemosiderin deposition (Chapter 11), particularly in parenchymal cells and bile duct epithelium, suggests hemochromatosis but is seen in alcoholic cirrhosis as well. Hepatic siderosis, fibrosis, and cirrhosis are inconstant findings in Zellweger's cerebrohepatic syndrome (Chapter 9). Although stains for copper may be suggestive of Wilson's disease, chemical analysis of fresh tissue for copper is a more reliable method to diagnose excessive hepatic copper deposition (Chapter 9). Abnormal stored materials, such as the carbohydrate of type IV

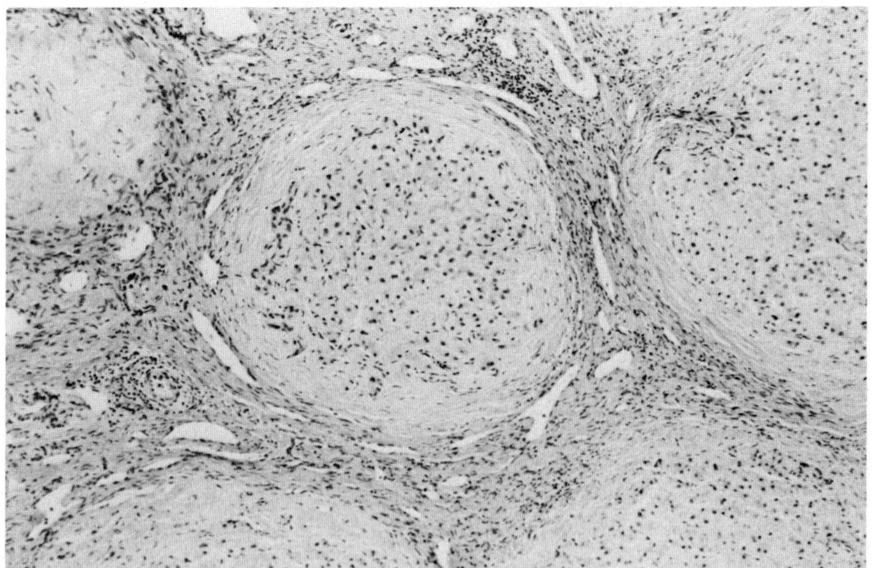

Figure 13. Micronodular cirrhosis in a 3-year-old child with alpha-1-antitrypsin deficiency. Note cellular, hyaline fibrosis surrounding the nodules in a circumferential manner. (Hematoxylin and eosin, ×34.)

glycogen and mucopolysaccharides in hepatocytes or Kupffer cells, suggest a metabolic disorder that must be confirmed by chemical analysis of fresh tissue. Among disorders of lipid metabolism, Gaucher's disease, Niemann-Pick disease, and Wolman's disease may be associated with portal fibrosis and micronodular cirrhosis (Chapter 10). Prominence of lipid-laden lipocytes suggests vitamin A intoxication (Chapter 6, Fig. 5). Fibrosis and cirrhosis may also occur in cystinosis (Chapter 10).

Cholestasis

Cholestasis can be a prominent morphologic feature in hepatic fibrosis and cirrhosis and can indicate activity of the causative hepatocellular lesion, including a broad range of hepatocellular disorders in adults (Chapter 7) or infants (Chapter 8). Cholestasis may also be the result of coexistent extrahepatic obstruction by such lesions as atresia, neoplasms, stones, or parasites. Such a coexistent extrahepatic obstruction may be extremely difficult to diagnose in cirrhosis, as the usual criteria for extrahepatic obstruction involve observation of portal bile ducts which are generally altered, damaged, or destroyed by the cirrhosis. The finding of such parasites as *Clonorchis sinensis* or *Fasciola hepatica* in intrahepatic bile ducts is, of course, of great importance diagnostically (47).

Parasites

Schistosoma mansoni, japonicum, or less commonly, *hematobium,* can cause hepatic lesions. These start as a granulomatous response to ova in the portal triads (Chapter 4). If the infection persists, portal fibrosis develops, probably centered around the portal vein branches. In its most advanced form, this has been called "pipestem cirrhosis" and is associated with portal hypertension. However, true cirrhosis probably does not develop in uncomplicated schistosomiasis. Capillaria hepatica is primarily a rat parasite but occasionally affects humans, usually children. Foreign-body granulomas develop around the ova, which are scattered diffusely through the hepatic parenchyma. Gradually a diffuse fibrosis develops in response to the granulomas. The fibrosis may be quite severe, but true cirrhosis does not seem to have been reported.

Among bacteria, syphilis is one of the few associated with hepatic fibrosis. However, syphilitic lesions of the liver are exceedingly rare nowadays. Congenital syphilis causes diffuse hepatic fibrosis in newborns and infants. The spirochetes are usually demonstrable by silver stains in congenital syphilis and in secondary syphilis in adults (Chapter 3). Tertiary syphilis may cause gummas of the liver. These may heal with the formation of deep, irregular scars.

Granulomatous Hepatitis

Hepatic granulomas (Chapter 4) generally resolve without scarring. Tuberculous and fungal granulomas in the liver rarely caseate and old calcified tubercles, presumably caused by these agents, are rarely found in the liver. Stains for acid-fast bacilli and fungi, as well as culture of biopsy specimens with granulomas, is indicated whenever material is available. Among hepatic granulomas, sarcoidosis appears to be the one most likely to lead to fibrosis, and more rarely to cirrhosis. As cirrhosis develops, the granulomas become less conspicuous and often the cirrhosis in such patients appears quite nonspecific. The diagnosis of cirrhosis related to sarcoidosis may, therefore, have to be made on the basis of previous biopsy specimens showing hepatic granulomas.

Hepatic Infiltrates

Hepatic infiltration with hemopoietic cells, as in lymphomas and leukemias (Chapter 14), is occasionally associated with fibrosis, particularly in Hodgkin's disease of the nodular sclerosis type. The fibrosis in these cases is generally portal. The hepatic extramedullary hemopoiesis of myelofibrosis (agnogenic myeloid metaplasia) is occasionally associated with portal and septal fibrosis and portal hypertension (48).

DEGREE OF ACTIVITY OF CIRRHOSIS

In every case of cirrhosis, the degree of activity of the pathologic process should be assessed. This is done by looking for hepatocellular necrosis or dropout, inflammatory cell infiltration, and Kupffer cell activation. Cirrhosis can thus be classified as inactive or active and activity graded subjectively as mild, moderate, or severe. This morphologic assessment usually corresponds quite well to the severity of the clinical features of liver damage and to the serum biochemistry, particularly the transaminase enzymes and cholestasis. Histologic assessment of activity thus provides some indication of the rate of progression of cirrhosis, and therefore of prognosis. It should be remembered, however, that the apparent activity may be influenced by sampling error and by therapy, particularly steroid administration in chronic active hepatitis.

RELATIONSHIP OF HEPATOCARCINOMA TO CIRRHOSIS

Hepatocellular carcinoma is far more common in patients with cirrhosis than in patients with a normal liver. The incidence of this neoplasm in cirrhosis varies in different parts of the world, with different types of cirrhosis, and with different etiologic factors. As an average figure, it appears that hepatocarcinoma develops in about 10% of cases of cirrhosis (49). It is more common in macronodular cirrhosis than in micronodular cirrhosis. Chronic infection with hepatitis B, alcoholism, and hemochromatosis are among the etiologic factors that have been incriminated. Primary hepatocellular carcinoma is relatively uncommon in primary biliary cirrhosis and in Wilson's disease (50). Because of the increased incidence of hepatocellular carcinoma in cirrhosis, it has been suggested that possible precursor lesions of hepatocarcinoma such as focal liver cell dysplasia (Chapter 14) (51) or hyperplasia (52) be looked for in cirrhotic livers. Metastatic carcinoma from a primary tumor outside the liver is relatively rare in cirrhosis

(53). Therefore, if a carcinoma without special distinguishing features is found in the liver of a patient with cirrhosis, the odds are in favor of its being a hepatocarcinoma rather than a metastasis.

HEPATIC NODULES IN THE NONCIRRHOTIC LIVER

Regenerative Nodules

Neoplastic hepatic nodules are described in Chapter 14. Nodules that do not appear to be neoplastic may be observed in patients with submassive hepatic necrosis, particularly in children (Fig. 14) (53a). Such nodules are usually multi-

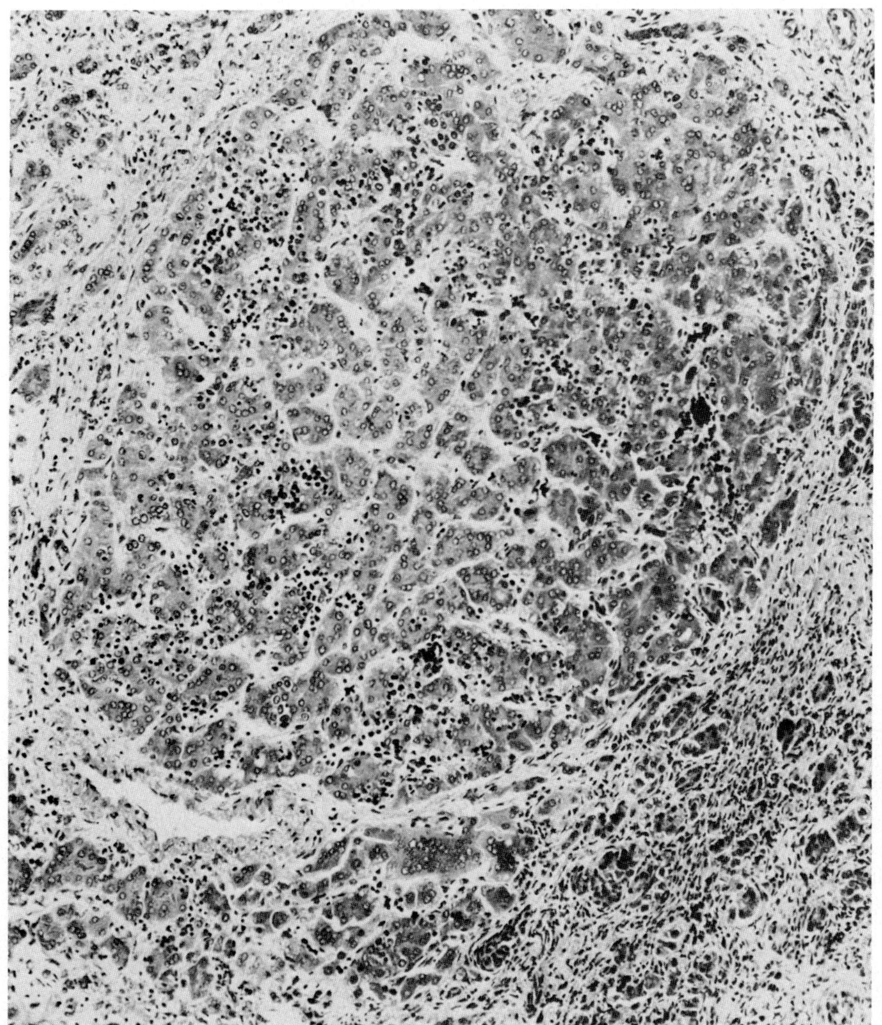

Figure 14. Regenerative nodule in an infant with massive hepatic necrosis. The nodule contains foci of extramedullary hemopoiesis. A multinucleated hepatic giant cell is seen to the left of the nodule (Hematoxylin and eosin, ×150.)

ple, and it seems fair to consider them regenerative in origin. The fate of these nodules is not clear, since most patients who recover from submassive necrosis do so without sequelae (Chapter 2). Similar nodules may also be seen in chronic active hepatitis (Chapter 2), where they probably represent precursors of cirrhosis. In fact, it may often be difficult to be certain whether a patient has chronic active hepatitis with regenerative nodules or cirrhosis with chronic active hepatitis.

Nodular Transformation

Nodular transformation of the liver in the absence of cirrhosis or obvious recent hepatic injury has also been called noncirrhotic nodulation (54), adenomatous hyperplasia (55) or nodular regenerative hyperplasia (55a). This condition is quite rare, but may be insufficiently diagnosed (56,56a). Although there may be a variable amount of fibrosis of the portal triads, there are no fibrous septa. Therefore, this condition or group of conditions does not meet the criteria for cirrhosis outlined above. This condition was probably first described by Steiner (57) as nodular regenerative hyperplasia, particularly in patients with cardiac decompensation. He was uncertain whether this type of nodular transformation might progress to cirrhosis. Similar changes have been observed in the Budd-Chiari syndrome (Chapter 12). More recently, nodular transformation has been reported in association with Felty's syndrome (58), rheumatoid arthritis (59),

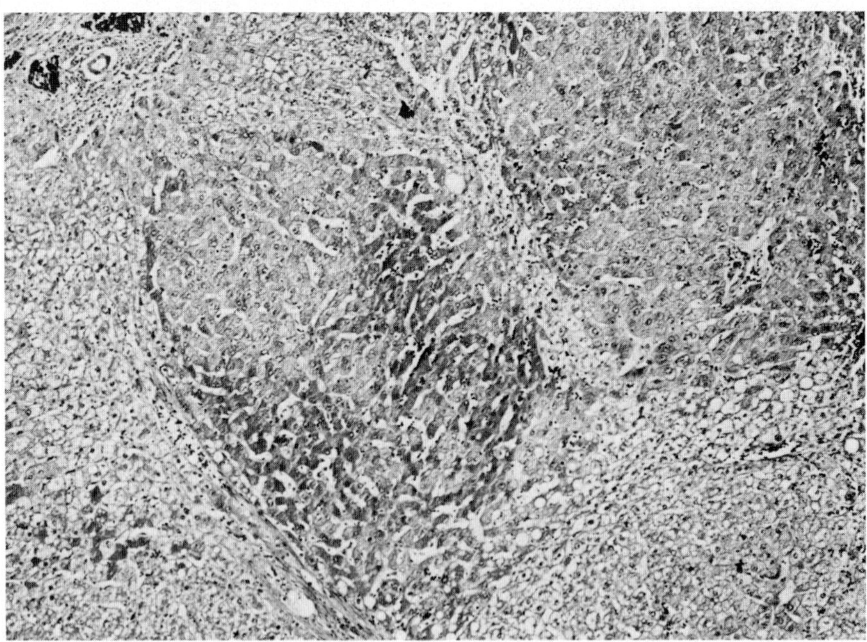

Figure 15. Nodular transformation of hepatocytes, showing two hepatocytic nodules, with no significant deposition of fibrous tissue between the nodules. (Hematoxylin and eosin, ×190.) (Contributed by K. Miyai, M.D., ref. 56.)

myelofibrosis (60), and renal transplantation (60a) in the absence of cardiac decompensation. Most cases have occurred in adults but the disease has been described in childhood (60b). In some cases, nodular transformation does not involve the entire liver, but only the hilar area (61–63). This condition has been termed partial nodular transformation and is of obscure etiology. Some cases may be intermediate between nodular transformation and partial nodular transformation (64). Nodular transformation of the liver may, in some cases, be unassociated with signs or symptoms pointing to hepatic involvement (54,57). However, both complete and partial nodular transformation have been accompanied by portal hypertension (55,58,59,61,63,65).

The liver in nodular transformation may be enlarged (58,61,63) or decreased in size (59). The surface is smooth or granular (66). Nodules up to 1 or 2 cm in diameter can generally be made out on cross section. The smaller nodules are the size of lobules or less, whereas some are much larger. Histologically, these nodules can be seen in hematoxylin and eosin-stained sections, but stand out better in reticulin preparations (Fig. 15). Portal areas are often located at the centers of the nodules. The hepatocytes in the nodules are arranged in plates more than one cell thick. Surrounding the nodules there is usually a rim of compressed hepatocytes. A precise anatomic diagnosis of nodular transformation may be difficult or impossible when only a needle biopsy specimen is available (59,66). This is particularly true in partial nodular transformation. In some cases the distinction of partial nodular transformation from multiple adenomas (Chapter 14) may be difficult (67).

REFERENCES

1. Rojkind M, Giambrone M, Biempica L: Collagen types in normal and cirrhotic liver. *Gastroenterology* 76:710, 1979.

1a. Scheuer PJ, Maggi G: Hepatic fibrosis and collapse. Histological distinction by orcein staining. *Histopathology* 4:487, 1980.

2. Hahn EG, Martini GA: Clinical parameters of fibroplasia. *Ital J Gastroenterol* 12:41, 1980.

3. Popper H, Piez K: Collagen metabolism in the liver. An annotated and supplemented report of a workshop at the National Institutes of Health on February 28th and March 1st, 1977. *Dig Dis* 23:641, 1978.

4. Biempica L, Morecki R, Wu CH, et al: Immunocytochemical localization of Type B collagen. *Am J Pathol* 98:591, 1980.

5. Remberger K, Gay S, Fietzek PP: Immunohistochemical characterization of collagen in cirrhosis. *Virchows Arch [Pathol Anat]* 367(3):231, 1975.

5a. Voss B, Rauterberg J, Allan S, et al: Distribution of collagen type I and type III and of two collagenous components of basement membranes in the human liver. *Pathol Res Pract* 170:50, 1980.

6. Anthony PP, Ishak KG, Nayak NC, et al: The morphology of cirrhosis. *J Clin Pathol* 31:395, 1978.

7. Popper H: Pathologic aspects of cirrhosis. *Am J Pathol* 87(1):228, 1977.

8. Takahashi T: Three-dimensional morphology of the liver in cirrhosis and related disorders. *Virchows Arch [Pathol Anat]* 377:97, 1978.

8a. Schlichting P, Fauerholdt L, Christensen E: Clinical relevance of restrictive morphological criteria for the diagnosis of cirrhosis in liver biopsies. *Liver* 1:56, 1981.

8b. Takahashi T: Topological analysis of the morphogenesis of liver cirrhosis. *Virchows Arch [Pathol Anat]* 377:189, 1978.

9. Galambos JT: Classification of cirrhosis. *Am J Gastroenterol* 64(6):437, 1975.

10. Rojkind M, Dunn MA: Hepatic fibrosis. *Gastroenterology* 76:849, 1979.

11. Campana HA, Park YS, Gourgoutis GD: Congenital hepatic fibrosis. Two cases simulating hepatic cirrhosis. *Dig Dis* 19:325, 1974.

12. Kerr DNS, Okonokwo S, Choa RG: Congenital hepatic fibrosis: the long-term prognosis. *Gut* 19:514, 1978.

12a. Naveh Y, Roguin N, Ludatscher R, et al: Congenital hepatic fibrosis with congenital heart disease. A family study with ultrastructural features of the liver. *Gut* 21:799, 1980.

13. Strayer DS, Kissane JM: Dysplasia of the kidneys, liver and pancreas: Report of a variant of Ivemark's syndrome. *Hum Pathol* 10(2):228, 1979.

13a. Ghishan FK, Younszai MK: Congenital hepatic fibrosis. A disease with diverse manifestations. *Am J Gastro* 75:317, 1981.

13b. Alvarez F, Bernard O, Brunelle F: Congenital hepatic fibrosis in children. *J Ped* 99:370, 1981.

14. Balázs M, Lukács VF, Dénes J, et al: Cholangiodysplastic pseudocirrhosis. *Virchows Arch [Pathol Anat]* 368:61, 1975.

15. Howlett SA, Shulman ST, Ayoub EM, et al: Cholangitis complicating congenital hepatic fibrosis. *Am J Gastroenterol* 73:113, 1980.

16. Daroca PJ, Tuthill R, Reed RJ: Cholangiocarcinoma arising in congenital hepatic fibrosis. *Arch Pathol Lab Med* 99:592, 1975.

17. Scott J, Shousha S, Thomas HC, et al: Bile duct carcinoma. A late complication of congenital hepatic fibrosis. *Am J Gastroenterol* 73:113, 1980.

18. Hodgson HJF, Davies DR, Thompson RPH: Congenital hepatic fibrosis. *J Clin Pathol* 29:11, 1976.

19. Averback P: Congenital hepatic fibrosis. Asymptomatic adults without renal anomaly. *Arch Pathol Lab Med* 101:260, 1977.

20. Habbick BF, Casey R, Zaleski WA, et al: Liver abnormalities in three patients with fetal alcohol syndrome. *Lancet* 1:580, 1979.

21. Lieberman E, Salinas-Madrigal L, Gwinn JL, et al: Infantile polycystic disease of the kidneys and liver: Clinical, pathological and radiological correlations and comparison with congenital hepatic fibrosis. *Medicine* 50:277, 1971.

22. Dupond J, Miguet J, Carbillet J, et al: Kidney polycystic disease in adult congenital hepatic fibrosis. *Ann Intern Med* 88(4):514, 1978.

23. Landing BH, Wells TR, Claireaux AE: Morphometric analysis of liver lesions in cystic diseases of childhood. *Hum Pathol* 11:549, 1980.

24. Nayak NC, Ramalingaswami V: Obliterative portal venopathy of the liver. *Arch Pathol Lab Med* 87:359, 1969.

25. Mikkelsen WP, Edmondson HA, Peters RL, et al: Extra- and intrahepatic portal hypertension without cirrhosis (hepatoportal sclerosis). *Ann Surg* 162:602, 1965.

25a. Kingham JGC, Levison DA, Stansfeld AG, et al: Non-cirrhotic intrahepatic portal hypertension: A long term follow-up study. *QJ Med NS* 199, 259, 1981.

26. Reisman T, Levi JU, Zeppa R, et al: Non-cirrhotic portal hypertension in Felty's syndrome. *Dig Dis* 22(2):145, 1977.

27. Sama SK, Bhargava S, Nath NG, et al: Non-cirrhotic portal fibrosis. *Am J Med* 51:160, 1971.

28. Boyer JL, Hales MR, Klatskin G: "Idiopathic" portal hypertension due to organized thrombi: A study based on postmortem vinylite—injection, corrosion and dissection of the intrahepatic vasculature in 4 cases. *Medicine* 53(1):77, 1974.

29. Bras G: Aspects of hepatic vascular diseases, in Gall EA, Mostofi FK (eds): *The Liver.* Baltimore, Williams & Wilkins, 1973, p 406.

30. Nakata K, Uehara Y, Wada K, et al: Sinusoidal stenosis—the causative anatomical lesion of portal hypertension. *Acta Pathol Jpn* 23(2):225, 1973.

31. Nataf C, Feldmann G, Lebrec D, et al: Idiopathic portal hypertension (perisinusoidal fibrosis) after renal transplantation. *Gut* 20:531, 1979.

32. Nakanuma Y, Yamatami M, Ohta G, et al: Intrahepatic bile duct lesions in idiopathic portal hypertension. *Jpn J Gastroenterol* 77:603, 1980.

33. Huet PM, Guillaume E, Côté J, et al: Non-cirrhotic presinusoidal portal hypertension associated with chronic arsenical intoxication. *Gastroenterology* 68(5):1270, 1975.

34. Morris JS, Schmid M, Newman S, et al: Arsenic and non-cirrhotic portal hypertension. *Gastroenterology* 66:86, 1974.

35. Blendis LM, Smith PK, Lawrie BW, et al: Portal hypertension in vinyl chloride monomer workers. *Gastroenterology* 75:206, 1978.

36. Smith PM, Crossley IR: Portal hypertension in vinyl-chloride production workers. *Lancet* 2:602, 1976.

37. Telles NC, Thomas LB, Popper H, et al: Evolution of thorotrast-induced hepatic angiosarcomas. *Environ Res* 18:74, 1979.

38. Lascari AD, Givler RL, Soper RT, et al: Portal hypertension in a case of acute leukemia treated with antimetabolites for 10 years. *N Engl J Med* 279:303, 1968.

39. Datta DV, Mitra SK, Chuttani PN, et al: Chronic oral arsenic intoxication as a possible aetological factor in idiopathic portal hypertension (noncirrhotic portal fibrosis) in India. *Gut* 20:378, 1979.

40. Rubin E, Krus S, Popper H: Pathogenesis of postnecrotic cirrhosis in alcoholics. *Arch Pathol Lab Med* 73:288, 1962.

41. Gall EA: Posthepatitic, postnecrotic, and nutritional cirrhosis. *Am J Pathol* 36:3241, 1960.

42. Falchuk KR, Fiske SC, Haggit RC, et al: Pericentral hepatic fibrosis and intracellular hyalin in diabetes mellitus. *Gastroenterology* 78:535, 1980.

42a. Psachrapoulos HT, Howard ER, Portmann B, et al: Hepatic complications of cystic fibrosis. *Lancet* i:78, 1981.

43. Roberts WC: The hepatic cirrhosis in cystic fibrosis of the pancreas. *Am J Med* 32:324, 1962.

44. Stern RC, Stevens DP, Boat TF, et al: Symptomatic hepatic disease in cystic fibrosis. Incidence, course and outcome of hepatic shunting. *Gastroenterology* 70:645, 1976.

45. Isenberg JN, L'Heureux PR, Warwick WJ, et al: Clinical observations on the biliary system in cystic fibrosis. *Am J Gastroenterol* 65:134, 1976.

46. Altman AR, Gottfried EB, Paronetto F, et al: Idiopathic familial cirrhosis and steatosis in adults. *Gastroenterology* 77:1211, 1979.

47. Sullivan WG, Koep LJ: Common bile duct obstruction and cholangiohepatitis in clonorchiasis. *JAMA* 243:2060, 1980.

48. Ruebner B: Myelosclerosis with serosal myeloid metaplasia and fatal liver involvement. *Ann Intern Med* 53:1075, 1960.

49. Miyai K, Ruebner BH: Acute yellow atrophy, cirrhosis and hepatoma. *Arch Pathol Lab Med* 75:609, 1963.

50. Sternlieb I: Copper and the liver. *Gastroenterology* 78:1615, 1980.

50a. Mallet L, Petite JP, Amat D, et al: Carcinome hepatocellulaire au cours de la cirrhose biliaire primitive. *Gastroent Clin Biol* 5:379, 1981.

51. Anthony PP: Precursor lesions for liver cancer in humans. *Cancer Res* 36:2579, 1976.

52. Peters RL: Pathology of hepatocellular carcinoma, in Okuda K, Peters RL (eds): *Hepatocellular Carcinoma.* New York, Wiley, 1976, p 107.

53. Ruebner BH, Green R, Miyai K, et al: The paucity of intrahepatic metastasis in cirrhosis of the liver. *Am J Pathol* 39:739, 1961.

53a. Ruebner BH, Bhagavan BS, Greenfield AJ, et al: Neonatal hepatic necrosis. *Pediatrics* 43:963, 1969.

54. Smith JC: Non-cirrhotic nodulation of the liver. *Arch Pathol Lab Med* 102:398, 1978.

55. Gindhart TD, Cimis RJ, Mosenthal WT, et al: Adenomatous hyperplasia of the liver. *Arch Pathol Lab Med* 103:34, 1979.

55a. Guarda LA, Hales MR: Nodular regenerative hyperplasia of the liver: Report of two cases and review of the literature. *J Clin Gastroenterol* 3:193, 1981.

56. Miyai K, Bonin ML: Nodular regenerative hyperplasia of the liver. Report of 3 cases and review of the literature. *Am J Clin Pathol* 73:267, 1980.

56a. Stromeyer FW, Ishak KG: Nodular transformation (nodular "regenerative" hyperplasia) of the liver. *Human Pathol* 12:60, 1981.

57. Steiner PE: Nodular regenerative hyperplasia of the liver. *Am J Pathol* 35(5):943, 1959.

58. Blendis L: Nodular regenerative hyperplasia of the liver in Felty's syndrome. *Q J Med* 169:25, 1974.

59. Harris M, Rash RM, Dymock IW: Nodular, non-cirrhotic liver associated with portal hypertension in a patient with rheumatoid arthritis. *J Clin Pathol* 27:963, 1974.

60. Shorey J, Weinberg MN, Frenkel EP, et al: Nodular regenerative hyperplasia of the liver in a case of myelofibrosis with extramedullary hematopoiesis and secondary portal venous hypertension. *Am J Clin Pathol* 72:122, 1979.

60a. Bredtfeldt JE, Havey AL: Nodular regenerative hyperplasia of the liver following renal transplantation. *Dig Dis Sci* 26:271, 1981.

60b. Alperstein G, Kahn E, Aiges H, et al: Nodular regenerative hyperplasia of the liver. An unusual cause of portal hypertension in childhood. *Am J Dis Child* 135:572, 1981.

61. Sherlock S, Feldman A, Moran B, et al: Partial nodular transformation of the liver with portal hypertension. *Am J Med* 4:195, 1966.

62. Variend S: An unusual nodular lesion of the liver: Probable partial nodular transformation. *Histopathology* 2:363, 1978.

63. Classen M, Elster K, Pesch HJ, et al: Portal hypertension caused by partial nodular transformation of the liver. *Gut* 11(3):245, 1970.

64. Shedlovski S, Koehler RE, DeSchriver-Kecskemeti K, et al: Non-cirrhotic nodular transformation of the liver with portal hypertension. Clinical, angiographic and pathological correlation. *Gastroenterology* 79:938, 1980.

65. Connolly CE, O'Brien MJ: Nodular transformation of the liver:Report of a case. *Hum Pathol* 8:350, 1977.

66. Rougier P, DeGott C, Reuff B, et al: Nodular regenerative hyperplasia of the liver. *Gastroenterology* 75:169, 1978.

67. Liu AK, Hiratzka LF, Hirose FM: Multiple adenomas of the liver. *Cancer* 45:1001, 1980.

14
Space-Occupying Lesions of the liver

GENERAL APPROACH

Space-occupying lesions in the liver are encountered clinically under a great variety of circumstances. No hepatic abnormality may be demonstrated either clinically or as judged by laboratory tests. In such patients, the lesion(s) tend to be found incidentally or when looking for metastases at laparotomy or when a hepatic scan is performed. In other patients, attention may be drawn to space occupying lesions by hepatomegaly; a mass, pain, discomfort, or tenderness in the liver. Jaundice with conjugated hyperbilirubinemia, although usually a relatively late finding, may also be the presenting feature (1,1a). Elevation of the serum alkaline phosphatase, however, is often seen relatively early. A vascular, space-occupying, hepatic lesion with an alpha-fetoprotein of more than 500 ng is virtually diagnostic of a hepatocarcinoma. Polycythemia, hypertension, hypoglycemia, hypercalcemia, precocious puberty, and gynecomastia in patients with a hepatic mass would suggest a malignant hepatocellular tumor with endocrine activity (2). The carcinoid syndrome, of course, is suggestive of a metastatic hepatic carcinoid tumor. However, a primary hepatocarcinoma producing the carcinoid syndrome has been described (3). If fever is present, this would suggest that the mass has an infectious etiology. A history of foreign travel as well as the duration of the illness may also be important in the differential diagnosis.

A hepatic space-occupying mass, detected and localized radiologically or by some other method, generally can be definitively diagnosed only by biopsy. If a percutaneous biopsy is performed, the site of entry and direction of the needle should be chosen carefully with regard both to the localization of the tumor, as well as to the hazards of the route selected (4). In one group of cancer patients, percutaneous-directed transthoracic right-lobe and subcostal left-lobe biopsies were performed after death, immediately before autopsy. The biopsies were serially sectioned. One of the two biopsies was positive in 58% of patients with hepatic neoplastic involvement. Multiple directed biopsies are, therefore, indicated when searching for a focal lesion. When a space occupying lesion is suspected but not found in the first sections, step sections at multiple levels should be obtained. Among the few contraindications to needle biopsy is the suspicion that one may be dealing with hydatid disease or with a highly vascular lesion, such as a hemangioma. Guided fine needle aspiration biopsy is highly recommended for the diagnosis of space-occupying lesions because of its accuracy and safety (4a).

Laparoscopy combined with liver biopsy in the hands of an experienced operator is undoubtedly preferable to percutaneous biopsy when a focal lesion is suspected. Bagley et al. (5) found that in patients with Hodgkin's disease, the yield of positive biopsies was doubled by performing peritoneoscopy or laparotomy after a negative percutaneous biopsy. Excisional or incisional biopsy is indicated when focal lesions are encountered during laparotomy. Excisional biopsy may be performed for benign lesions and partial hepatectomy for malignant tumors, once a diagnosis has been made by previous needle biopsy or by frozen section while the patient is undergoing laparotomy. Space-occupying hepatic lesions are most commonly neoplastic (6–9). A unified approach to hepatic resection has been described by Joishy and Balasegaram (10) (Chapter 1).

NEOPLASTIC SPACE-OCCUPYING LESIONS

Metastatic Tumors

Undoubtedly, the most common malignant neoplasms encountered are metastatic carcinomas, particularly from the gastrointestinal tract. Most frequently these manifest themselves as multiple nodules in a noncirrhotic, although often greenish, liver. Occasionally, however, there may be a single solitary, metastatic nodule. Such nodules are now frequently diagnosed early enough to be still resectable (Fig. 1). Diffuse metastatic spread to the liver is rare. It results in a finely granular appearance that grossly resembles cirrhosis and may be associated with portal hypertension (11,12). Whitish fibrous tumors are most likely metastatic carcinoma or cholangiocarcinoma, rather than hepatocarcinoma. Hemorrhagic tumors are most likely hepatocarcinoma, hemangiosarcoma, or metastatic choriocarcinoma. Metastatic colonic adenocarcinoma may undergo calcification and may be visible on x-ray films (8). Melanomas are often intensely black. Biliary cirrhosis is rare in association with hepatic cancers, probably because patients with extrahepatic biliary obstruction due to carcinoma do not survive long enough to develop biliary cirrhosis. Surgical staging systems for cancer of the liver, both primary and metastatic, have been developed 13,13a). In one of these (13a) stage I disease is limited to the resected portion of the liver without involvement of the margins of resection, vascular, or biliary structures. In stage II there is residual hepatic disease, vascular or biliary involvement, direct extension to adjacent structures, or tumor rupture. Stage III disease is defined as distant metastasis.

The histologic distinction of primary malignant hepatic tumors from metastatic lesions is generally relatively easy. This is particularly true if the lesion is of hepatocellular origin, or if it is obviously metastatic, as in a mucin-secreting colonic adenocarcinoma (Fig. 2). Sometimes a complete metastatic workup with laparotomy is required to find the primary tumor. On a purely histologic basis the distinction between cholangiocarcinomas and metastatic pancreatic duct tumors, for instance, is virtually impossible. Because of recent improvements in surgery, chemotherapy, radiation, and hormonal therapy, the identification of

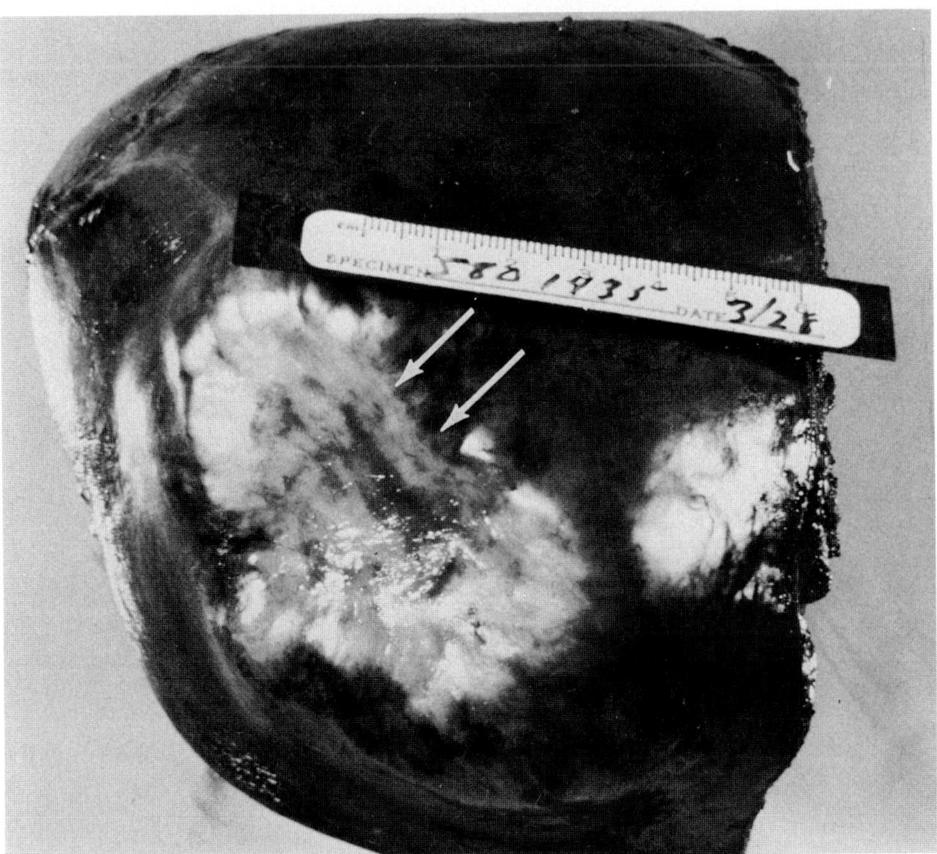

Figure 1. Gross photograph of a specimen from right hepatectomy for a solitary metastasis (arrows) from a colonic carcinoma. Note the centrally depressed (umbilicated) appearance of the metastasis. The white spot on the right of the metastatic deposit is a reflected highlight. The liver between the nodules appears normal, and the margin of excision seems uninvolved.

the site of origin of hepatic metastatic tumors has become much more crucial. The pathologist is frequently asked to suggest, on histologic grounds, the most probably primary sites so that the metastatic workup can be directed at the organs most likely to be involved. Morphologic identification of a hepatic neoplasm often requires special stains such as mucicarmine or PAS. The Grimelius stain is positive in many hormone secreting tumors, particularly metastatic carcinoids. In addition, immunohistochemistry for B-cell surface markers is very helpful in non-Hodgkin's lymphoma. Lymphomas very rarely involve only the liver, but such cases have been described (14,15). Immunohistochemical demonstration of alpha-fetoprotein and antitrypsin may be very helpful in identifying hepatocellular neoplasms. Fresh tissue from hepatic tumors should always be fixed for electron microscopy and embedded and sectioned if this approach seems likely to prove helpful. One group of tumors in which electron microscopy is particularly helpful are apudomas, including carcinoids, since they contain characteristic granules.

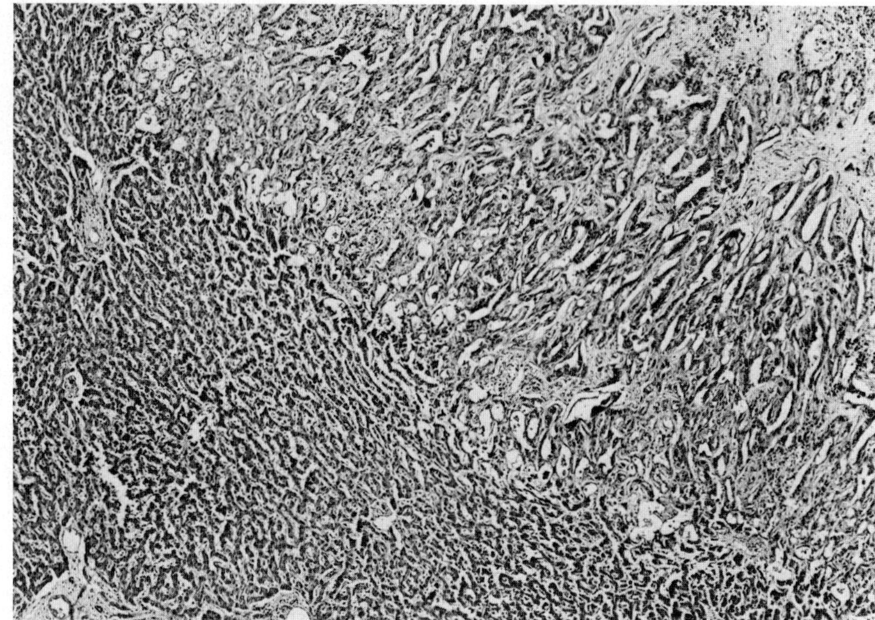

Figure 2. Metastatic adenocarcinoma from the gastrointestinal tract. (Hematoxylin an eosin, ×40.)

Hepatocellular Neoplasms and Neoplasm-like Lesions

Since our understanding of the nature of many of these lesions is inadequate, a generally accepted nomenclature for them is lacking (6,7,16–18). There has been much confusion because many synonyms exist for several of these lesions. This is particularly true of benign hepatocellular lesions, such as hepatocellular adenoma and focal nodular hyperplasia. It seems likely that these two hepatic lesions have sometimes been confused in the literature. Perhaps it would be better to adapt to human hepatic pathology a nomenclature devised for the rat that divides proliferations of hepatocytes into neoplastic nodules and hepatocarcinoma (19). Until such time as a rational nomenclature for hepatic tumors can be devised, an empirical classification has to be adopted, using those terms that are currently most popular. Several excellent reviews have dealt with the subject of hepatocellular neoplasia (6,7,17,18).

Benign Hepatocellular Nodules

Scattered regenerative nodules may be seen after submassive necrosis (Chapter 13, Fig. 14). Diffuse nodular transformation of virtually the entire liver is most commonly seen in cirrhosis. Complete and partial nodular transformation without fibrosis is quite rare. These lesions have been described earlier (Chapter 13, Fig. 15).

Hepatocellular Adenomas

These are focal lesions that apparently have become more frequent recently. They usually occur in women during the reproductive years, and most patients are known to have been on steroid contraceptives (20–25). Some of these lesions, however, are not associated with contraceptive use. A few have been reported in patients with glycogen storage disease (26), diabetes (27), and iron overload (27a). However, it has been claimed that the lesions associated with glycogen storage are not adenomas but represent focal nodular hyperplasia (28).

Attention may be drawn to adenomas by a mass or pain in the region of the liver or by intra-abdominal hemorrhage and shock. This last presentation is the result of tumor necrosis and rupture and is seen typically in women on contraceptive steroids. Rupture of the liver in the absence of neoplasia may also occur in eclampsia or as a complication of oral anticoagulants (29). Adenomas may also be found incidentally at laparotomy. These lesions may appear as a defect on hepatic scintiscans but occasionally may show normal uptake. Adenomas are usually single (Figs. 3,4), but in a quarter of the cases they are multiple (8,8a). The number of nodules, however, is generally much less than in partial nodular transformation (Chapter 13). Sometimes, however, there may be so many nodules that this distinction becomes difficult (30). The nodules rarely measure more than 25 cm in diameter and are yellow to light brown and well circumscribed. They have an abundant blood supply. Areas of hemorrhage and necrosis are quite common but are virtually limited to adenomas in women who had been on contraceptives.

Microscopically, the tumors consist of hepatocytes that resemble quite closely those of the surrounding normal liver (Fig. 5) (31). Because of this, and because a capsule is usually lacking, it may be difficult to define clearly the border between the adenoma and normal liver. The neoplastic hepatocytes, as well as their nuclei and nucleoli, tend to be slightly larger than normal hepatocytes, and their cytoplasm frequently is rather pale because of increased glycogen or fatty change. Mitotic figures are very rare. The neoplastic hepatocytes are arranged in plates one to three cells thick, separated by sinuses lined by inconspicuous sinusoidal lining cells. Occasionally they are arranged in a pseudoglandular or acinar pattern. Bile plugs may be seen in these tumors. Eosinophilic droplets of PAS-positive diastase resistant material, identified histochemically as alpha-1-antitrypsin, have been demonstrated in the hepatocytes composing many of these lesions, even though the patients did not have alpha-1-antitrypsin deficiency (32). The significance of this finding is not clear (33). Extramedullary hemopoiesis may occasionally be seen in these neoplasms (34). Whereas they have no true capsule, they are often surrounded by a pseudocapsule of compressed normal liver lobules. Arteries, veins, and occasional slender fibrous septa have been seen within the lesions, but bile ducts and ductules are absent.

Hemorrhagic necrosis is often seen in the centers of the adenomas (Fig. 4). In the great majority of cases, hepatocellular adenomas can be distinguished with confidence from hepatocarcinomas. Hepatocellular adenomas differ from well-differentiated hepatocellular carcinomas in the scarcity of nuclear atypism or mitotic figures in only slight enlargement of nucleoli and, most importantly, in the absence of a true trabecular pattern (see p. 246) and vascular invasion. Withdrawal of the hormone responsible usually, but not always, induces regression of the adenoma (35,36). Although these lesions may recur after resection, malignant transformation is rare (25).

The hepatic lesions seen in patients on androgenic anabolic hormones differ

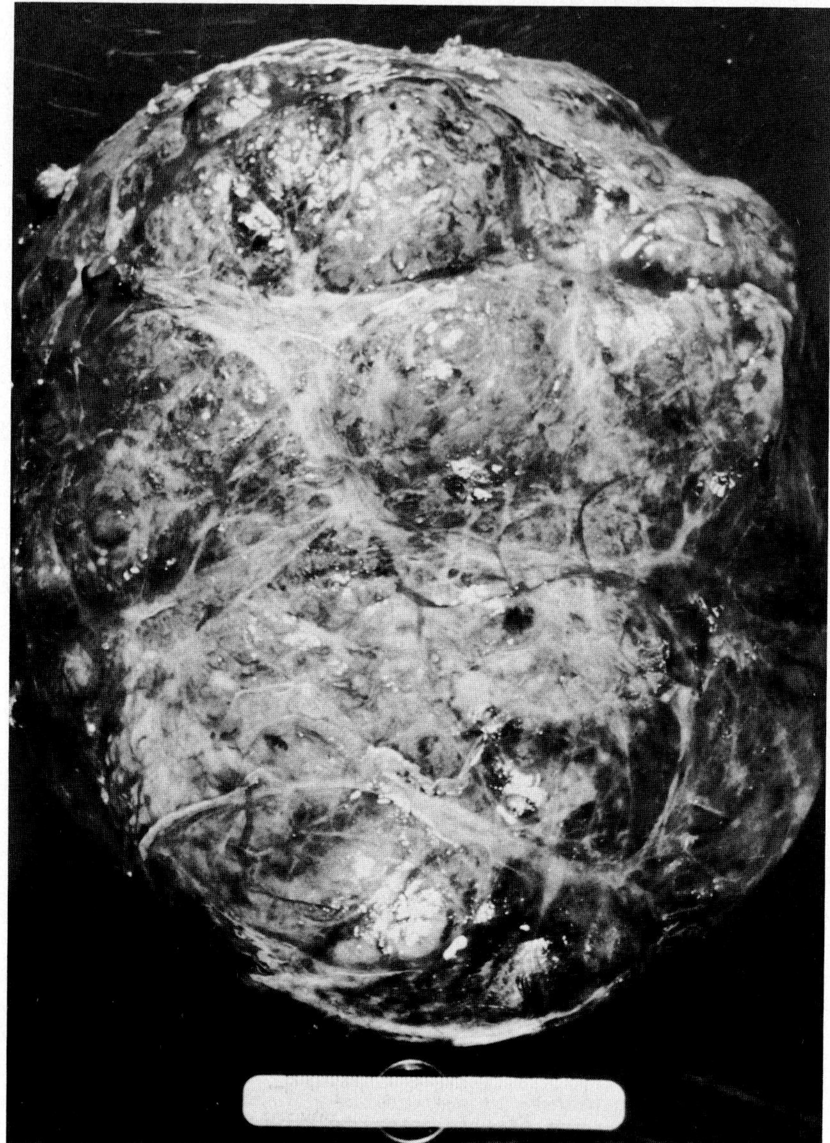

Figure 3. Gross photograph of a hepatic adenoma from a 14-year-old girl. (Contributed by W. M. Christopherson, M.D.)

from those associated with contraceptives in several respects. Grossly, they tend to be greenish, and histologically, they frequently show atypia and a trabecular or glandular pattern. However, some of these tumors appear to have regressed after hormone withdrawal, and metastases have been very rare. Nevertheless, because of their histology (Fig. 6), most of these lesions have been called hepatocarcinomas (25,37–40).

Focal Fatty Change

Nodules have been described measuring up to 4 cm in diameter and composed of hepatocytes showing marked fatty change. Their pathogenesis is obscure but

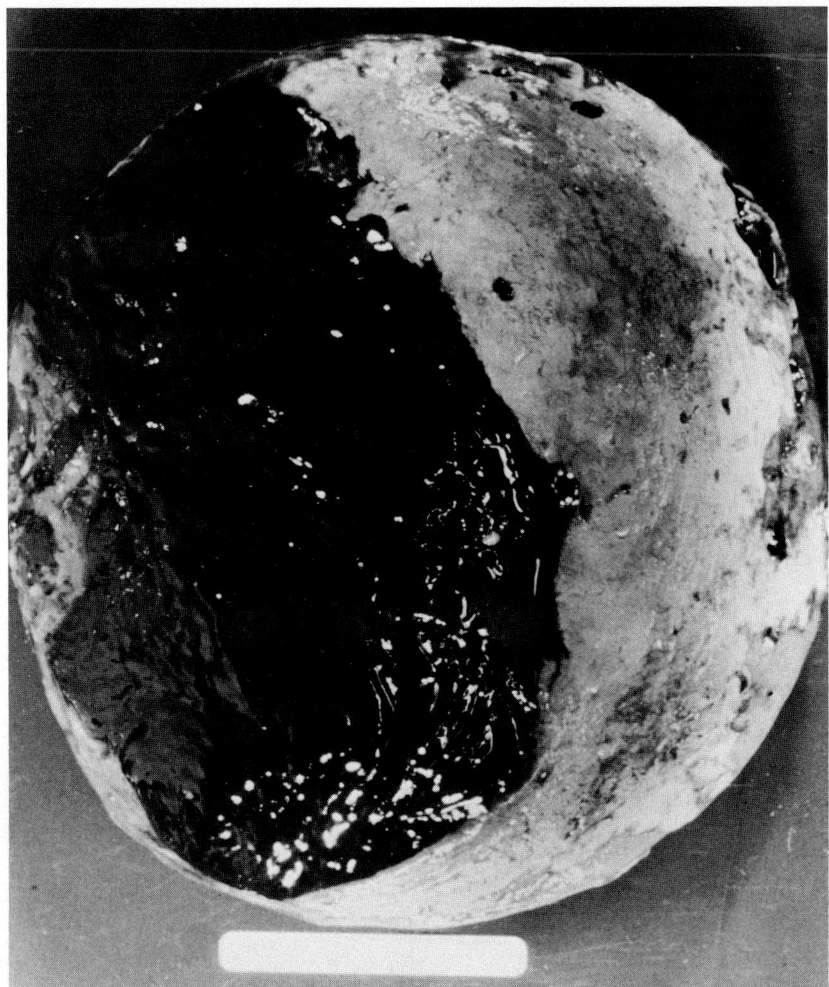

Figure 4. Gross photograph of same tumor shown in Figure 3 in a cross section showing hemorrhage. (Contributed by W. M. Christopherson, M.D. (8a).

they have to be considered in the differential diagnosis of space-occupying lesions (41).

Focal Nodular Hyperplasia

The origin of this lesion is uncertain. It may be congenital, in which case the correct name for this lesion might be epithelial hamartoma. The occasional finding of hemangiomas or other vascular anomalies in this lesion suports the congenital theory, at least in some cases (42,42a). Alternatively, the lesion may be acquired. The hepatic nodules not uncommonly seen in glycogen storage disease may be focal nodular hyperplasia (28). Because of the uncertain etiology of this lesion, the noncommital term focal nodular hyperplasia is preferred over others. such as focal cirrhosis, hepatic hamartoma, and adenoma (8,20–24). The age range of focal nodular hyperplasia is wider than that of hepatic adenoma. Its female to male ratio is 2:1 and it is observed from infancy to old age (42b). In the

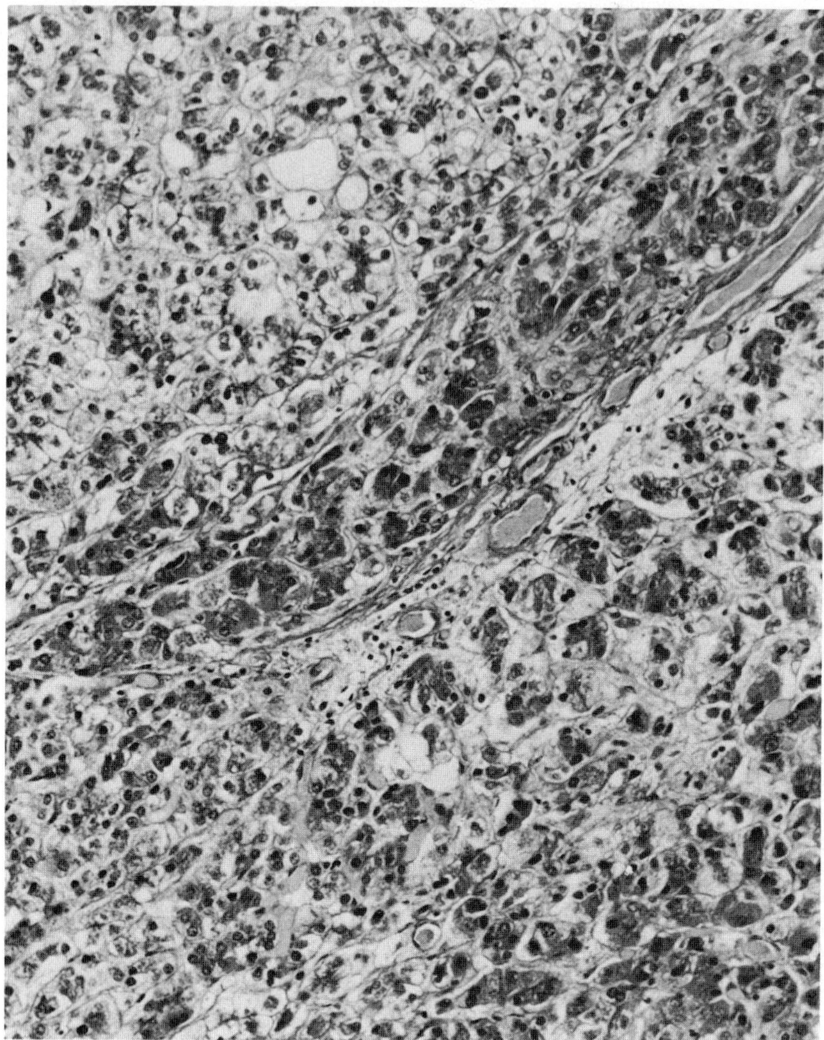

Figure 5. A hepatic adenoma is shown in the upper part of this micrograph. Note the general resemblance of this lesion to normal liver, except for the absence of a normal lobular and plate pattern. Note the compressed normal liver at the periphery of the adenoma, lower right. (Hematoxylin and eosin, ×197.) (Contributed by W. M. Christopherson, M.D.)

great majority of cases, this lesion is discovered incidentally at laparotomy and may be mistaken grossly for a hepatic metastasis in a patient with a carcinoma. Only 20% of patients with this lesion have symptoms, usually pain, tenderness, or a mass. One patient with this lesion had hypertension and renin secretion (43). The relationship of focal nodular hyperplasia to contraceptive steroids is disputed (16,21,44,45). However, if there is a relationship, it must be less close than that between hepatic adenoma and contraceptives. Eighty percent of these lesions are single (8). Grossly, they are gray-white to tan and tend to be paler and more firm than the surrounding liver. The nodules are generally located just

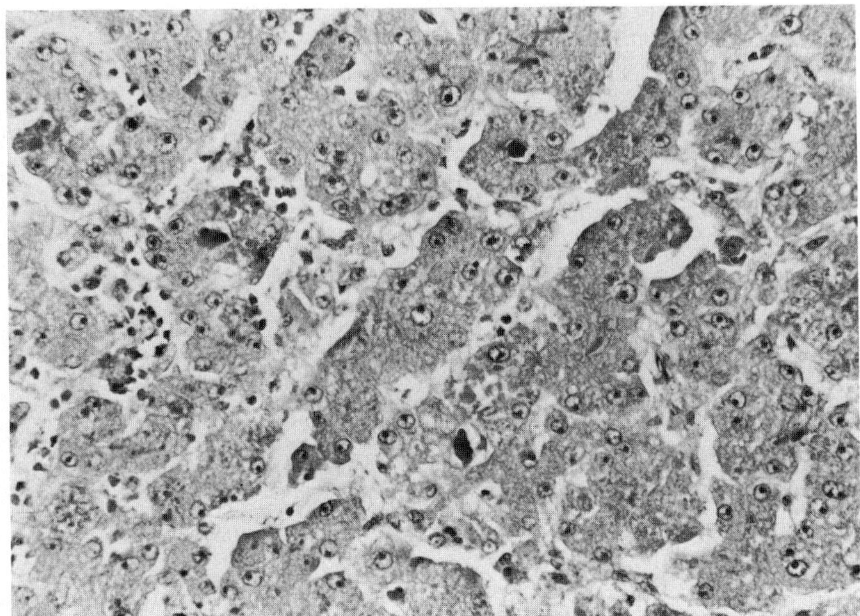

Figure 6. Hepatocellular tumor associated with androgen administration for Fanconi's anemia. The tumor shows an abnormal hepatic plate pattern, suggestive of a trabecular arrangement, as well as some cytologic atypia. (Hematoxylin and eosin, ×85.)

beneath the capsule (Fig. 7). They may measure up to 15 cm in diameter and rarely weigh more than 700 g. On cut section the nodules bulge slightly above the cut surface. They generally have a central scar from which fine septa radiate to the periphery to subdivide the lesion.

Microscopically, focal nodular hyperplasia differs from hepatic adenoma in having wide collagenous septa radiating from a central scar (Fig. 8). Another difference is that the septa contain not only veins and arteries, but bile ducts or ductules as well. Scanty inflammatory cells are often seen in the septa as well as in the parenchyma. Occasionally, however, focal inflammation is intense and is associated with piecemeal necrosis (Chapter 2). The hepatocytes are generally quite similar to those of the surrounding normal liver, but a few cases with cytologic atypia and Mallory's hyalin have been reported. In some cases the atypia has been severe enough for a diagnosis of hepatocellular carcinoma (46). Alpha-1-antitrypsin droplets have been demonstrated in many of these lesions, just as in hepatic adenomas (32). Necrosis and hemorrhage, which are frequent in adenomas, do not usually occur in focal nodular hyperplasia. Because of the limited amount of tissue available, this diagnosis may be very difficult if only a needle biopsy specimen is available.

Hepatocellular Carcinoma

This is the most common malignant hepatocellular neoplasm, except in the pediatric age group, in which hepatoblastoma is more frequent. The terms hepatocellular carcinoma or hepatocarcinoma (HCC) are more precise than are such designations as liver carcinoma or hepatoma and are, therefore, preferred.

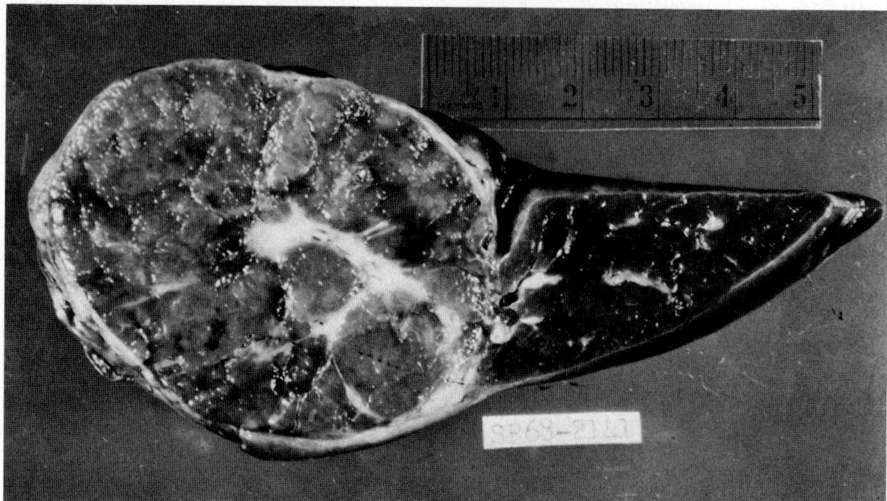

Figure 7. Gross photograph of focal nodular hyperplasia.

Etiology. Hepatocarcinoma, like cirrhosis, differs strikingly in incidence in different areas of the world. For example, it is particularly common in certain parts of Africa and Asia (47). The incidence of this tumor may differ strikingly, even in populations of identical ethnic backgrounds located in different countries. It seems clear that environmental factors must be responsible for these striking differences. Cirrhosis, predominantly of the postnecrotic variety, is found in 60% (48) or more of patients with hepatocarcinoma. Those patients who do not have cirrhosis generally have at least some fibrosis and inflammation, but lack regenerative nodules (48). It seems probable that it is not the cirrhosis that predisposes to hepatocarcinoma, but that the same etiologic factors may produce cirrhosis and HCC in some patients and HCC with fibrosis but without cirrhosis in others.

The environmental factors responsible for the great majority of hepatocarcinomas have not yet been conclusively identified. In Africa and Asia, the principal suspects are type B hepatitis (49) and aflatoxins (50), toxic substances produced by *Aspergillus flavus*, a food spoilage fungus. The United States and Western Europe are areas of relatively low incidence, and there hepatitis B (51) and alcohol (52) appear, at present, the most likely etiologic agents. Autoimmune chronic active hepatitis is rarely associated with this tumor (52a,b). Hepatocellular carcinoma has also been reported after hepatic irradiation (53), thorotrast (54), and methotrexate therapy (55). A few cases have been reported in women on long term oral contraceptives (25,56–59). Hepatocellular tumors, most of which were considered to be malignant, have also been observed in patients with anemia treated with androgens. These neoplasms are often multiple and develop in normal livers (p. 237–238).

A relatively small proportion of hepatocarcinomas develop in patients with a variety of congenital hepatic anomalies, metabolic errors, and neonatal liver disease (Chapters 9–11). The most common of these appears to be deficiency of alpha-1-antitrypsin, particularly the severe homozygous variety. However, the heterozygous types, such as MZ, have also been suspected (60,61). There is little

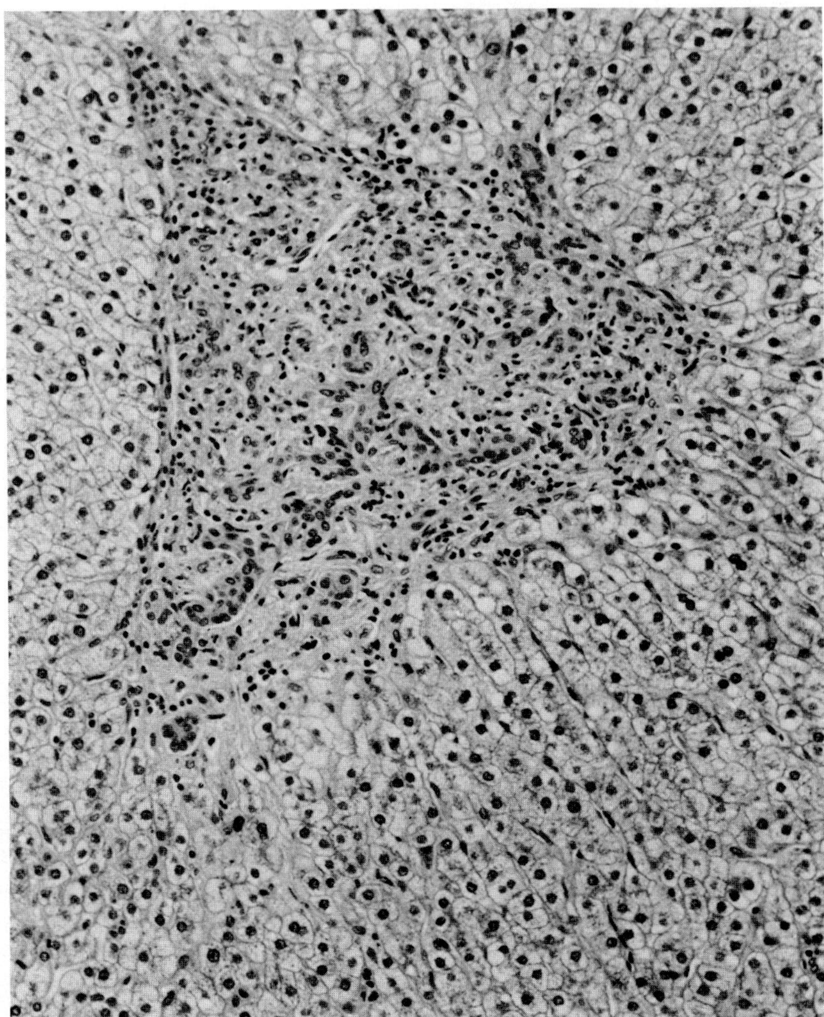

Figure 8. Focul nodular hyperplasia. Note the fibrous strand in the center of the lesion containing blood vessels and bile ductules. (Hematoxylin and eosin, ×197.) (Contributed by W. M. Christoperson, M.D.)

doubt that patients with hemochromatosis have a high risk of developing hepatocarcinoma. Even venesection, which can deplete hepatic iron stores and induce regression of hepatic fibrosis, seems incapable of preventing the development of hepatocarcinoma (62). Tyrosinemia (63), cystinosis (9), hemihypertrophy (6), cerebral gigantism (64), ataxia-telangiectasia (64a), glycogenosis type 1 (26), biliary atresia (65), neonatal hepatitis (65), Byler's disease (66,66a) and, rarely, Wilson's disease (9,67) and primary biliary cirrhosis (67a) have also been reported in association with hepatocarcinoma.

Preneoplastic Changes. Preneoplastic microscopic changes have frequently been described in hepatocytes during experimental carcinogenesis (19). Altered microscopic foci and grossly visible nodules are diffusely distributed throughout

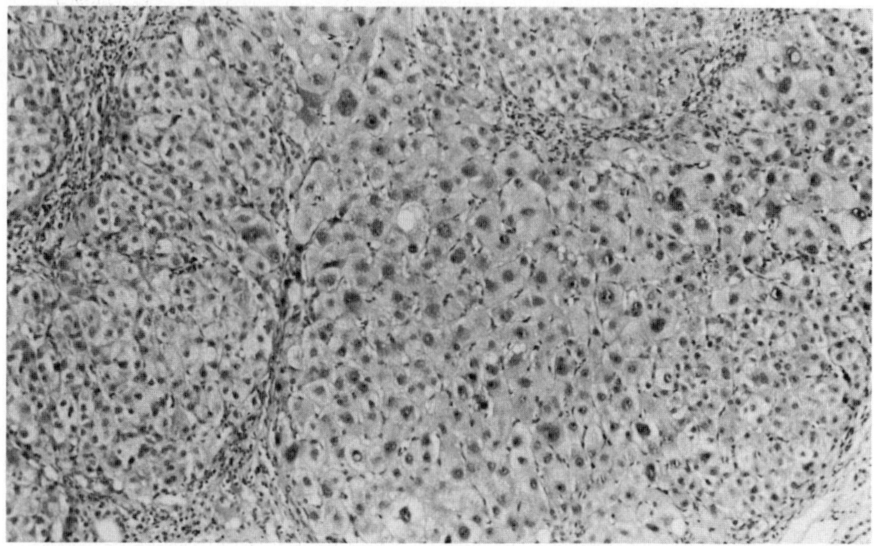

Figure 9. Liver cell dysplasia in a patient with cirrhosis. Note nuclear enlargement with prominent nucleoli and pleomorphism affecting many of the nuclei in this cirrhotic nodule. (Hematoxylin and eosin, ×85.)

such livers before the development of hepatocarcinomas, which may be single or multiple. Preneoplastic hepatocellular changes in man are less clearly established. Anthony has defined liver cell dysplasia as hepatocellular enlargement, nuclear pleomorphism, and multinucleation of liver cells in foci or in entire cirrhotic nodules. This change has been considered precancerous (Fig. 9) (68,69). Peters has described a different type of focal change, which he termed adenomatous. These foci are rounded but poorly defined and contain eosinophilic hepatocytes with relatively uniform nuclei. We have seen somewhat similar scattered foci composed of clear hepatocytes in a patient on androgens in whom hepatocellular neoplasms developed (38). Further studies are required to clarify the morphology of human hepatic preneoplasia.

Symptoms. The most common early symptoms in patients with hepatocarcinoma are abdominal discomfort, pain, and malaise. In about 10% of cases, jaundice is present (70,71). The clinical picture of hepatocarcinoma may, therefore, resemble closely that of chronic hepatitis or cirrhosis. An abdominal mass is felt in only 10% of cases. In patients known to have cirrhosis, sudden clinical deterioration must always make one suspect the development of hepatocarcinoma. Portal hypertension may develop in patients with hepatocellular carcinoma, even in the absence of cirrhosis (71a).

Hepatocarcinomas are accompanied not uncommonly by systemic manifestations (6,72), such as hypercalcemia (particularly in the sclerosing type), polycythemia, precocious puberty, gynecomastia, hypoglycemia, hypercholesterolemia, hypertriglyceridemia, porphyria cutanea tarda, abnormalities of fibrinogen or alkaline phosphatase, aldolase, and even the carcinoid syndrome. For diagnosis, the most important manifestation is the secretion of alphafetoprotein. Significant elevations of this protein are found in 50–70% of patients with hepatocarcinoma. It is generally accepted that a significant elevation of 500 ng/ml (73,74) or more in a patient with a vascular hepatic tumor is virtually diagnostic of hepatocarcinoma.

Gross Findings. Most hepatocarcinomas arise in livers with cirrhosis, predominantly of the macronodular type. The liver is frequently green because of cholestasis. Hepatocarcinomas may vary in gross appearance (7). They may present as a single mass or several adjacent masses (Fig. 10), most commonly in the right lobe. If the tumor is located near the hilum, it may present with obstructive jaundice. The tumor may also be multinodular at the time of diagnosis, again most frequently in the right lobe. The third type is diffuse and hardly ever occurs in a noncirrhotic liver. In this variety, the tumor nodules are dispersed among the cirrhotic nodules, from which they are difficult to distinguish. Generally, the tumors are grey to light brown or hemorrhagic but may also appear green. A few hepatocarcinomas are grossly pale and hard because of diffuse fibrosis (6). Grossly, this sclerosing type resembles a metastatic scirrhous carcinoma or a cholangiocarcinoma. The gross features of metastatic cancer are discussed in more detail on p. 234 and those of cholangiocarcinoma on p. 255. Attempts to classify hepatocarcinoma grossly according to the above classification into massive, nodular, and diffuse are frequently difficult, frustrating, and ultimately arbitrary. This may be explained by the fact that human hepatocarcinomas are rarely studied grossly until they are quite advanced. Our ignorance of the early stages of hepatocarcinogenesis in humans is profound. We are still uncertain, for instance, whether hepatocarcinoma most commonly arises in a single nodule or whether it may have a multifocal origin, as seems to be usual in experimental chemical hepatocarcinogenesis. A method of surgical staging for hepatic tumors has been described above (see p. 234).

Microscopic Structure. Hepatocarcinomas vary considerably from one another and also frequently from one area to another in the same tumor. In spite of these

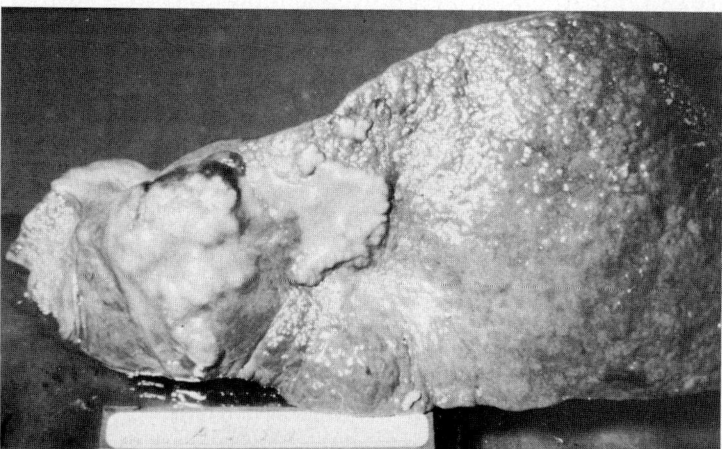

Figure 10. Gross appearance of a hepatocellular carcinoma arising in a patient with cirrhosis and hemochromatosis. The tumor appears to consist of two adjacent whitish nodules. Note the granularity of the cirrhotic liver.

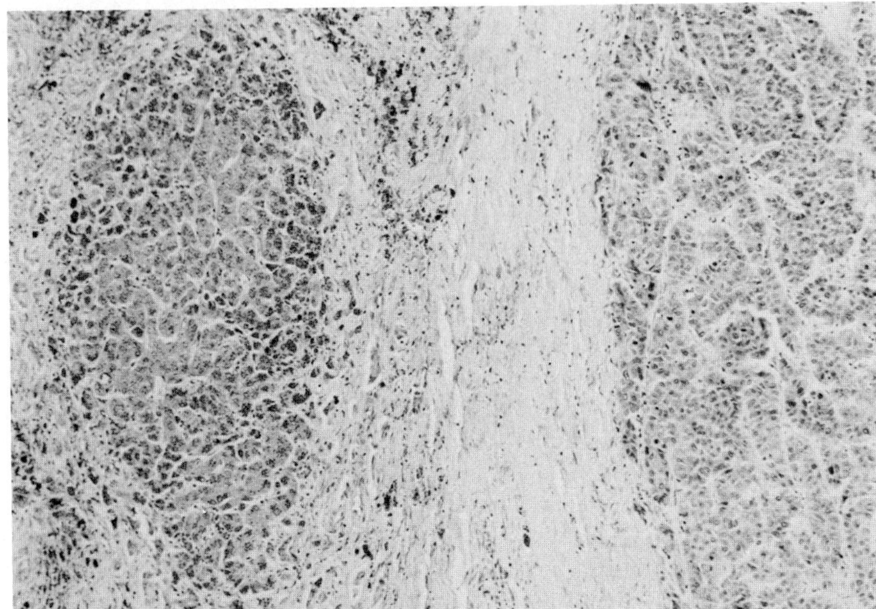

Figure 11. Microscopic section of the same liver shown in Figure 10. A cirrhotic nodule is seen on the left and the hepatocarcinoma on the right. Note the trabecular pattern in the tumor. (Hematoxylin and eosin, ×100.)

variations, morphologic features characteristic of hepatocarcinoma can generally be found (Figs. 11–18). The first and most important feature in differentiating hepatocellular carcinomas from other neoplasms is the resemblance of individual tumor cells to non-neoplastic hepatocytes. In the great majority of cases of hepatocarcinoma, the neoplastic cells appear more immature (anaplastic) than non-neoplastic hepatocytes, and have prominent eosinophilic nucleoli, as well as significant mitotic activity (Fig. 13). Bizarre pleomorphic cells are plentiful in some tumors and rare or absent in others; Edmondson (7) introduced a grading system for hepatocarcinomas, grade I being the best differentiated and grade IV the most anaplastic. The recent WHO classification has only three grades. Most hepatocarcinomas are clearly malignant cytologically. However, a small proportion (grade I) are very difficult to distinguish cytologically from benign lesions, such as adenomas. Spread of tumor cells into portal or hepatic veins is distinctly unusual in these low-grade neoplasms. A trabecular arrangement of the tumor cells is a characteristic feature of hepatocellular carcinomas, particularly in differentiating benign from malignant hepatocellular neoplasms. Instead of being arranged in plates one or two cells thick like non-neoplastic hepatocytes, neoplastic hepatocytes in hepatocarcinomas are most frequently arranged in trabeculae varying in width from one to ten or more cells (Figs. 11–15). Trabeculae differ from hepatic plates in non-neoplastic liver not only in the width they may attain, but also in a more haphazard arrangement of hepatocytes. Cells of the peripheral layer of trabeculae frequently are smaller and more hyperchromatic than those in the interior (7). Unlike hepatic plates in non-neoplastic liver, trabeculae may appear papillary or branching (Fig. 14). Vascular spaces between

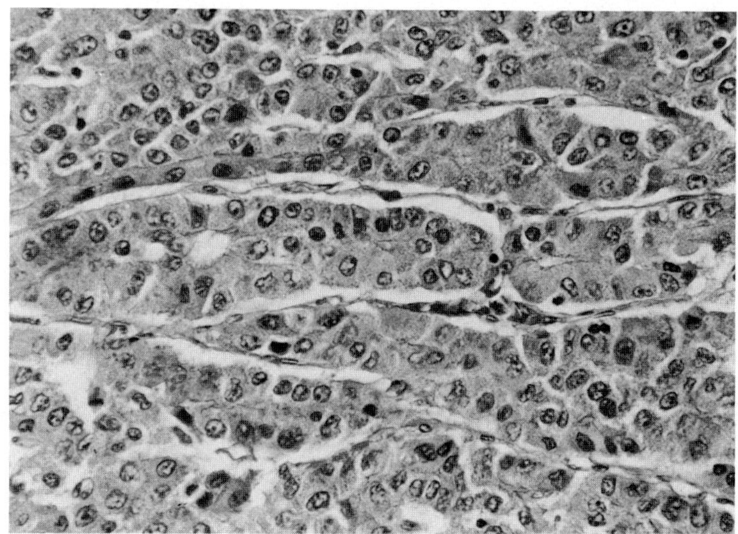

Figure 12. Higher-power view of a hepatocarcinoma. The trabecular pattern is clearly seen. (Hematoxylin and eosin, ×250.)

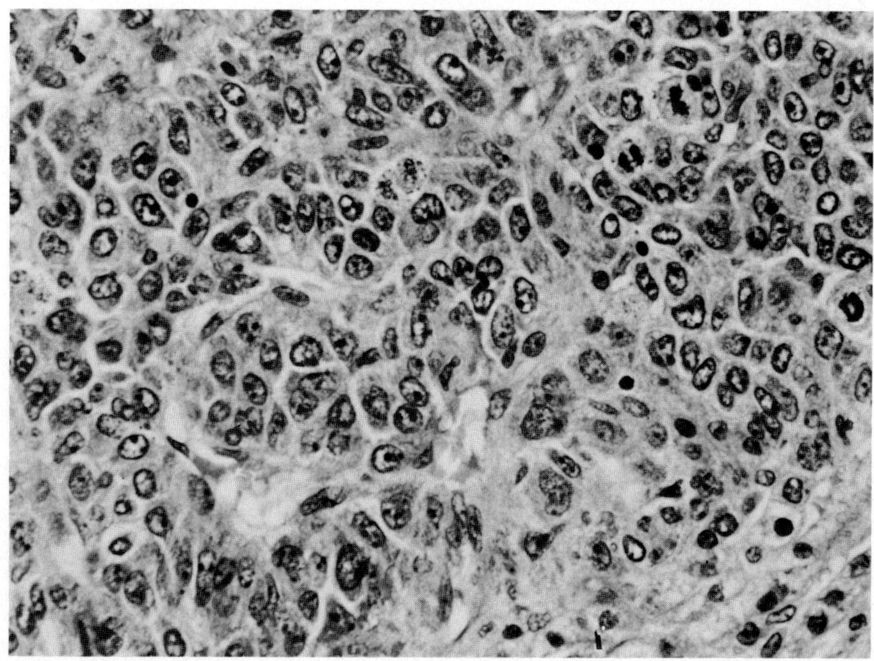

Figure 13. Hepatocellular carcinoma. The trabecular pattern is less distinct, particularly on the right, where the tumor appears to have a sheetlike pattern and contains several mitotic figures. (Hematoxylin and eosin, ×400.)

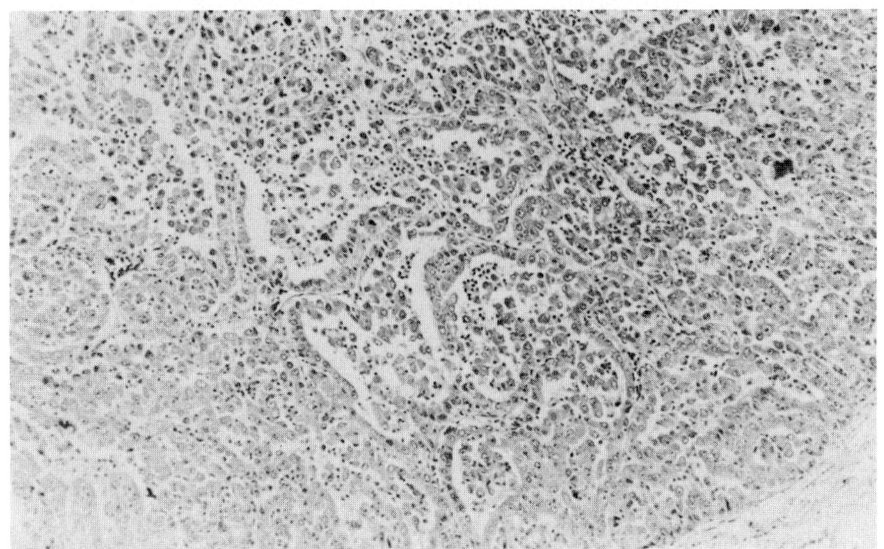

Figure 14. Hepatocellular carcinoma. Note anastomosing pattern of trabeculae. (Hematoxylin and eosin, ×85.)

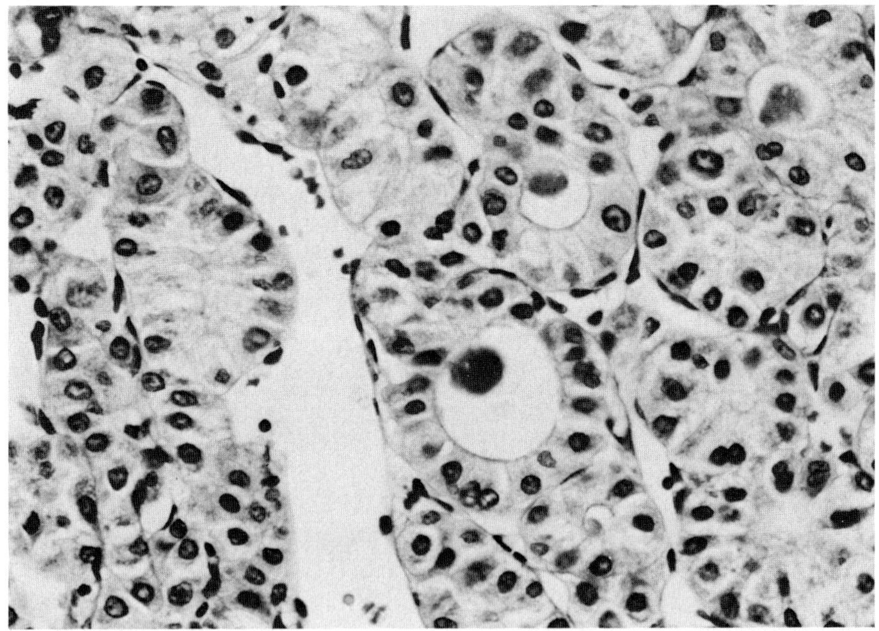

Figure 15. Hepatocellular carcinoma. A trabecular pattern is seen on the left, and a pseudoglandular pattern with bile thrombi in the center. (Hematoxylin and eosin, ×400.)

the trabeculae are not lined by Kupffer cells with the easily discernible, often quite plump, cytoplasm characteristic of such cells in non-neoplastic liver. Instead, trabeculae are lined by an extremely inconspicuous, often incomplete layer of slender endothelial cells. The trabecular pattern is brought out well by reticulin stains. This is particularly true in the "compact" type of hepatocellular carcinoma. In hematoxylin and eosin-stained sections, this type seems to consist of sheets of tumor cells (Fig. 13). However, reticulin stains may reveal closely packed trabeculae without intervening sinusoids separated only by scanty connective tissue (47).

In some predominantly trabecular hepatocarcinomas, there are pseudoductal or pseudoglandular areas (Fig. 15); a few hepatocarcinomas have a predominantly pseudoglandular pattern. These pseudoglandular spaces may contain bile or, rarely, PAS-positive mucinous material. Tumors with this pattern resemble cholangiocarcinomas in their overall growth pattern. However, the neoplastic cells are hepatocytic, rather than biliary in type. Another characteristic of most hepatocarcinomas is the relatively scanty intercellular stroma separating groups of neoplastic cells from each other. Exceptional in this respect are a small group of sclerosing hepatocarcinomas with a prominent fibrous stroma (see below). The recent WHO classification has subdivided hepatocellular carcinomas according to their predominant pattern into four types: trabecular, pseudoglandular, compact, and scirrhous. The classification of Peters (6) is more complex and takes into account some of the less frequent variants of HCC.

Poorly differentiated hepatocarcinomas are composed of immature cells with large nuclei and relatively little cytoplasm, generally arranged in trabeculae, Although immature (anaplastic), these cells often do not necessarily vary greatly from each other and display little pleomorphism. Pleomorphic hepatocarcinomas are composed of extremely bizarre cells. Some hepatocarcinomas are composed of multinucleated cells and are therefore called giant cell hepatocarcinomas (75). Another variant is the clear cell type (Figs. 16,17) (75a,76). Such tumors contain a variable proportion of clear polygonal cells with nuclei resembling those of more classic hepatocarcinoma. The clear cytoplasm contains lipid or glycogen or both, and such tumors may be associated with hypoglycemia or hypercholesterolemia (76a). These clear cell variants form a variety of patterns including trabecular and pseudoglandular arrangements. Clear cell hepatocarcinomas used to be thought to arise from adrenal rests in the liver (76b). However, it seems more likely that they are of hepatocellular origin. Clear cell hepatocarcinomas may be difficult to distinguish, on light microscopy, from clear cell tumors metastatic to the liver, particularly certain renal cell carcinomas. However, finding areas of typical hepatocarcinoma in a clear cell tumor usually clinches the diagnosis. Hepatic clear cell tumors seem to have a relatively good prognosis (77). The rare sclerosing variant of hepatocellular carcinoma composed of granular eosinophilic neoplastic hepatocytes (Fig. 18) with abundant fibrous stroma usually occurs in a noncirrhotic liver, predominantly in young adults. Like the clear cell variant, it seems to have an unusually good prognosis (6,20,78,79). It may be associated with hypercalcemia (79a). Electron microscopically, it contains abundant mitochondria (78) and may be considered an oncocytic neoplasm.

A variety of antigens can be identified immunohistochemically in HCC. These

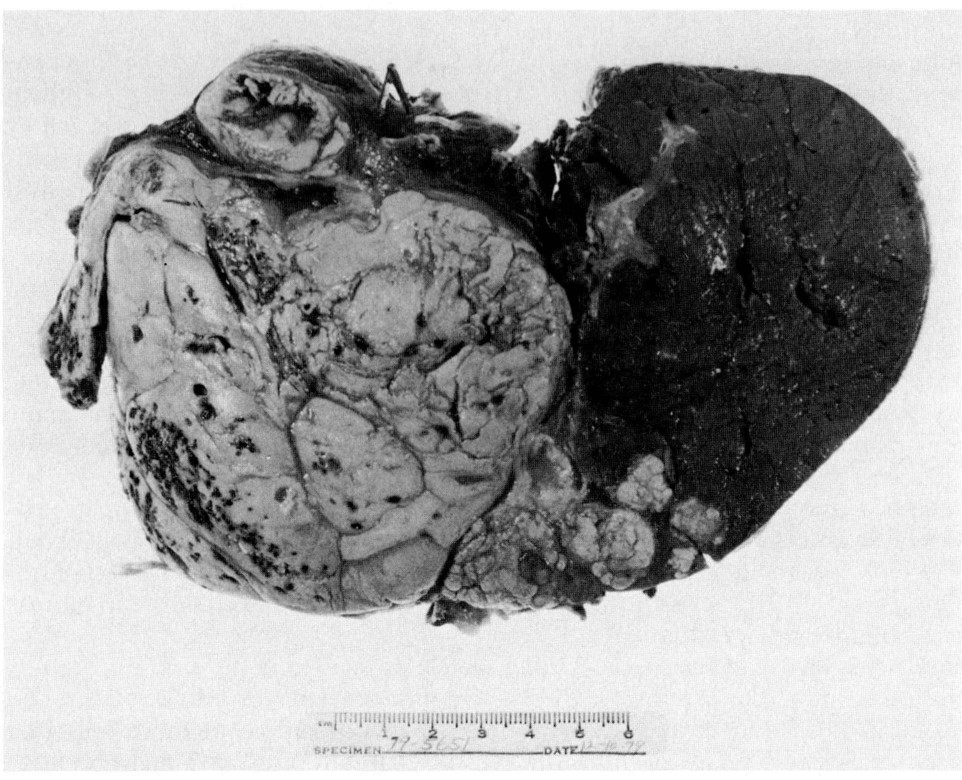

Figure 16. Hepatocellular carcinoma arising in a normal liver. Lobectomy specimen in a young woman who had been on contraceptives. (Contributed by H. Tesluk, M.D.) (75a)

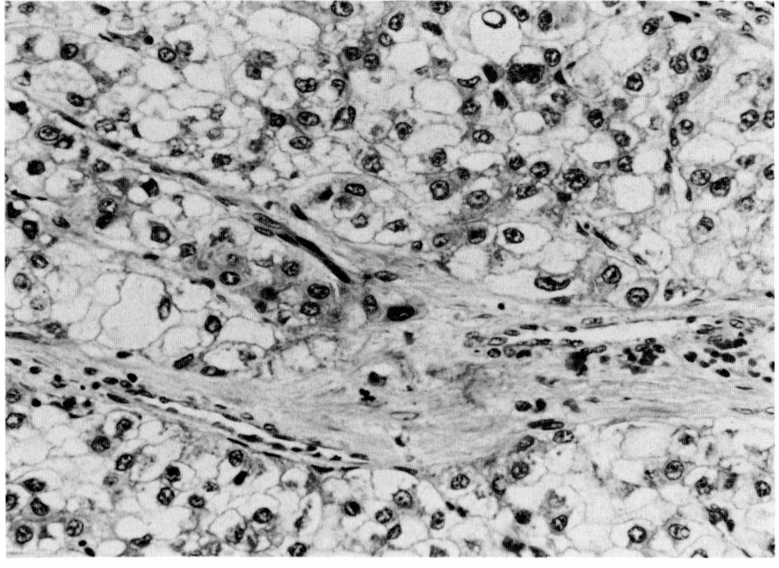

Figure 17. Same tumor shown in Figure 16. Note that the tumor is composed predominantly of clear-appearing hepatocytes arranged in trabecular and sheetlike patterns. (Hematoxylin and eosin, ×250.) (Contributed by H. Tesluk, M.D.) (75a)

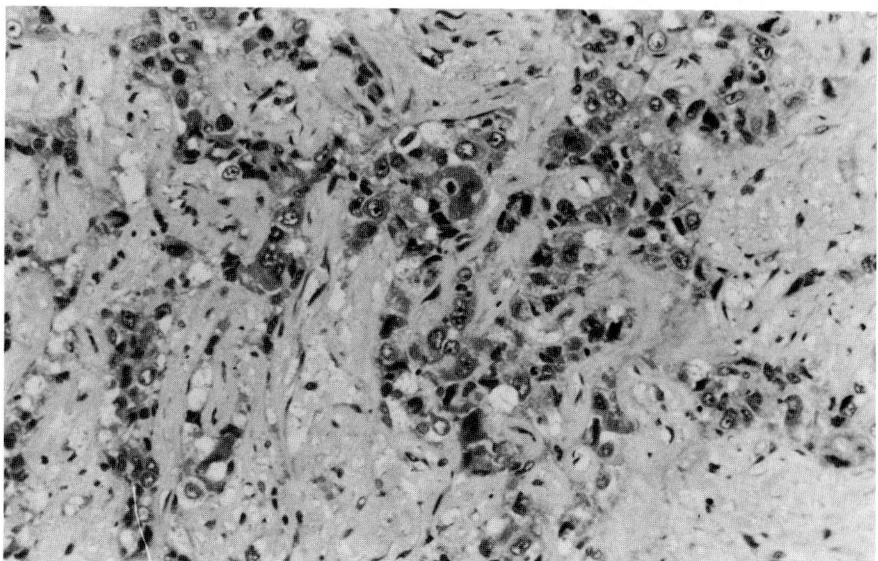

Figure 18. Sclerosing hepatocarcinoma with fibrous stroma. Note groups of eosinophilic hepatocytes separated by lamellae of fibrous connective tissue. (Hematoxylin and eosin, ×214.)

include alpha-1-antitrypsin, alpha fetoprotein, carcinoembryonic antigen, albumin (79b), and hepatitis B antigens. Orcein is not as sensitive an indicator for HB_sAg as immunoperoxidase (80). Hepatitis HB_sAg was often found in the same cell as the other antigens (81). In some cases antigens other than HB_sAg are associated with strongly PAS-positive cytoplasmic droplets composed of different constituents in different cases. In patients with alpha-1-antitrypsin deficiency, both homo- and heterozygous, the droplets contain alpha-1-antitrypsin only, while in patients who do not have this disease, the droplets contain alpha fetoprotein and alpha-2-macroglobulin, as well as alpha-1-antitrypsin (60,82,83). Some tumors that do not contain PAS-positive droplets stain diffusely for alpha-l-antitrypsin (84). Weakly PAS-positive inclusions of uncertain composition may also be present in HCC. Although hepatitis B surface antigen has been detected in HCC associated with hepatitis B infection, ground-glass cells have only rarely been described in this tumor. While the ground glass cells of HCC may contain HB_sAg, they may also contain fibrinogen rather than HB_sAg, particularly in eosinophilic hepatocarcinomas with abundant fibrous stroma (78,85). HB_sAg is generally more scanty in the tumors than in the nontumorous livers of the same cases (80,87–89). Occasionally, HB_sAg is found in a tumor, but not in the serum (80). Among the PAS-negative inclusions, some have the characteristic light and electron microscopic morphology of reticular Mallory's alcoholic hyalin (Chapter 5) (90). Other PAS-negative inclusions are globular and not characteristic of Mallory's hyalin by light microscopy; however, ultrastructurally, they have its characteristic fibrillar morphology. Both types of Mallory's hyalin are seen virtually exclusively in hepatocarcinomas of alcoholics (6). Michaelis-Gutmann bodies have been identified in one case of HCC (91).

Spread of hepatocarcinoma is mostly by the intravascular route. Histologically, sinusoidal invasion is difficult to diagnose, but involvement of portal or hepatic veins is easily diagnosed and quite frequent. Grossly, involvement of the hepatic veins and vena cava are not uncommon. Metastasis is most often to the lungs. Involvement of the portal lymph nodes is almost as common (6). Peritoneal dissemination is rare (91a).

Embryonal Tumors

Hepatoblastoma is an embryonal neoplasm corresponding to, but less common than, nephroblastoma and neuroblastoma. Hepatoblastoma virtually always manifests itself before the age of 3 years, an age at which hepatocellular carcinoma is quite rare (9,9a). The tumor is more common in males than in females. A few cases of a somewhat similar tumor have been reported in adults as mixed malignant tumors (9,92–92b). The dysontogenetic nature of hepatoblastoma is supported by its association with congenital malformations, such as hemihypertrophy (93) and the Wiedemann-Beckwith syndrome (9). Hepatoblastoma most commonly presents with abdominal enlargement with or without a palpable mass. Pallor and loss of weight may also be present. Jaundice is unusual. Onset may also be an acute abdominal emergency with rupture of the neoplasm and consequent hemoperitoneum. Alpha-fetoprotein is positive in the great majority of cases, particularly the well-differentiated (fetal) type. Hepatoblastoma is a rare cause of precocious puberty (94). The ultrastructure of only a few of these tumors has been studied (95,95a).

Grossly, hepatoblastomas usually form a single mass up to 20 cm in diameter, which generally appears well circumscribed. The weight of the liver may be up to 20 times that of normal. The neoplasms are tan to gray in color and may have yellowish red areas of hemorrhage and necrosis. The tumors may appear lobulated and, occasionally, may be bile stained.

Histologically, hepatoblastomas have been subdivided into pure epithelial and mixed epithelial and mesenchymal types (93). The pure epithelial type seems to be the more frequent (9). The mesenchymal tissues in mixed hepatoblastomas are benign and include not only fibromyxoid mesenchyme, but often osteoid, and, rarely, chondroid or squamous foci. The epithelial element in hepatoblastoma varies in differentiation. The cells of the immature embryonal type are small, dark, and poorly cohesive and have marked mitotic activity. They are arranged in ribbons, glandlike formations, or pseudorosettes (Fig. 19). The more mature fetal type cells are larger, but still smaller than adult hepatocytes. They are pale or dark staining, according to their content of fat and glycogen. The cells of the fetal type are arranged in cords two cells thick with little mitotic activity. Bile plugs are found occasionally. Fibrous septa with occasional bile ducts may be seen, and groups of ductular cells may be found in these tumors (95b). Foci of squamous epithelium are not uncommon. Occasionally, melanin-containing cells and respiratory or intestinal epithelium are seen, which may make it difficult to distinguish these tumors from teratomas. Most hepatoblastomas are composed of both fetal and embryonal elements. Hepatoblastomas differ from most hepatocarcinomas in the frequency with which they show hemopoiesis in the sinusoids, particularly in the fetal cell areas, and in the usual absence of cellular pleomorphism. Hepatic cirrhosis or fibrosis are uncommon in

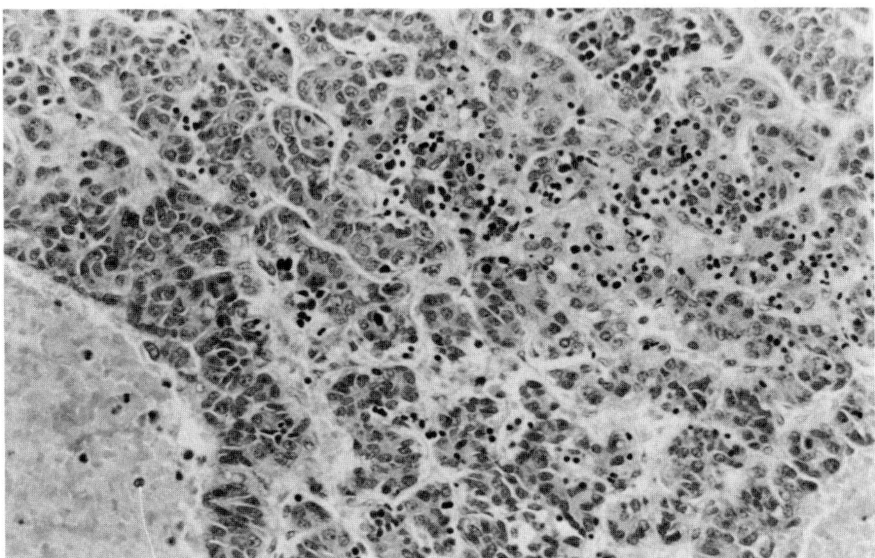

Figure 19. Hepatoblastoma, exhibiting an epithelial area. The cells in this fetal area have relatively little cytoplasm and are arranged in an indistinct trabecular pattern. Foci of hemopoietic cells are scattered through the tumor. (Hematoxylin and eosin, ×215.)

hepatoblastoma, as well as in HCC in childhood (9). An endodermal sinus tumor of the liver has also been reported (96).

Proliferative Biliary Epithelial Lesions

Diffuse lesions involving virtually the entire intrahepatic biliary system, such as polycystic disease of the liver and congenital hepatic fibrosis, were described in Chapter 13. This chapter deals with focal neoplastic or hamartomatous biliary epithelial lesions.

Bile Duct Adenomas (Bile Duct Hamartomas, Meyenburg's Complexes)

These structures are composed of proliferated bile ducts embedded in a fibrous stroma. They are usually multiple and most likely represent developmental anomalies (hamartomas). However, it has been suggested that at least in some cases they may be acquired (97). Bile duct adenomas are generally microscopic, but in a few cases are large enough (up to 0.5 cm) to be observed as single or multiple, tan to green, hepatic subcapsular nodules mimicking metastatic tumor at laparotomy (98,99). When these lesions are very extensive, they may be difficult to distinguish from those of hepatic polycystic disease and congenital hepatic fibrosis (Chapter 13). Bile duct adenomas, unlike polycystic disease and congenital hepatic fibrosis, usually do not produce clinical signs or symptoms. However, multiple duct adenomas may be associated with other biliary tract abnormalities, such as simple intrahepatic biliary cysts or polycystic bile ducts (Chapter 17). Not infrequently, these patients also have renal cysts.

Microscopically, bile ducts adenomas are located in interlobular and supcapsu-

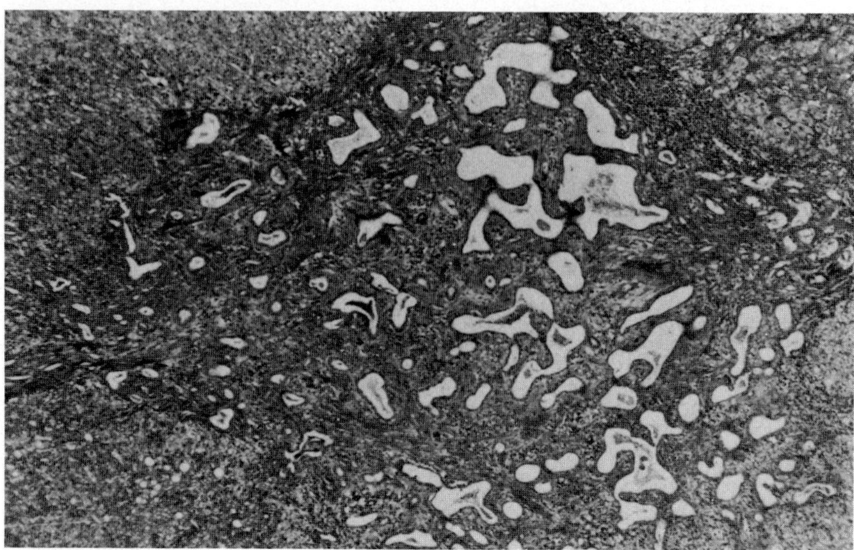

Figure 20. Bile duct adenoma (Von Meyenburg complex). Note proliferated bile ducts in fibrous stroma. This was a single incidental lesion found at autopsy. (Hematoxylin and eosin, ×34.)

lar zones. The lesions are irregularly shaped, multiple cystic spaces lined by benign cuboidal or columnar epithelium resembling that of bile ducts. These ductlike spaces are embedded in a fibrous stroma and may be empty or may contain bile (Fig. 20). Very rarely, one of these bile duct adenomas may undergo malignant change resulting in adenocarcinoma (100).

Simple Biliary Cysts

Simple cystic malformations of the bile ducts are described in Chapter 17. Biliary cysts (101–104) are relatively rare and often completely asymptomatic. When symptoms are present, there may be abdominal discomfort, distention, and, occasionally, jaundice. Simple cysts are most often found in adult females and are probably congenital. These lesions must be differentiated from biliary cystadenomas.

On gross examination, simple cysts are usually solitary. They may be up to 30 cm in diameter and are unilocular or multilocular. Generally, the contents are clear and yellow, but they may be bile stained. The inner surface of the cyst wall is usually smooth but may be trabeculated. Histologically, the cysts are lined by simple biliary epithelium with underlying loose fibrous tissue frequently containing blood vessels, nests of hepatic cells, or groups of bile ducts. Aggregates of these ducts in the cyst wall may form bile duct adenomas. Not infrequently, these cysts may be very closely related anatomically to the bile ducts. Occasionally, these patients also have hepatic bile duct adenomas (see above), benign bile duct polyps, polycystic disease of the liver (Chapter 17), or congenital hepatic fibrosis (Chapter 13) (105). Malignant transformation of biliary cysts is a rare complication (106).

Biliary Cystadenomas and Cystadenocarcinomas

Primary cystic neoplasms of the biliary system are rare. Cystadenomas usually present as abdominal masses in middle-aged women. There may be some abdominal discomfort (107). Cystadenocarcinomas have a more equal sex incidence. Their clinical presentation generally is similar to that of cystadenoma.

Grossly, cystadenomas may be as large as 25 cm in diameter with a smooth external surface. On cut section, they are usually multiloculated with thin walls and a smooth inner lining. Unilocular cystadenomas and cystadenomas with polypoid areas have also been reported. Cystadenocarcinomas are similar in size and general configuration, but their wall may vary in thickness and the lining may be smooth or rough. There is considerable variation in the appearance of the liquid contents of these lesions. Hemorrhage is more common in cystadenocarcinomas.

Microscopically, cystadenomas consist of cysts lined by a single layer of cuboidal to columnar cells with occasional papillary projections. The epithelium shows no atypia and has round to oval nuclei with faintly eosinophilic and vacuolated cytoplasm. Mitotic figures are inconspicuous. The cytoplasmic vacuoles stain for mucin. The stroma underlying the epithelium is compact and cellular, resembling ovarian stroma. In most cases cystadenomas can be distinguished from simple cysts. Papillary epithelial projections favor a cystadenoma while bile-stained contents, a close anatomic relationship to biliary structures and associated biliary anomalies, such as bile duct adenomas, polycystic disease of the liver, or congenital hepatic fibrosis, favor a simple biliary cyst.

Cystadenocarcinomas consist of cysts lined by an epithelium that is often multilayered and papillary. The lining epithelium shows considerable loss of polarity with variation in size and shape of the cells and of their nuclei. Some of these lining cells may be multinucleated. The nuclei are hyperchromatic, and mitotic figures are present but not abundant. The neoplastic cells may infiltrate into the adjacent liver. Cystadenomatous epithelium is found in most cystadenocarcinomas, suggesting that a benign precursor lesion underwent malignant transformation. This has been documented in one case (106a). Although cystadenocarcinomas can metastasize (106b), some of these patients have survived as long as 13 years after resection (106a,107,108). This tumor, therefore, seems to have a relatively good prognosis, certainly better than that for cholangiocarcinoma.

Cholangiocarcinoma

These tumors are composed of cells with malignant criteria, still having some resemblance to biliary epithelium. The signs and symptoms produced by the lesions depend on their location. If situated in the hilum of the liver, cholangiocarcinomas usually produce biliary obstruction and cholestasis (109,110). However, the jaundice may be intermittent, and the clinical picture may appear to be that of chronic liver disease (111). If the tumor is located asymmetrically, it may obstruct only one of the main bile ducts. Histologic evidence of biliary obstruction will, therefore, be limited to one lobe before the onset of jaundice. This is one reason why hilar cholangiocarcinomas have been notoriously difficult to diagnose. Lesions proximal to the junction of the left and right hepatic ducts have the clinical features of space occupying lesions. The symptoms and signs of this type of tumor resemble those of hepatocellular carcinoma. Most common are abdominal swelling, pain, and loss of weight. Jaundice usually is not an early feature (112).

In western countries, the sex incidence of cholangiocarcinoma, unlike that of hepatocarcinoma, is equal, and it usually develops in a normal liver. No etiologic factors can be established for most cases of cholangiocarcinoma. A few may perhaps be related to contraceptive or anabolic steroids (113). While hemangiosarcoma appears to be the most common consequence of thorotrast injection, cholangiocarcinoma has also been reported (54,115,116). The livers of these patients generally show considerable diffuse scarring. In endemic areas such as Hong Kong, *Clonorchis sinensis* appears to be another known etiologic factor (116). Patients with this parasitic infection develop mucinous metaplasia of the ductal epithelium, duct proliferation, and periductal fibrosis before the development of cholangiocarcinoma (Chapter 7, Fig. 20) (117). Cystic malformations of the biliary system, such as choledochal cyst and congenital hepatic fibrosis, may be complicated by the development of adenocarcinoma resembling cholangiocarcinoma, or, rarely, by squamous carcinoma (Chapter 17). Alpha-fetoprotein is not elevated in the serum of patients with cholangiocarcinoma.

Cholangiocarcinomas, like hepatocellular carcinomas, may consist grossly of a single mass or multiple nodules or may be diffuse (Fig. 21) (7). The tumors are usually grayish white and generally firmer than hepatocarcinoma, since cholangiocarcinomas usually have more fibrous stroma. Tumor nodules beneath Glis-

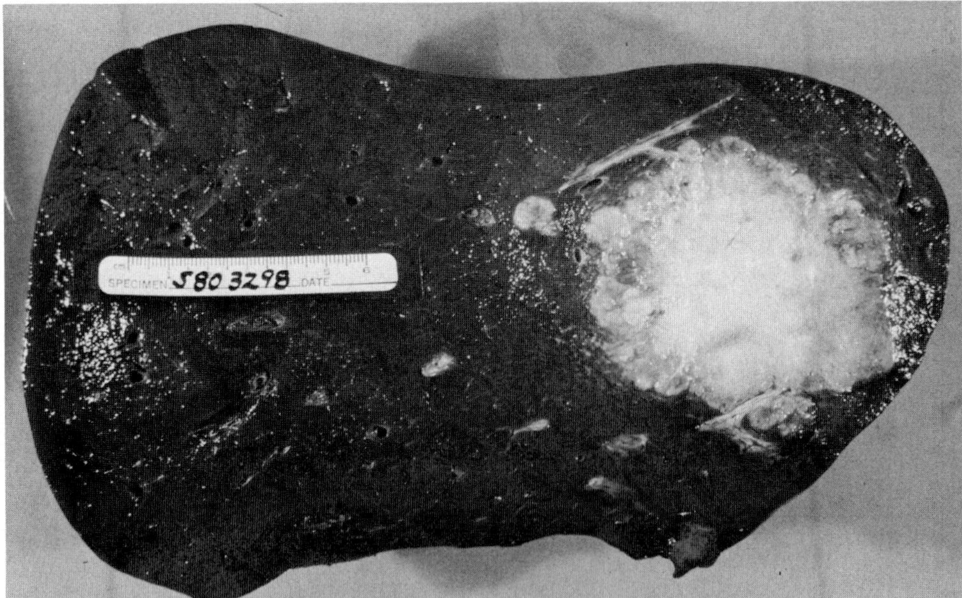

Figure 21. Gross photograph of a right hepatic lobectomy specimen removed for cholangiocarcinoma. The tumor is close to the margin of excision. A small satellite nodule is seen to the left of the main tumor. Note that the liver is neither cirrhotic nor fibrotic.

son's capsule are often umbilicated. Vascular invasion by tumor is less common than in HCC. Hilar cholangiocarcinomas cause obstruction of the main bile ducts at the hilum with dilatation of the intrahepatic biliary system. The liver is usually severely bile stained. These hilar tumors may appear grossly as a fibrous collar constricting a duct or ducts, as a mass constricting ducts and invading parenchyma, or as a spongy friable mass within the biliary lumen (109,110). Biliary cirrhosis (Chapter 13) may develop if these patients survive long enough.

Histologically, cholangiocarcinomas usually have a ductal pattern and are embedded in a dense fibrous stroma (Figs. 22,23). More rarely, these neoplasms have a papillary or microcystic pattern. The cells lining the ductal, microcystic, and papillary structures are cuboidal to columnar and are usually quite well differentiated. Their nuclei are smaller and less variable than those of HCC. The cytoplasm is usually clear but may be faintly granular. Bile is never seen in the cells or lumens. However, the presence of mucin can frequently be demonstrated in the tumor cells and in the lumens (118). A papillary pattern is more common in cholangiocarcinomas than in HCC. Blood vessels are not invaded as frequently as in HCC, but when this occurs, cholangiocarcinomas tend to line the vascular basement membrane in an acinar-like pattern. Histologically, primary hepatic cholangiocarcinomas cannot be distinguished from adenocarcinomas of the gallbladder or pancreatic ducts metastatic to the liver. Clinical data are usually required to determine the origin of such ductal adenocarcinomas. Electron microscopically, the tumor cells of cholangiocarcinomas generally resemble duct cells, and in particular have a prominent basement membrane. Compared with HCC, cholangiocarcinomas metastasize somewhat more frequently to the hilar

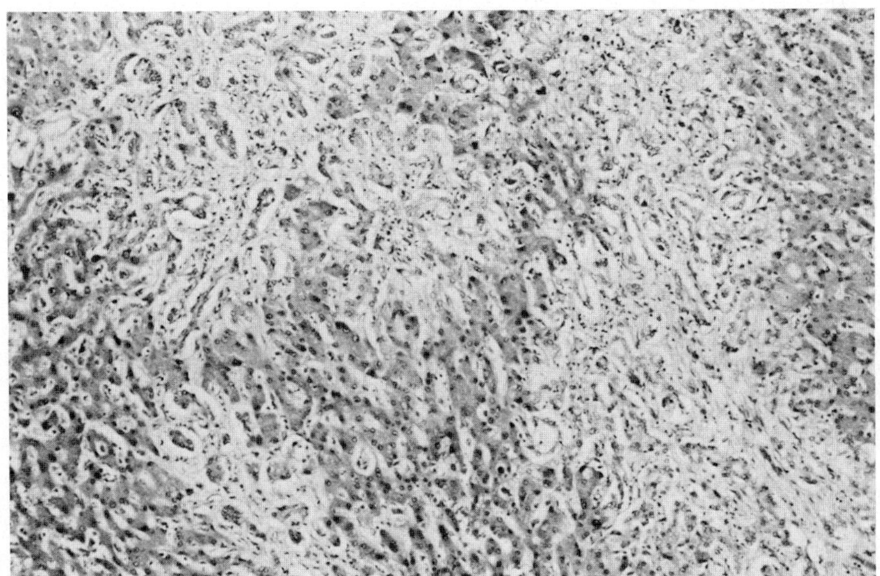

Figure 22. Moderately differentiated cholangiocarcinoma. Note tumor cells arranged in ductlike structures infiltrating among groups of normal hepatocytes. (Hematoxylin and eosin, ×85.)

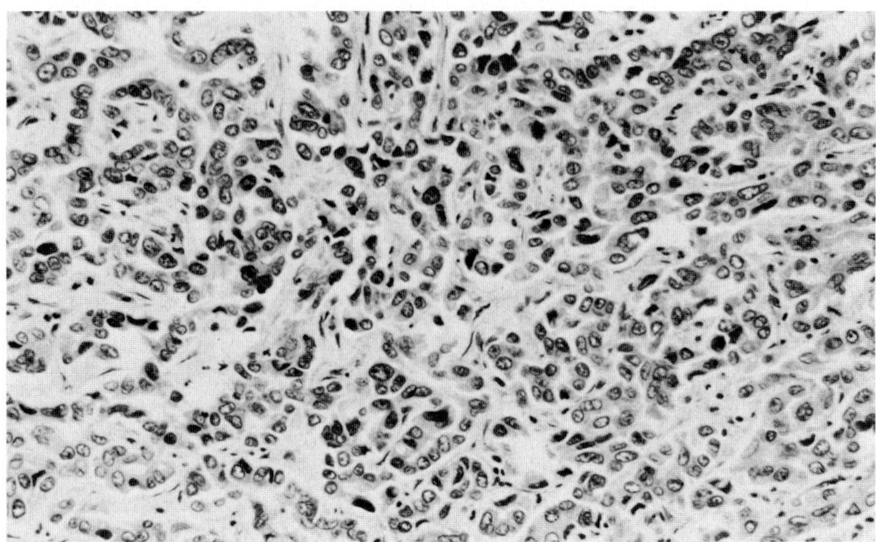

Figure 23. Less well-differentiated cholangiocarcinoma than that shown in Figure 22. The tumor is arranged in irregular ductlike structures and composed of pleomorphic cells. (Hematoxylin and eosin, ×215.)

and abdominal lymph nodes and less frequently to the lungs (6). Average survival of patients with cholangiocarcinomas seems to be slightly longer than that of patients with HCC (7).

Cholangiolocarcinoma
A malignant hepatic tumor composed of structures resembling cholangioles (ductules of Hering) (119), cholangiolocarcinoma represents about 1% of liver cancers (6). Too few cases have been described to be sure whether in sex incidence and etiology this neoplasm resembles cholangiocarcinoma or HCC. Grossly, these neoplasms are usually scirrhous and resemble cholangiocarcinoma. Microscopically, they consist largely of cuboidal cells with small nuclei and clear cytoplasm arranged in a double row. A tiny lumen may be visible between the rows (Fig. 24). Such well-differentiated areas closely resemble proliferating non-neoplastic cholangioles, both in their cytology and in their arrangement. Less well-differentiated, more anaplastic areas can usually be found in these tumors, enabling one to diagnose them as carcinomas.

Other Carcinomas

Primary hepatic squamous (7,106) and mucoepidermoid (120,120a) carcinomas have been reported. Most likely these originated from metaplastic ductal epithelium of biliary cysts.

Combined Hepatocellular and Cholangiocarcinomas

Hepatocellular carcinomas frequently show a variety of patterns in the same tumor. In addition to trabecular areas, which are usually the predominant type,

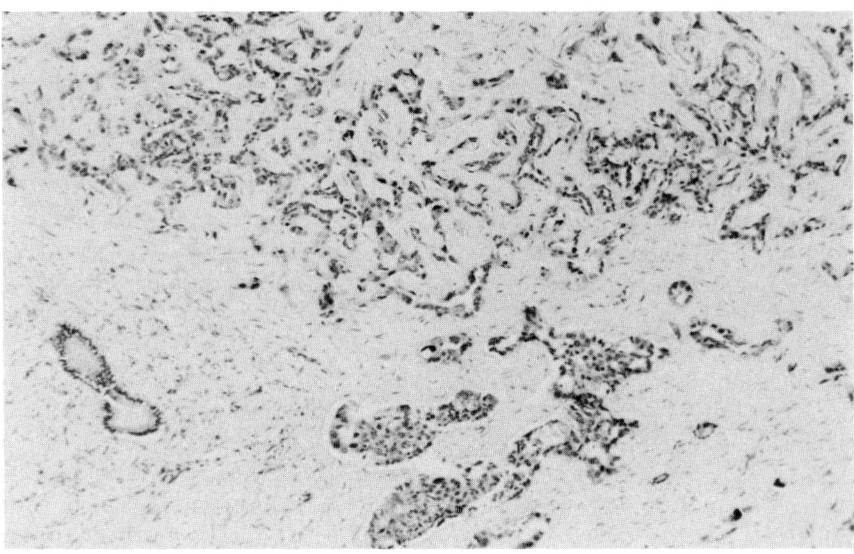

Figure 24. Cholangiolocarcinoma? Note regularly arranged infiltrating small ductal structures, many without a lumen in the upper part of this illustration. A surviving normal portal bile duct is seen at the lower left. (Hematoxylin and eosin, ×85.)

ductal or glandular arrangements of the tumor cells are frequently seen. Papillary formations also ocur occasionally. Such neoplasms are not truly combined carcinomas, because the various patterns are all composed of malignant hepatocytes. The most common type of combined hepatic carcinoma is that of HCC with cholangiocarcinoma. Three subtypes can be recognized: (*1*) separate tumors, each of which is composed of one cell type; (*2*) contiguous tumors, which may be grossly and histologically distinguishable as two different, yet adjacent, tumors; and (*3*) single lesions composed of an intimate mixture of the two cell types (7). This last group is the most frequent and important subtype. These tumors are composed of typical HCC and typical cholangiocarcinoma interspersed in varying proportions. Apparently, they usually occur in male patients with cirrhosis (7) and have been reported to constitute about 4% of primary hepatic cancers (112). Such figures would seem to be rather subjective, since they depend on adequacy of sampling of each tumor and on the diagnostic criteria employed to differentiate HCCs with ductal or glandular patterns from HCC combined with cholangiocarcinoma.

Proliferative Vascular Lesions

Diffuse vascular lesions involving virtually all portal triads, such as Osler-Weber-Rendu disease, as well as arteriovenous shunts, infarcts, and peliosis hepatis, were described in Chapter 12. This chapter deals with focal proliferative vascular lesions.

Benign Cavernous Hemangioma

The most common benign hepatic tumor of the liver, benign cavernous hemangioma, may be a malformation (hamartoma), rather than a neoplasm. It has been reported in up to 8% of autopsies (6,8). Cavernous hemangiomas are seen more often in women than men.

Most cavernous hemangiomas are asymptomatic and are incidental findings at laparotomy or at autopsy. When they do cause symptoms, there may be an abdominal mass, swelling, or pain. A few patients develop an acute abdominal emergency due to rupture of a hemangioma. Thrombocytopenia, hypofibrinogenemia, and anemia may develop, possibly due to intravascular coagulation in these tumors (121). Some cases in childhood have been reported that were probably not hemangiomas, but hemangioendotheliomas (8,122). Needle biopsy is contraindicated if this lesion or another vascular hepatic lesion is suspected. The treatment is steroid administration, hepatic artery ligation, or partial hepatectomy (123).

Cavernous hemangiomas may be single or multiple and may be pedunculated. They measure from a few millimeters to 30 cm in diameter. The lesions are well circumscribed, reddish purple, and spongy in consistency. Thrombi and fibrosis may develop in them. Microscopically, the hemangiomas consist of multiple channels of varying sizes lined by a singly layer of flattened endothelium. The endothelium is supported by a delicate fibrous stroma (Fig. 25). Thrombi, which may be in the process of organization, are common. Fibrosis and calcification may also develop. Peliosis hepatis differs from a hemangioma in the absence of a fibrous stroma (Chapter 12) (Fig. 11).

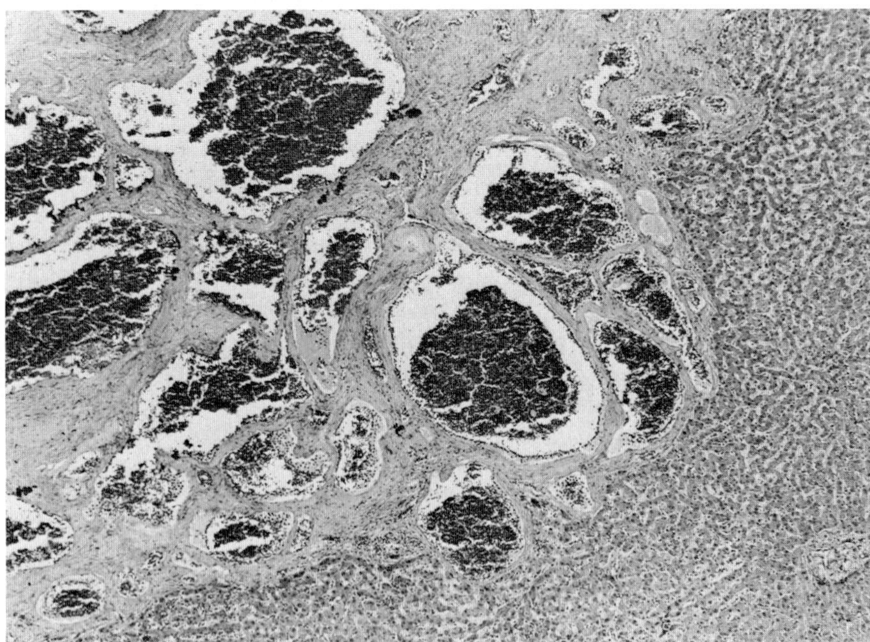

Figure 25. Benign cavernous hemangioma. Note large vascular spaces lined by endothelium embedded in fibrous connective tissue. (Hematoxylin and eosin, ×40.)

Infantile Hemangioendothelioma

Overall, this is a rare lesion, although it is relatively common in childhood. The great majority become manifest by the age of 6 months (9,9a) and almost always by the age of 4 years (124). However, a few cases have been described in adults(125). In approximately half the patients in one series, the lesion was an incidental finding at laparotomy or autopsy. The others manifested themselves by hepatomegaly with or without an abdominal mass and congestive cardiac failure. Heart failure in these patients probably results from arteriovenous shunting between the hepatic artery and hepatic vein. About half these patients have multiple cutaneous hemangiomas, and jaundice is seen in about one-third. Occasionally, rupture of such a lesion occurs, resulting in an acute abdominal catastrophy. Thrombocytopenia and a microangiopathic hemolytic anemia may also occur.

These tumors may be solitary or multifocal and may vary in size from a few millimeters to 15 cm in diameter. The lesions are reddish brown to grayish tan and may be hemorrhagic. They are spongy in consistency, but can contain fibrotic areas and yellowish foci of calcification. Two basic histologic patterns have been described (126). The lesions of type I, the commoner variant, consist of vascular channels lined by a single layer of plump endothelial cells (127). The vascular channels are usually of capillary size but, focally, may be larger and are surrounded by reticulin fibers. Focal extramedullary hemopoiesis is frequently found in these vessels (Fig. 26). Focal hemorrhage, thrombosis, myxomatous degeneration, fibrosis, and calcification may be seen. Small type I lesions tend to be intimately related to portal tracts. Numerous bile ducts are seen among the

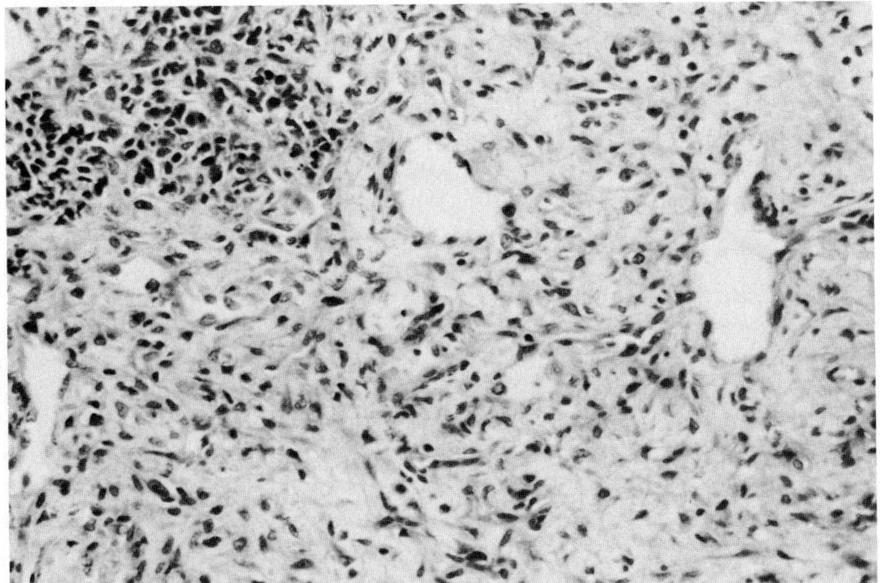

Figure 26. Infantile hemangioendothelioma. The vascular pattern is clearly evident in some areas. A focus of extramedullary hemopoiesis is seen in the upper left corner. (Hematoxylin and eosin, ×214.)

vascular channels. Nests of hepatocytes may also be present. In type II lesions (8) the endothelial cells are multilayered with occasional irregular papillary tufting and branching so that the basic vascular pattern may be difficult to discern in the absence of a PAS or silver stain to demonstrate the basement membranes. The neoplastic cells are larger and more pleomorphic. Their nuclei are hyperchromatic and rarely show mitotic figures. Many endothelial cells appear to be outside vascular channels and seem to be invading the surrounding liver. Invasion of veins, however, is not observed. Unequivocal distinction of types I and II is not always possible.

These neoplasms may undergo spontaneous involution, and, unlike hepatic angiosarcomas in adults, they are usually considered to be benign. Nonetheless, they may infiltrate locally and do have the potential, albeit limited, to metastasize (8). Treatment is similar to that of cavernous hemangioma and survival is about 50% (124). Frank hemangiosarcoma in association with infantile hemangioendothelioma has recently been described (127a).

Hemangiosarcoma (Malignant Hemangioendothelioma, Kupffer Cell Sarcoma)

Hemangiosarcoma is a malignant tumor of endothelial lining cells (127b) or Kupffer cells (128), occurring considerably less frequently than HCC or cholangiocarcinoma. During the last few years, it has become clear that hemangiosarcoma of the liver may follow exposure to certain carcinogens, such as thorotrast (54,129,130), vinyl chloride (130–131a), arsenic (130,132), and perhaps even diethylstilbestrol (133), contraceptive steroids (133a), and androgen-anabolic steroids (134). An association with hydrazine compounds (phenelzine, isoniazid, procarbazine, hydralazine) has also been suggested (135). Hemangiosarcoma has also been reported in hemochromatosis (136).

Clinically, these patients complain of weight loss, abdominal swelling due to hepatomegaly or ascites, abdominal pain, anorexia, vomiting, or jaundice. On palpation there may be tenderness or irregularity of the liver or an actual hepatic mass. Hepatic coma may also develop. Intraperitoneal rupture of the tumor with hemorrhage may occur. This produces an acute abdominal emergency. Some abnormalities of liver function test are usually present, but are nonspecific.

Most of these lesions are multicentric and involve both lobes of the liver, varying from a few millimeters to several centimeters in diameter. Frequently, the larger subcapsular lesions produce some bulging of the overlying capsule. On cut section, the lesions are hemorrhagic and consist of spongy tissue or of blood-containing cavities with a shaggy lining. Microscopically, these tumors generally have a variety of patterns that may be sinusoidal, capillary, cavernous, or solid (Figs. 27–29) (137). Different patterns are usually seen in different areas of the same tumor. In particular, the solid type is hardly ever seen alone. The sinusoidal pattern resembles normal liver in that the normal liver plate pattern remains intact. Interspersed among the hepatocytes, however, there are vascular spaces composed of the sinusoidal lining cells with large hyperchromatic anaplastic nuclei. Both the capillary and sinusoidal areas may be lined by one or more layers of anaplastic endothelial cells, arranged in a papillary pattern, and supported by fibrous connective tissue. The anaplastic endothelial cells have faintly

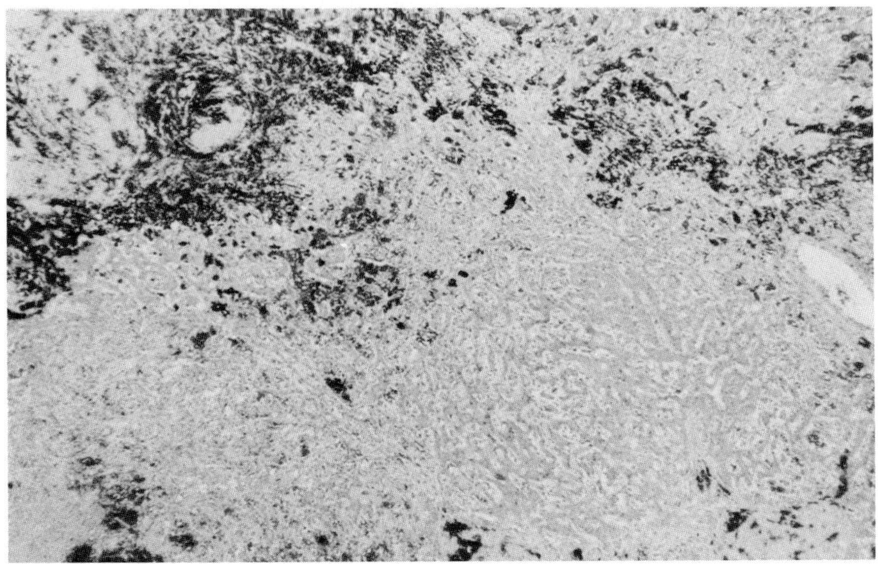

Figure 27. Hemangiosarcoma after injection of thorotrast. Note dense granular thorotrast deposits, particularly in the tumorous areas. (Hematoxylin and eosin, ×34.)

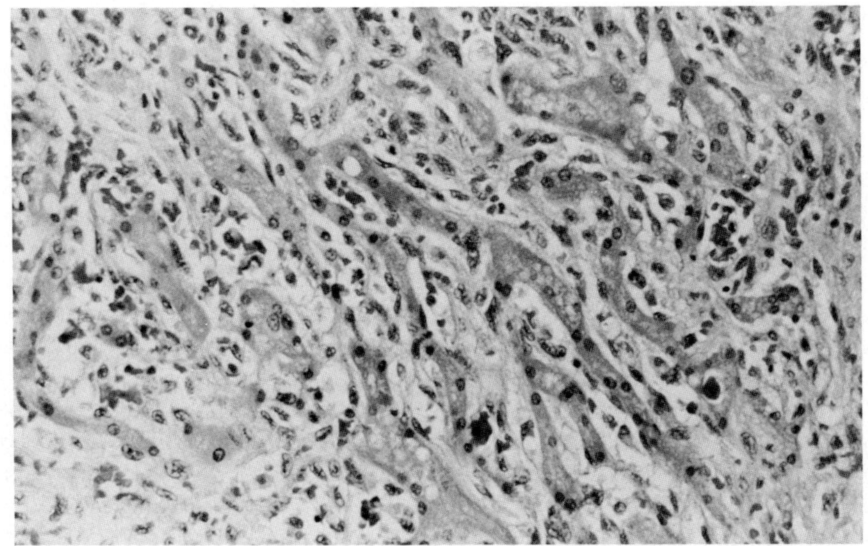

Figure 28. Hemangiosarcoma after injection of thorotrast. Note tumor cells interspersed between plates of hepatocytes. (Hematoxylin and eosin, ×215.)

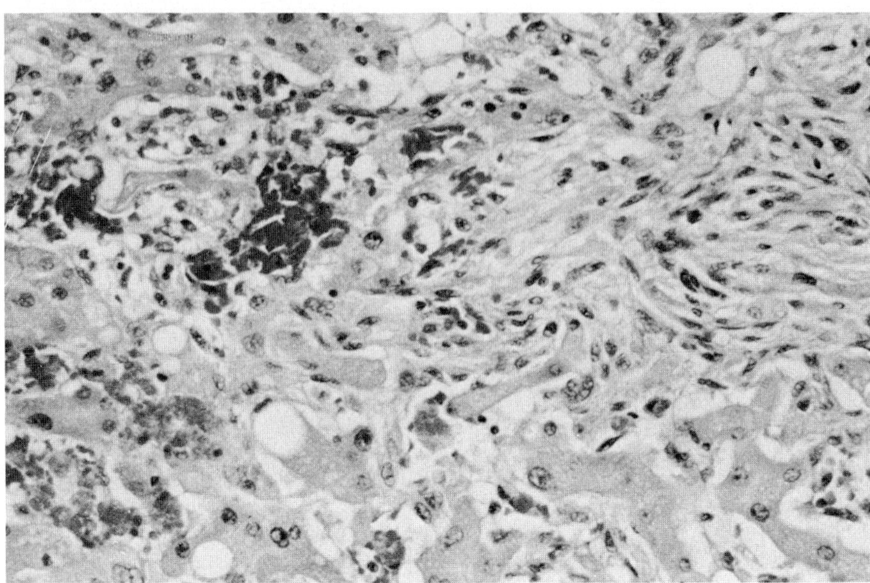

Figure 29. Hemangiosarcoma after injection of thorotrast. Note dense granular thorotrast deposits and areas displaying sheets of spindle-shaped tumor cells at upper right. (Hematoxylin and eosin, ×545.)

eosinophilic cytoplasm, are elongated and have ill-defined cell borders. The nuclei are elongated and hyperchromatic and have small nucleoli. There is a variable amount of nuclear pleomorphism, mitotic activity, and giant cell formation in different tumors and even in different areas of the same tumor. Solid areas consist of masses of these cells, often arranged in a fibrosarcoma-like pattern. In such areas, the tumor cells may have a considerable amount of cytoplasm and bizarre outlines. Foci of extramedullary hemopoiesis are commonly seen in these tumors. They may also show hemorrhage, necrosis, and fibrosis.

Hemangiosarcoma differs from infantile hemangioendothelioma in having more nuclear atypia, mitotic acitvity, and giant cell formation. Invasion of intrahepatic veins is also characteristic of hemangiosarcoma. Tumors consisting of infantile hemangioendothelioma and hemangiosarcoma have been described (127a). Diagnosis of the solid portions of hemangiosarcomas may be impossible beyond "undifferentiated sarcoma," particularly on biopsy. Other neoplasms to be considered in the differential diagnosis are vascular HCCs and metastatic hypernephroma, choriocarcinoma, and Kaposi's sarcoma. Metastatic hemangiosarcoma is indistinguishable from primary hemangiosarcoma. Peliosis hepatis also must be considered. This lesion differs from hemangiosarcoma in the benign appearance of its endothelial lining cells (Chapter 12, Fig. 11).

The non-neoplastic areas of these livers frequently show portal fibrosis and ductular proliferation, particularly in patients with a history of arsenic, thorotrast, or vinyl chloride ingestion (Chapter 13). In thorotrast cases, the granules of thorotrast can usually be found fairly easily (Fig. 24), and their radioactivity can be demonstrated by autoradiography and micro-X-ray analysis (Chapter 11).

Tumors of Fibrous Tissue

There are very few acceptable cases of hepatic fibroma. These are usually large tumors in elderly people (138). Grossly, they consist of large masses, white to tan, which may appear lobulated, and may be either firm or soft. Histologically, they consist of interlacing bundles of fibroblasts and collagen in varying proportions. Mitotic figures are absent.

Fibrosarcomas are quite rare and usually occur in elderly males. While most patients complain of an abdominal mass; hypoglycemia may be the presenting feature. Fibrosarcomas are usually large, white, firm masses. Often there are foci of hemorrhage and necrosis (138,139). Microscopically, they consist of spindle-shaped cells surrounded by reticulin fibers and varying amounts of collagen. The nuclei show varying degrees of pleomorphism, hyperchromasia, and mitotic activity. Some of these tumors have been associated with cirrhosis (139).

Tumors of Smooth Muscle

Primary smooth muscle tumors are also quite rare, particularly if stringent criteria for this diagnosis are met. The tumor must be composed of smooth muscle cells, and a uterine or gastrointestinal origin should be excluded (140). Only a minority of these tumors in the liver are benign (140). Among these, leiomyoma and leiomyoblastoma have been encountered (138). As in the uterus, the most important criterion for distinguishing the benign neoplasms from leiomyosarcomas appears to be the number of mitotic figures. Leiomyosarcomas may arise within the liver or from the ligamentum teres. They occur in middle-aged patients, most frequently presenting as an abdominal mass (138,141–143). The prognosis is somewhat better than that of HCC and of cholangiocarcinoma.

Grossly, these lesions resemble smooth muscle tumors elsewhere. They may be single or multiple and may reach a very large size. Microscopically, also, they resemble smooth muscle sarcomas of the uterus and gastrointestinal tract. In uterine leiomyosarcoma, five or more mitotic figures per 10 high-power fields are required by most investigators to make a diagnosis of sarcoma (144). The finding of atypical mitotic figures is also helpful. For such counts, the most active areas of the tumor should be studied. The same standards should, at present, probably also be applied to smooth muscle tumors of the liver. However, because experience with these tumors is limited, these criteria should be applied with discretion.

Lipomatous Tumors

The few lipomas described have been benign, and the great majority have been incidental findings at autopsy (138,145). Microscopically, the major component of these lesions is mature adipose tissue. Depending on the presence of other elements, myelolipomas, angiomyolipomas, and angiolipomas have been described. A liposarcomatous component has been described in a mesenchymoma (146).

Pseudolipomas are encapsulated lesions embedded on a concavity on the surface of the liver. They are thought to represent appendices epiploicae that have lost their attachment to the large bowel and become fixed in the liver capsule.

Tumors of Bone and Cartilage

Benign osteoid and chondroid areas are common in mixed epithelial and mesenchymal hepatoblastomas (see p. 252), as well as in infantile mesenchymal hamartomas (see below). Osteosarcomatous and chondrosarcomatous areas have apparently been described only as parts of a malignant mesenchymoma (146,147).

Osteoclastoma

An osteoclastoma-like giant cell tumor of the liver has been reported in a patient with macronodular cirrhosis (148).

Benign Mesothelioma

Only two benign mesotheliomas appear to have been reported (7,138). Grossly, they are fibrous tumors attached to the capsule of the liver by a broad stalk. Microscopically, they consist of spaces lined by flat or cuboidal cells with occasional papillary projections and a fibrous stroma. Malignant hepatic mesotheliomas have not been reported.

Myxoma

A single case of a benign myxoma has been described (7). Myxomatous stroma may be seen in infantile mesenchymal hamartoma and in mesenchymal sarcoma.

Tumors of Neural Crest Origin

The most common of the tumors of neural crest origin, at least in children, is metastatic neuroblastoma. Neurofibroma and ganglioneuroma are rarely found in the liver and may represent a matured metastatic neuroblastoma (150). Hepatic carcinoids, islet cell tumors, and other members of the APUD system are also usually metastatic. However, apparently primary carcinoids (7), and other apparently primary apudomas with and without endocrine manifestations (150,151), have been reported. Tumors composed of hepatocellular carcinoma and carcinoid elements have been observed and an hepatocellular carcinoma associated with the carcinoid syndrome has been reported (3).

Infantile Mesenchymal Hamartoma

An uncommon mass lesion, usually diagnosed in the first two years of life (9), infantile mesenchymal hamartoma also occurs in adolescents and young adults (152). Although this lesion may enlarge rapidly, most investigators consider it a hamartoma composed predominantly of mesenchyme, rather than classifying it as a true neoplasm. Alternative terms that have been applied to this lesion are bile duct fibroadenoma and lymphangioma. Complete resection is curative. Malignant transformation has never been observed. The lesion is more common in males (8). Patients generally have abdominal enlargement or a palpable mass. Rarely is this an incidental lesion at necropsy.

The lesions are generally solitary and may measure up to 20 cm in diameter. They are well demarcated but are nonencapsulated. A few are pedunculated. On cut section, they consist of grayish white solid tissue and usually of multiple cysts containing serous or mucinous fluid (153). Histologically, the principal component is loose immature mesenchyme with stellate cells in a myxomatous stroma that may resemble osteoid (154). Cystic degeneration accounts for the cysts seen grossly. Scattered through the mesenchyme are bile ducts that may appear normal or branched, tortuous, and dilated. The pattern of ducts and stroma may resemble fibroadenoma of the breast. Islands of normal hepatocytes and hemopoietic cells may also be present. Vascular spaces, including lymphatics, are generally inconspicuous.

Benign Mesenchymoma

Such a tumor has been described as consisting of myxomatous, fibrous, and hemangiomatous tissues but without any epithelial components (155).

Teratoma

Only a few cases of hepatic teratoma have been reported (156,157), most of which were considered benign. However, successful resection with long-term survival was rare.

Undifferentiated Sarcoma and Malignant Mesenchymoma

The term *malignant mesenchymoma* has been applied to undifferentiated hepatic sarcomas in children (9), although only a few of the cases reported (146,147) fit Stout's definition (158) of a mesenchymal neoplasm differentiating into two or more unrelated malignant neoplasms, such as osteogenic sarcoma and liposarcoma. Most of these tumors actually occurred in adults. Since the great majority of these tumors do not fit Stout's criteria, the term undifferentiated sarcoma (159) seems preferable. The term fibromyxosarcoma has also been used for these tumors. In the largest series (160), ages varied from a few months to 28 years. The usual complaints were abdominal swelling or a mass. Upper abdominal pain and fever were also encountered. Anemia and leukocytosis were common.

Undifferentiated sarcomas are usually solitary masses (9), most frequently in the right lobe, which may be pedunculated and measure up to 20 cm in diameter. They are roughly spherical, soft, and well demarcated. On cut surface they are variegated, and gray, tan, or pink tissue alternates with hemorrhagic, mucinous, and yellowish necrotic areas.

Histologically, the predominant cells are poorly differentiated anaplastic mesenchymal tumor cells. They may be tightly packed or embedded in a myxoid stroma, and mitoses are easily found. PAS-positive, diastase-resistant droplets have been observed in these tumors (161). Structures resembling bile ducts are generally also found, particularly at the periphery. The lining cells of these ducts are hyperchromatic but not clearly malignant. Foci of necrosis with inflammatory cells and fibrotic stroma usually surround the lesion. A few tumors have been studied ultrastructurally (161,161a). Metastases are composed of the mesenchymal tumor cells, but a case has been reported in which the metastases also contained ducts (160). The principal feature differentiating these tumors from mesenchymal hamartomas is the atypical and anaplastic quality of the stromal cells. Lack of cross-striations distinguishes them from rhabdomyosarcomas. Rhabdomyosarcomas usually arise in the common bile duct but may involve the hepatic duct. They are rarely predominantly intrahepatic.

Rhabdomyosarcoma

Most of the hepatic rhabdomyosarcomas reported (126) were of the embryonal type and have to be distinguished particularly from undifferentiated hepatic sarcoma. Embryonal rhabdomyosarcoma also occurs in childhood. It usually arises in the vicinity of extrahepatic or intrahepatic bile ducts. Because of this location, jaundice with or without fever and malaise are the usual presenting symptoms.

The tumor has a grayish tan, mucoid appearance. There is complete or partial occlusion of the ducts by tumor. The tumor has a characteristic gross appearance of sarcoma botryoides and may extend throughout the hepatobiliary tract. The tumor may be so necrotic and hemorrhagic that a frozen section is requested to make sure there is adequate tissue for diagnosis. Microscopically, the tumor cells are elongated or plump and have eosinophilic cytoplasm. Cross-striations are often not detected. The nuclei show hyperchromasia, pleomorphism, and mitoses. A simultaneous liver biopsy specimen may show cholestasis and cholangitis.

Malignant Mixed Tumor (Carcinosarcoma)

The diagnosis of carcinosarcoma requires the demonstration of malignancy in both epithelial and mesenchymal components. Few of the cases reported with this diagnosis meet such strict criteria. Those that do usually contained hepatocellular carcinoma with rhabdomyosarcoma (162,163) or fibrosarcoma (164). In the absence of a malignant cartilaginous, osteoid, neural, or muscular element, it may be difficult to be entirely certain that the "fibrosarcoma" is not actually a spindle cell carcinoma.

Lymphoma, Leukemia, and Other Lymphoreticular Neoplasms

Few cases of lymphoma, apparently primary in the liver, have been reported (14,15,165). One of these (165) was associated with an hepatocarcinoma. Lymphomatous involvement of the liver generally indicates advanced systemic dissemination (166), and is, therefore, encountered relatively rarely in patients not already known to have the disease. Staging laparotomy with splenectomy and wedge biopsy of the liver has provided much important information on the natural history of the lymphomas, particularly Hodgkin's disease (166). Review of previous liver scans and of the liver surface during laparotomy by the surgeon is most important, so as to obtain tissue from the area that grossly seems most likely to be involved (167).

Hodgkin's Disease

Hepatic lymphomatous involvement occurs in 50% of patients with Hodgkin's lymphoma who have massive splenic disease but is hardly ever seen in the absence of splenic involvement (166,168). Wedge biopsy obtains a higher yield of lymphomas in these patients than needle biopsy, even if needle biopsy is aimed at a lesion seen on liver scan or if it is combined with peritoneoscopy (166). Rarely, hepatic involvement may be a presenting manifestation of Hodgkin's disease (169). At autopsy, about 60% of cases have hepatic involvement (170). However, at staging laparotomy, the corresponding figure is 15% (170). Grossly, Hodgkin's disease may be characterized by bulky single or multiple irregular whitish yellow nodules or by a focal miliary infiltrate. A combination of the two patterns is not uncommon (166).

Microscopically, the lesions of Hodgkin's disease are generally not difficult to identify when the lesions consist of large nodules. However, the diagnosis of hepatic involvement may be quite difficult when the lesions are small, as they frequently are in patients undergoing staging laparotomy. Hepatic Hodgkin's disease generally involves portal triads (166). In patients with diagnosed Hodgkin's disease, cellular infiltrates are occasionally found that have the stromal pattern of Hodgkin's disease (lymphocytes, plasma cells, eosinophils, and histiocytes), but that lack the characteristic multinucleated Reed-Sternberg cells (Fig. 30). There is some dispute whether in such cases the strict criteria appropriate for lymph node biopsies should be applied (166,170). We agree with the recommendation that in such cases identification of mononuclear cells with the nuclear features of Reed-Sternberg cells should be regarded as sufficient to indicate hepatic involvement. When the lesions are large, it may be possible to subclassify them according to the Rye classification. However, in small lesions this is rarely possible, except in the lymphocytic depletion types. Hepatic epithelioid cell granulomas resembling those of sarcoidosis are not uncommon (12%) in Hodgkin's disease. Such granulomas may occur in the presence, as well as the absence, of hepatic involvement by Hodgkin's disease, and, therefore, do not prove spread of Hodgkin's disease to the liver (166,167). They must be distinguished from foreign body lipogranulomas (Chapter 4, Fig. 11) (170a).

Non-Hodgkin's Lymphoma

As in Hodgkin's disease, hepatic involvement at autopsy is seen in approximately 50% of cases. At staging laparotomy, however, the incidence of hepatic involvement is higher in non-Hodgkin's lymphoma than in Hodgkin's disease. If staging laparotomy is not done, needle biopsy with peritoneoscopy, rather than percutaneous biopsy is indicated (171). Hepatic involvement is more frequent in poorly differentiated lymphocytic lymphoma than in the other types. Histiocytic lymphomas tend to produce large masses while lymphocytic lymphomas usually produce a uniform miliary pattern (166).

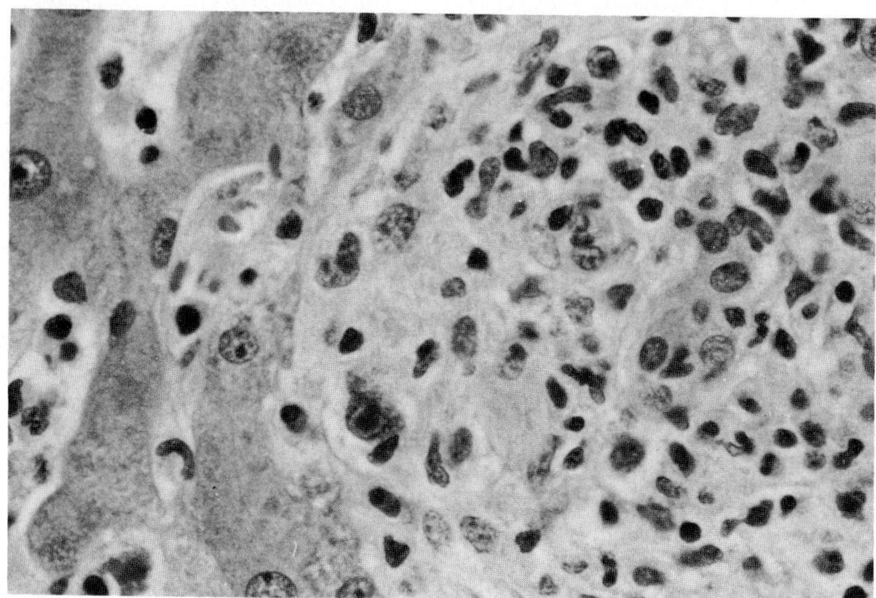

Figure 30. Hodgkin's disease. A portal infiltrate is present, composed of a variety of cells, including a mononuclear cell with nuclear features characteristic of a Reed-Sternberg cell. (Hematoxylin and eosin, ×545.)

In non-Hodgkin's lymphomas, as in Hodgkin's disease, the portal triads represent the site of initial hepatic involvement (Fig. 31). Microscopically, the hepatic lesions generally closely resemble those in the lymph nodes. Lymphocytic lymphomas generally remain localized to portal triads. However, diffuse infiltration of the sinusoids may occur in patients with involvement of the bone marrow or peripheral blood. Histiocytic lymphomas tend to infiltrate from the portal triads into the adjacent parenchyma in patients with advanced disease, occasionally mimicking piecemeal necrosis (166,172). Immunohistologic identification of surface markers in lymphomas is of increasing interest and potential usefulness in diagnosis. Mycosis fungoides and Sezary syndrome are T-cell lymphomas that may involve the liver. Characteristic "mycosis cells" with large hyperchromatic indented nuclei were found in the portal triads of about one-third of these patients (166).

The differentiation of lymphomatous lesions from nonspecific round cell inflammation (nonspecific reactive hepatitis) depends on the relative uniformity of the infiltrate, the atypical cytology of the infiltrating cells, and the tendency of lymphomas to expand portal triads and sometimes to invade the adjacent hepatic lobules. Nonspecific infiltrates consist of a mixed cellular population, frequently containing eosinophils and/or histiocytes, and may contain follicles with germinal centers. These infiltrates are particularly common in the subcapsular region and are, therefore, common in wedge biopsy specimens. Among the inflammatory lesions most likely to simulate lymphoma or leukemia are infectious mononucleosis, Felty's syndrome, and tropical splenomegaly (173). Cases of massive hepatic infiltration with mature lymphocytes in immunodeficiency states have been reported as pseudolymphoma (174,174a).

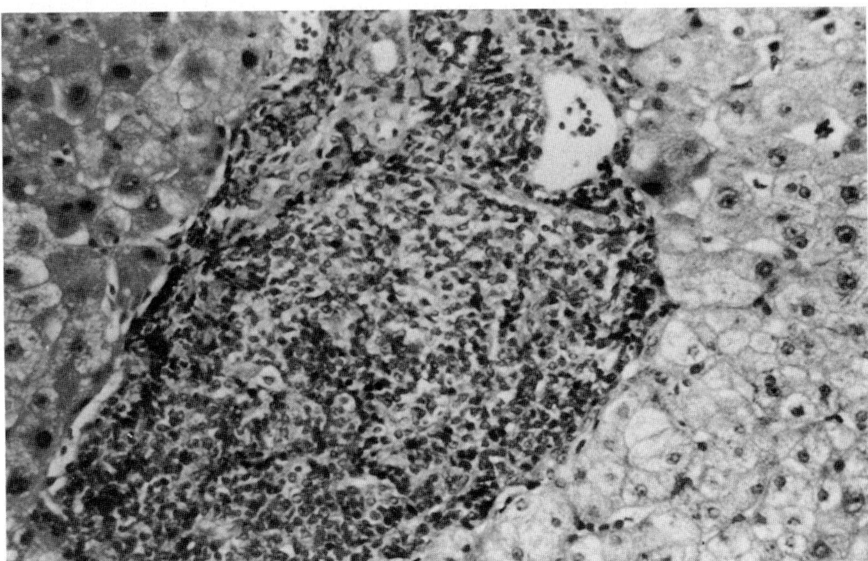

Figure 31. Well-differentiated lymphocytic lymphoma. A monotonous infiltrate of rather uniform lymphocytic cells is confined to a portal triad. (Hematoxylin and eosin, ×214.)

Hepatic epithelioid cell granulomas resembling those of sarcoidosis are much less common (2%) than in Hodgkin's disease.

Leukemias and Other Lymphoreticular Neoplasms

Leukemic involvement of the liver only rarely takes the form of space-occupying lesions. Acute leukemia and chronic myeloid leukemia generally produce diffuse infiltration of the sinusoids and hepatomegaly, rather than hepatic nodules. This is also true for most of the other reticuloendothelial neoplasms, such as hairy cell leukemia and histiocytic medullary reticulosis (173). The diagnosis of such involvement depends on finding a monomorphic infiltrate in patients with the appropriate clinical and hematologic picture. In identifying infiltrating cells, fresh frozen sections and touch preparations stained by the Wright-Giemsa and Papanicolaou techniques are helpful in addition to routine paraffin sections. Enzyme histochemistry, immunohistochemistry, and electron microscopy are frequently also useful in the identification of the infiltrating cells. B-cell leukemia can often be shown to carry immunoglobulin markers, and hairy cell leukemia has a tartrate resistant acid phosphatase (172). As described in the section on lymphomas, these infiltrates have to be differentiated particularly from nonspecific reactive hepatitis, infectious mononucleosis, Felty's syndrome, and tropical splenomegaly.

In chronic lymphocytic leukemia, the liver usually has a finely mottled, whitish, miliary pattern. Histologically, this is seen to be the result of a lymphocytic infiltrate which fills and expands the portal areas but usually does not invade into the lobules.

Hepatic extramedullary hemopoiesis is a normal feature in the newborn (Chapter 8) but disappears very soon after birth. Its persistence in infants indicates anoxia, most usually caused by the pulmonary distress syndrome or may be associated with neonatal cholestasis (Chapter 8). In adults, extramedullary hemopoiesis is also called myeloid metaplasia. It usually consists of focal infiltrates. in the lobules consisting predominantly of normoblasts and megakaryocytes. Myeloid precursors are not seen as often and tend to be localized in portal triads. Hepatic myeloid metaplasia, particularly normoblastic, is not uncommon in patients with hemolysis. Myeloid metaplasia is also part of the myeloproliferative syndrome and suggests myelofibrosis, also termed agnogenic myeloid metaplasia (Fig. 32). Very rarely in patients with the myeloproliferative syndrome, the foci of extramedullary hemopoiesis in the liver and elsewhere attain a diameter of several centimeters and undergo fibrosis. They thus become hard nodules that grossly resemble a scirrhous carcinoma but can generally be easily distinguished microscopically (175). Occasionally, the megakaryocytes of extramedullary hemopoiesis resemble Reed-Sternberg cells and suggest a diagnosis of Hodgkin's disease. These two cell types can be distinguished by the PAS reaction, which stains megakaryocytes but does not stain Reed-Sternberg cells.

Multiple myeloma frequently involves the liver (176). In such patients there is either infiltration of portal spaces by plasma cells of varying maturity, diffuse sinusoidal infiltration, or formation of tumor nodules. When the plasma cells are undifferentiated, they can generally be identified by their ultrastructure. Im-

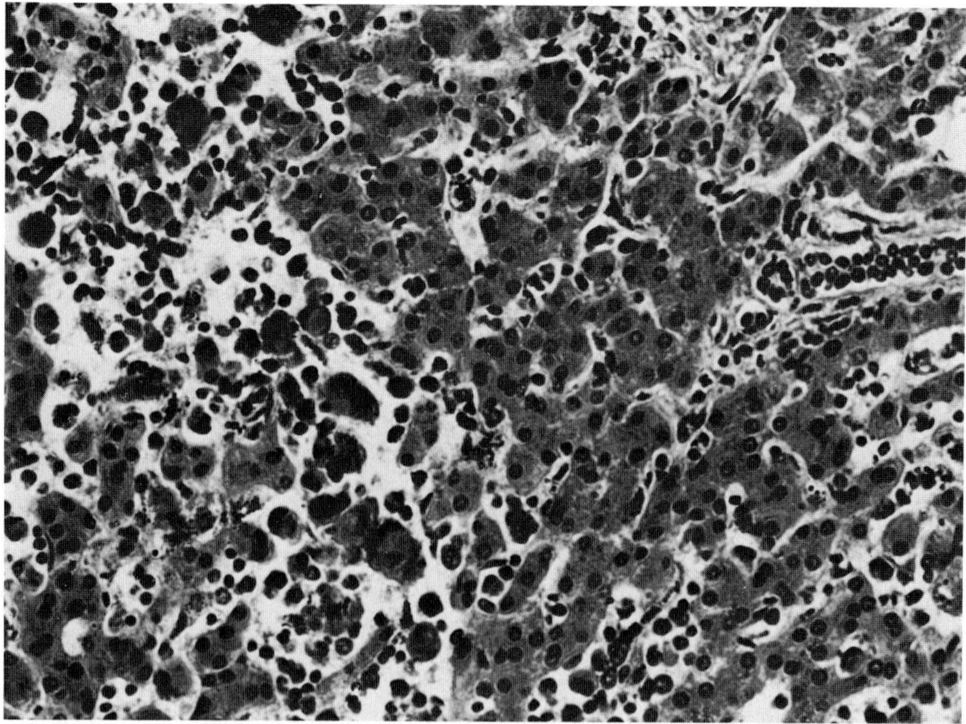

Figure 32. Myelofibrosis, exhibiting a focus of extramedullary hemopoiesis with large atypical megakaryocytes among the parenchymal cells. (Hematoxylin and eosin, ×230.)

munohistochemistry can establish whether the plasma cells are likely to be neoplastic by showing that they are monoclonal with respect to immunoglobulin secretion.

Rarely, other proliferative diseases of the lymphoreticular system may become disseminated and form tumor masses in the liver and other organs. An example is generalized mastocytosis. Mast cells can be identified by their metachromatic staining with toluidine blue or Giemsa, as well as their electron microscopic morphology. Cases with portal hypertension have been reported (177,178). Letterer-Siwe disease and histiocytosis X may also occasionally involve the liver, particularly the biliary tract (Chapter 17). Immunohistochemistry for muramidase is a useful marker for histiocytes. Electron microscopy is also helpful in their identification. Patients with successfully treated histiocytosis X have developed cirrhosis and portal hypertension (179).

SPACE-OCCUPYING INFLAMMATORY LESIONS

Pyogenic Abscess

Pyogenic liver abscesses may be single or multiple. Solitary abscesses often have no obvious source of infection, that is, they are cryptogenic. They have an insidious protracted course. Multiple abscesses tend to be associated with an obvious acute infection, such as cholangitis, appendicitis, diverticulitis, or chronic inflammatory bowel disease (180,181). In patients with an intestinal inflammatory disease, the infection travels to the liver via the portal vein (pylephlebitis). Liver abscesses have also been reported as a complication of metastases (182) and of chemotherapy for the treatment of malignant tumors (183). The principal symptoms of pyogenic liver abscess are pain in the right upper abdominal quadrant, sweating, vomiting, anorexia, malaise, and weight loss (184). The serum alkaline phosphatase is generally raised. Liver scan, angiogram, and ultrasound are very likely to be diagnostically useful. Diagnosis and therapy generally require surgical drainage. Smears and cultures for aerobes and anaerobes must be obtained from the aspirate. If a specimen of abscess wall is obtained, histologic examination will show a layer of pus toward the lumen surrounded by a zone of granulation tissue with acute inflammation (Fig. 33). Sections must be stained by Gram's stain as well as Wright Giemsa. Stains for fungi and AFB are also indicated, although caseation is rare in hepatic granulomas (Chapter 4). Culture of ground-up abscess wall is more likely to be diagnostic than culture of the pus. Hepatic actinomycosis is suggested by the finding of sulfur granules and confirmed by anaerobic culture (Fig. 34) (185–187). Hepatic botryomycosis (188) and yersinia have also been reported (188a). An inflammatory hepatic "pseudotumor" or plasma cell granuloma of uncertain etiology has also been described (189). If the liver tissue removed includes areas remote from the abscess, then the portal triads should be studied carefully to search for evidence of cholangitis as well as for inflammatory and thrombotic changes in the portal vein branches which would suggest pylephlebitis.

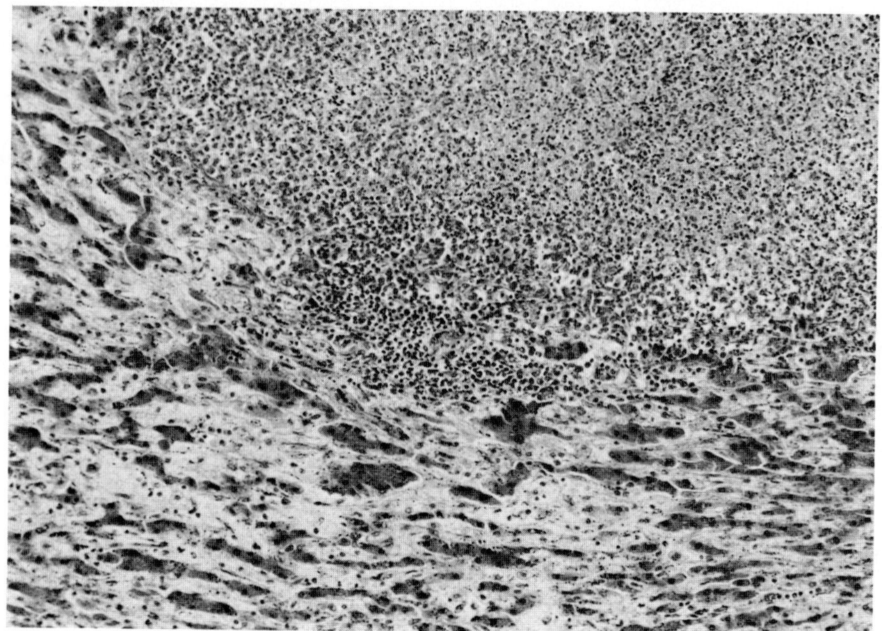

Figure 33. Pyogenic abscess, displaying a mass of necrotic tissue infiltrated by neutrophils at the upper right and surrounded by compressed hepatocytes. (Hematoxylin and eosin, ×100.)

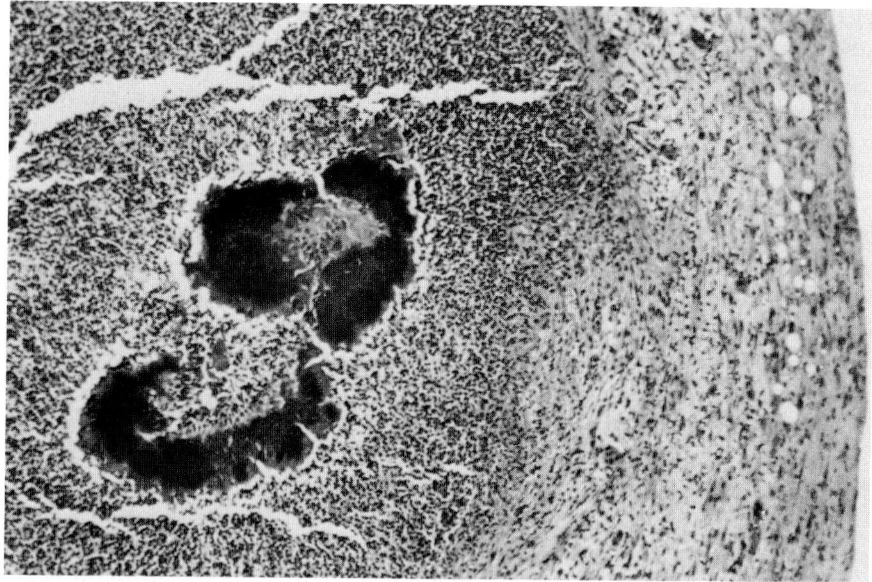

Figure 34. Actinomycosis, showing a "sulfur granule" in a hepatic abscess. (Hematoxylin and eosin, ×35.)

Amebic Abscess

Amebic liver abscesses are most often single lesions up to 15 or more cm in diameter and occur most often in the right lobe (190–192). As the disease progresses, pain, tenderness in the right upper quadrant, and hepatomegaly develop, frequently with high fever, chills, and leukocytosis. Cough and hemoptysis suggest erosion through the diaphragm. Patients with such clinical features should always be asked about foreign travel. Intestinal amebiasis may or may not be manifest clinically. Stools should always be studied for amebae, and serum specimens should be investigated for antibodies.

Aspiration of the abscess usually yields brown "anchovy-sauce"-type material that rarely contains viable cells or amebae. Once these serum and stool tests are obtained and the abscess has been aspirated, antiamebic therapy may be commenced. Alternatively, the abscess may be drained surgically. Grossly, the abscess wall has a yellowish, shaggy appearance. Microscopically, it consists of eosinophilic necrotic material that may contain amebae if the patient has not been treated. The necrotic material is generally surrounded by granulation tissue with scanty inflammatory cells, and sometimes foreign body giant cells. Portal inflammation and fibrosis may be seen in the adjacent liver. The vegetative forms of *Entamoeba histolytica* are approximately 40 μm in diameter with vacuolated cytoplasm containing occasional phagocytosed red blood cells. If necrotic, they may stain poorly with hematoxylin and eosin, but their cell cytoplasm usually remains strikingly positive by the PAS reaction. Any aspirated material or cyst wall, obtained surgically, should also be investigated as described above for pyogenic abscesses. Secondarily infected amebic abscesses differ from uncomplicated amebic abscesses by containing pus and showing polymorph infiltration. Hepatic venous thrombosis producing the Budd-Chiari syndrome may be a complication of amebic abscesses.

Echinococcosis

The liver is the organ most commonly affected by this disease. Most cases in the United States occur among immigrants (193). Symptoms may not appear for many years after the primary infection, which usually occurs in childhood. The patient may accidentally discover an asymptomatic abdominal mass or present with right upper quadrant pain. Cysts may rupture into the biliary tract and present a clinical picture compatible with cholecystitis and cholelithiasis or cholangitis (194). Daughter cysts or scolices in the stool or vomitus will confirm this diagnosis. Cysts may also rupture into the peritoneal cavity. Rupture of echinococcal cysts may be associated with urticaria and eosinophilia (194). The diagnosis is suggested by hepatic scans and angiography. Serologic tests are positive in a high percentage of cases.

The mean diameter of echinococcal cysts is 15 cm, but they may reach up to 35 cm (Fig. 35) (195). *Echinococcus granulosus* produces unilocular cysts and is more common than E. *multilocularis,* which produces more solid masses (196–199). Surgical removal or marsupialization remain the treatment of choice. On the inside of the cysts is the germinative layer composed of epithelial cells, which give rise to the scolices (Figs. 35–37). The intermediate layer consists of a hyalinized

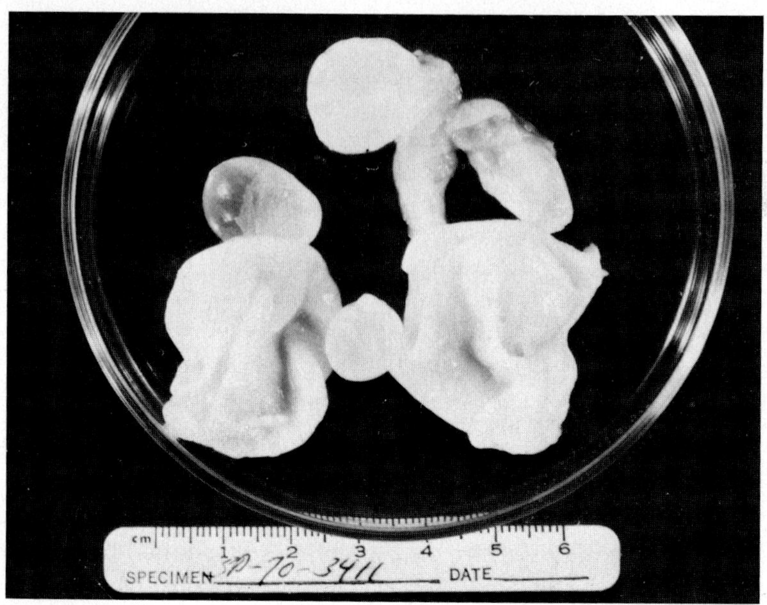

Figure 35. Echinococcosis. Gross picture of hydatid cysts removed surgically.

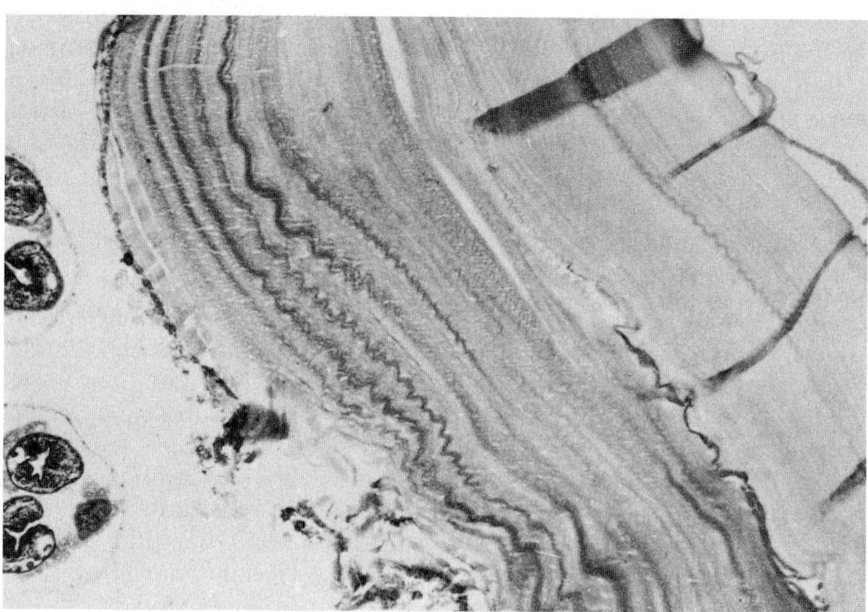

Figure 36. Echinococcosis. View of cyst wall and brood capsules containing scolices. (Hematoxylin and eosin, ×85.)

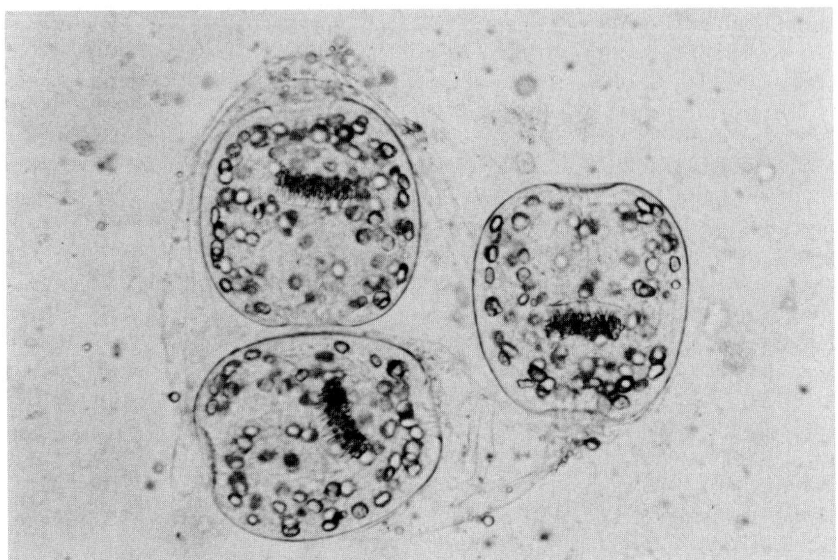

Figure 37. Echinococcosis. High-power microscopic view of three scolices from a hydatid cyst. Each scolex has a row of hooklets.

laminated membrane formed by the parasite. The adventitia that may calcify is composed of fibroblasts, chronic inflammatory cells, and compressed hepatic tissue. The daughter cysts average 5 cm in diameter and contain hooklets, scolices, and fragments of the germinative and laminated membranes. Hooklets and scolices can generally be identified quite easily in aspirates and in sections of cyst wall, particularly with polarized light. The hooklets are 20–40 μm in length.

REFERENCES

1. Cleland PG, Adjukewicz A: Hepatoma and obstructive jaundice. *Postgrad Med J* 56:371, 1980.

1a. Jurco S, Kim H-S:Extrahepatic biliary obstruction by hepatocellular carcinoma. *Am. J. Gastroenterol* 74:176, 1980.

2. Butenandt O, Knorr D, Hecker WC, et al: Precocious puberty in a boy with hCG-producing hepatoma. *Helv Paediatr Acta* 35:155, 1980.

3. Primack A, Wilson J, O'Connor GT, et al: Hepatocellular carcinoma with the carcinoid syndrome. *Cancer* 27:1182, 1971.

4. Conn HO: Rational use of liver biopsy in the diagnosis of hepatic cancer. *Gastroenterology* 62:142, 1972.

4a. Schwerk WB, Schmitz-Moormann P: Ultrasonically guided fine-needle biopsies in neoplastic liver disease: Cytohistologic diagnoses and echo pattern of lesions. *Cancer* 48:1469, 1981.

5. Bagley CM Jr, Roth JA, Thomas LB, et al:Liver biopsy in Hodgkin's disease. *Ann Intern Med* 76:219, 1972.

6. Peters RL: Pathology of hepatocellular carcinoma, in Okuda K, Peters RL (eds): *Hepatocellular Carcinoma.* New York, Wiley, 1976, p 107.

7. Edmondson HA: Tumors of the liver and intrahepatic bile ducts. *Atlas Tumor Pathology,* Armed Forces Institute of Pathology, 1958, section 7, part 25.

8. Ishak KG, Rabin L: Benign tumors of the liver. *Med Clin North Am* 59:995, 1975.

8a. Christopherson WM, Mays ET: Liver tumors and contraceptive steroids: Experience with the first one hundred registry patients. *J NCI* 58:171, 1977.

9. Dehner LP: Hepatic tumors in the pediatric age group. A distinctive clinicopathologic spectrum, in Rosenberg HS, Bolande RP (eds): *Pediatric Pathology*. Chicago, Year Book Medical Publishers, 1978, vol 4, p 217.

10. Joishy SK, Balasegaram M: Hepatic resection for malignant tumors of the liver. Essentials for a unified surgical approach. *Am J Surg* 39:360, 1980.

11. Borja ER, Hori JM, Pugh RP: Metastatic carcinomatosis of the liver mimicking cirrhosis: Case report and review of the literature. *Cancer* 35:445, 1975.

12. Breitfellner G, Dirschmid K: Leberzirrhose infolge Metastasierung bei Mammakarzinom. *Schweiz Med Wochenschr* 107:241, 1977.

13. El-Domeiri AA, Huvos AG, Goldsmith HS, et al: Primary malignant tumors of the liver. *Cancer* 27(1):7, 1971.

13a. Fortner JG, Maclean BJ, Dong KK, et al: The Seventies evolution in liver surgery for cancer. *Cancer* 47:2162, 1981.

14. Chambers TJ, O'Donoghue DP, Stansfeld AG: A case of primary lymphoma of the liver. *J Clin Pathol* 29:967, 1976.

15. Strayer DS, Reppun TS, Levin M, et al: Primary lymphoma of the liver. *Gastroenterology* 78:1571, 1980.

16. Mays ET: Standard nomenclature for primary hepatic tumors. *JAMA* 236:1469, 1976.

17. Lapis K, Johannessen JV: Pathology of primary liver cancer. *J Toxicol Environ Health* 5:315, 1979.

18. Hruban Z: Ultrastructure of hepatocellular tumors. *J Toxicol Environ Health* 5:403, 1979.

19. Squire RA, Levitt MH: Report of a workshop on classification of specific hepatocellular lesions in rats. *Cancer Res* 35:3214, 1975.

20. Christopherson WM, Mays ET, Barrows GH: Liver tumors in young women. A clinical pathologic study of 201 cases in the Louisville registry. *Prog Surg* 2:187, 1980.

21. Klatskin G: Hepatic tumors: Possible relationship to use of oral contraceptives. *Gastroenterology* 73:386, 1977.

22. Fechner RG: Benign hepatic lesions and orally administered contraceptives. *Hum Pathol* 8:255, 1977.

23. Foster JH: Primary benign solid tumors of the liver. *Am J Surg* 133:536, 1977.

24. Gold JH, Guzman IJ, Rosai J: Benign tumors of the liver. Pathologic examination of 45 cases. *Am J Clin Pathol* 70:6, 1978.

25. Ishak KG: Hepatic neoplasms associated with contraceptive and anabolic steroids. *Rec Results Cancer Res* 66:73, 1979.

26. Howell RR, Stevenson RE, Ben-Menachem Y, et al: Hepatic adenomata with type 1 glycogen storage disease. *JAMA* 236:1481, 1976.

27. Foster JH, Donohue TA, Berman MM: Familial liver-cell adenomas and diabetes mellitus. *N Engl J Med* 299:239, 1978.

27a. Cannon RO, DuSheiko GM, Long JA, et al: Hepatocellular adenoma in a young woman with beta-thalassemia and secondary iron overload. *Gastroenterology* 81:352, 1981.

28. Pizzo CJ: Type 1 glycogen storage disease with focal nodular hyperplasia of the liver and vasoconstrictive pulmonary hypertension. *Pediatrics* 65:341, 1980.

29. Dizadji H, Hammer R, Strzyz B, et al: Spontaneous rupture of the liver. *Arch Surg* 114:734, 1979.

30. Liu AK, Hiratzka LF, Hirose FM: Multiple adenomas of the liver. *Cancer* 45:1001, 1980.

31. Balazs M: Comparative electron-microscopic studies of benign hepatoma and icterus in patients on oral contraceptives. *Virchows Arch [Pathol Anat]*381:97, 1978.

32. Palmer PE, Christopherson WM, Wolfe HJ: Alpha-1-antitrypsin, protein marker in oral contraceptive-associated hepatic tumors. *Am J Clin Pathol* 68:736, 1977.

33. Kelly JK, Davies JS, Jones AW: Alpha-1-antitrypsin deficiency and hepatocellular carcinoma. *J Clin Pathol* 32:373, 1979.

34. Stenwig AE, Solgaard T: Ruptured benign hepatoma associated with an oral contraceptive. *Virchows Arch [Pathol Anat]* 367:337, 1975.

35. Edmondson HA, Reynolds TB, Henderson B, et al: Regression of liver cell adenomas associated with oral contraceptives. *Ann Intern Med* 86:180, 1977.

36. Mariani AF, Livingstone AS, Pereiras RV, et al: Progressive enlargement of an hepatic cell adenoma. *Gastroenterology* 77:1319, 1979.

37. Coombes GB, Reiser J, Paradinas FJ, et al: An androgen-associated hepatic adenoma in a trans-sexual. *Br J Surg* 65:869, 1978.

38. Shapiro P, Ikeda RM, Ruebner BH, et al: Multiple hepatic tumors and peliosis hepatis in Fanconi's anemia treated with androgens. *Am J Dis Child* 131:1104, 1977.

39. Sale G, Lerner K: Multiple tumors after androgen therapy. *Arch Pathol Lab Med* 101:600, 1977.

40. Obeid DA, Hill FGH, Harnden D, et al: Fanconi anemia. Oxymetholone hepatic tumors and chromosome aberrations associated with leukemic transition. *Cancer* 46:1401, 1980.

41. Brawer MK, Austin GE, Lewin KJ: Focal fatty change of the liver, a hitherto poorly recognized entity. *Gastroenterology* 78:247, 1980.

42. Benz FJ, Baggenstoss AH: Focal cirrhosis of the liver: Its relation to so-called hamartoma (adenoma; benign hepatoma). *Cancer* 6:743, 1953.

42a. Lough J, Spicer P, Kinch R: Focal nodular hyperplasia of the liver. An electron microscopic study of the vascular lesions. *Human Path* 11:181, 1980.

42b. Stocker JT, Ishak, KG: Focal nodular hyperplasia of the liver. A study of 21 pediatric cases. *Cancer* 48: 336, 1981.

43. Cox JN, Paunier L, Vallotton MB et al: Epithelial liver hamartoma, systemic arterial hypertension and renin hypersecretion. *Virchows Arch [Pathol Anat]* 366:15, 1975.

44. Moesner J, Baunsgaard P, Starklint H, et al: Focal nodular hyperplasia of the liver. *Acta Pathol Microbiol Scand [A]* 85:113, 1977.

45. Knowles D II, Wolff M: Focal nodular hyperplasia of the liver. A clinicopathologic study and review of the literature. *Hum Pathol* 7(5):533, 1976.

46. Wetzel WJ, Alexander RW: Focal nodular hyperplasia of the liver with alcoholic hyalin bodies and cytologic atypia. *Cancer* 44:1322, 1979.

47. Norredam K: Primary carcinoma of the liver. *Acta Pathol Microbiol Scand [A]* 87:227, 1979.

48. Miyai K, Ruebner BH: Acute yellow atrophy, cirrhosis and hepatoma. *Arch Pathol Lab Med* 75:609, 1963.

49. Anthony PP: Primary carcinoma of the liver: A study of 282 cases in Ugandan Africans. *J Pathol* 110:37, 1973.

50. Wogan GN: Aflatoxins and their relationship to hepatocellular carcinoma, in Okuda K, Peters RL (eds): *Hepatocellular Carcinoma.* New York, Wiley, 1976 p 25.

51. Joske RA, Laurence BH, Matz LR: Familial active chronic hepatitis with hepatocellular carcinoma. *Gastroenterology* 62:441, 1972.

52. Dourdourekas D, Villa F, Szanto PB, et al: Hepatocellular carcinoma: Relation to alcohol, HB-antigen and alpha-fetoprotein. *Am J Gastroenterol* 48:307, 1975.

52a. Jenkins PJ, Melia WM, Portmann B, et al: Hepatocellular carcinoma in HB_sAg negative chronic active hepatitis. *Gut* 22:332, 1981.

52b. Jacobovits AW, Gibson PR, Dudley FJ: Primary liver cell carcinoma complicating autoimmune chronic active hepatitis. *Dig Dis Sci* 26:686, 1981.

53. Moore TA, Ferrante WA, Crowson TD: Hepatoma occurring two decades after hepatic irradiation. *Gastroenterology* 71:128, 1976.

54. Battifora HA: Thorotrast and tumors of the liver, in Okuda K, Peters RL (eds): *Hepatocellular Carcinoma.* New York, Wiley, 1976, p 83.

55. Ruymann FB, Mosijczuk AD, Sayers RJ: Hepatoma in a child with methotrexate-induced hepatic fibrosis. *JAMA* 238:2631, 1977.
56. Pryor AC, Cohen RJ, Goldman RL: Hepatocellular carcinoma in a woman on long-term oral contraceptives. *Cancer* 40:884, 1977.
57. Alpert E, Ferrucci J, Athanasoulis C, et al: Primary hepatic tumor. Clinical conference. *Gastroenterology* 74(4):759, 1978.
58. Trias R, Rius X, Autonell J, et al: Hepatocarcinoma and oral contraceptives. *Lancet* 1:821, April 1978.
59. Neuberger J, Nunnerley HB, Davis M, et al: Oral-contraceptive-associated liver tumors: Occurrence of malignancy and difficulties in diagnosis. *Lancet* 1:273, 1980.
60. Lieberman J, Silton RM, Agliozzo CM, et al: Hepatocellular carcinoma and intermediate alpha-l-antitrypsin deficiency (MZ phenotype). *Am J Clin Pathol* 64:304, 1975.
61. Reintoft I, Hagerstrand IE: Does the Z gene variant of alpha-1-antitrypsin predispose to hepatic carcinoma. *Hum Pathol* 10:419, 1979.
62. Hurst P, Kakulas B, Walters M: Hepatoma developing in treated hemochromatosis. Report of a case. *Med J Aust* 48(II):18, 1961.
63. Weinberg AG, Worthen HG: The occurrence of hepatoma in the chronic form of hereditary tyrosinemia. *J Pediatr* 88:434, 1976.
64. Sugarman GI, Heuser ET, Reed WB: A case of cerebral gigantism and hepatocarcinoma. *Am J Dis Child* 131:631, 1977.
64a. Yoshitomi F, Zaitsu Y, Tanaka K: Ataxia-telangiectasia with renal cell carcinoma and hepatoma. *Virchows Arch [Pathol Anat]* 389:119, 1980.
65. Montgomery CK, Ruebner BH: Neonatal hepatocellular giant cell transformation, a review, in Rosenberg HS, Bolande RP (eds): *Perspectives in Pediatric Pathology*. Chicago, Year Book Medical Publishers, 1976, p 85.
66. Dahms BB: Hepatoma in familial cholestatic cirrhosis of childhood. Its occurrence in twin brothers. *Arch Pathol Lab Med* 103:30, 1979.
66a. Ugarte N, Gonzalez-Crussi F: Hepatoma in siblings with progressive familial cholestatic cirrhosis of childhood. *Am J Clin Pathol* 76:172, 1981.
67. Sternlieb I: Copper and the liver. *Gastroenterology* 78:1615, 1980.
67a. Mallet L, Petite JP, Amat D, et al: Carcinome hepatocellulaire au cour de la cirrhose primitive. *Gastroent Clin Biol* 5:379, 1981.
68. Anthony PP, Vogel CL, Barker LF: Liver cell dysplasia: A premalignant condition, *J Clin Pathol* 26:217, 1973.
69. Cohen C, Berson SD, Geddes EW: Liver cell dysplasia. Association with hepatocellular carcinoma, cirrhosis and hepatitis B antigen carrier status. *Cancer* 44:1671, 1979.
70. Okuda K: Clinical aspects of hepatocellular carcinoma—analysis of 134 cases, in Peters RL, Okuda K (eds): *Hepatocellular Carcinoma.* New York, Wiley, 1976, p 387.
71. Tsuzuki T, Ogata Y, Shuhei I, et al: Hepatoma with obstructive jaundice due to the migration of a tumor mass in the biliary tract: Report of a successful resection. *Surgery* 85:593, 1979.
71a. Cooney TG, Bauer DC, Knauer CM: Portal hypertension associated with hepatocellular carcinoma without cirrhosis. *Am J Gastroenterol* 74:436, 1980.
72. Cochrane M, Williams R: Humoral effects of hepatocellular carcinoma, in Okuda K, Peters RL (eds): *Hepatocellular Carcinoma.* New York, Wiley, 1976, p 333.
73. Chen DS, Sung JL: Serum alpha fetoprotein in hepatocellular carcinoma. *Cancer* 40(2):779, 1977.
74. Wepsic HT, Kirkpatrick A: Alpha-fetoprotein and its relevance to human disease. *Gastroenterology* 77:787, 1979.
75. Stolinsky DC, Sun MVC: Giant cell carcinoma of the liver: Occurrence in a patient with ileal carcinoid, medullary breast carcinoma and pulmonary aspergillosis. *CA* 29(6):373, 1979.
75a. Tesluk H, Lawrie J: Hepatocellular adenoma: Its transformation to carcinoma in a user of oral contraceptives. *Arch Pathol Lab Med* 105:296, 1981.

76. Buchanan TF Jr, Huvos AG: Clear-cell carcinoma of the liver. *Am J Clin Pathol* 61:529, 1973.

76a. Sasaki K, Okuda S, Takahashi M, et al: Hepatic clear cell carcinoma associated with hypoglycemia and hypercholesterolemia. *Cancer* 47:820, 1981.

76b. Wallace EZ, Leonidas JR, Stanek AE, et al: Endocrine Studies in a patient with functioning adrenal rest tumor of the liver. *Am J Pathol* 70:1122, 1981.

77. Lai LC, Wu PC, Lam KC, et al: Histologic prognostic indicators in hepatocellular carcinoma. *Cancer* 44:1677, 1979.

78. Craig JR, Peters RL, Edmundson HA, et al: Fibrolamellar carcinoma of the liver. *Cancer* 46:372, 1980.

79. Berman MM, Libby NP, Foster JH: Hepatocellular carcinoma. Polygonal cell type with fibrous stroma—An atypical variant with a favorable prognosis. *Cancer* 46:1448, 1980.

79a. Omata M, Peters RL, Tatter D: Sclerosing hepatic carcinoma. Relationship to hypercalcemia. *Liver* 1:33, 1981.

79b. Kojiro M, Kawano Y, Isomura T, et al: Distribution of albumin and/or α-fetoprotein positive cells in hepatocellular carcinoma. *Lab invest* 44:221, 1981.

80. Kew MC, Ray MB, Desmet VJ, et al: Hepatitis B surface antigen in tumor tissue and non-tumorous liver in black patients with hepatocellular carcinoma. *Br J Cancer* 41:399, 1980.

81. Thung SN, Gerber MA, Sarno E, et al: Distribution of five antigens in hepatocellular carcinoma. *Lab Invest* 41(2):101, 1979.

82. Palmer PE, Wolfe HJ: Alpha-1-antitrypsin deposition in primary hepatic carcinomas. *Arch Pathol Lab Med* 100:232, 1976.

83. Palmer PE, Ucci AA, Wolfe HJ: Expression of protein markers in malignant hepatoma. *Cancer* 45:1424, 1980.

84. Reintoft I, Hagerstrand IE: Demonstration of alpha-1-antitrypsin in hepatomas. *Arch Pathol Lab Med* 103:495, 1979.

85. Strohmeyer FW, Ishak KG, Gerber MA, et al: Ground-glass cells in hepatocellular carcinoma may contain fibrinogen (meeting abstract). *Gastroenterology* 77(5):A42, 1979.

86. Trevisan A, Realdi G, Losi C, et al: Hepatitis B virus antigens in primary hepatic carcinoma: Immunofluorescent techniques of fixed liver tissue. *J Clin Pathol* 31:1133, 1978.

87. Omata M, Ashcaval M, Liew C, et al: Hepatocellular carcinoma in the U.S.A., etiologic considerations. Localization of hepatitis B antigens. *Gastroenterology* 76:279, 1979.

88. Wu P: Patterns of hepatitis B surface antigen. Localization on cells of hepatocellular carcinoma. *Arch Pathol Lab Med* 103:165, 1979.

89. Theodoropoulos G, Nakopoulou L, Repanti M, et al: Detection of hepatitis B surface antigen in fixed tissues of patients with cirrhosis and hepatoma. *Virchows Arch [Pathol Anat]* 382:293, 1979.

90. Keeley AF, Iseri OA, Gottlieb LS: Ultrastructure of hyaline cytoplasmic inclusions in a human hepatoma: Relationship to Mallory's alcoholic hyalin. *Gastroenterology* 62:280, 1972.

91. Ho KJ: Michaelis-Gutman bodies. *Arch Pathol Lab Med* 103:488, 1979.

91a. Millicua JM, Scapa MAM, Ranz, FH, et al: Peritoneal Metastases of Hepatocarcinoma. Report of 2 cases. *Gastroenterol Hepatol* 4:132, 1981.

92. Ludwig J, Grier WW, Hoffman HN, et al: Calcified mixed malignant tumor of the liver. *Arch Pathol Lab Med* 99:162, 1975.

92a. Honan RP, Haqqani MT: Mixed hepatoblastoma in the adult. Case report and review of the literature. *J Clin Pathol* 33:1058, 1980.

92b. Popper H: Bidermales hepatoblastom in an adult. *Zentralblatt f. Allg Pathol* 124:403, 1980.

93. Ishak KG, Glunz PR: Hepatoblastoma and hepatocarcinoma in infancy and childhood. *Cancer* 20:396, 1967.

94. Kumar EV, Kumar L, Pathak IC, et al: Clinical, hormonal and ultrastructure studies of a virilizing hepatoblastoma. *Acta Paediatr Scand* 67:389, 1978.

95. Horie A, Kotoo Y, Hayashi I: Ultrastructural comparison of hepatoblastoma and hepatocellular carcinoma. *Cancer* 44:2184, 1979.

95a. Rosa F and Grases PJ: Ultrastructural studies in a case of hepatoblastoma. *Human Path* 11:70, 1980.

95b. Ruebner BH, Gonzalez-Licea A, Slusser RJ: Electron microscopy of some human hepatomas. *Gastroenterology* 53:18, 1967.

96. Hart WR: Primary endodermal sinus (yolk sac) tumor of the liver. *Cancer* 35:1453, 1975.

97. Popovsky MA, Costa JC, Doppman JL: Meyenburg complexes of the liver and bile cysts as a consequence of hepatic ischemia. *Hum Pathol* 10(4):425, 1979.

98. Levin SE, Dail DH, Saik RP, et al: Bile duct adenomatosis of the liver; a misleading finding on surgical exploration of the abdomen. *Am Surg* 41(2):106, 1975.

99. Cho C, Rullis I, Rogers L: Bile duct adenomas as liver nodules. *Arch Surg* 113:272, 1978.

100. Homer L, White H, Read R: Neoplastic transformation of v. Meyenburg complexes of the liver. *J Pathol* 96:499, 1968.

101. Santman FW, This LG, Van Der Veen EA, et al: Intermittent jaundice: A rare complication of a solitary non-parasitic liver cyst. *Gastroenterology* 72:325, 1977.

102. Wellwood J, Madara J, Cady B, et al: Large intrahepatic cysts and pseudocysts. *Am J Surg* 135:57, 1978.

103. Williamson RCN, Ramus NI, Shorey BA: Congenital solitary cysts of the liver and spleen. *Br J Surg* 65:871, 1978.

104. Martin ME, Baker DA, Vanagunas A, et al: Solitary nonparasitic cyst causing obstructive jaundice. *Am J Gastroenterol* 73:434, 1980.

104a. Austin EH, Mitchell GE, Oliphant M, et al: Solitary hepatic cyst and benign bile duct polyp. A heretofore unheralded association. *Surgery* 89:359, 1981.

105. Strayer DS, Kissane JM: Dysplasia of the kidneys, liver and pancreas: Report of a variant of Ivemark's syndrome. *Hum Pathol* 10:228, 1979.

106. Greenwood N, Orr NW: Primary squamous cell carcinoma arising in a solitary non-parasitic cyst of the liver. *J Pathol* 107:145, 1972.

106a. Woods GL: Biliary cystadenocarcinoma: Case report of hepatic malignancy originating in benign cystadenoma. *Cancer* 47:2936, 1981.

106b. Iemoto Y, Kondo Y, Fukamachi S: Biliary cystadenocarcinoma with peritoneal carcinomatosis. *Cancer* 48:1664, 1981.

107. Ishak JG, Willis GW, Cummins SD, et al: Biliary cystadenoma and cystadenocarcinoma. *Cancer* 38:322, 1977.

108. Azizah N, Paradinas FJ: Cholangiocarcinoma coexisting with developmental liver cysts: A distinct entity different from liver cystadenocarcinoma. *Histopathology* 4:391, 1980.

109. Klatskin G: Adenocarcinoma of the hepatic duct at its bifurcation within the porta hepatis. *Am J Med* 38:241, 1965.

110. Fortner JG, Kallum BO, Kim DK: Surgical management of carcinoma of the junction of the main hepatic ducts. *Ann Surg* 184:68, 1976.

111. Pellya-Kouri R, Dusol M, Orta D, et al: Bile duct carcinoma mimicking chronic liver disease. *Arch Intern Med* 136:1051, 1976.

112. Mori W, Nagasako K: Cholangiocarcinoma and related lesions, in Okuda K, Peters RL (eds): *Hepatocellular Carcinoma.* New York, Wiley, 1976, p 227.

113. Littlewood ER, Barrison IG, Murray-Lyon IM, et al: Cholangiocarcinoma and oral contraceptives. *Lancet* 1:311, 1980.

114. Johnson PK, Babb RR: Cholangiocarcinoma in a patient previously given thorotrast. *Dig Dis* 20:384, 1975.

115. Winberg CID, Rachod M: Thorotrast induced hepatic cholangiocarcinoma and angiosarcoma. *Hum Pathol* 10:108, 1979.

116. Hou PC: The relationship between primary carcinoma of the liver and infestation with *Clonorchis sinensis. J Pathol* 72:239, 1956.

117. Hou PC: The pathology of *Clonorchis sinensis* infection of the liver. *J Pathol* 70:53, 1955.

118. Alpert LI, Zak FG, Werthamer S, et al: Cholangiocarcinoma. A clinicopathologic study of five cases with ultrastructure observations. *Hum Pathol* 5:709, 1974.

119. Steiner PE, Higginson J: Cholangiolocellular carcinoma of the liver. *Cancer* 12:753, 1959.

120. Pianzola LE, Drut R: Mucoepidermoid carcinoma of the liver. *Am J Clin Pathol* 56:758, 1971.

120a. Ho JCI: Two cases of mucoepidermoid carcinoma of the liver in Chinese. *Pathology* 12:123, 1980.

121. Somppi E, Niemi K, Ruuskanen O, et al: Cavernous hepatic hemangioma in the newborn infant: Case report of a successful resection. *J Pediatr Surg* 9(2):239, 1974.

122. Wishnick MM: Multinodular hemangiomatosis with partial biliary obstruction. *J Pediatr* 92:960, 1978.

123. Starzl TE, Koep LJ, Weil R, et al: Excisional treatment of cavernous hemangioma of the liver. *Ann Surg* 192:25, 1980.

124. Alrenga DP: Primary angiosarcoma of the liver. Review article. *Int Surg* 60(4):198, 1975.

125. Chowdhury AR, Black M, Lorber SH, et al: Hemangioendotheliomatosis of the liver. A 12-year follow-up. *Gastroenterology* 72:157, 1977.

126. Dehner LP, Ishak KG: Vascular tumors of the liver in infants and children. A study of 30 cases and review of the literature. *Arch Pathol Lab Med* 92:101, 1971.

127. Feldman PS, Shneidman D, Kaplan C: Ultrastructure of infantile hemangioendothelioma of the liver. *Cancer* 42:521, 1978.

127a. Falk H, Herbert JT, Edmonds L: Review of four cases of childhood hepatic angiosarcoma—elevated environmental arsenic exposure in one case. *Cancer* 47:382, 1981.

127b. Fortwengler HP Jr, Jones D, Espinosa E, et al: Evidence for endothelial cell origin of vinyl chloride induces hepatic angiosarcoma. *Gastroenterology* 80:1415, 1981.

128. Jennings RC, Priestley SE: Hemangioendothelioma (Kupffer cell angiosarcoma), myelofibrosis, splenic atrophy and myeloma paraproteinemia after parenteral thorotrast administration. *J Clin Pathol* 31:1125, 1978.

129. Telles NC, Thomas LB, Popper H, et al: Evolution of thorotrast-induced hepatic angiosarcomas. *Environ Res* 18(1):74, 1979.

130. Popper H, Thomas LB, Telles NC, et al: Development of hepatic angiosarcoma in man induced by vinyl chloride, thorotrast, and arsenic. *Am J Pathol* 92:349, 1978.

131. Berk PD, Martin JF, Young RS, et al: Vinyl chloride-associated liver disease. NIH conference. *Ann Intern Med* 84:717, 1976.

131a. Popper H, Maltoni C, Selikoff IJ: Vinyl chloride induced hepatic lesions in man and rodents. A comparison. *Liver* 1:7, 1981.

132. Lander JJ, Stanley RJ, Sumner HW, et al: Angiosarcoma of the liver associated with Fowler's solution (potassium arsenite). *Gastroenterology* 68:1582, 1975.

133. Hoch-Ligeti C: Angiosarcoma of the liver associated with diethyl stilbestrol *JAMA* 240:1510, 1978.

133a. Monroe PS, Riddell RH, Siegler, M, et al: Hepatic angiosarcoma. Possible relationship to long-term oral contraceptive ingestion. *J Am Med Ass* 246:64, 1981.

134. Falk H, Thomas LB, Popper H, et al: Hepatic angiosarcoma associated with androgenic-anabolic steroids. *Lancet* 2:1120, 1979.

135. Daneshmend TK, Bradfield JWB: Hepatic angiosarcoma associated with androgenic-anabolic steroids. *Lancet* 2:1249, 1979.

136. Sussman EB, Nydick I, Gray GF, et al: Hemangioendothelial sarcoma of the liver and hemochromatosis. *Arch Pathol Lab Med* 97:39, 1974.

137. Weinbren K: Histopathology of liver lesions associated with exposure to vinyl chloride monomer. *Proc R Soc Med* 60(4):299, 1976.

138. Ishak KG: Mesenchymal tumors of the liver, in Okuda K, Peters RL (eds): *Hepatocellular Carcinoma.* New York, Wiley, 1976, p 247.

139. Nishisato T, Iharak, Onodera Y: A case of primary fibrosarcoma of the liver. *Acta Hep Jap* 22:1184, 1981.

140. Hawkins EP, Jordan GL, McGavran MH: Primary leiomyoma of the liver. Successful treatment by lobectomy and presentation of criteria for diagnosis. *Am J Surg Pathol* 4:301, 1980.

141. Fong JA, Ruebner BH: Primary leiomyosarcoma of the liver. *Hum Pathol* 5:115, 1974.
142. Masur H, Sussman EB, Molander DW: Primary hepatic leiomyosarcoma. *Gastroenterology* 69:994, 1975.
143. Echevarria RA, Arean VM, Galindo L: Hepatic tumors of long duration with eventual metastases. *Am J Clin Pathol* 69:624, 1978.
144. Scully RE, Kempson RL, Norris HJ: Mitosis counting. *Hum Pathol* 7:481, 1976.
145. Hubener KH, Hippeli R: Das Leberlipom. *Fortschr Roentgenstr* 133:176, 1980.
146. Hattori N, Arima M, Hasegawa H, et al: Malignant mesenchymoma of the liver with hypercalcemia. Report of a case. *Jpn J Clin Oncol* 2:139, 1972.
147. Sumiyoshi A, Nicho Y: Primary osteogenic tumor of the liver. Report of an autopsy case. *Acta Pathol Jpn* 21:305, 1971.
148. Monoz PA, Rao MS, Reddy JK: Osteoclastoma-like giant cell tumor of the liver. *Cancer* 46:771, 1980.
149. Knapp WA, Ruebner BH: Electron microscopy of a hepatic ganglioneuroblastoma with special reference to long spacing collagen and to portal hypertension. *Beitr Pathol* 157:200, 1976.
150. Ali M, Fayemi AO, Braun EV: Malignant apudoma of the liver with symptomatic intractable hypoglycemia. *Cancer* 42:686, 1978.
151. Warner TFCS, Seo IS, Madura JA, et al: Pancreatic polypeptide producing apudoma of the liver. *Cancer* 46:1146, 1980.
152. Grases PJ, Matos-Villalobos M, Arcia-Romero F, et al: Mesenchymal hamartoma of the liver. *Gastroenterology* 76:1466, 1979.
153. Rhodes RH, Marchildon MB, Luebke DC, et al: A mixed hamartoma of the liver: Light and electron microscopy. *Hum Pathol* 9:211, 1978.
154. Srouji MN, Chatten J, Schulman WM, et al: Mesenchymal hamartoma of the liver in infants. *Cancer* 42:2483, 1978.
155. Ichida T, Tomizawa M, Ozaki T, et al: A case of a surgically resected giant mesenchymoma of the liver in an adult. *Acta Pathol Jpn* 21:1229, 1980.
156. Dische MR, Gardner HA: Mixed teratoid tumors of the liver and neck in trisomy 13. *Am J Clin Pathol* 69:631, 1978.
157. Watanabe I, Kasai M, Suzuki S: True teratoma of the liver. Report of a case and review of the literature. *Acta Hepatogastroenterol* 25:40, 1978.
158. Stout AP: Tumors of the soft tissues. *Atlas of Tumor Pathology*, Washington, D.C., Armed Forces Institute of Pathology, 1953, section 2, pt 5, p 118.
159. Ishak KG: Primary hepatic tumors in childhood, in Popper H, Schaffner F (eds): *Progress in Liver Diseases.* New York, Grune & Stratton, 1976, vol 5, p 636.
160. Stocker JT, Ishak KG: Undifferentiated (embryonal) sarcoma of the liver. *Cancer* 42:336, 1978.
161. Abramowski CR, Cebelin M, Choudhuri A, et al: Undifferentiated embryonal sarcoma of the liver with alpha-1-antitrypsin deposits. Immunohistochemical and ultrastructural studies. *Cancer* 45:3108, 1980.
161a. Cozzuto C, De Bernardi B, Comelli A, et al: Malignant mesenchymoma of the liver in children. A clinicopathologic and ultrastructural study. *Human Pathol* 12:481, 1981.
162. Goldman RL, Friedman NB: Rhabdomyosarcohepatoma in an adult and embryonal hepatoma in a child. *Am J Clin Pathol* 51:137, 1969.
163. Watanabe I, Kasai M, Watanaki T, et al: Malignant mixed tumor of the liver, report of a case and a review of the literature. *Acta Hepatogastroenterol* 22:158, 1975.
164. Ladaga L, Kay S, Melcher M, et al: Combined epithelial and sarcomatous elements in a liver cancer associated with oral contraceptive use. *Am J Surg Pathol* 3(2):185, 1979.
165. Talamo TS, Dekker A, Gurecki J, et al: Primary hepatic malignant lymphoma. *Cancer* 46:336, 1980.
166. Kim H, Dorfman RF, Rosenberg SA: Pathology of malignant lymphomas in the liver. Application in staging, in Popper H, Schaffner F (eds): *Progress in Liver Diseases.* New York, Grune & Stratton, 1976, vol 5, p 683.

167. Abt AB, Kirschner RH, Belliveau RE, et al: Hepatic pathology associated with Hodgkin's disease. *Cancer* 33:1564, 1974.

168. Fialk MA, Jarowski CI, Coleman M, et al: Hepatic Hogkin's disease without involvement of the spleen. *Cancer* 43:1146, 1979.

169. Trewby PN, Portmann B, Brinkley DM, et al: Liver disease as presenting manifestation of Hodgkin's disease. *Q J Med* 189:137, 1979.

170. Givler RL, Brunk SF, Hass CA, et al: Problems of interpretation of liver biopsy in Hodgkin's disease. *Cancer* 5:1335, 1971.

170a. Pak HY, Friedman NB: Pseudosarcoid granulomas in Hodgkin's disease. *Human Pathol* 12:832, 1981.

171. Huberman MS, Bunn PA, Mathews MJ, et al: Hepatic involvement in the cutaneous T cell lymphomas. Results of percutaneous biopsy and peritoneoscopy. *Cancer* 45:1683, 1980.

172. Grouls V, Stiens R: Pathology of liver lesions in non-Hodgkin's lymphoma. *Leber, Magen, Darm* 10:83, 1980.

173. Schnitzer B: Sinusoidal hepatic infiltrates. *Lancet* 2:258, July 1976.

174. Snover DC, Filipovitch AH, Dehner LP et al: "Pseudolymphoma." Case associated with primary immunodeficiency disease and polyglandular failure syndrome. *Arch Pathol Lab Med* 105:46, 1981.

174a. Snover D, Dehner LP: Atypical hepatic lymphoid infiltrates occurring in primary immunodeficiency states—another instance of pseudolymphoma. *Lab Invest* 44:8, 1981.

175. Ruebner B: Myelosclerosis with serosal myeloid metaplasia and fatal liver involvement. *Ann Intern Med* 53:1075, 1960.

176. Thomas FB, Clausen KP, Greenberger NJ: Liver disease in multiple myeloma. *Arch Intern Med* 132:195, 1973.

177. Capron J, Lebrec D, Degott C, et al: Portal hypertension in systemic mastocytosis. *Gastroenterol* 74:595, 1978.

178. Grundfest S, Cooperman AM, Ferguson R, et al: Portal hypertension associated with systemic mastocytosis and splenomegaly. *Gastroenterology* 78:370, 1980.

179. Grosfeld JL, Fitzgerald JF, Wagner VM, et al: Portal hypertension in infants and children with histiocytosis X. *Am J Surg* 131(1):108, 1976.

180. Watts HD: Multiple hepatic abscesses complicating regional enteritis: The importance of prior surgery or corticosteroid therapy. *Dig Dis* 23:41s, 1978.

181. Nelson A, Frank HD, Taubin HL: Liver abscess. A complication of regional enteritis. *Am J Gastroenterol* 72:282, 1979.

182. Trump D, Fahnestock R, Cloutier C, et al: Anaerobic liver abscess and intrahepatic metastases. *Cancer* 41:682, 1978.

183. Jochimsen P, Zike W, Shirazi S, et al: Iatrogenic liver abscesses. *Arch Surg* 113:141, 1978.

184. Anonymous: Pyogenic abscess—A continuing problem of management. *Lancet* 1:1170, 1976.

185. Golematis B, Hatzitheofilou C, Melissas J: Liver actinomycosis. *Am J Gastroenterol* 65:148, 1976.

186. Meade RH: Primary hepatic actinomycosis. *Gastroenterology* 78:355, 1980.

187. Langewitz W, Grouls V, Schumacher B et al: Actinomycosis of the liver. *Leber Magen Darm* 10:107, 1980.

187a. Cedermark B, Sundblad R, Willems JS: Suspected neoplasm of the liver with pulmonary metastases cured by surgery and penicillin. Disseminated actinomycosis revisited. *Am J Surg* 141:384, 1981.

188. Bagby GC Jr, Gunning JJ: Botryomycosis as an obstructive hepatic disease. *Arch Intern Med* 138(3):472, 1978.

188a. Viteri AL, Howard PH, May JL, et al: Hepatic abscess due to Yersinia enterocolitica without bacteremia. *Gastroenterology* 81:592, 1981.

189. Someren A: "Inflammatory pseudotumor" of the liver with occlusive phlebitis. Report of a case in a child and review of the literature. *Am J Clin Pathol* 69(2):176, 1978.

190. Aikat BK, Bhusnurmath SR, Pal AK, et al: Amoebic liver abscess—A clinicopathological study. *Indian J Med Res* 67:381, 1978.
191. Brandt H, Tamayo RP: Pathology of human amebiasis. *Hum Pathol* 1:351, 1970.
192. Scully RE, McNeely BU: Amebic abscess of left lobe of liver. *N Engl J Med* 291:617, 1974.
193. Katz A, Pan C: Echinococcus disease in the United States. *Am J Med* 25:759, 1958.
194. Lewis JW, Koss N, Kerstein MD: A review of echinococcal disease. *Ann Surg* 181:390, 1975.
195. Amir-Jahed AK, Fardin R, Farzad A, et al: Clinical echinococcosis. *Ann Surg* 182(5):541, 1975.
196. Gamble WG, Segal M, Schantz PM, et al: Alveolar hydatid disease in Minnesota. First human case acquired in the contiguous United States. *JAMA* 241:904, 1979.
197. Singh G, Lee RE: Ultrastructure of hydatid cyst. *Arch Pathol Lab Med* 103:459, 1979.
198. Khuroo MS, Datta DV, Khoshy A, et al: Alveolar hydatid disease of the liver with Budd-Chiari syndrome. *Postgrad Med J* 56:197, 1980.
199. Majdandzic J, Kremer G, Langer KH: Echinococcus multilocularis. *Med Welt* 32:1060, 1981.

15
Liver Injury Induced by Drugs and Other Chemicals

GENERAL APPROACH

Drug-induced hepatic injury has been the subject of many recent reviews (1–12a). Irey (13) outlined the steps required to confirm, deny, or admit the possibility that there may be a connection between exposure to chemicals, particularly drug intake, and clinicopathologic findings. His approach includes a careful analysis of clinical and pathologic observations with respect to time of drug administration. It also tries to distinguish findings related to the original disease or to an intercurrent condition from those possibly related to the chemical. To assist in such an analysis, with respect to hepatic injury, this chapter presents an overview of the types of morphologic change reported to be associated with drugs and chemicals. A listing of compounds considered responsible for hepatic injury (Table 1) is included, as well as the various types of lesion with which each chemical is associated. This listing is not all-inclusive. If a certain chemical is not mentioned, other sources should be consulted (2,8,9). Those who interpret liver biopsy specimens should be aware that liver injury not previously reported may complicate recently introduced, as well as old, established drugs. Stopping the suspected drug should generally be considered, not only for its possible therapeutic value, but also as a step in deciding whether a drug is responsible for the patient's condition. Under certain circumstances, rechallenge with the suspected drug may be considered as a final step in proving whether the drug is responsible for a clinicopathologic picture. Liver injury induced by chemicals may be divided into predictable and unpredictable types. Individual chemicals can, with varying degrees of assurance, be classified as belonging to one or the other of these. Some compounds, such as halothane, actually seem to produce both predictable and unpredictable reactions.

PREDICTABLE (HEPATOTOXIC) REACTIONS

Although this chapter describes the effects of some toxic chemicals, most of the substances discussed are drugs. Relatively few drugs in current use are hepatotoxic, since they are used clinically only if their hepatotoxicity is minimal

Table 1. Chemicals Reported to Have Produced Hepatic Injury with Characterization of the Hepatic Lesions (For key to abbreviations and symbols see p. 291)

Analgesics and antipyretics		
Acetaminophen (Tylenol, paracetamol)	TH (Chr?)	(14,15,52–54, 54a)
Clomethacin	CH	(54b)
Phenacetin	Lipofuscin	(49,52)
Propoxyphene (Darvon)	CH	(55)
Salicylates (aspirin)	T(?) Reye's(?) H (Act + Chr)	(42,52,56–61a)
Anesthetics		
Chloroform	T	(62)
Enflurane	H (A Act)	(70, 70a)
Fluoroxene (Fluoromar)	T	(63)
Halothane*	H (Act + Chr)	(4,40,41,64–67)
Methoxyfluorane	H	(68,69)
Antiarthritics and muscle relaxants		
Allopurinol* (Zyloprim)	H CH	(2,71–75)
Carisprodol (relaxant)	H	(2)
Cinchophen	H	(76)
Dantrolene	H (Act + Chr)	(77–80)
Desacetylmethycolchicine (Democolcine)	CH	(81)
Gold	CH, H	(82–84)
Indomethacin (Indocin)	H, CH	(85,86)
Naproxen	H	(87)
Oxyphenbutazone*		(38)
Phenylbutazone* (Butazolidine)	H, CH	(52,88–90)
Probenecid (Benemid)	H	(91)
Zoxazolamine (Flexin)	H	(92)
Antibiotics		
Erythromycin estolate (Ilosone)	CH	(93–97)
Erythromycin ethyl succinate	CH	(98)
Carbenicillin	H	(99,99a)
Cephalexin*	H	(42)
Griseofulvin	CH	(100)
Novobiocin	H	(101)
Oxacillin* (Prostaphlin)	CH, H	(102,103)
Penicillin*	H, CH	(42,104,105,105a)
Rifampin	CH, H (Act + Chr)	(106,107)
Tetracycline	T (small-droplet fat)	(108–110)
Triacetyl oleandomycin (Cyclamycin)	T (Cholestatic)	(111,111a)
Anticoagulants		
Coumarin	H, CH	(112)
Phenindione (Hedulin)	CH	(113)
Warfarin sodium	T (Cholestatic)	(114)
Anticonvulsants and sedatives		
Carbamazepine (Tegritol)*	CH	(115,115a)
Diphenylhydantoin* (Dilantin)	H, CH (Reaction may resemble infectious mononucleosis)	(42,116–118)
Phenacemide (Phenurone)	H	(119)
Phenobarbital	H, CH	(120)
Trimethadione (Tridione)	H	(121)
Valproate	H, CH	(122–125)
Antihistamines		
Cimetidine	H	(125a)
Trimethobenzamide (Tigan)	H	(126)
Tripelennamine (Pyribenzamine)	CH	(127)
Antihypertensive and diuretic agents		
Alpha-Methyldopa* (Aldomet)	H (Act + Chr)	(4,128–130)
Chlorothiazide (Hygroton)	CH	(131,132)
Ethacrynic acid	H, CH	(132,133)
Hydralazine*	H, CH	(42,132,134–137b)
Hydrochlorothiazide	H	(137c)

Table 1. (Continued)

Metahydrin*		(42)
Metolazone*		(42)
Quinethazone (Hydromox)	CH	(138)
Tienilic acid (Ticrynafen)	CH	(138a)
Cardiovascular drugs		
Aprindin	H	(139,140)
Bis-Diethylaminoethoxyhexestrol (Coralgil)	T, Myeloid bodies by EM (secondary phospholipidosis),	(32)
Quinidine*	H	(141–145)
Papaverine	H	(146)
Perhexiline maleate	T "alcoholic hepatitis" Myeloid bodies by EM (secondary phospholipidosis and gangliosidosis)	(33,34,147,148–150)
Prajmulium bitartrate (Aymaline)	CH (bile duct necrosis)	(12a,150a)
Procainamide*	H	(42,151)
Pyridinol carbamate	H	(152,153)
Chemotherapeutic agents		
Azulphidine	H	(154)
Arsphenamine	CH	(155)
Carbarsone	H	(156)
Ethionamide	T, H	(157,158)
Fowler's solution (inorg. arsenical)	T (fibrosis, cirrhosis, hepatocarcinoma, hemangiosarcoma)	(159) (Chapters 13 and 14)
Hycanthone	T	(160)
Isoniazid*	H (Act + Chr)	(4,42,161–163)
Ketoconazole	H	163a
Nitrofurantoin (Furadantin)	(CH, H (Act + Chr)	(4,41,164–167)
Para-aminosalicylic acid (PAS)	H	(168)
Piperazine	H	(169)
Pyrazinamide	H	(170)
Quinacrine (Atabrine)	H	(171)
Sulfonamides*	H (Act + Chr)	(4,41,42,172,173,173a)
Sulfamethopyrazine	CH(Chr)	(174)
Thiobendazole	H	(175)
Trimethoprium sulfamethoxazole	CH,H	(176–179a)
Cytotoxic and immunosuppressive agents		
Azathioprine (Imuran)	CH T (veno-occlusive; peliosis)	(10,25,26)
Bischloroethylnitrosourea	T, veno-occlusive	(26a)
Busulfan	T (veno-occlusive)	(27,28)
Chlorambucil (Leukeran)	H	(180)
Cytosine arabinoside	T (veno-occlusive)	(29,30)
Dacarbazine (DTIC)	T (veno-occlusive)	(31,31a)
Methotrexate	T (fatty change; cirrhosis)	(21)
6-Mercaptopurine	T, CH	(181)
Mithramycin	T	(182)
Procarbazine*	H	(42)
Thioguanine	T (veno-occlusive)	(29)
Hormones		
Androgenic anabolic steroids	Cholestasis nodular transformation	(22,183,184) (184a)
	Hepatocellular tumors	(185–188)
	Cholangiocarcinoma	(189)
	Peliosis	(190,191)
	Angiosarcoma	(191a)

Table 1. (Continued)

Contraceptive steroids*	Cholestasis	(185,192–194)
	Hepatic adenoma	(187,195)
	Hepatocarcinoma	(187,195,196)
	Angiosarcoma	(196a,196b)
	Sinusoidal dilatation	(197,198)
	Budd-Chiari syndrome	(184a)
	Granuloma	(42,199)
	Nodular transformation	(184a)
Cortisone	Fatty change	(200)
	Peliosis	(201)
Diethyl stilbestrol (DES)	Peliosis	(202)
	Angiosarcoma	(191a,203)
	Hepatocarcinoma	(203a)
Laxatives		
Normolaxol	CH	(204)
Oxyphenisatin	H (Act + Chr)	(4,41,205–207)
Metabolic drugs		
Antithyroid drugs		
Methimazole (Tapazole)	CH	(208)
Carbimazole	CH	(209)
Propylthiouracil	H (Act + Chr)	(210–212)
Hypoglycemic agents		
Acetohexamide	CH	(213)
Carbutamide	H	(214)
Chlorpropamide* (Diabenese)	CH	(215,216)
Metahexamide (Euglycin)	H, CH	(217)
Sulfonylurea*	H	(38)
Tolazamide	CH	(218)
Tolbutamide (Orinase)	CH	(219)
Hypolipidemic agents		
Clofibrate	CH	(220)
Nicotinic acid	CH, H	(221–223)
Tranquilizers		
Phenothiazines		
Chlorpromazine (Thorazine)	Lipofuscin H, CH (Act + Chr)	(50,224,225)
Fluphenazine	CH	(8)
Prochlorperazine (Compazine)	CH	(224,226)
Trancyl promine	H, CH	(227)
Monamine oxidase (MAO) Inhibitors		
Amitryptilene	CH, H	(228,229)
Iproclozide	H	(230)
Iproniazid (Marsilid)	H	(231,232)
Nialamide	H	(232)
Phenelzine (Nardil)	H	(232,233)
Pheniprazine (Latron)	H	(232)
Trifluoroperazine	CH	(234)
Other Tranquilizers		
Chlordiazepoxide (Librium)	H, CH	(235,236)
Desipramine (Pertofrane)	H, CH	(237)
Diazepam* (Valium)	CH	(2,42)
Ectylurea (Nostyn)	CH	(238)
Fluorazepam hydrochloride (Dalmane)	CH	(239)
Haloperidol (Haldol)	H, CH	(240)
Imipramine (Tofranil)	H, CH (Act + Chr)	(237,241,242)
Iprindole (Prondol)	CH	(243)
Lergotrile mesylate	T (mitochondria)	(244)
Meprobamate (Equanil)	CH	(2)
Pemoline	H	(245)
Vitamins		
Vitamin A	T (fibrosis, cirrhosis)	(246–250) (Chapter 6)
Nicotinamide	T	(251)

Table 1. (Continued)

Miscellaneous drugs		
Cromolyn (antiasthmatic)	T (with bile duct necrosis)	(252)
Cyanamide	Lafora bodies	(35)
Disulfiram (Antabuse)	H, Lafora bodies	(35,253–255)
Ferrous sulfate	T	(18,256)
Iopanoic acid (Telepaque)	CH	(2)
Megluminioglycamide (Biligram)	T	(257)
Penicillamine	CH	(258, 258a)
Phenazopyridine (Pyridium), a urinary analgesic	H	(259)
Tromethamine (Tris)	T	(260)
Miscellaneous toxins		
Aflatoxin	T (Reye's syndrome?)	(261)
Amanita phalloides	T	(16,17)
Carbon tetrachloride	T	(262)
Chlorinated naphthalene	T	(19)
Copper salts*	T	(263,264)
DDT	T	(19)
Dichlorethane	T	(265)
Glue thistle	T	(266)
Kepone	SER induction	(267)
Lead	H	(267a)
Paraquat	T (hepatocellular and bile duct necrosis)	(23,268,268a)
Phosphorus	T	(20,269)
Pennyroyal oil (a cyclohexanone)	T	(98)
Pyrrolizidine alkaloids	T (veno-occlusive)	(270,271)
Toluene (Glue sniffing)	T	(10)
Trichlorethylene (solvent sniffing)	T	(10)
Tetrachlorethylene	T	(19)
Trinitrotoluene	T	(19)
Tetrachlorethane	T	(19)
Thorotrast	(Fibrosis, angiosarcoma)	(Chapters 13 and 14)
Vinyl chloride	(Fibrosis, angiosarcoma)	(Chapters 13 and 14)

*, Granulomas; T, toxic injury; H, hepatitic reaction; CH, cholestatic hepatitis; Act, acute; Chr, chronic.

at therapeutic doses, or if they possess unique therapeutic properties. Three features characterize hepatotoxic substances: (*1*) if a sufficient dose is given, a reaction is invariable and predictable in humans, generally after a latent period of a few hours or days; (*2*) similar lesions are reproducible in experimental animals; and (*3*) the severity of the lesions in humans and experimental animals is generally directly proportional to the dose. However, the severity of the lesion may be modified by various factors, many of which probably act by modifying the activity of the drug-metabolizing enzymes of the smooth endoplasmic reticulum (3).

Hepatocellular Necrosis

In large doses, most hepatotoxic drugs, such as chloroform and acetaminophen (14,15) and hepatic poisons, such as the mushroom *Amanita phalloides* (16,17), produce uniformly distributed centrilobular hepatocellular necrosis (Fig. 1). This may be associated with variable hydropic and hyaline hepatocellular degen-

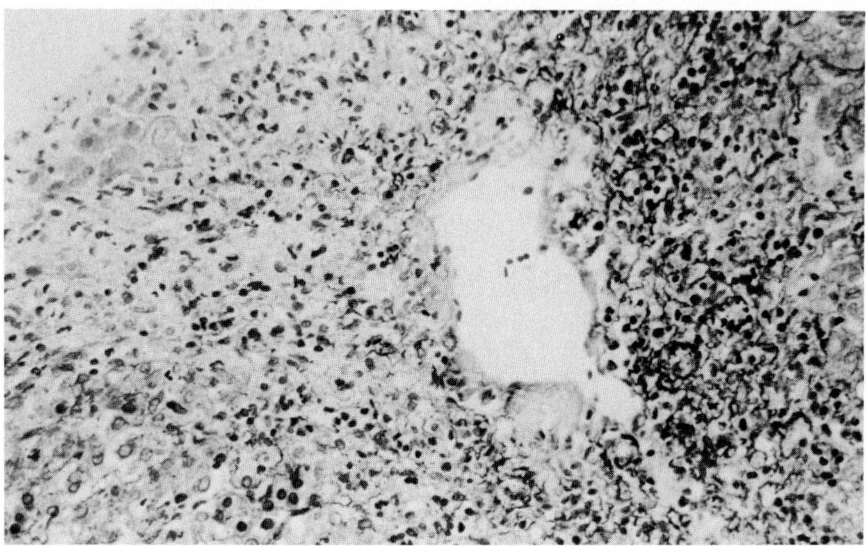

Figure 1. Centrilobular necrosis produced by ingestion of *Amanita phalloides* several days previously. A central vein is shown surrounded by a necrotic zone. The necrosis to the right of the central vein is hemorrhagic. Surviving periportal hepatocytes are seen at the left lower corner. (Hematoxylin and eosin, ×214.)

eration and fatty change in hepatocytes adjacent to the area of necrosis. The inflammatory reaction to these changes is generally quite mild. Ferrous sulfate (18) and phosphorus, particularly the yellow form (19,20), are among the few chemicals that cause periportal necrosis. Depending on the dose, most of these drugs can cause fatal massive necrosis. Periportal necrosis is also seen in eclampsia (Chapter 3) and in occasional cases of Reye's syndrome (Chapter 6). Repeated administration of small therapeutic doses of certain hepatotoxic drugs, such as methotrexate, is characterized by small scattered foci of hepatocellular necrosis or degeneration, fatty change of variable severity, and portal inflammation and fibrosis (21). If therapy is continued, such lesions may progress to cirrhosis. Azathioprine and 6-mercaptopurine have also been reported to cause cirrhosis (9). Ethanol is considered a hepatotoxin by many and can produce acute and chronic liver injury (Chapter 5).

The clinical manifestations of acute hepatocellular necrosis resemble those of viral hepatitis, except for the absence of preicteric fever. Clinical manifestations do not become evident for a variable interval after exposure to hepatotoxins. In acute poisoning, as for instance with acetaminophen, it is usually only a matter of hours, or at most, 2 or 3 days. Following repeated exposure to small doses, as in the case of methotrexate, clinical manifestations may be delayed for weeks or months.

Fatty Change

Large-droplet fatty change is not uncommon in toxic liver injury and is frequently seen in association with toxic hepatic necrosis. Chemicals particularly associated with fatty change are carbon tetrachloride, methotrexate, and ethanol (Chapter 5). A picture resembling alcoholic hepatitis has been reported after administration of perhexilene maleate, an antianginal drug.

Small-droplet fatty change, the lesion produced by tetracycline, usually in relatively large doses given intravenously, is quite unusual among hepatotoxins. It resembles those of Reye's syndrome and of acute fatty liver of pregnancy (Chapter 6, Fig. 3). There is extensive fine-droplet fatty change without displacement of the nucleus to the periphery. Although histologically evident hepatocellular necrosis is rare in this type of hepatic injury, its clinical manifestations are those of severe hepatic injury.

Administration of excessive amounts of vitamin A leads to focal lipid accumulation in Ito cells, followed by fibrosis and even cirrhosis (Chapter 6, Fig. 5).

Cholestasis

"Pure cholestasis" is characterized histologically by bile plugs in canaliculi and bile granules in hepatocytes, particularly in central zones, without significant inflammation or hepatocellular damage other than that related to the cholestasis (Chapter 7). This type of reaction is seen particularly in patients taking anabolic or contraceptive steroids (Fig. 2). This lesion is considered to be hepatotoxic by many observers because the electron microscopic and serum biochemical changes of cholestasis, though not the jaundice, occur in all patients on a sufficiently high dose and because the ultrastructural lesion (canalicular dilatation and loss of microvilli) can be reproduced in animals. This lesion may be

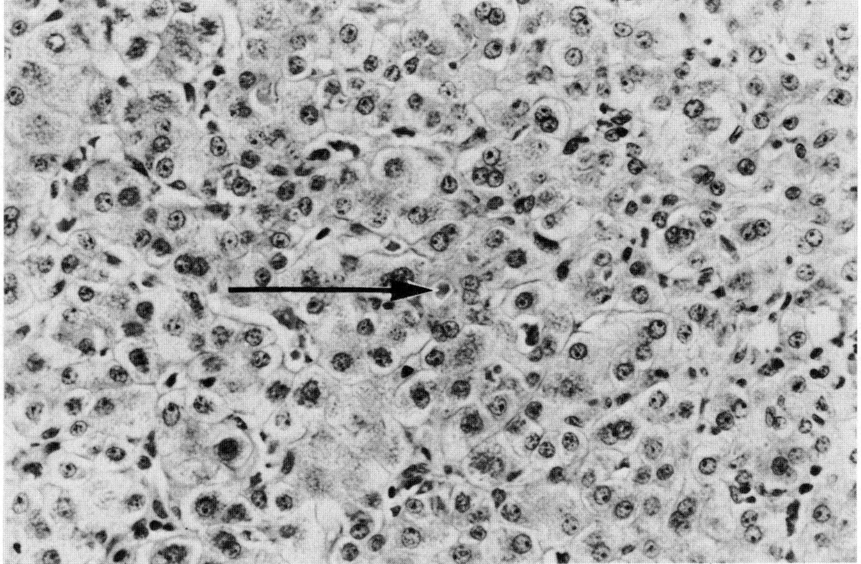

Figure 2. 'Pure" cholestasis after administration of the anabolic steroid, methandrostenolone (Dianabol). Note the bile plug, indicative of cholestasis (arrow). In addition, there is mild swelling of the hepatocytes with some irregularity of the hepatic plates. (Hematoxylin an eosin, ×325.)

difficult or impossible to differentiate from early, partial, or intermittent extrahepatic biliary obstruction when the characteristic microscopic changes of extrahepatic obstruction have not yet developed (Chapter 7). When the responsible drug is stopped, the cholestasis clears spontaneously in the vast majority of cases. However, very rarely, biliary cirrhosis may supervene (22).

Paraquat (23) and prajmulium bitartrate (12a,150a) have been reported to produce necrosis of portal bile ducts and cholestasis with little hepatocellular necrosis, resembling the lesions produced by the graft-versus-host reaction (23) and of primary biliary cirrhosis (Chapter 7).

Veno-Occlusive Disease

Pyrrolizidine alkaloids, derived from senecio and crotelaria plants, are contained in "bush tea," a popular drink in Jamaica, where veno-occlusive disease was first described in children. The disease has now been described in many other parts of the world (Chapter 12). In humans and in nonhuman primates, these compounds produce fibrous obliteration of central veins, which may progress to cirrhosis. These chemicals often also have some hepatocellular effects, but hepatocellular degeneration and necrosis are inconspicuous in humans and nonhuman primates. However, hepatocellular changes predominate in rodents. Drugs such as azathioprine, urethane, and dimethyl busulfan have also been found to be associated with veno-occlusive disease (10,24–31). The lesions of radiation damage also closely resemble those of veno-occlusive disease (Chapter 12, Figs. 7 and 8).

Budd-Chiari Syndrome

Contraceptive corticosteroids appear to be associated with an increased tendency to venous thrombosis. Thrombosis of the hepatic veins and/or the inferior vena cava producing the Budd-Chiari syndrome (Chapter 12, Fig. 3) is a rare complication of contraceptive steroid administration. Although this type of injury does not fulfill all the criteria, particularly predictability, it is probably best classified as hepatotoxic.

Hepatoportal Sclerosis

Inorganic arsenicals, such as Fowler's solution, given for prolonged periods to patients with psoriasis, have been reported to be associated with portal hypertension unaccompanied by cirrhosis (idiopathic portal hypertension). Only relatively slight periportal fibrosis may be seen (Chapter 13, Fig. 4). Thorotrast and vinyl chloride have also been found to be associated with this condition, as well as with angiosarcomas.

Storage Phenomena

Phospholipid accumulation may be the result of drug administration or of an inborn metabolic error. A coronary vasodilator (bis-diethyl-amino-ethoxyhexestrol) has been implicated in one type of fatal phospholipidosis (32).

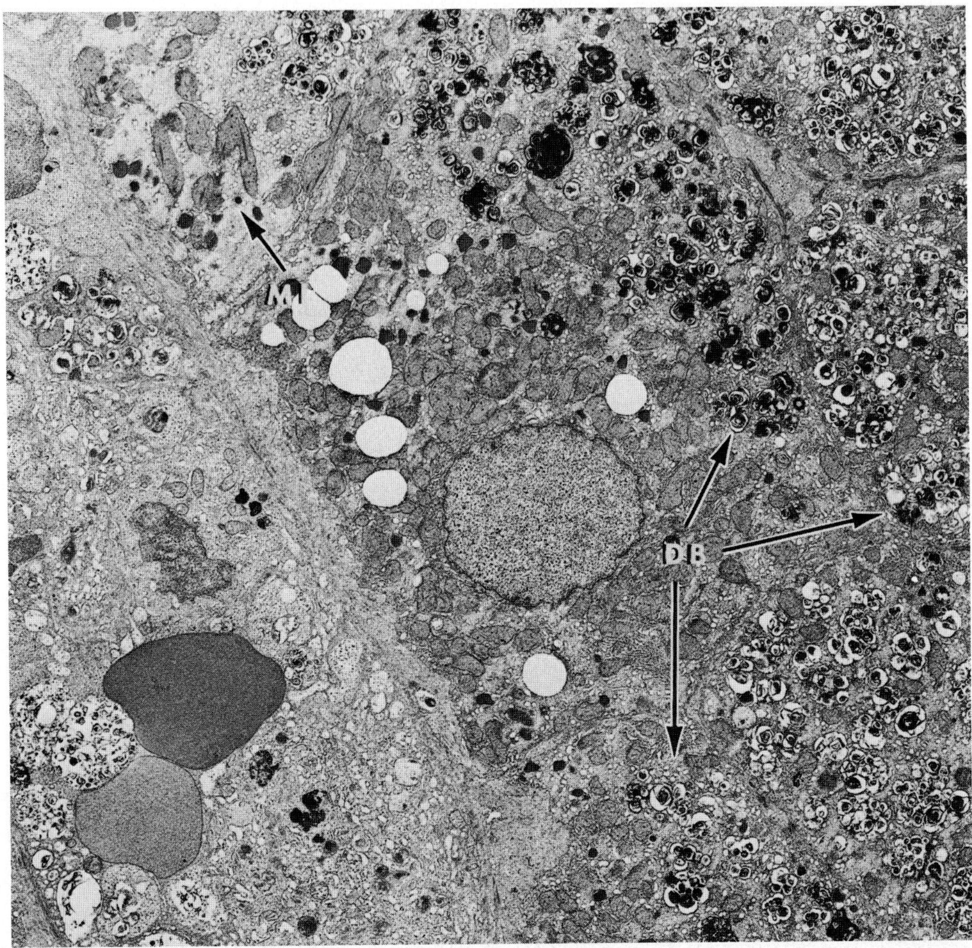

Figure 3. Drug-induced phospholipidosis. Note the curlicue-type myeloid dark bodies (DB) in hepatocytes. (×3,500.) The arrows point to mitochondria. (Contributed by F. de la Iglesia, M.D., ref. 32.)

In these patients, the hepatocytes and Kupffer cells appear foamy and enlarged. Ultrastructurally, there are many lamellated myeloid bodies (Fig. 3). Similar morphologic and biochemical observations have been reported after perhexilene maleate (33,34). Lafora-like inclusions in hepatocytes resembling light microscopically those seen in type IV glycogen storage disease (Chapter 10, Fig. 2) have been reported after cyanamide and antabuse (35,36).

UNPREDICTABLE (HYPERSENSITIVITY) REACTIONS

Many drugs in current use have, on occasion, been reported to cause hepatic injury. However, the frequency of such unpredictable side effects varies with different drugs, and each drug tends to have a predominant pattern of reactions. Even with drugs known to cause this type of liver injury, only a small proportion of patients are affected, and it is not currently possible to predict which patients are at risk. Drug-induced hepatic injury of this kind is uncommon in children, except possibly for aspirin hepatitis (37,38). Unpredictable hepatic reactions are only exceptionally reproduced in animals. There is no correlation between the dose and the severity of the lesions. The latent period is variable and may be quite long. The hepatic lesions may be accompanied by manifestations of hypersensitivity such as fever, rash, arthralgia, and eosinophilia. Readministration of the drug following recovery from a reaction usually induces a prompt recurrence. Patients with atopy, and those with a history of reactions to other drugs, are particularly susceptible. While hypersensitivity is generally considered responsible for unpredictable reactions, the evidence in many cases is incomplete and circumstantial. Two principal types of unpredictable hepatic lesions are induced by drugs: hepatocellular and cholestatic. Neither of these lesions resembles the effects of hepatotoxic drugs. Some drugs may produce both types in different patients and some patients may show a combination of both.

Since there are at present no absolute histologic criteria for unpredictable drug induced reactions, the lesions must be interpreted in the light of all the clinical data (13). Particular care should be taken with small biopsy specimens, in which examination of multiple levels is highly desirable. This may permit the detection of focal changes helpful in differential diagnosis. For instance, the typical changes of extrahepatic obstruction that must be differentiated from those of drug induced cholestasis (Chapter 7) generally do not involve every portal tract.

Hepatitic Reactions

Acute Hepatitis

In the milder cases, the hepatocellular unrest characteristic of acute viral hepatitis is lacking. However, there is focal necrosis with ballooning and acidophilic bodies which may vary considerably in severity. An inflammatory reaction is seen in the necrotic foci and in the portal triads. Histologically, the mildest of these lesions resemble focal nonspecific reactive hepatitis (Chapter 3). More severe reactions may resemble hepatitis produced by viruses such as herpes (Chapter 3). However, there are no intranuclear inclusions. Fatty change, polymorphs, and eosinophils are more prominent in drug-induced lesions than in hepatocellular injury produced by viruses. A marked portal inflammatory reaction resembling that seen in infectious mononucleosis and CMV infection may be produced by diphenylhydantoin (Dilantin). In some patients, drug-induced lesions may be indistinguishable from classic acute viral hepatitis. However, the parenchymal damage tends to be rather severe, frequently producing central necrosis rather sharply delimited from surviving parenchyma, bridging necrosis, submassive, or even massive necrosis. Lesions of this type are encountered following the use of a wide variety of drugs including isoniazid, iproniazid, pyrazinamide, cinchophen, zoxazolamine, and halothane (Fig. 4). Bridging necrosis (Chapter 2) in drug-induced hepatitis may not be be associated with an increased risk of chronic active liver disease (39). In viral hepatitis, bridging necrosis has been thought to indicate a group of cases with a poor prognosis

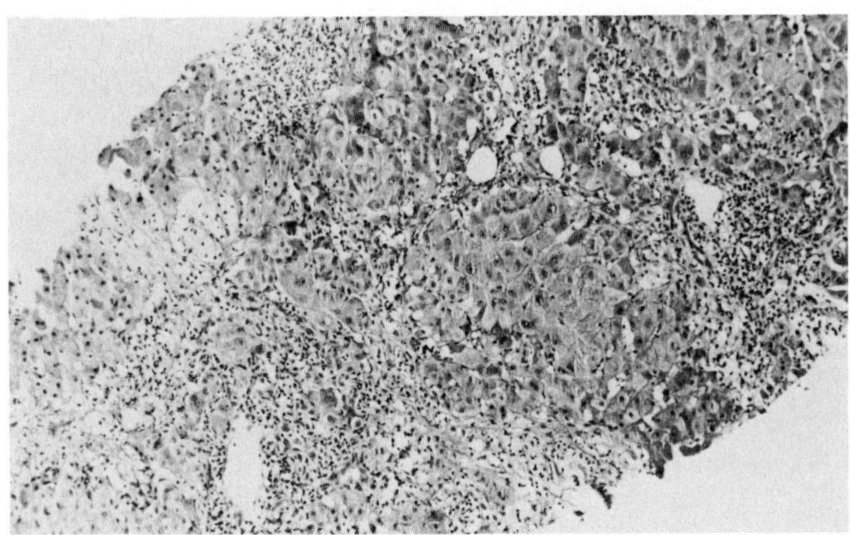

Figure 4. Marked hepatitic reaction after administration of halothane. Necrosis is particularly severe in the pericentral zones. (Hematoxylin and eosin, ×85.)

(Chapter 2). Death from massive necrosis is seen most frequently in patients given halothane or isoniazid. However, those who recover from massive necrosis generally do so without sequelae (Chapter 2) (40).

Chronic Hepatitis

In the case of some drugs, such as acetohexamide, oxyphenisatin, aspirin, isoniazid, halothane and methyldopa, sulfonamides, nitrofurantoin, propylthiouracil, phenyl butazone, and dantrolene, the lesions may appear abruptly and resemble those of a generally rather mild, acute viral hepatitis. Alternatively, the lesion may develop more insidiously, giving rise to a picture indistinguishable from chronic active hepatitis with or without the development of cirrhosis (4,9,41). Once the responsible drug has been stopped, drug-induced chronic active hepatitis has a better prognosis than chronic active hepatitis not related to drugs.

Granulomas

Drug-induced noncaseating hepatic granulomas, composed of epithelioid cells, giant cells, or histiocytes, and sometimes containing eosinophils, may be increasing in incidence and may or may not be associated with a hepatitic reaction (42). Of course, other etiologic factors that may be responsible for granulomas, such as foreign material or infections, must always be excluded (Chapter 4). Granulomas have been reported in patients on halothane, sulfonamides, phenylbutazone, and some other drugs (Table 1).

Cholestatic Hepatitis

The cholestatic type of unpredictable reaction to drugs is more common and less serious than the hepatitic type (2). It is most important to distinguish drug-

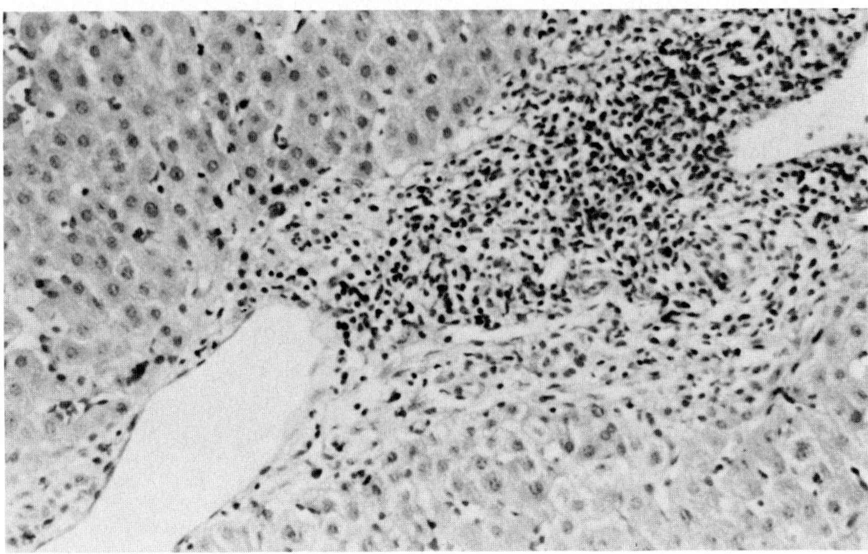

Figure 5. Cholestatic hepatitis after administration of chlorpromazine. Note marked portal inflammatory infiltrate with mild activation of sinusoidal lining cells of some damage to the hepatocytes. (Hemotoxylin and eosin, ×215.)

induced cholestasis from extrahepatic obstruction (Chapter 7). Among the many agents that may be responsible for drug-induced cholestatic hepatitis, the phenothiazines are the most frequent offenders, particularly chlorpromazine. Others are chlordiazepoxide, thorazine, antibiotics such as erythromycin estolate and oleandomycin, sulfonyl urea derivatives such as tolbutamide, chlorpropamide, and metaheximide, as well as oxyphenisatin, and 6-mercaptopurine.

Canalicular bile plugs are usually prominent, especially in central zones (Fig. 2). With time, scattered foci of liver cell damage develop, particularly in relation to the bile plugs. This damage consists of swelling of the hepatocytes, scattered acidophilic bodies, variation in size and number of nuclei, scattered acidophilic bodies, and eventually dropout of hepatocytes. There are a few scattered inflammatory cells in cholestatic, and to a lesser extent, in noncholestatic areas. If jaundice persists for some time, the cholestasis and hepatocellular damage may extend to the periportal zones. There is usually a marked mixed portal inflammatory infiltrate composed mostly of lymphocytes (Fig. 5). Large numbers of eosinophils in portal triads and sinusoids, in the absence of a parasitic infestation, suggest drug-induced cholestasis but are not pathognomonic. Eosinophils may be seen in other conditions, such as viral hepatitis and extrahepatic biliary obstruction. Portal edema may sometimes be quite striking (Fig. 6) and has to be differentiated from that of extrahepatic obstruction. While eosinophilic infiltration favors hypersensitivity to drugs, a neutrophilic infiltrate in the vicinity of the bile ducts, bile duct proliferation, and periductal fibrosis, as well as bile infarcts, favor extrahepatic obstruction. Drug-induced cholestasis usually heals without significant residual damage, once the offending drug has been stopped. However, rare cases have been said to progress to biliary cirrhosis, despite drug withdrawal (2). Phenothiazines, tolbutamide, and organic arsenicals have been implicated.

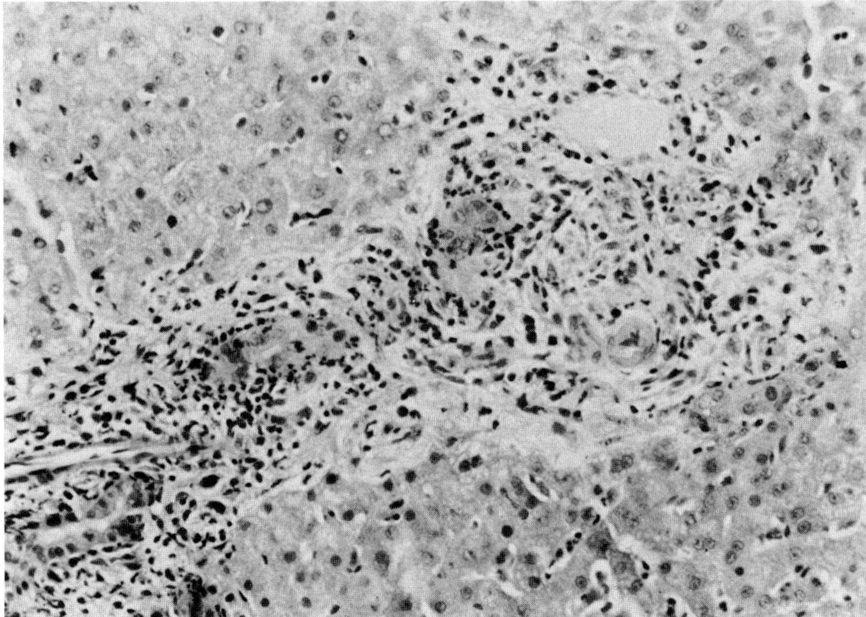

Figure 6. Cholestatic hepatitis after administration of haloperidol. Note periductal edema and infiltration by inflammatory cells, many of which are eosinophils, in the vicinity of a portal bile duct. (Hematoxylin and eosin, ×245.)

Mixed Reactions

Many drugs cause a combination of cholestatic and hepatitic types of injury. A number of drugs that produce reactions with overt cholestatic and/or hepatitic features are also mildly hepatotoxic under some conditions. The following drugs may fall in this category: isoniazid, rifampin, and methyldopa. Under certain conditions, halothane causes predictable lesions in animals and seems then to belong in this category. In general, either the cholestatic or hepatitic or toxic reaction will predominate in a patient with each drug at one point in time (5).

Peliosis Hepatis

The lesion consists in the formation of abnormal hepatic vascular spaces (Chapter 12, Fig. 10). It is not established whether the initial lesion is vascular dilatation or necrosis. The best documented etiologic agents are anabolic steroids.

Hepatocellular Neoplasms

Hepatocarcinoma with cirrhosis, particularly macronodular cirrhosis (Chapter 13), is frequently seen in alcoholics in the United States and Europe. Whether there is a direct etiologic relationship betwen ethanol and hepatocarcinoma is not clear (43,44). Hepatocarcinoma with cirrhosis is much more common in Africa south of the Sahara. This has been attributed to ingestion of mycotoxins, such as aflatoxin, plant products such as cycad nuts, and pyrrolizidine alkaloids. All these compounds have been shown to be carcinogenic in experimental animals but their importance in humans remains uncertain, and it may be that hepatitis B is actually the most important etiologic factor in those areas.

During the past few years, hepatocellular neoplasms in patients without cirrhosis have been increasingly reported in patients on contraceptive steroids or synthetic androgens, given usually for aregenerative anemia. So far there is rather scanty epidemiologic proof of these associations, and experimental evidence that these compounds are carcinogenic is weak. Nonetheless, the association between a history of taking these steroid compounds and the development of hepatocellular neoplasms in humans is difficult to attribute to chance. The nature of the hepatic nodular lesions associated with these two types of steroids remains somewhat uncertain. It seems likely that most are benign neoplasms. Contraceptive steroids have been found to be associated particularly with hepatocellular adenomas (Chapter 14), possibly with focal nodular hyperplasia (Chapter 14), and apparently with a few hepatocarcinomas. Synthetic androgens have been reported to be associated mostly with hepatocarcinomas, but few of these have metastasized and the actual malignancy of most of the reported cases has been disputed (45).

Hemangiosarcoma has been shown in a significant proportion of cases to be related to exposure to vinyl chloride, arsenic, or thorotrast (Chapter 14).

OTHER UNTOWARD EFFECTS OF THERAPY

Total Parenteral Nutrition

In some cases parenteral feeding has been shown to be associated with cholestasis and hepatic failure. Histologically, there is a combination of fatty change (Chapter 5), cholestasis (Chapter 7), hepatocellular injury with fibrosis, and cirrhosis. This picture was first described in infants (46,47) but is also seen in adults (48).

Pigments

Excessive accumulation of a lipofuscin-like pigment in hepatocytes (Chapter 11) has been reported to follow prolonged ingestion of a number of drugs, particularly phenacetin and chlorpromazine (49,50).

Foreign Material

Accumulation in Kupffer cells of foreign pigmented materials, such as polyvinyl pyrrolidine, thorotrast, carbon, and silver is also discussed in Chapter 11. Fragments of silicone rubber may be found in Kupffer cells as a result of the fracture of prosthetic cardiac valves (51). Talc and starch accumulation are discussed under "hippie hepatitis" (Chapter 2) and granulomas (Chapter 4).

REFERENCES

1. Bianchi L, De Groote J, Desmet V, et al: Guidelines for diagnosis of therapeutic drug-induced liver injury in liver biopsies. *Lancet* 1:854, 1974.

2. Klatskin G: *Toxic and Drug Induced Hepatitis in Diseases of the Liver*, ed 4. Philadelphia, Lippincott, 1975, p 604.
3. Mitchell JR, Lauterburg BH: Drug-induced liver injury. *Hosp Pract* 12:95, 1978.
4. Maddrey W, Boitnott J: Progress in hepatology: Drug-induced chronic liver disease. *Gastroenterology* 72:1348, 1977.
5. Schaffner F, Popper H: Adverse drug reactions involving the liver: Probable mechanisms. *Mt. Sinai J Med* 44(6):813, 1977.
6. Scheuer PJ: Long term effects on the liver. *J Clin Pathol* 28:71, 1975.
7. Talbot IC: Acute liver injury. *J Clin Pathol* 28:66, 1975.
8. Zimmerman HJ: Hepatotoxicity. *The Advserse Effects of Drugs and Other Chemicals on the Liver.* New York, Appleton-Century-Crofts, 1978.
9. Ludwig J: Drug effect on the liver. A tabular compilation of drugs and drug-related hepatic diseases. *Dig Dis Sci* 24:785, 1979.
10. Sherlock S: Progress report. Hepatic reactions to drugs. *Gut* 20:634, 1979.
11. Rubin E: Iatrogenic hepatic injury. *Hum Pathol* 11:312, 1980.
12. Davidson CS, Leevy CM, Chamberlayne EC (eds): Guidelines for detection of hepatotoxicity due to drugs and chemicals. NIH 79-313:11. Washington, D.C., US Department of Health, Education, and Welfare, 1979.

12a. Popper H, Geller SA: Pathogenetic considerations in the histologic diagnosis of drug-induced liver injury. *Prog Surg Pathol* 3:233, 1981.

13. Irey NS: Teaching monograph: Tissue reactions to drugs. *Am J Pathol* 82:617, 1976.
14. Williams R, Davis M: Pathology and biochemistry of paracetamol-induced liver damage. *Proc Eur Soc Toxicol* 18:27, 1977.
15. Ferguson DR, Snyder SK, Cameron AJ: Hepatotoxicity in acetaminophen poisoning. *Mayo Clin Proc* 52:246, 1977.
16. Panner BJ, Hanss RJ: Hepatic injury in mushroom poisoning. *Arch Pathol Lab Med* 87:35, 1969.
17. Wepler W, Opitz K: Histologic changes in the liver biopsy in amanita phalloides intoxication. *Hum Pathol* 3:249, 1972.
18. Luongo MA, Bjornson SS: The liver in ferrous sulphate poisoning. *N Engl J Med* 251:995, 1954.
19. Popper H, Gerber MA, Schaffner F, et al: Environmental hepatic injury in man, in Popper H, Schaffner F (eds): *Progress In Liver Diseases.* New York, Grune & Stratton, 1979, vol 6, p 605.
20. Greenberger NJ, Robinson WL, Isselbacher KJ: Toxic hepatitis after the ingestion of phosphorus with subsequent recovery. *Gastroenterology* 47:179, 1964.
21. Podurgiel BJ, McGill DB, Ludwig J, et al: Liver injury associated with methotrexate therapy for psoriasis. *Mayo Clin Proc* 48:787, 1973.
22. Globea GA, Wilkerson JA: Biliary cirrhosis following the administration of methyltestosterone. *JAMA* 204:170, 1968.
23. Mullick FG, Ishak KG, Mahabir R, et al: Hepatic injury associated with paraquat toxicity in humans. *Lab Invest* 42:138, 1980.
24. Brodsky I, Johnson H, Killman SA, et al: Fibrosis of central and hepatic veins and perisinusoidal spaces of the liver following prolonged administration of urethane. *Am J Med* 30:976, 1961.
25. Marubbio AT, Danielson B: Hepatic veno-occlusive disease in a renal transplant patient receiving azathioprine. *Gastroenterology* 69:739, 1975.
26. DeGott C, Rueff B, Kreisch CA, et al: Peliosis hepatis in recipients of renal transplants. *Gut* 19:748, 1978.

26a. McIntyre RE, Magidson JG, Austin GE, et al: Fatal veno-occlusive disease of the liver following high dose 1-3 Bis (2-chloroethyl) 1-Nitrosourea (BCNU) and autologous bone marrow transplantation. *Am J Clin Path* 75:614, 1981.

27. Beschorner WE, Pino J, Boitnott JK, et al: Pathology of the liver with bone marrow transplantation. *Am J Pathol* 99:369, 1980.

28. Shulman HM, McDonald GB, Mathews D, et al: An analysis of hepatic veno-occlusive disease and centrilobular hepatic degeneration following bone marrow transplantation. *Gastroenterology* 79:1178, 1980.
29. Griner PF, Elbadawi A, Packman CH: Veno-occlusive disease of the liver after chemotherapy of acute leukemia. *Ann Intern Med* 85:578,1976.
30. Woods WG, Dehner LP, Nesbit ME, et al: Fatal veno-occlusive disease of the liver following high dose chemotherapy, irradiation and bone marrow transplantation. *Am J Med* 68:285, 1980.
31. Asbury RF, Rosenthal SN, Descalzi ME, et al: Hepatic veno-occlusive disease due to DTIC. *Cancer* 45:2670, 1980.
31a. Voigt H, Caselitz J, Janner M: Veno-occlusive syndrome following dacarbazine. *Klin Wschr* 59:229, 1981.
32. De La Iglesia F, Feller G, Takada A, et al: Morphologic studies on secondary phospholipidosis in human liver. *Lab Invest* 30:539, 1974.
33. Lageron A, Poupon R, de Saint-Maur PP, et al: Liver ganglioside storage after perhexiline maleate. *Lancet* 1:483, 1977.
34. Le Gal JY, Guillouzo A, Glaise D, et al: Perhexilene maleate toxicity on human liver cell lines. *Gut* 21:977, 1980.
35. Vazquez JJ, Cervera S: Cyanamide-induced liver injury in alcoholics. *Lancet* 1:361, 1980.
36. Vazquez JJ, Pardo-Mindan J: Liver cell injury. Bodies similar to Lafora's in alcoholics treated with disulfiram (antabuse). *Histopathology* 3:377, 1979.
37. Mullick F, Drake R, Irey N: Morphologic changes in adverse drug reactions in infants and children. *Hum Pathol* 8:361, 1977.
38. Zimmerman HJ: Drug induced chronic hepatic disease. *Med Clin North Am* 63:567, 1979.
39. Spitz RD, Keren DF, Boitnott JK, et al: Bridging hepatic necrosis. Etiology and prognosis. *Dig Dis* 23(12):1076, 1978.
40. Miller DH, Dwyer J, Klatskin G: Halothane hepatitis: Benign resolution of a severe lesion. *Ann Intern Med* 89:212, 1978.
41. Maddrey WC, Boitnott JK: Drug-induced chronic hepatitis and cirrhosis, in Popper H, Schaffner F (eds): *Progress in Liver Diseases.* New York, Grune & Stratton, 1979, vol 6, p 595.
42. McMaster KR, Hennigar GR: Drug induced granulomatous hepatitis. *Lab Invest* 44:61, 1981.
43. Miyai K, Ruebner BH: Acute yellow atrophy, cirrhosis and hepatoma. *Arch Pathol* 75:609, 1963.
44. Peters RL: Pathology of hepatocellular carcinoma, in Okuda K, Peters RL (eds): *Hepatocellular Carcinoma.* New York, Wiley, 1976, p 107.
45. Anthony PP: Hepatoma associated with androgenic steroids. *Lancet* 1:685, 1975.
46. Bernstein J, Chang CH, Brough AJ, et al: Conjugated hyperbilirubinemia in infancy associated with parenteral alimentation. *J Pediatr* 90:361, 1977.
47. Postuma R, Trevenen CL: Liver disease in infants receiving total parenteral nutrition. *Pediatrics* 63:110, 1979.
48. Sheldon G, Petersen S, Sanders R: Hepatic dysfunction during hyperalimentation. *Arch Surg* 113:504, 1978.
49. Abrahams C, Wheatley A, Rubenstein AH, et al: Hepatocellular lipofuscin after excessive ingestion of analgesics. *Lancet* 2:621, 1964.
50. Greiner AC, NicolsonGA: Pigment deposition in viscera associated with prolonged chlorpromazine therapy. *Can Med Assoc J* 91:627, 1964.
51. Ridolfi RL, Hutchins GM: Detection of ball variance in prosthetic heart valve by liver biopsy. *Johns Hopkins Med J* 134:131, 1974.
52. Prescott LF: Hepatotoxicity of mild analgesics. *Br J Clin Pharm* 10:373s, 1980.
53. McClain CJ, Kromhout JP, Peterson FJ, et al: Potentiation of acetaminophen hepatotoxicity by alcohol *JAMA* 244:251, 1980.
54. Bonkowski HL, Mudge GH, McMurtrie RJ: Chronic hepatic inflammation and fibrosis due to low doses of paracetamol *Lancet* 1:1016, 1978.

54a. Gerber MA, Kaufmann H, Klion F: Acetaminophen induced hepatic injury. Report of two cases showing unusual portal tract reactions. *Human Path* 11:37, 1980.
54b. Mamou P, Levy VG: Atteintes hepatiques après clometacine. *Nouve Presse Med* 10:2719, 1981.
55. Klein NC, Magida MG: Propoxphene (Darvon) hepatotoxicity. *Am J Dig Dis* 16:467, 1971.
56. O'Gorman T, Koff RS: Salicylate hepatitis. *Gastroenterology* 72(4):726, 1977.
57. Sbarbara JA, Bennett RM: Aspirin hepatotoxicity and disseminated intravascular coagulation. *Ann Inern Med* 86:183, 1977.
58. Saltzman D, Gall E, Robinson S: Aspirin induced hepatic dysfunction in a patient with adult rheumatoid arthritis. *Dig Dis* 21(9):815, 1976.
59. Seaman WE, Ishak KG, Plotz PH: Aspirin-induced hepatotoxicity in patients with systemic lupus erythematosus. *Ann Intern Med* 80:1, 1974.
60. Ulshen MH, Grand RJ, Crain JD, et al: Hepatotoxicity with encephalopathy associated with aspirin therapy in rheumatoid arthritis. *J Pediatr* 93:1034, 1978.
61. Gitlin N: Salicylate hepatotoxicity. The potential role of hypoalbuminemia. *J Clin Gastroenterol* 2:281, 1980.
61a. Partin JS, Partin JC, Schubert WK, et al: Serum salicylate concentrations in Reye's disease. *Lancet* i:191, 1982.
62. Whipple GH, Sperry JA: Chloroform poisoning, liver necrosis and repair. *Johns Hopkins Med J* 20:278, 1909.
63. Reynolds ES, Brown BR Jr, Vandam LD: Massive hepatic necrosis after fluoroxene anesthesia—A case of drug interaction? *N Engl J Med* 286:530, 1972.
64. Dordal E, Glagov S, Orlando RA, et al: Fatal halothane hepatitis with transient granulomas. *N Engl J Med* 283:357, 1970.
65. Kaplan HG, Bakken J, Quadracci L, et al: Hepatitis caused by halothane sniffing. *Ann Intern Med* 90(5):797, 1979.
66. Schlippert W, Anuras S: Recurrent hepatitis following halothane exposures. *Am J Med* 65:25, 1978.
67. Peters RL, Edmondson HA, Reynolds TB, et al: Hepatic necrosis associated with halothane anesthesia. *Am J Med* 47:748, 1969.
68. Brenner AI, Kaplan MM: Recurrent hepatitis due to methoxyflurane anesthesia. *N Engl J Med* 284:961, 1971.
69. Rubinger D, Davidson JT, Melmed RN: Hepatitis following the use of methoxyflurane in obstetric analgesia. *Anesthesiology* 43:593, 1975.
70. Kline MA: Enflurane associated hepatitis. *Gastroenterology* 79:126, 1980.
70a. White LB, De Tarnowski GO, Mir JA: Hepatotoxicity following enflurane anesthesia. *Dig Dis Sci* 26:466, 1981.
71. Alkawas FH, Seeff LB, Berendson RA: Allopurinol hepatotoxicity. Report of two cases and review of the literature. *Ann Int Med* 95:588, 1981.
72. Swank LA, Chejfec G, Nemchausky BA: Allopurinol-induced granulomatous hepatitis with cholangitis and sarcoid-like reaction. *Arch Intern Med* 138:997, 1978.
73. Espiritu C, Alalu J, Glueckauf L, et al: Allopurinol-induced granulomatous hepatitis. *Dig Dis* 21(9):804, 1976.
74. Simmons F, Feldman B, Gerety D: Granulomatous hepatitis in a patient receiving allopurinol. *Gastroenterology* 62:101, 1972.
75. Butler RC, Shah M, Grunow WA, et al: Massive hepatic necrosis in a patient receiving allopurinol. *JAMA* 237(5):473, 1977.
76. Lenzer AR, Lockie ML, Becker CR: Acute yellow atrophy following cinchophen administration. Report of a case. *N Engl J MEd* 236:500, 1947.
77. Ogburn RM, Myers RL, Burdick GE: Hepatitis associated with dantrolene sodium. *Ann Intern Med* 84:53, 1976.
78. Utili R, Boitnott JK, Zimmerman HJ: Dantrolene-associated hepatic injury. *Gastroenterology* 72:610, 1977.

79. Schneider R, Mitchell D: Dantrolene hepatitis. *JAMA* 235:1590, 1976.

80. Donegan JH, Donegan WL, Cohen EB: Massive hepatic necrosis associated with dantrolene therapy. *Dig Dis* 23:48s, 1978.

81. Velasco HA, Sokal JE: Cholestatic jaundice in association with desacetylmethyl colchicine. *N Engl J Med* 260:1280, 1959.

82. Hartfall SJ, Garland HG: Further observations on the gold treatment of rheumatoid arthritis. *Lancet* 1:1459, June 1936.

83. Ghishan FK, La Brecque DR, Younoszai K: Intrahepatic cholestasis after gold therapy in juvenile rheumatoid arthritis. *J Pediatr* 93:1042, 1978.

84. Favreau M, Tannebaum H, Lough J: Hepatic toxicity associated with gold therapy. *Ann Intern Med* 87:717, 1977.

85. Fenech FP: Hepatitis with biliverdinemia in association with indomethacine therapy. *Br Med J* 3:155, 1967.

86. Kelsey WM, Scharyj M: Fatal hepatitis probably due to indomethacin. *JAMA* 199:586, 1967.

87. Victorino RMM, Silveira JCB, Baptista A, et al: Jaundice associated with naproxen. *Postgrad Med J* 56:368, 1980.

88. Mauer EF: The toxic effects of phenylbutazone (butazolidin). Review of the literature and report of the twenty-third death following its use. *N Engl J Med* 253:404, 1955.

89. Benjamin SB, Ishak KG, Zimmerman HJ, et al: Phenylbutazone liver injury. A clinicopathologic survey of 23 cases and review of the literature. *Hepatology* 1:255, 1981.

90. Lebacq EG, Desmet V: Sarcoid granulomas associated with phenylbutazone treatment. *Mt Sinai J Med* 44:778, 1977.

91. Reynolds ES, Schlant RC, Gonick HC: Necrosis of the liver as a manifestation of hypersensitivity to probenecid. *N Engl J Med* 256:592, 1957.

92. Carr HJ, Knauer QF: Death due to hepatic necrosis in a patient receiving zoxazolamine. Report of a case and review of the literature. *N Engl J Med* 264:977, 1961.

93. Lloyd-Still JD, Sherman JO, Boggs J, et al: Erythromycin estolate hepatotoxicity. *Am J Dis Child* 132:320, 1978.

94. Cooksley W, Powell L: Erythromycin jaundice: Diagnosis by an in vitro challenge test. *Aust NZ J Med* 7:291, 1977.

95. Lunzer MR, Huang SN, Ward KM, et al: Jaundice due to erythromycin estolate. *Gastroenterology* 68:1284, 1975.

96. Zafrani ES, Ishak KG, Rudzki C: Cholestatic and hepatocellular injury associated with erythromycin esters: Report of nine cases. *Am J Dig Dis* 24:385, 1979.

97. Krowchuk D, Seashor JH: Complete biliary obstruction due to erythromycin estolate administration in an infant. *Pediatrics* 64:956, 1979.

98. Sullivan JB, Rumack BH, Thomas H, et al: Pennyroyal oil poisoning and hepatotoxicity. *JAMA* 242:2873, 1979.

99. Wilson FM, Belamaric J, Lauter CB, et al: Anicteric carbenicillin hepatitis. *JAMA* 232:818, 1975.

99a. Nakamura T, Shioufu M, Seko A: Two cases of hepatic injury due to cephalexin. *Acta Hepatogastroenterol (Jpn)* 21:1545, 1980.

100. Chiprut RO, Viteri A, Jamroz C, et al: Intrahepatic cholestasis after griseofulvin administration. *Gastroenterology* 70:1141, 1976.

101. Bridges RA, Berendes H, Good RA: Serious reaction to novobiocin. *J Pediatr* 50:579, 1957.

102. Goldstein LI, Granoff M, Waisman J: Hepatic injury due to oxacillin administration. *Am J Gastroenterol* 70:171, 1978.

103. Bruckstein A, Attia A: Oxacillin hepatitis. Two patients with liver biopsy. *Am J Med* 64:519, 1978.

104. Goldstein LI, Ishak KG: Hepatic injury associated with penicillin therapy. *Arch Pathol Lab Med* 98:114, 1974.

105. Murphy ES, Mireles M: Shock, liver necrosis, and death after penicillin injection. *Arch Pathol Lab Med* 73:355, 1962.

105a. Williams CN, Macatjalian DA: Severe penicillin-induced cholestasis in a 91-year-old woman. *Dig Dis Sci* 26:470, 1981.

106. Thompson JE: The effect of rifampicin on liver morphology in tuberculous alcoholics. *Aust NZ J Med* 6(2):111, 1976.

107. Scheuer PJ, Summerfield JA, Lal S, et al: Rifampicin hepatitis. *Lancet* 1:421, 1974.

108. Lloyd-Still JD, Grand RJ, Vawter GF: Tetracycline hepatotoxicity in the differential diganosis of postoperative jaundice. *J Pediatr* 84(3):366, 1974.

109. Peters RL, Edmondson HA, Mikkelsen WP: Tetracycline-induced fatty liver in nonpregnant patients. *Am J Surg* 113:622, 1967.

110. Schenker S, Lewis M, Combes B: Studies on the pathogenesis of tetracycline-induced fatty liver. *Am J Dig Dis* 12(5):429, 1967.

111. Ticktin HE, Zimmerman HJ: Hepatic dysfunction and jaundice in patients receiving triacetyloleandomycin. *N Engl J Med* 267:964, 1967.

111a. Haber I, Hubens A: Cholestatic jaundice after triacetyloleandomycin and oral contraceptives. *Acta Gastroenterol [Belg]* 43:475, 1980.

112. Slagbom G, Loeliger EA: Coumarin associated hepatitis. *Arch Intern Med* 140:1028, 1980.

113. Portal RW, Emmanuel RW: Phenindione hepatitis complicating anticoagulant therapy. *Br Med J* 2:1318, 1961.

114. Rehnquist N: Intrahepatic jaundice due to Warfarin therapy. *Acta Med Scand* 204:335, 1978.

115. Ramsay ID: Carbamazepine induced jaundice. *Br Med J* 4:155, 1967.

115a. Levy M, Goodman MW, Van Dyne BJ, et al: Granulomatous hepatitis secondary to carbamazepine. *Ann Int Med* 95:64, 1981.

115b. Hopen G, Nesthus I, Laerum OD: Fatal Carbamazepine-associated hepatitis. Report of two cases. *Acta Med Scand* 210:333, 1981.

116. Speckler SJ, Sperber H, Doos WG, et al: Cholestasis and toxic epidermal necrolysis associated with penytoin sodium ingestion: The role of bile duct injury. *Ann Int Med* 95:455, 1981.

117. Lee TJ, Carney CN, Lapis JL, et al: Diphenylhydantoin-induced hepatic necrosis. *Gastroenterology* 70:422, 1976.

118. Mullick FG, Ishak KG: Hepatic injury associated with diphenyl hydantoin therapy. A clinicopathologic study of 20 cases. *Am J Clin Pathol* 74:442, 1980.

119. Levy RW, Simons DJ, Aronson S: Fatal hepatorenal syndrome associated with phenurone therapy. *N Engl J Med* 242:933, 1950.

120. Pagliaro L, Campesi G, Aguglia F: Barbiturate jaundice. Report of a case due to a barbital containing drug, with positive rechallenge to phenobarbital. *Gastroent* 56:938, 1969.

121. Leard SE, Greer WER, Kaufman CI: Hepatitis, exfoliative dermatitis and abnormal bone marrow occurring during tridione therapy. Report of a case with recovery. *N Engl J Med* 240:962, 1949.

122. Suchy FJ, Balistreri WF, Buchino JJ, et al: Acute hepatic failure associated with the use of sodium valproate. *N Engl J Med* 300:962, 1979.

123. Sussman NM, McLain LW: A direct hepatotoxic effect of valproic acid. *JAMA* 242:1173, 1979.

124. Ware S, Millward-Sadler GH: Acute liver disease associated with sodium valproate. *Lancet* 2:1110, 1980.

125. Anonymous: Sodium valproate and the liver. *Lancet* 2:1119, 1980.

125a. Lorenzini I, Jezequel AM, Orlandi F: Cimetidine induced hepatitis. Electron microscopic observations and clinical pattern of liver injury. *Dig Dis Sci* 26:275, 1981.

126. Borda I, Jick H: Hepatitis following the administration of trimethobenzamide hydrochloride. *Arch Intern Med* 120:371, 1967.

127. Bjorneboe M, Iversen O, Olsen S: Infective hepatitis and toxic jaundice in municipal hospital during a five-year period. *Acta Med Scand* 182:491, 1967.

128. Miller AC Jr, Reid WM: Methyldopa-induced granulomatous hepatitis. *JAMA* 235:2001, 1976.

129. Arranto AJ, Sotaniemi EA: Morphologic alterations in patients with alpha-methyldopa induced liver damage after short- and long-term exposure. *Scand J Gastroent* 16:853, 1981.

130. Arranto AJ, Sotaniemi EA: Histologic follow-up of alpha-methyl dopa induced liver injury. *Scand J Gastroent* 16:865, 1981.
131. Huseby KO: Jaundice with persisting pericholangitic inflammation in a patient treated with chlorothiazide. Report of a case. *Am J Dig Dis* 9:439, 1964.
132. Olsson R: Liver damage due to antihypertensive drugs. *Acta Med Scand* 628:53, 1978.
133. Datey KK, Deshmukh SN, Dalvi CP, et al: Hepatocellular damage with ethacrynic acid. *Br Med J* 3:152, 1967.
134. Jori GP, Peschile C: Hydralazine disease associated with transient granulomas in the liver. *Gastroenterology* 64:1163, 1973.
135. Bartoli E, Massarelli G, Solinas A, et al: Acute hepatitis with bridging necrosis due to hydralazine intake. *Arch Intern Med* 139:698, 1979.
136. Barnett DB, Hudson JA, Golightly PW: Hydralazine induced hepatitis. *Br Med J* 280:1165, 1980.
137. Forster HS: Hepatitis from hydralazine. *N Engl J Med* 302:1362, 1980.
137a. Itoh S, Ichione Y, Tsuruday Y, et al: Hydralazine-induced hepatitis *Hepatogastroenterology* 28:13, 1981.
137b. Stewart GW, Peart WS, Boylston AW: Obstructive jaundice, pancytopenia and hydralazine. *Lancet* 1:1207, 1981.
137c. Anez MS, Dickson G, Zabala R: Acute hepatitis due to hydrochlorothiazide. *Gastro y Hep* 4, 476, 1981.
138. Hutchison JC, Roediger PM, Werblin M: Cholestatic jaundice following administration of quinethazone. *Curr Ther Res* 6:199, 1964.
138a. Schumacher R, Lobeck H: Cholestatic hepatitis after tienilic acid. *Med Welt* 32:402, 1981.
139. Brandes JW, Schmitz-Moormann P, Lehmann FG, et al: Jaundice after aprindine. A hepatitis-like hepatic damage. *Dtsch Med Wochenschr* 101(4):111, 1976.
140. Herlong HF, Reod PF, Boitnott JK, et al: Aprindine hepatitis. *Ann Intern Med* 89:359, 1978.
141. Alam M, Duvernoy WFC, Pickard SD, et al: Quinidine-induced hepatitis and thrombocytopenia. *Henry Ford Hosp Med J* 25:53, 1977.
142. Koch MJ, Seeff LB, Crumley CE, et al: Quinidine hepatotoxicity. A report of a case and review of the literature. *Gastroenterology* 70:1136, 1976.
143. Handler SD, Hirsch NR, Haas K, et al: Quinidine hepatitis. *Arch Intern Med* 135(6):871, 1975.
144. Chajek T, Lehrer B, Geltner D, et al: Quinidine-induced granulomatous hepatitis. *Ann Intern Med* 81:774, 1974.
145. Geltner D, Chajek T, Rubinger D, et al: Quinidine hypersensitivity and liver involvement. A survey of 32 patients. *Gastroenterology* 70:650, 1976.
146. Ronnov JV, Tjernlund A: Hepatotoxicity due to treatment with papaverine. *N Engl J Med* 281:1333, 1969.
147. Pessayre C, Eichara M, Feldmann G, et al: Perhexiline maleate-induced cirrhosis. *Gastroenterology* 76:170, 1979.
148. Paliard P, Vitrey D, Rournier G, et al: Perhexiline maleate-induced hepatitis. *Digestion* 17:419, 1978.
149. Kopelman P, Morgan PGM: Liver damage after perhexiline maleate. *Lancet* 1:705, 1977.
150. Forbes GB, Rake MO, Taylor DJE: Liver damage due to perhexiline maleate. *J Clin Pathol* 32:1282, 1979.
150a. Rotmensch H, Liron M, Yust I: Cholestatic jaundice: An immune response to prajmulium bitartrate. *Postgrad Med J* 56:738, 1980.
151. Rotmensch HH, Yust I, Siegman-Igra Y, et al: Granulomatous hepatitis: A hypersensitivity response to procainamide. *Ann Intern Med* 89:646, 1978.
152. Litvin Y, Lubovsky E, Brezis M: Liver damage induced by pyridinol carbamate. *Lancet* 1:1257, 1977.
153. Enat R, Barzilai D, Gellei B: Hepatic injury due to pyridinol carbamate. *Isr J Med Sci* 14(3):333, 1978.

154. Rafoth RJ: Systemic granulomatous reaction to salicylazosulfapyridine (azulfidine) in a patient with Crohn's disease. *Dig Dis* 19:465, 1974.

155. Hanger FM, Gutman AB: Post-arsphenamine jaundice apparently due to obstruction of intrahepatic biliary tract. *JAMA* 115:263, 1940.

156. Radke RA, Baroody WG: Carbarsone toxicity. A review of the literature and report of 45 cases. *Ann Intern Med* 47:418, 1957.

157. Kuntz E, Liehr H, Pfingst W: Toxische Leberschädigung durch Athinomid. *Dtsch Med Wochenschr* 92:1718, 1967.

158. Conn HO, Binder HJ, Orr HD: Ethionamide induced hepatitis. A review with a report of an additional case. *Am Rev Respir Dis* 90:542, 1964.

159. Morris JS, Schmid M, Scheuer PJ, et al: Arsenic and non-cirrhotic portal hypertension. *Gastroenterology* 66(1):86, 19764.

160. Cohen C: Liver pathology in hycanthone hepatitis. *Gastroenterology* 75:103, 1978.

161. Black M, Mitchell J, Zimmerman H, et al: Isoniazid-associated hepatitis in 114 patients. *Gastroenterology* 69:289, 1975.

162. Mitchell JR, Zimmerman HJ, Ishak KG, et al: Isoniazid liver injury: Clinical spectrum, pathology, and probable pathogenesis. *Ann Intern Med* 84(2):181, 1976.

163. Vanderhoof JA, Ament ME: Fatal hepatic necrosis due to isoniazid chemoprophylaxis in a 15-year-old girl. *J Pediatr* 88:867, 1976.

163a. Heiberg JK, Svejgaard E: Toxic hepatitis during ketoconazole treatment. *Br Med J* 283:825, 1981.

164. Engel JJ, Vogt TR, Wilson DE: Cholestatic hepatitis after administration of furan derivatives. *Arch Intern Med* 135:733, 1975.

165. Goldstein LI, Ishak KG, Burns W: Hepatic injury associated with nitrofurantoin therapy. *Dig Dis* 19:987, 1974.

166. Sharp J: Chronic active hepatitis and severe hepatic necrosis associated with nitrofurantoin. *Ann Intern Med* 92(1):14, 1980.

167. Black M, Rabin L, Schatz N: Nitrofurantoin-induced chronic active hepatitis. *Ann Intern Med* 92(1):62, 1980.

168. Simpson DG, Walker JH: Hypersensitivity to para-aminosalicylic acid. *Am J Med* 29:297, 1960.

169. Hamlyn AN, Morris JS, Sarkany I, et al: Piperazine hepatitis. *Gastroenterology* 70:1144, 1976.

170. Danan G, Pessayre D, Larrey, et al: Pyrazinamide fulminant hepatitis: an old hepatotoxin strikes again. *Lancet* ii, 1056, 1981.

171. Livingood CS, Diemaide FR: Untoward reactions attributable to atabrine. *JAMA* 129:1091, 1945.

172. Fries J, Siraganian R: Sulfonamide hepatitis—Report of a case due to sulfamethoxazole and sulfisoxazole. *N Engl J Med* 274(2):95, 1966.

173. Sotolongo RP, Neefe LI, Rudzki C, et al: Hypersensitivity reaction to sulfasalazine with severe hepatotoxicity. *Gastroenterology* 75:95, 1978.

173a. Namias A, Bhalotra R, Donowitz M: Reversible sulfasalazine-induced granulomatous hepatitis. *J Clin Gastro* 3:198, 1981.

174. Koike Y, Nagata A, Kiyosawa K, et al: Pathohistological studies on the bile ducts in an autopsied case with drug-induced intrahepatic cholestasis. *Acta Hepatogastroenterol (Jpn)* 21:55, 1980.

175. Jalota R, Freston JW: Severe intrahepatic cholestasis due to thiabendazole. *Am J Trop Med Hyg* 23(4):676, 1974.

176. Colucci CR, Cicero ML: Hepatic necrosis and trimethoprim-sulfamethoxazole. *JAMA* 233:952, 1975.

177. Stevenson DK, Christie DL, Haas JE: Hepatic injury in a child caused by trimethoprim-sulfamethoxazole. *Pediatrics* 61:964, 1978.

178. Ogilvie AL, Toghill PJ: Cholestatic jaundice due to co-trimoxazole. *Postgrad Med J* 56:202, 1980.

179. Nair SS, Kaplan JM, Levine LH, t al: Trimethoprim-sulfamethoxazole induced intrahepatic cholestasis. *Ann Intern Med* 92:511, 1980.

179a. Ransohoff DF, Jacobs G: Terminal hepatic failure following a small dose of sulfamethoxazole-trimethoprim. *Gastroenterology* 80:816, 1981.

180. Amromin GD, Deliman RM, Shanbrom E: Liver damage after chemotherapy for leukemia and lymphoma. *Gastroenterology* 42:401, 1962.

181. Einhorn M, Davidsohn I: Hepatotoxicity of mercaptopurine. *JAMA* 188:802, 1964.

182. Ream NW, Perlia CP, Wolter J, et al: Mithramycin therapy in disseminated testicular cancer. *JAMA* 204:1030, 1968.

183. Schaffner F, Popper H, Chestrow E: Cholestasis produced by the action of norethandrolone. *Am J Med* 26:249, 1959.

184. Almaden PJ, Ross SW: Jaundice due to methyl testosterone therapy. *Ann Intern Med* 40:146, 1954.

184a. Ishak KG: Hepatic lesions caused by anabolic and contraceptive steroids. *Semin Liv Dis* 1:116, 1981.

185. Shapiro P, Ikeda RM, Connors MH, et al: Multiple hepatic tumors and peliosis hepatis in Fanconi's anemia treated with androgens. *Am J Dis Child* 131:1104, 1977.

186. Treuner J, Niethammer D, Flach A, et al: Hepatozelluläres Karzinom nach Oxymetholonbehandlung. *Med Welt* 31:952, 1980.

187. Ishak KG: Hepatic neoplasms associated with contraceptive and anabolic steroids. *Rec Results Cancer Res* 66:73, 1979.

188. Christopherson WM, Mays ET: Relation of steroids to liver oncogenesis. *J Toxicol Environ Health* 5:207, 1975.

189. Littlewood ER, Barrison IG, Murray Lyon IM, et al: Cholangiocarcinoma and oral contraceptives. *Lancet* 1:310, 1980.

190. Nadell J, Kosek S: Peliosis hepatis: Twelve cases associated with oral androgen therapy. *Arch Pathol Lab Med* 101:405, 1977.

191. Usatin MS, Wigger SA: Peliosis hepatis in a child. *Arch Pathol Lab Med* 100:419, 1976.

191a. Ham JM, Pirola RC, Crouch RL: Hemangioendothelial sarcoma of the liver associated with long-term estrogen therapy in a man. *Dig Dis Sci* 25:879, 1980.

192. Larsson-Cohn A, Stenram A: Jaundice during treatment with oral contraceptive agents. Report of 2 cases. *JAMA* 193:422, 1965.

193. Donner HP, Hoyl C, Aliaga C et al: Jaundice and oral contraceptives. *Acta Hepatogastroenterol* 18:84, 1971.

194. Thulin KE, Nermark J: Seven cases of jaundice in women taking an oral contraceptive, anovlar. *Br Med J* 1:584, 1966.

195. Klatskin G: Hepatic tumors. Possible relationship to use of oral contraceptives. *Gastroenterology* 73:386, 1977.

196. Neuberger J, Nunnerley HB, Davis M, et al: Oral contraceptive associated liver tumors. Occurrence of malignancy and difficulties in diagnosis. *Lancet* 1:273, 1980.

196a. Monroe RS, Riddell RH, Siegler M, et al: Hepatic angiosarcoma. Possible relationship to long term oral contraceptive ingestion. *J Am Med Ass* 246:64, 1981.

196b. Shi EC, Fischer A, Crouch R, et al: Possible association of angiosarcoma with oral contraceptive agents. *Med J Aust* 1:473, 1981.

197. Balazs M, Kovach G, Winkler G, et al: Dilatation of hepatic sinusoids after use of oral contraceptives. *Dtsch Med Wschr* 106:1345, 1981.

198. Winkler K, Poulson H: Liver disease with periportal sinusoidal dilatation. A possible complication to contraceptive steroids. *Scand J Gastroenterol* 10:699, 1975.

199. Wu SM, Spurny OM: Budd-Chiari syndrome after taking oral contraceptives; a case report and review of 14 reported cases. *Am J Dig Dis* 22:623, 1977.

200. Steinberg H, Webb WM, Rafsky HA: Hepatomegaly with fatty infiltration secondary to cortosone therapy. *Gastroenterology* 21:304, 1952.

201. Taxy JB: Peliosis. A morphologic curiosity becomes an iatrogenic problem. *Hum Pathol* 9:331, 1978.

202. Puppala AR, Ro JA: Possible association between peliosis hepatis and diethylstilbestrol. *Postgrad Med J* 65(5):277, 1979.

203. Hoch-Ligeti C: Angiosarcoma of the liver associated with diethyl stilbestrol. *JAMA* 240:1510, 1978.

203a. Rosinus V, Maurer R: Diethyl stilbestrol induced hepatocellular carcinoma. *Schweiz Med Wschr* 111:1139, 1981.

204. Trulzsch D, Klinge O, Zilly W, et al: Cholestatic jaundice following ingestion of the laxative, normolaxol. *Med Klin* 70(17):771, 1975.

205. Pearson AJG, Grainger JM, Scheuer PJ, et al: Jaundice due to oxyphenisatin. *Lancet* 1:994, 1971.

205a. Kotha P, Rake MO, Willat D: Liver damage induced by oxyphenisatin. *Br Med J* 281:1530, 1980.

206. Reynolds TB, Peters RL, Yamada S: Chronic active and lupoid hepatitis caused by a laxative, oxyphenisatin. *N Engl J Med* 285:813, 1971.

207. Kotha P, Rake MO, Willat D: Liver damage induced by oxyphenisatin. *Br Med J* 281:1530, 1980.

208. Fischer MG, Miller A, Nayer HR: Methiomazole induced jaundice. *JAMA* 223:1028, 1973.

209. Lunzer M, Huang SN, Ginsburg J, et al: Jaundice due to carbimazole. *Gut* 16:913, 1975.

210. Fedotin MS, Lefer LG: Liver disease caused by propylthiouracil. *Arch Intern Med* 135(2):319, 1975.

211. Mihas AA, Holley P, Koff RS, et al: Fulminant hepatitis and lymphocyte sensitization due to propylthiouracil. *Gastroenterology* 70:770, 1976.

212. Weiss M, Hassin D, Bank H: Propylthiouracil induced hepatic damage. *Arch Intern Med* 140:1184, 1980.

213. Goldstein WJ, Rothenberg AJ: Jaundice in a patient receiving acetohexamide. *N Engl J Med* 275:97, 1966.

214. Camerini DR, Root HF, Marble A: Clinical experience with carbutamide (BZ 55). A progress report. *Diabetes* 6:74, 1957.

215. Reichel J, Goldberg SB, Ellenberg M, et al: Intrahepatic cholestasis following administration of chlorpropamide. Report of a case with electron microscopic observations. *Am J Med* 28:654, 1960.

216. Rigberg LA, Goldberg SB, Ellenberg M, et al: Chlorpropamide induced granulomas: A probable hypersensitivity reaction in liver and bone marrow. *JAMA* 235:409, 1976.

217. Dolger H: An assessment of oral antidiabetic therapy. *Ann NY Acad Sci* 82:531, 1959.

218. Van Thiel DH, de Belle R, Mellow M, et al: Tolazamide hepatotoxicity. *Gastroenterology* 67:506, 1974.

219. Gregory DH, Zaki GF, Sarcos GA, et al: Chronic cholestasis following prolonged tolbutamide administration associated with destructive cholangitis and cholangiolitis. *Arch Pathol Lab Med* 84:194, 1967.

220. Valdes M, Jacobs WH: Intrahepatic cholestasis following the use of atromid-S. *Am J Gastroenterol* 66(1):69, 1976.

221. Parsons WB Jr: Studies of nicotinic acid use in hypercholesterolemia: Changes in hepatic function, carbohydrate tolerance and uric acid metabolism. *Arch Intern Med* 107:653, 1961.

222. Kohn RW, Montes M: Hepatic fibrosis following long-acting nicotinic acid therapy. *Am J Med Sci* 258:94, 1969.

223. Berge KG, Achor RWP, Christenson NA, et al: Hypercholesterolemia and nicotinic acid. *Am J Med* 31:24, 1961.

224. Ishak KG, Irey NS: Hepatic injury associated with the phenothiazines. *Arch Pathol Lab Med* 93:283, 1972.

225. Russell RI, Allan JG, Patrick R: Active chronic hepatitis after chlorpromazine ingestion. *Br Med J* 1:655, 1973.
226. McFarland RB: Fatal drug reaction associated with prochlorperazine (Compazine). *Am J Clin Pathol* 40:284, 1963.
227. Bandt C, Hoffbauer FW: Liver injury associated with trancylpromine therapy. *JAMA* 188:752, 1964.
228. Yon J, Anuras S: Hepatitis caused by amitriptyline therapy. *JAMA* 232:833, 1975.
229. Biagi RW, Bapat BN: Intrahepatic obstructive jaundice from amitryptilene. *Br J Psychiatry* 113:1113, 1967.
230. Pessayre D, De Saint-Louvent P, DeGott C, et al: Iproclozide fulminant hepatitis. Possible role of enzyme induction. *Gastroenterology* 75:492, 1978.
231. Popper H: Pathologic findings in jaundice associated with iproniazid therapy. *JAMA* 168:2235, 1958.
232. Holdsworth CD, Atkinson M, Goldie W: Hepatitis caused by the newer amine-oxidase-inhibiting drugs. *Lancet* 2:621, 1961.
233. Jones EA, Clain D, Clink HM, et al: Hepatic coma due to acute hepatic necrosis treated by exchange blood transfusion. *Lancet* 2:169, 1967.
234. Kohn N, Tiyerson RM: Cholestatic hepatitis associated with trifluoperazine. *N Engl J Med* 264:549, 1961.
235. Abbruzese A, Swanson J: Jaundice after therapy with chlorodiazepoxide hydrochloride. *N Engl J Med* 273:321, 1965.
236. Pickering D: Hepatic necrosis after chlorodiazepoxide therapy. *N Engl J Med* 274:1449, 1966.
237. Powell WJ Jr, Koch-Weser J, Williams RA: Lethal hepatic necrosis after therapy with imipramine and desipramine. *JAMA* 206:642, 1968.
238. Hochman R, Robbins JJ: Jaundice due to ectylurea. *N Engl J Med* 259:583, 1958.
239. Fang MH, Ginsberg AL, Dobbins WO: Cholestatic jaundice associated with fluorazepam hydrochloride. *Ann Intern Med* 89:363, 1978.
240. Nagasaka K, Kuwabara T, Takezawa J, et al: A case of drug-induced liver injury caused by haloperidol with a positive LE-cell test. *Acta Hep Jap* 22:1176, 1981.
241. Andersen H, Kristiansen ES: Tofranil treatment of endogenous depressions. *Acta Psychiatr Scand* 34:387, 1959.
242. Horst DA, Grace ND, LeCompte PM: Prolonged cholestasis and progressive hepatic fibrosis following imipramine therapy. *Gastroenterology* 79:550, 1980.
243. Ajdukiewicz AB, Grainger J, Scheuer PJ, et al: Jaundice due to iprindole. *Gut* 12(9):705, 1971.
244. Teychenne PF, Jones EA, Ishak KG, et al: Hepatocellular injury with distinctive mitochondrial changes induced by lergotrile mesylate: A dopaminergic ergot derivative. *Gastroenterology* 76:575, 1979.
245. Tolman KG, Freston JW, Berenson MM, et al: Hepatotoxicity due to pemoline. *Digestion* 9:532, 1973.
246. Russell RM, Boyer JL, Bagheri SA, et al: Hepatic injury from chronic hypervitaminosis A resulting in portal hypertension and ascites. *N Engl J Med* 291:435, 1974.
247. Rubin E, Florman AL, Degnan T, et al: Hepatic injury in chronic hypervitaminosis A. *Am J Dis Child* 119:132, 1970.
248. Babb R, Kieraldo J: Cirrhosis due to hypervitaminosis A. *West Med J* 128:244, 1978.
249. Fleischmann R, Schlote W, Schomerus H, et al: Small nodular liver cirrhosis with marked portal hypertension due to vitamin A intoxication resulting from psoriasis treatment. *Dtsch Med Wochenschr* 102(45):1637, 1977.
250. Jacques EA, Buschmann RJ, Layden TJ: The histopathologic progression of vitamin A induced hepatic injury. *Gastroenterology* 76:599, 1979.
251. Winter SL, Boyer JL: Hepatic toxicity from large doses of vitamin B_3 (nicotinamide). *N Engl J Med* 289:1180, 1973.
252. Rosenberg JL, Edlow D, Sneider R: Liver disease and vasculitis in a patient taking cromolyn. *Arch Intern Med* 138:989, 1978.

253. Keefe EB, Smith FW: Disulfiram hypersensitivity hepatitis. *JAMA* 230:435, 1974.

254. Morris SJ, Kanner R, Chiprut RO, et al: Disulfiram hepatitis. *Gastroenterology* 75:100, 1978.

255. Ranek L, Andreasen PB: Side effects of drugs: Disulfiram hepatotoxicity. *Br Med J* 2:94, 1977.

256. Jacobs J, Greene H, Gendel BR: Acute iron intoxication. *N Engl J Med* 273:1124, 1965.

257. Winckler K: Hepatic necroses after infusion cholangiography. *Dtsch Med Wochenschr* 103(10):420, 1978.

258. Barzilai D, Dickstein G, Enat R, et al: Cholestatic jaundice caused by D-penicillamine. *Ann Rheumatol Dis* 37:98, 1978.

258a. Multz CV: Cholestatic hepatitis caused by penicillamine. *JAMA* 246:674, 1981.

259. Goldfinger JE, Marx S: Hypersensitivity hepatitis due to phenazopyridine. *N Engl J Med* 286:1090, 1972.

260. Goldenberg VE, Wiegenstein L, Hopkins GB: Hepatic injury associated with tromethamine. *JAMA* 205:81, 1968.

261. Krishnamachari KAVR, Nagarajan V, Bhat RV, et al: Hepatitis due to aflatoxicosis: An outbreak in western India. *Lancet* 1(7915):1061, 1975.

262. Jennings RB: Fatal fulminant acute carbon tetrachloride poisoning. *Arch Pathol* 55:269, 1955.

263. Stein RS, Jenkins D, Korns ME: Death after use of cupric sulfate as emetic. *JAMA* 235:801, 1976.

264. Pimentel JC, Menezes AP: Liver disease in vineyard sprayers. *Gastroenterology* 72:275, 1977.

265. Yodaiken RE, Babcoch JR: 1,2-dichloroethane poisoning. *Arch Environ Health* 26(5):281, 1973.

266. Lemaigre G, Tebbi Z, Galinsky R, et al: Fulminant hepatitis due to the "glue thistle" (atractylis gummifera l): An anatomic-pathologic study of four cases. *Nouv Presse Med* 4(40):2865, 1975.

267. Guzelian PS, Vranian G, Boylan JJ, et al: Liver structure and function in patients poisoned with chlordecone (Kepone). *Gastroenterology* 78:206, 1980.

267a. Beattie AD, Mullin PJ, Baxter RH, et al: Acute lead poisoning: An unusual cause of hepatitis. *Scot Med J* 24:318, 1979.

268. Bullivant CM: Accidental poisoning by paraquat. Report of two cases in man. *Br Med J* 1:1272, 1966.

268a. Matsumoto T: A histopathological study of the liver in paraquat poisoning. An analysis of 20 autopsy cases with emphasis on bile duct injury. *Acta Hep Jap* 22:637, 1981.

269. Fletcher GF, Galambos JT: Phosphorus poisoning in humans. *Arch Intern Med* 112:846, 1963.

270. Fox DW, Hart MC, Bergeson PS, et al: Pyrrolizidine (senecio) intoxication mimicking Reye's syndrome. *J Pediatr* 93:980, 1978.

271. Stillman AE, Huxtable R, Consroe P, et al: Hepatic veno-occlusive disease due to pyrrholizidine (senecio) poisoning in Arizona. *Gastroenterology* 73:349, 1977.

16
The Gallbladder

GENERAL APPROACH TO THE SPECIMEN

Although biopsies of the gallbladder are occasionally performed (1), cholecystectomy remains the standard operation on the gallbladder. Usually it is performed for chronic cholecystitis and cholelithiasis. In a relatively small proportion of cholecystectomy specimens, additional lesions, such as a carcinoma, or entirely different lesions, such as congenital anomalies or unusual neoplasms, are found. Routine needle biopsy of the liver during abdominal surgery has been advocated, since it frequently provides useful information (2). The finding of cholangitis or other evidence of sepsis in such biopsy specimens would be of particular interest (Chapter 7).

The decision to perform a cholecystectomy is made on the basis of a combination of clinical features, radiologic investigations, and the observations of the surgeon at laparotomy. Clinically, the possibility of gallbladder diseases is raised by indigestion with intolerance of fat or spicy foods, belching, flatulence, postprandial fullness, nausea, and, in some cases, vomiting, often coupled with right upper quadrant pain and tenderness. However, clinical symptoms are unreliable indicators of the type and severity of gallbladder disease. In fact, severe disease of the gallbladder, such as chronic cholecystitis with cholelithiasis and complete obstruction of the cystic duct by gallstones, may be totally asymptomatic and may be discovered only by finding abdominal opacities on a plain x-ray film of the abdomen. Radiologic investigations of the biliary tract, including plain x-ray films, cholangiography, and body scanning, are steadily improving in accuracy and in their ability to diagnose preoperatively the location, and sometimes the nature, of lesions of the gallbladder. Pathologic observations are usually necessary to make a definite diagnosis. Frozen sections are indicated if a malignant tumor is suspected by the surgeon or the pathologist, as such a finding would be an indication for a more extensive operation.

Specimen Handling

Most commonly the gallbladder is received after cholecystectomy without any attached structures, except for the cystic duct. Sometimes, particularly for malignant neoplasms of the gallbladder, varying amounts of contiguous hepatic tissue are removed as well. The gallbladder may also be included in a hepatic lobectomy specimen. If attached hepatic tissue is removed, it should be described and processed as described in the liver section. We prefer to receive the gallbladder unfixed and unopened in the surgical pathology laboratory as soon as possible after cholecystectomy. If the specimen cannot be processed at once, it should be nicked and immersed in formalin to give the fixative access to the mucosa. Often the specimen is received already opened by the surgon and placed in fixative in the operating room. This is not advised because if calculi are present, their location can be confidently identified by the pathologist only if the gallbladder is received intact.

Gross Anatomy, Dissection, and Description

The gallbladder lies in a shallow bed on the inferior surface of the liver in the plane dividing the liver into true right and left lobes (Fig. 1, Chapter 1). Just to the right of the gallbladder is the anterior segment of the right lobe; to the left is the quadrate lobe, a subsegment of the medial segment of the left lobe. Inferiorly, the gallbladder is covered by peritoneum reflected off the liver. The normal gallbladder is a pear-shaped, whitish, thin-walled structure consisting of a fundus, body, and neck. The fundus points forward and is continuous with the body. At the porta hepatis, the body narrows into an infundibular portion that curves anteroinferiorly to form a short neck, which becomes the cystic duct. The gallbladder should be measured in three dimensions if received unopened, in two if opened. It varies in size, averaging 9 cm in length and 4 cm in width. A giant gallbladder measuring 18 × 4 cm has been reported (3). The cystic duct is 0.3 cm in diameter and runs a convoluted sigmoid course for 2–4 cm before usually joining the common hepatic duct to form the common bile duct. The cystic duct is difficult to open because its diameter is so small and its mucosa is thrown into a dozen or more oblique crescentic folds, the spiral valves of Heister (4).

The arterial blood supply to the gallbladder comes from the cystic artery, most frequently a branch of the right hepatic artery. The cystic artery usually passes behind the common hepatic or bile duct to reach the neck of the gallbladder, where it divides into anterior and posterior branches. Occasionally, the cystic artery arises from the left hepatic or gastroduodenal artery. The venous drainage of the gallbladder has an inconstant relationship to the arterial supply. Most of the venous blood drains by small veins directly into the liver. However, some blood also drains into the cystic branch of the portal vein. Lymphatic drainage from the gallbladder is via the cystic node at its neck and the pericholedochal nodes on the right side of the common bile duct to the pancreaticoduodenal and preaortic nodes. Afferent sympathetic and efferent parasympathetic nerves are found chiefly in the subserosa of the gallbladder, both supplemented by branches from the right phrenic nerve.

The gallbladder should be opened with blunt scissors from fundus to neck, including the cystic duct. The contents are then measured and described. Normally bile is a viscous, greenish-brown fluid, varying considerably in quantity but averaging 30 ml. Three organic solutes comprise 80–90% of the total solids: conjugated bile salts, phospholipids (predominantly lecithin), and cholesterol. The most abundant inorganic cations are Cl^- and HCO^{3-}. The color of bile is due principally to bilirubin, most of which is conjugated. Bile is normally bacteriologically sterile. If cholangitis is suspected, if the bile looks abnormal, or if there is gangrene or perforation of the wall, the bile should be cultured. The size, shape, color, and approximate number of any stones should be recorded. Small calculi impacted in the cystic duct should be particularly watched for. After cutting or sawing through the center of a representative stone, the characteristic colors seen on cross section will usually elucidate the composition of the stone (see p. 316). Rarely, when a metabolic disorder is suspected, chemical analysis of a calculus may be indicated.

The normal gallbladder wall is 0.2–0.3 cm thick. Most of this is mucosa, which has a plush velvet pile appearance, a reticulated surface pattern, and a brown or green color due to bile staining. Color, average as well as maximum thickness of the wall, and appearance of serosa and mucosa should be described. Mucosal ulceration, hemorrhage, necrosis, or fibrosis should be noted. The entire mucosal surface should be examined for small polyps, which may easily escape detection. Palpation of the specimen, particularly at the neck and fundus, assists in detecting small intramural lesions. The cystic lymph node should be dissected off the neck and bisected before fixation.

Anomalies of Number, Location, and Shape

Congenital anomalies of the gallbladder are rare and generally attributed to abnormal budding of the hepatic diverticulum from the primitive gut or to failure of formation of a lumen in the diverticulum. Usually, such anomalies are functionally insignificant, but they may predispose to cholecystitis, cholangitis, and carcinoma of the biliary tract (5–9).

The gallbladder may be congenitally absent (8,10,11), or at the other extreme, there may be two or even three gallbladders with independent cystic ducts and peritoneal investments (12,13). True duplication of the gallbladder is distinguished from an accessory gallbladder by the presence of separate cystic ducts (13). Bilobed gallbladders have also been described (14). Absence of the gallbladder may be associated with other congenital anomalies (11). A small gallbladder is more apt to represent a sequel to chronic cholecystitis than an anomaly. Stones, mucosal atrophy, scarring, and dystrophic calcification of the wall ("porcelain" gallbladder) support such a diagnosis. A peritoneal sheet or "congenital adhesion" may attach the gallbladder to the small or large bowel or to the right hepatic lobe.

The gallbladder may be totally intrahepatic or, conversely, free floating, completely invested by peritoneum, and attached to the liver only by a mesentery. This "floating" gallbladder occurs in about 10% of the population and is susceptible to torsion with ischemia, hence may present a clinical problem on occasion (15). Other variations in position, such as retrodisplacement, transverse lie, and a suprahepatic location (16), have also been noted. These are more of a problem for the surgeon than for the surgical pathologist, as are the not-too-infrequent anomalies of the cystic duct (17).

The Phrygian cap, or "folded fundus," is the most common anomaly of shape. The term is derived from a pointed headgear worn with its apex turned forward by the ancient Phrygians. It is usually diagnosed by the radiologist and was detected in 18% of one series of cholecystograms, while at autopsy its incidence was only 4% in otherwise normal gallbladders (14). The Phrygian cap anomaly is probably caused by adherence of redundant fundal serosa to the body of the gallbladder (18). Septa of fibromuscular connective tissue, sometimes inapparent on external examination, may give rise to "hourglass" or bilobed gallbladders. Multiseptate gallbladders have also been reported (19).

True diverticula, carrying with them muscularis, are usually asymptomatic and probably originate from persistent cystohepatic ducts. Pulsion-type diverticula may be present in the fundus distal to transverse septa.

Preparation of Microscopic Sections

The gallbladder is notoriously susceptible to autolysis and must, therefore, be fixed as soon as possible in buffered formalin. Smooth flat sections can be obtained if the fresh unfixed opened gallbladder is gently stretched and pinned, serosa down, on cardboard while fixing for at least 1 hour. Longer periods of fixation are desirable if scarring or mucosal lesions are present. Full-thickness routine sections, one each from fundus, body, neck (coronal), and cystic node, are recommended. All will fit easily on one slide. If a neoplasm is suspected, multiple full-thickness blocks through mucosa and serosa are essential. Margins in such cases should be evaluated by sections of the cystic and any other available extrahepatic ducts, as well as of any attached hepatic parenchyma.

Frozen sections of the gallbladder are indicated when there are localized mucosal lesions suspicious of malignancy or marked generalized thickening of the gallbladder wall, which can be caused either by chronic cholecystitis or by scirrhous carcinoma. It is most desirable to make a diagnosis of carcinoma during laparotomy so that a more extensive cancer operation may be done at that time. If a tumor is suspected, a part of the lesion should be fixed for transmission electron microscopy. If light microscopy shows an unusual appearance, then electron microscopy may be helpful.

Enzyme histochemistry has been applied to the gallbladder as a research technique, but at present seems to have little to offer the diagnostic histopathologist. Scanning electron microscopy gives a very good view of the mucosal surface of the gallbladder and may well become useful diagnostically.

Normal Histology

The mucous membrane consists of columnar absorptive cells. A faint brush border may be detected by light microscopy if the section is well prepared, and microvilli can be seen by electron microscopy (20). The mucosal layer is thrown into frequent folds or rugae, but apart from the neck region, the normal gallbladder contains no mucus-producing glands (Fig. 1). The mucosal lining cells rest on a rather scanty layer of connective tissue, the lamina propria. There is no muscularis mucosae and no submucosa. The fibers of the muscular wall (muscularis propria) are admixed with elastic tissue and are arranged into oblique circular and longitudinal layers, most prominent at the neck of the gallbladder. Outside the muscular wall is subserosal fat with arteries, veins, lymphatics, nerves, and paraganglia (21). The serosa proper consists of flattened mesothelial cells, the peritoneal investment. Small aberrant bile ducts (Luschka's Ducts) are seen in about 10% of cholecystectomies. They are located in the

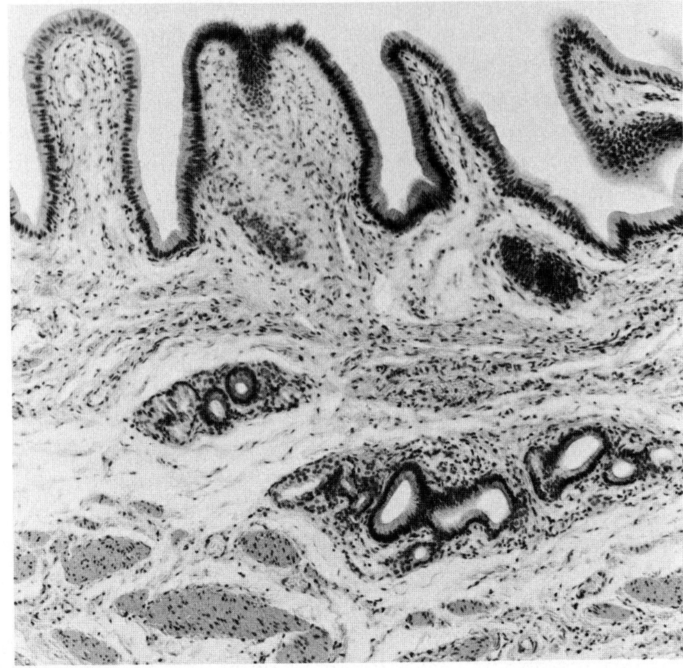

Figure 1. Normal gallbladder (neck region). The columnar epithelium is thrown into folds. Groups of glands are seen in the lamina propria. (Hematoxylin and eosin, ×40.)

connective tissue bed between liver and gallbladder and communicate directly with the liver (22).

ABNORMALITIES OF CONTENT

Gallstones

Calculi are, of course, the most important abnormality with respect to gallbladder content. They are usually associated with chronic cholecystitis and are quite rare in a normal gallbladder. Calculi represent precipitated, normally solubilized, bile components and are classified according to their composition into cholesterol, pigment, and mixed types. Their pathogenesis has been greatly clarified in recent years and elegant microstructure studies have also been done (23–31). The vast majority of stones are mixed and associated with chronic cholecystitis. There may be a few or literally hundreds; often "crops" or several "families" of stones of different sizes are present. They vary in color and are multifaceted, with smooth surfaces. Most cut fairly easily, are laminated and of a different color inside than out. They contain appreciable amounts of both cholesterol and pigment. The latter consists of calcium bilirubinate and related hemoglobin derivatives, as well as a variety of poorly characterized insoluble compounds. Very large cylindrical single stones up to 3 cm are most frequently of the combined or compound type. On cut section, there is a central cholesterol nidus of typical laminated, yellow, crystalline translucency, or dark bilirubinate, and an outer darker shell of mixed composition (various combinations of cholesterol, calcium bilirubinate, and calcium carbonate). Conversely, there may be a mixed nucleus surrounded by a coat of cholesterol or bilirubinate. Large single spherical stones are more often yellowish and composed of pure cholesterol. Innumerable dark brown to jet black stones of multifaceted or mulberry appearance and measuring 0.2–0.8 cm in diameter are characteristic of calcium bilirubinate. They cut or crumble easily and are of uniform color. They are usually associated with hemolytic anemias, but are also seen in cirrhosis, in elderly patients, and in the bile ducts of patients in the Orient (28–32). Multiple small, chalk white, very hard stones of variable contour are typically composed of calcium carbonate or calcium phosphate. They are seen infrequently and may be associated with chronic, low-grade, biliary obstruction (24).

Mucocele

Mucocele or hydrops is probably the most familiar anomaly of the bile itself. The gallbladder contains colorless mucoid fluid. Usually, there is chronic cystic duct obstruction with distention of the gallbladder. However, idiopathic acute hydrops without stones or inflammation has also been reported (33). This change is also seen in some cases of cystic fibrosis of the pancreas. In a more acute setting of high-grade cystic duct obstruction, the gallbladder may be tensely filled with a sterile but puslike, milky emulsion of $CaCO_3$ and cholesterol. The refractile cholesterol crystals may be seen grossly with oblique lighting. Secondary bacterial invaders may cause suppuration, and the pus may contain blood and debris.

Empyema

A gallbladder full of pus (empyema) is one possible consequence of acute cholecystitis (33a).

Hemobilia

Hemobilia is a diagnosis that can be made if blood is found in the biliary tract, including the gallbladder. It is not often diagnosed preoperatively. If the bleeding arises from the gallbladder, this is called hemocholecyst (33b). Most frequently hemocholecyst occurs in conjunction with hemorrhagic cholelithiasis or erosion of the cystic artery near the neck of the gallbladder. Trauma (including needle biopsy), aneurysms, neoplasms, or abscesses may also be responsible (34–38a). The clinical picture may be that of upper gastrointestinal bleeding, biliary colic, cholecystitis, or obstructive jaundice, which may recur because of repetitive hemorrhage. Cord-like blood clots mixed with bile may be vomited or passed in the stool (39,40). Hemorrhage may be acute and dramatic, although chronic, low-grade mucosal bleeding is more common (41).

Parasites

Round worms (ascaris) may be found in the gallbladder and biliary tract, where they may produce pseudotumors (42), and ascaris eggs have been found to constitute the nidus for calcium bilirubinate stones in the gallbladder (33). Apart from this, it is unusual to find parasites within the gallbladder proper, although flukes may infest the intrahepatic biliary passages (*Opisthorchis sinensis* and *Fasciola hepatica*) (43,44). Some cases of cholecystitis and cholangitis have been attributed to *Giardia lamblia* (44a). Amebic abscesses or hydatid cysts may also extend to and involve the gallbladder.

ABNORMALITIES OF THE WALL

Cholecystitis

Chronic Cholecystitis

If the gallbladder wall is opaquely white, firm, gritty, and thickened, with a smooth, atrophic, or ulcerated mucosa, the diagnosis is most likely chronic cholecystitis. Extreme dystrophic calcification gives rise to the "porcelain" gallbladder (45). Mixed stones are usually associated with chronic cholecystitis and may burrow into the wall and form a pseudodiverticulum. Most carcinomas of the gallbladder are scirrhous and grossly may simulate chronic cholecystitis perfectly. In one large series of cholecystectomies, 1.9% proved, histologically, to be carcinoma (46). A firm, thickened gallbladder, therefore, requires more than routine sections. The microscopic picture of chronic cholecystitis varies (47). Minimal requirements for such a diagnosis probably are Rokitansky-Aschoff sinuses and some mononuclear inflammatory cells including plasma cells (Figs. 2–5). Eosinophils may also be present. Smooth muscle hypertrophy is also commonly seen. Rokitansky-Aschoff sinuses are mucosal pseudodiverticula lined by cuboidal epithelium penetrating into or through the muscular wall. They may contain bile pigment, cholesterol crystals, or true biliary calculi. A synonym for Rokitansky-Aschoff sinuses is Luschka crypts, which must be distinguished from Luschka ducts. These are quite different structures (see above). Because of this possible confusion, it would probably be desirable to drop both the terms Rokitanski-Aschoff sinus and Luschka crypt and to use only the term mucosal pseudodiverticulum (48). The pseudodiverticula may be large enough to produce palpable nodules (Fig. 6). Such lesions have been called adenomyosis (p. 325). In addition, there may be ulceration and atrophy of the mucosa with fibrosis, endarteritis obliterans, and neural hypertrophy in the lamina propria. A variety of epithelial changes may be seen in many of these gallbladders. These include flattening of the epithelium and hyperplasia with papillary formation, as well as metaplasia with the formation of intestinal and gastric epithelium and of argentaffin cells (49,50). Mucous glands may be seen just deep to the gallbladder epithelium (Fig. 2). In one series of cholecystectomies for chronic cholecystitis and cholelithiasis, 80% of the specimens showed epithelial hyperplasia, 13% atypical hyperplasia, and 3% carcinoma in situ (51). Fistulae or abscesses may be present as focal areas of suppuration in a scarred wall. If epithelioid tubercles are seen, the possibility of tuberculosis (52) or fungal infection should be considered. Granulomas have also been reported in sclerosing cholangitis (52a).

Eosinophilic Cholecystitis

Eosinophilic cholecystitis is a condition of obscure etiology, clinically resembling chronic cholecystitis. Calculi are usually absent (53,54).

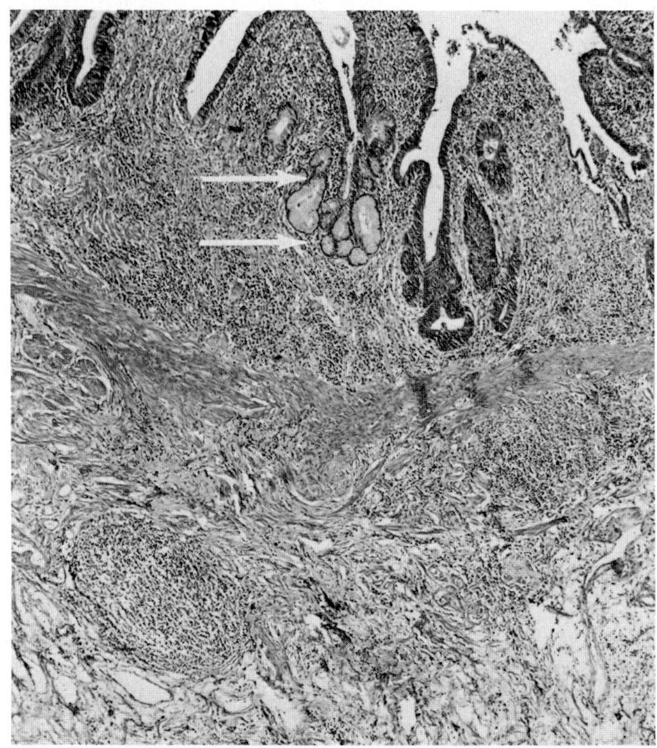

Figure 2. Chronic cholecystitis, showing chronic inflammation and fibrosis of the gallbladder wall. Metaplastic, mucus-secreting glands (arrows) are seen immediately underlying the mucosa, and a lymphoid follicle deeper in the wall. (Hematoxylin and eosin, ×40.)

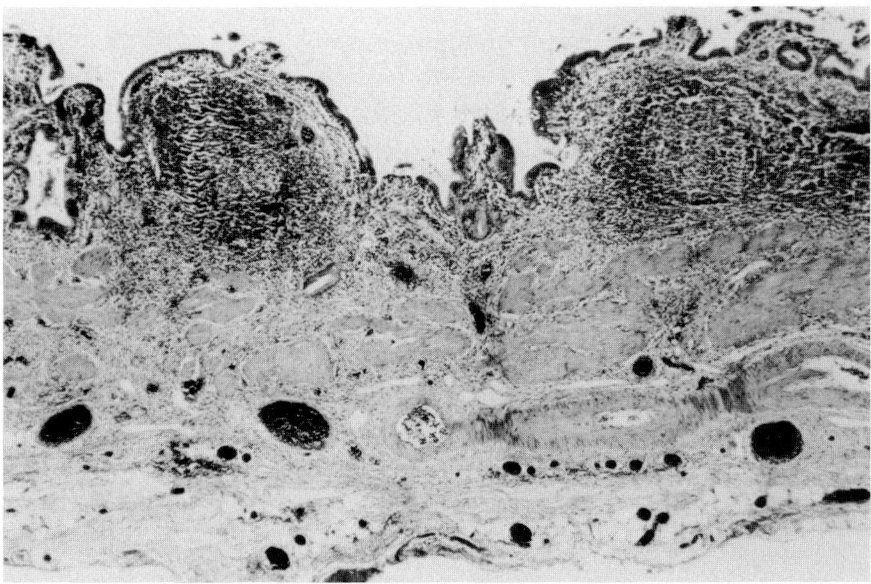

Figure 3. Chronic cholecystitis, displaying lymphoid follicles with germinal centers in the lamina propria. (Hematoxylin and eosin, ×34.)

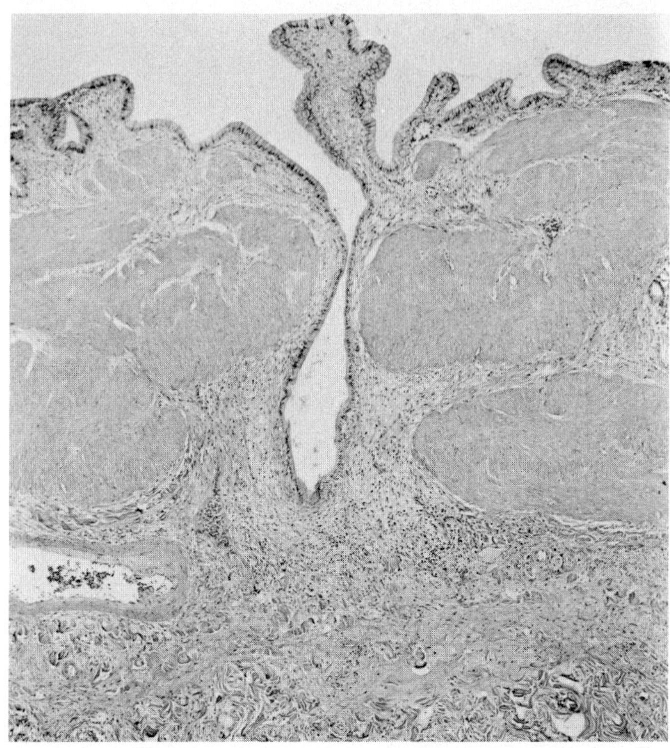

Figure 4. Chronic cholecystitis, showing an Rokitansky-Aschoff sinus as a diverticular protrusion into the muscular wall. (Hematoxylin and eosin, ×40.)

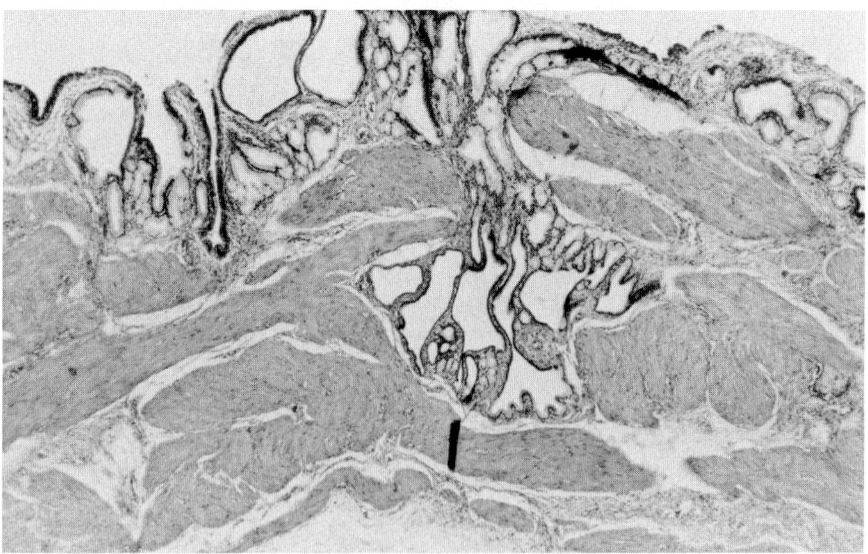

Figure 5. Chronic cholecystitis, showing a more deeply invaginated, more complex Rokitansky-Aschoff sinus. (Hematoxylin and eosin, ×34.)

Acute Cholecystitis

A shaggy, fibrinous, dull serosa with vascular engorgement denotes either acute cholecystitis or acute pericholecystitis, most commonly associated with peptic ulceration and perforation. Microscopic examination distinguishes these entities, since acute inflammatory cells in acute pericholecystitis are virtually limited to the gallbladder serosa. Diffuse transmural acute inflammation of the gallbladder wall with edema, hyperemia, variable degrees of scarring, and often stones with mucosal ulcers or exudate typify acute cholecystitis.

Most cases of acute cholecystitis are related to cystic duct obstruction by one or more stones and frequently occur in a gallbladder that already shows chronic cholecystitis. Concentrated bile is a chemical irritant and probably initiates the inflammatory process. Should obstruction continue unrelieved for more than 72 hours, secondary bacterial infection almost always ensues. The usual organisms are *Escherichia coli* or *Streptococcus faecalis*, and less often, *Clostridium welchii* or *Salmonella typhi.* The bacteria probably gain access to the gallbladder from the gut via the lymphatics or the portal venous system (55). Shreds of necrotic inflamed mucosa may form inflammatory pseudopolyps adjacent to ulcers. In severe cases the wall is greenish black and fragile, indicative of gangrene. Free perforation into the abdominal cavity may develop, or more infrequently, internal biliary fistulae involving the gastrointestinal tract. Radiologically, an internal biliary fistula may be suspected if air is seen in the gallbladder. If a stone of at least 2.5 cm diameter passes through such a fistula into the small bowel, intestinal obstruction may ensue. The stone may simply be too large to pass, produce intussusception, or embed itself in the intestinal wall and evoke an inflammatory mass (56).

Microscopic examination of the inflamed gallbladder may produce some clue as to etiology. When pyogenic bacterial infection is present, polymorphonuclear leukocytes dominate the histologic picture (Fig. 7); eosinophils may be fairly numerous. In some cases they are so numerous that eosinophilic cholecystitis has been suggested as a separate entity (see above). In typhoid carriers, typhoid nodules (nodular collections of mononuclear cells, chiefly macrophages) may be found within the mucosa; the muscular coat and subserosa are spared.

Acalculous Cholecystitis

Acalculous cholecystitis accounts for only 2–10% of acute cholecystitis. It is seen in patients with burns, dehydration, bacteremia, diabetes, and in persons with anomalies of the biliary system or its blood supply (9,57). It is also a recognized complication of other illnesses in childhood (58) and of intravenous hyperalimentation (59). There probably is cystic duct obstruction in many cases of acalculous cholecystitis, but its mechanism remains unclear (60,61).

Emphysematous Cholecystitis

In emphysematous cholecystitis, which is usually acalculous, the wall of the gallbladder is focally or diffusely filled with air bubbles. These may be visualized or palpated as crepitus. Far more often air is demonstrated radiologically in the gallbladder wall, the patient is given antibiotics, and the pathologist receives a black gangrenous gallbladder. This condition is probaby commoner in older diabetic males (62). Obliterative vascular disease within the branches of the cystic

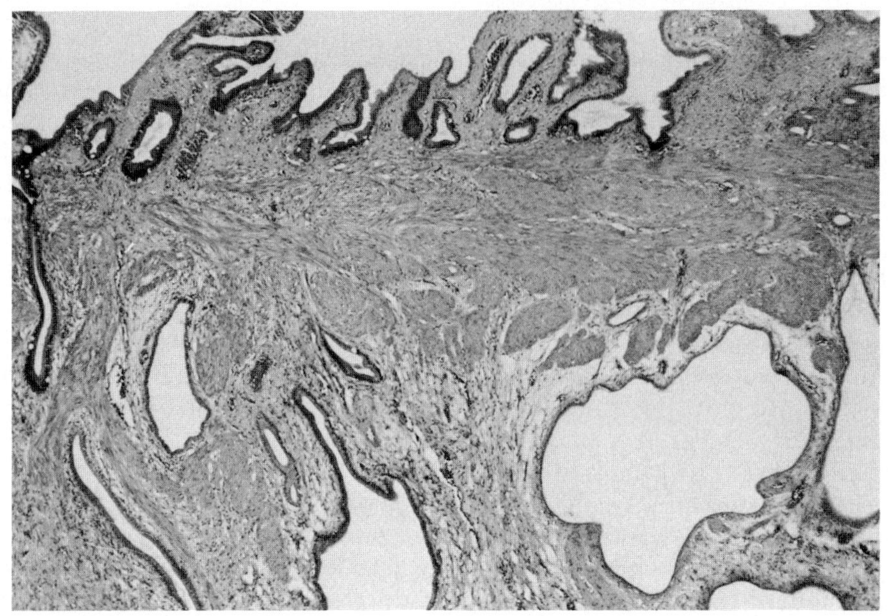

Figure 6. Adenomyosis (cholecystitis glandularis), with large dilated glandular spaces deep in the muscular wall. (Hematoxylin and eosin, ×34.)

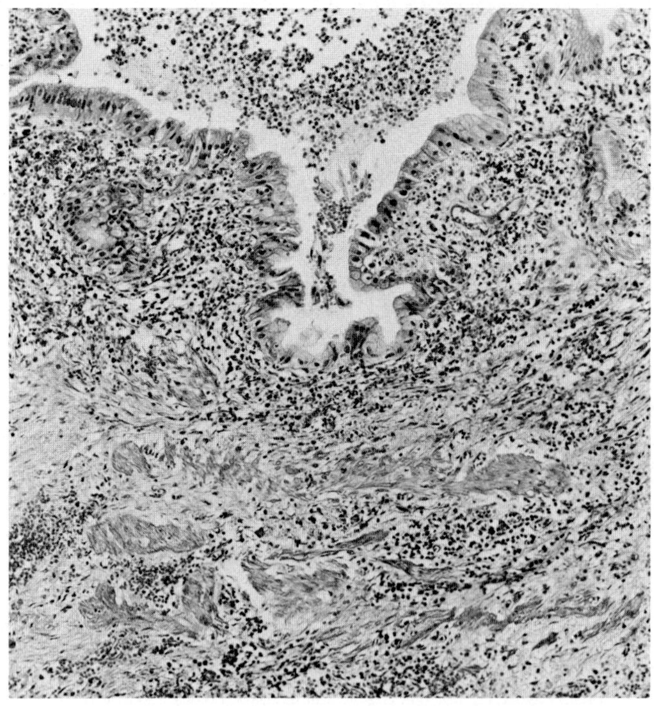

Figure 7. Acute cholecystitis, showing intense acute and chronic inflammation in the gallbladder wall and lumen. (Hematoxylin and eosin, ×100.)

artery has been incriminated (63). Others blame impacted stones for impaired venous drainage (64). Whatever the primary factors, ischemia and subsequent growth of anaerobic organisms such as *Cl. welchii,* are probably responsible for the gas formation (65).

Vascular Lesions

Polyarteritis nodosa of the gallbladder may mimic acute cholecystitis, clinically. These patients almost always progress to generalized vasculitis (66,67). Pathologically, there may be focal necrosis with erosion or ulceration of the mucosa or infarction of the entire gallbladder. The small and medium-sized muscular arteries in the gallbladder wall show eccentric fibrinoid necrosis with neutrophil infiltration of their wall. There may also be older lesions showing thrombotic occlusion of vascular lumens, organization, or recanalization. However, such changes may be seen adjacent to any inflammatory process, and in the absence of destruction of the elastica, are not diagnostic of a primary vasculitis. Patients with rheumatoid arthritis may develop a clinical and histologic picture very similar to polyarteritis. Other types of occlusive vascular disease may also lead to infarction of the gallbladder (68). Torsion of the gallbladder also may produce ischemic necrosis and gangrene. This generally occurs in anatomically abnormal gallbladders (15,69). Hyalinization of arterioles in the adventitia of the gallbladder is not uncommon. However, the correlation of this lesion with significant vascular disease elsewhere in the body is not clear. Amyloidosis of small arteries resembles hyaline arteriosclerosis and is easily missed in sections stained with hematoxylin and eosin. If suspected, amyloidosis should be looked for in sections stained with Congo red and viewed with polarized light (see liver section). Amyloidosis in the gallbladder is almost always part of generalized amyloidosis.

Nodules and Tumors

Cholesterolosis

"Strawberry" gallbladder or cholesterolosis is quite common. Grossly, yellow spots are seen on the mucosa (Fig. 8). These lesions may be distributed in an irregular "salt-and-pepper" pattern or they may be concentrated along mucosal folds as ridges or streaks. Rarely, large aggregates of such spots form nodules or polyps. In sections stained with hematoxylin and eosin, formy macrophages are present in the lamina propria (Fig. 9). Fat stains on frozen sections viewed with polarized light or specific stains demonstrate that these cells contain cholesterol. Occasionally, such cholesterol nodules become detached and float free within the viscus. Polyps composed of foamy macrophages in the lamina propria are also seen in metachromatic leukodystrophy. These cells stain positively with cresyl violet, toluidine blue, and the PAS stain (69a).

Inflammatory Polyps

Inflammatory polyps are composed of a fibrous stroma infiltrated with chronic inflammatory cells and covered by normal or mildly hyperplastic epithelium. They are usually associated with chronic cholecystitis and generally form sessile

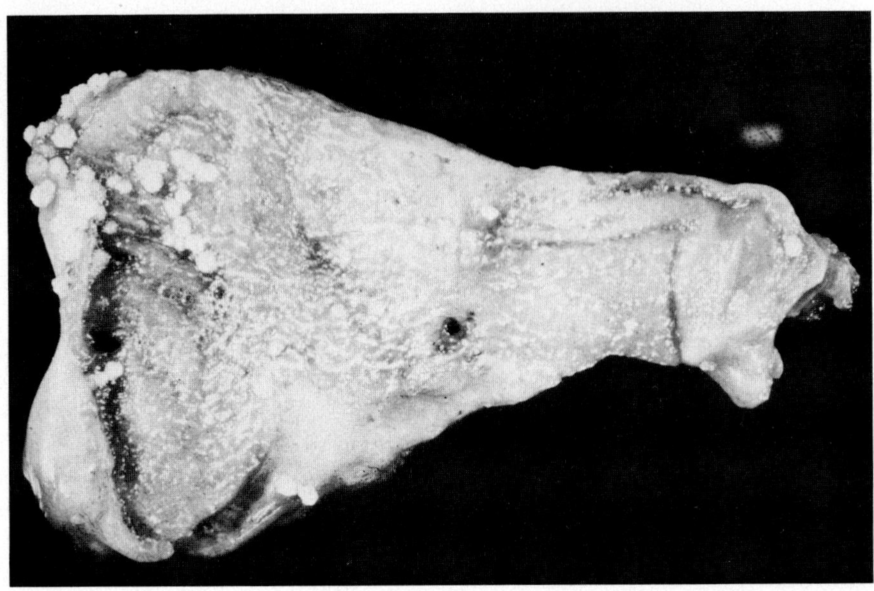

Figure 8. Gallbladder with cholesterol stones and cholesterolosis. Note pale spots arranged in an irregular pepper-and-salt pattern, forming linear streaks in some areas.

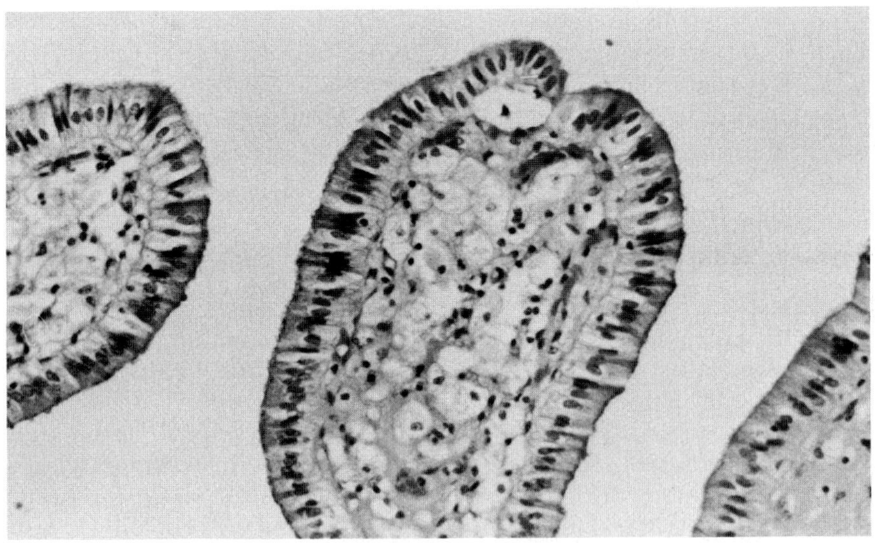

Figure 9. Cholesterolosis of gallbladder, showing a nodule composed of foamy macrophages immediately underlying the columnar epithelium. (Hematoxylin and eosin, ×24.)

rather than stalked nodules. They may be single or multiple (42). Nodules composed of foamy histiocytes, often containing brown pigment granules characteristic of lipofuscin or ceroid (Chapter 11), which usually also contain chronic inflammatory cells, have been described in chronic cholecystitis (70,70a). Such lesions may extend through the entire thickness of the gallbladder wall and may contain foreign-body giant cells. They have been called fibroxanthogranulomas. One such nodule contained Michaelis Gutmann bodies typical of malakoplakia (70b). Tumor-like nodules, containing eggs of ascaris and paragonimus, have also been observed.

Adenomyosis

A large single, palpable, intramural nodule in the fundus is most likely an adenomyoma. The overlying mucosa may be umbilicated, and on cut section the nodule is grey and multicystic. Microscopically, one sees cystic and glandlike spaces resembling Rokitansky-Aschoff sinuses or Luschka crypts lined by normal gallbladder mucosa and surrounded by hyperplastic smooth muscle (Fig. 6). These lesions may be only extreme examples of mucosal diverticula of the gallbladder (see above). However, the prominence of the muscular component has led to the suggestion that the adenomyoma may be a hamartoma rather than a sequel to an inflammatory process. Gallstones are found in only about 50% of cases of adenomyomas. When it is more diffuse, this lesion has been called adenomyomatosis. The term cholecystitis glandularis proliferans (71) is often used almost synonymously with adenomyosis, particularly when muscular hypertrophy is not conspicuous. These diverticula in the gallbladder wall may extend into the subserosa and may simulate carcinoma. Their organization, bland cytologic appearance, and absence of desmoplasia or perineural invasion should help one avoid such a diagnostic error (72). Submucosal cysts may be found in the gallbladder of children with cystic fibrosis (72a).

Heterotopia and Metaplasia

Nodules composed of epithelium not found in the normal gallbladder are most frequent in the neck region and may be palpable or discernible only microscopically. Gastric tissue that might contain both parietal and chief cells (42) is most common, but intestinal, pancreatic, argentaffin, and argyrophil cells or thyroid may be present (49,50). Deposition of melanin (73) and of a lipofuscin-like pigment (73a) in the epithelial cells have also been described. Whether these lesions are congenital or acquired is not always clear and their malignant potential is uncertain (74–76a). Nodules of ectopic liver tissue have been described on the inferior peritoneal surface of the gallbladder, entirely separated from the liver (77).

Benign Neoplasms

Benign neoplasms of the gallbladder are uncommon and generally symptomatic only if large enough and located so as to obstruct bile flow. Adenomas are the most frequent of these (42). They are soft, red, occasionally multiple, and usually found in the body of the gallbladder. Approximately one-half are microscopically villous or papillary. The remainder are lobulated and have an adenomatous microscopic configuration with crowded acini lined by cuboidal or columnar epithelium (42). Most of the villous and adenomatous polyps possess a stalk (42). A chloride-secreting papillary adenoma with heterotopic small intestinal epithelium has been reported (78). Adenomatous polyps have also been reported in a patient with the Peutz-Jeghers syndrome (79). The malignant potential of adenomas in the gallbladder is controversial. Adenomas with carcinoma in situ have been reported (78,80). Other benign tumors are rarely seen; these include hemangiomas (80), granular cell tumors (81), leiomyomas (78), lipomas (80), and pseudolymphomas (82). A benign mixed tumor containing cartilage and duct-like structures has been described (83). A traumatic neuroma of the gallbladder has also been reported (42).

Malignant Neoplasms

Carcinoma of the gallbladder is detected in approximately 1.5% of cholecystectomies for presumed benign disease, usually chronic cholecystitis with cholelithiasis (84). In patients over age 70 (85), the incidence of primary carcinoma has been reported to be 7% of all surgically removed gallbladders. In most series, the female-to-male ration is 3 : 1, and there is almost always a history, sometimes long standing, of antecedent gallbladder disease. Dystrophic calcification ("porcelain gallbladder") is associated with a particularly high incidence of carcinoma (up to 22%) and indicates prolonged inflammation with dysfunction of the gallbladder (86). Concomitant cholelithiasis is present in about three-fourths of the patients with carcinoma (87).

In scirrhous carcinoma, the gallbladder wall is firm, thickened, and gritty, and because in this type of cancer a discrete mucosal mass is generally absent, a gross diagnosis of chronic inflammation and scarring is usually made (Fig. 10). Adequate microscopic sections, however, will disclose an atypical, frequently papillary pattern of neoplastic glands (Fig. 11). Infiltrating tumors often show perineural invasion. Vascular invasion is rare (88). Localized hepatic invasion of the gallbladder bed and regional node involvement are almost the rule. Contiguous organs, such as duodenum, colon, and stomach, may also be involved. Larger papillary carcinomas form grossly obvious mucosal lesions, and, therefore, are most likely to alert the pathologist to the possibility of malignancy. They tend to be soft, erythematous, broad-based polypoid lesions.

Eighty-five percent of primary gallbladder neoplasms are quite well-differentiated adenocarcinomas (89). More than one-half are scirrhous; the papillary type is next in frequency, and the mucinous variety is least common. Squamous, adenosquamous, and anaplastic carcinomas are much less common (89a). Among the unusual types reported are the intestinal type (90,90a), giant cell adenocarcinoma with choriocarcinoma-like areas (90a), and oat cell carcinomas (90a), which may represent malignant carcinoid tumors. Epithelial hyperplasia, metaplasia, atypical hyperplasia, and carcinoma in situ are frequent in mucosa adjacent to these carcinomas (49–51). The prognosis for invasive tumors is poor (91). A staging and grading method has been developed by Nevin et al. (92). His stage I was confined to the mucosa, stage II also involved muscularis, stage III involved all layers, stage IV also the cystic lymph node, and stage V spread to other organs. Histologic grading from I to III was based on the differentiation of the tumor. Lymphatic spread and involvement of contiguous

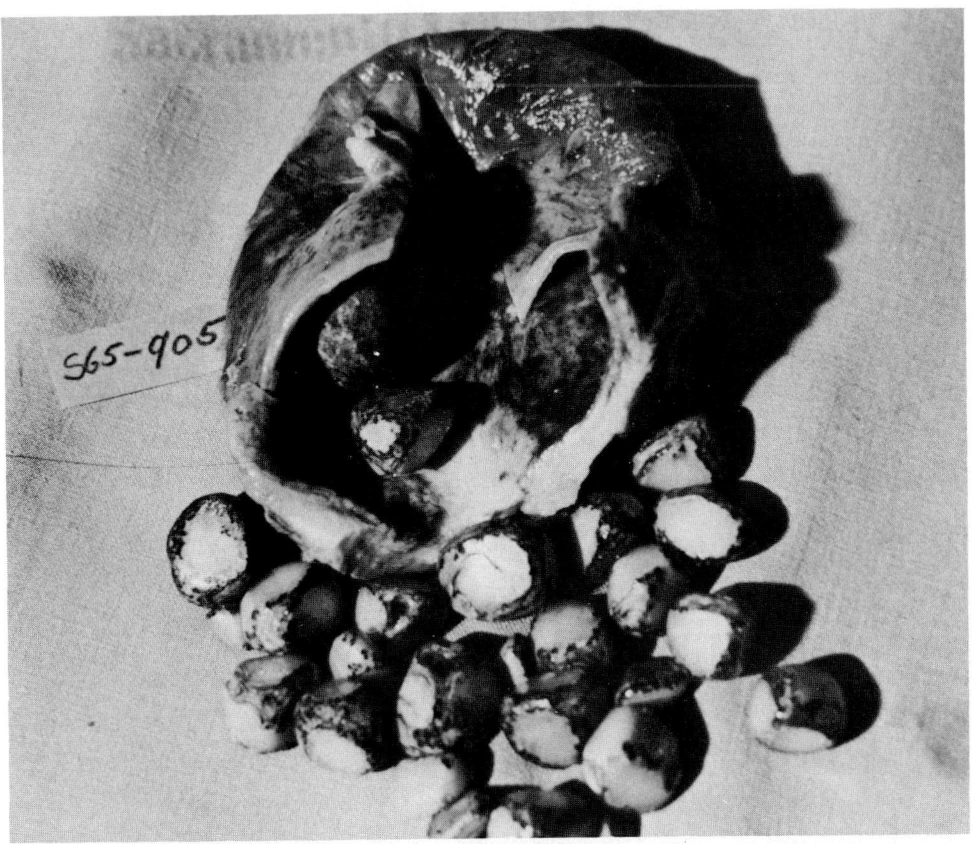

Figure 10. Gallbladder with thickened wall containing multiple mixed stones. Histologically, this specimen proved to be a carcinoma.

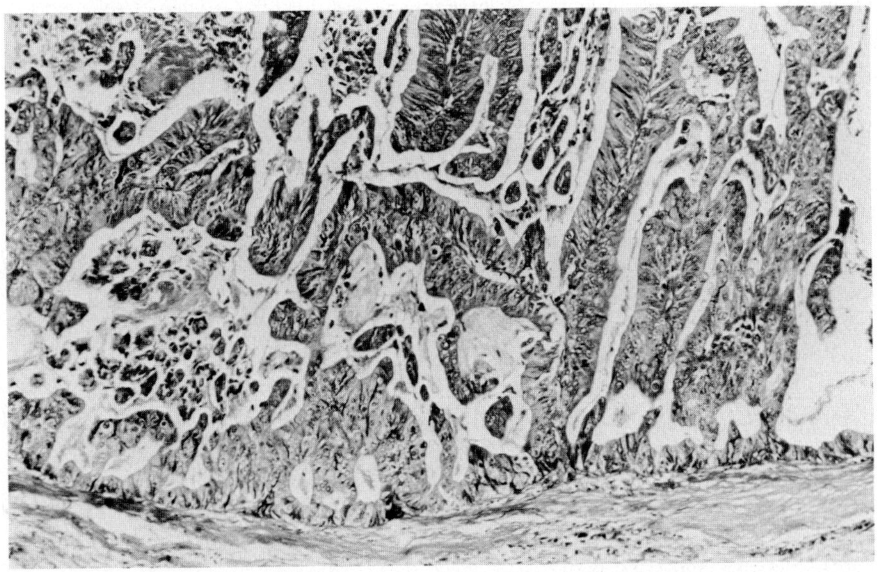

Figure 11. Papillary adenocarcinoma of gallbladder. (Hematoxylin and eosin, ×24.)

organs may occur, as may intraductal extension. Clinically inapparent carcinomas discovered only as incidental histologic lesions, usually small papillary carcinomas, undoubtedly have the best prognosis (93–96).

Malignant tumors of the gallbladder, other than carcinomas, are rare. Melanomas (90,97,98) and carcinoids (78,99), as well as an ACTH-secreting apudoma (100) have been reported. The "oat cell" tumors of the gallbladder may also be apudomas (90a). Connective tissue tumors primary in the gallbladder are particularly rare. Leiomyosarcoma (78), rhabdomyosarcoma (78), and undifferentiated sarcoma (101) have been described. Sometimes the distinction between a poorly differentiated carcinoma and a sarcoma may be difficult. Electron microscopy is of help in making this distinction. Malignant mixed tumors and carcinosarcomas (78,102,103), as well as a nodular lymphoma, apparently primary in the gallbladder, have also been observed (104).

REFERENCES

1. Vinnard RT: The acalculous gallbladder. *Am J Surg* 133:153, 1977.
2. Michel SL, Lipsky R, Morgenstern L: Routine liver biopsy in upper abdominal surgery. *Arch Surg* 112:959, 1977.
3. Maeda Y, Setoguchi T, Yoshida T, et al: A giant gallbladder. *Gastroenterol Jpn* 14(6):621, 1979.
4. Wood M: Eponyms in biliary tract surgery. *Am J Surg* 138:746, 1979.
5. Gross RE: Congenital anomalies of the gallbladder; review of 146 cases with report of a double gallbladder. *Arch Surg* 32:131, 1936.
6. Lockwood BC: Congenital anomalies of the gallbladder. *JAMA* 36:678, 1948.
7. Palmisano DJ: Double gallbladder. *Am J Surg* 118:463, 1969.
8. Hatfield PM, Wise RE: Anatomic variation in the gallbladder and bile ducts. *Roentgen* 11(3):157, 1976.
9. Schoenfield LJ: *Diseases of the Gallbladder and Biliary System.* New York, Wiley, 1977, p 1.
10. Sachdeva HS, Agrawal BK, Mittal VK: Agenesis of the gallbladder. *Am Surg* 41:109, 1975.
11. Martinoli S, Schmitt HE, Allgower M: Eine ungewöhnliche Trias: Gallen-blasenagenesie, Pancreas annulare und Pfortaderanomalie. *Helv Chir Acta* 46:767, 1979.
12. Harlaftis N, Gray SW, Skandalakis JE: Multiple gallbladders. *Surg Gynecol Obstet* 745(6):928, 1977.
13. Diserens H, Jost A, Mostmann R: Duplication vesiculaire et vesicules accessoires. *Helv Chir Acta* 46:779, 1979.
14. Boyden EA: "Phrygian cap" in cholecystography: Congenital anomaly of the gallbladder. *Am J Roent Rad Ther* 33:589, 1935.
15. Neher RG, Warner GW: Torsion of the gallbladder. *Abd Surg* 17:32, 1975.
16. Faintuch J, Machado MCC, Raia AA: Suprahepatic gallbladder with hypoplasia of the right lobe of the liver. *Arch Surg* 115:658, 1980.
17. Goor DA, Ebert PA: Anomalies of the biliary tree: Report of a repair of an accessory bile duct and review of the literature. *Arch Surg* 104:302, 1972.
18. Ober WB, Wharton RN: On the "Phrygian Cap." *N Engl J Med* 255:571, 1956.
19. Okuda K, Nakajima M, Nakayama M, et al: Multiseptate gallbladder. Report of a case with a review of literature. *Acta Hepatogastroenterol* 26:70, 1979.
20. Elias H, Sherrick JC: *Morphology of the Liver.* New York, Academic Press, 1969, p 137.
21. Fine G, Rajdu UB: Paraganglia in the human gallbladder. *Arch Pathol Lab Med* 104:265, 1980.
22. Jones AL, Spring-Mills E: The liver and gallbladder, in Weiss L, Greep RO (eds): *Histology.* New York, McGraw-Hill, 1977, p 701.

23. Been JM, Bills PM, Lewis D: Microstructure of gallstones. *Gastroenterology* 76:548, 1979.

24. Wosiewitz U: Limy bile and radio-opaque calcified gallstones. A combined analytical, radiographic and micromorphologic investigation. *Pathol Res Pract* 167:273, 1980.

25. Admirand WH, Small DM: The physicochemical basis of cholesterol gallstone formation in man. *J Clin Invest* 47:1043, 1968.

26. Holzbach RT, Pak CYC: Metastabile supersaturation: Physicochemical studies provide new insights into formation of renal and biliary tract stones. *Am J Med* 56:141, 1974.

27. Trotman BW, Soloway RD: Pigment vs. cholesterol cholelithiasis: Clinical and epidemiological aspects. *Dig Dis* 20:735, 1975.

28. Soloway RD, Trotman BW, Ostrow JD: Pigment gallstones. *Gastroenterology* 72(1):167, 1977.

29. Pearlman BJ, Schoenfield LJ: Gallstones: The present and future of medical dissolution. *Med Clin North Am* 62:87, 1978.

30. Trotman BW, Morris TA, Cheney HM, et al: Pigment gallstone composition in cirrhotic and noncirrhotic subjects. *Dig Dis* 23:872, 1978.

31. Bennion LJ, Grundy SM: Risk factors for the development of cholelithiasis in man. *N Engl J Med* 299:1161, 1978.

32. Bouchier IAD: Post-mortem study of the frequency of gallstones in patients with cirrhosis of the liver. *Gut* 10:705, 1969.

33. Admirand W, Way LW: Bile formation and biliary tract function, in Sleisinger MH, Fordtran JS (eds): *Gastrointestinal Disease. Pathophysiology, Diagnosis, Management.* Philadelphia, Saunders, 1973, p 352.

33a. Fry DE, Cox RA, Harbrecht PJ: Empyema of the gall bladder. A complication in the natural history of acute cholecystitis. *Am J Surg* 141:366, 1981.

33b. Broderick NJ, Cullen MH, Jones SP, et al: Death from a sharp stone. A fatal case of hemobilia. *Postgrad Med J* 57:396, 1981.

34. Sandblom P: *Hemobilia (Biliary Tract Hemorrhage), History, Pathology, Diagnosis, Treatment.* Springfield, Ill, Charles C. Thomas, 1972.

35. Goldberg MD, Waye JD: Traumatic hemobilia. *Am J Gastroenterol* 71:605, 1977.

36. Koshy A, Khuroo MS, Suri S, et al: Amebic liver abscess with hemobilia. *Am J Surg* 138:453, 1979.

37. Schubert GE, Hoehler LW, Roth A, et al: Leberarterien Aneurysma in der Gallenblase. *Med Welt* 31:315, 1980.

38. Schultz F, Fritsch A: Hemobilia after intraoperative liver biopsy. *Dtsch Med Wochenschr* 105:645, 1980.

38a. Thomas WEG, May RE: Hepatic artery aneurysm following cholecystectomy. *Postgrad Med J* 57:393, 1981.

39. Shah VR, Clegg JF: Haemorrhagic cholecystitis. *Br J Surg* 66:404, 1979.

40. Van der Linden W: Hemobilia: A case with recurrent jaundice cured by removal of a blood clot from the common bile duct. *Acta Chir Scand* 141:445, 1975.

41. Angres G, Srikantaswamy S, Zarnow H: Hemocholecyst: An angiographic demonstration. *JAMA* 228:1026, 1974.

42. Christensen AH, Ishak KG: Benign tumors and pseudotumors of the gallbladder: Report of 180 cases. *Arch Pathol Lab Med* 90:423, 1970.

43. Acosta-Ferreira W, Vercelli-Retta J, Falconi LM: Fasciola hepatica human infection. *Virchows Arch [Pathol Anat]* 383:319, 1979.

44. Hou PL: The pathology of *Clonorchis sinensis* infestation of the liver. *J Pathol* 70:53, 1955.

44a. McGowen JM, Nussbaum CC, Burroughs EW: Cholecystitis due to *Giardia lamblia* in a left sided gallbladder. *Ann Surg* 128:1032, 1948.

45. Ashur H, Siegal B, Oland Y, et al: Calcified gallbladder (porcelain gallbladder). *Arch Surg* 113(5):594, 1978.

46. Russell PW, Brown CH: Primary carcinoma of the gallbladder. *Ann Surg* 132:121, 1950.

47. Nahrwold DL, Rose RC, Ward SP: Abnormalities in gallbladder morphology and function in patients with cholelithiasis. *Ann Surg* 184(4):415, 1976.
48. Robertson HE, Ferguson WJ: The diverticula (Luschka's crypts) of the gallbladder. *Arch Pathol Lab Med* 40:312, 1945.
49. Azadeh B, Parai SK: Argentaffin cells, intestinal metaplasia and antral metaplasia in carcinoma of the gallbladder. *Histopathology* 4:653, 1980.
50. Laitio M: Morphology and histochemistry of non-tumorous gallbladder epithelium. A series of 103 cases. *Pathol Res Pract* 167:335, 1980.
51. Albores-Saavedra J, Alcantra-Vazquez A, Cruz-Ortiz H, et al: The precursor lesions of gallbladder carcinoma. Hyperplasia, atypical hyperplasia and carcinoma in situ. *Cancer* 45:919, 1980.
51a. Black WC: The morphogenesis of gall bladder carcinoma. *Prog Surg Pathol* 2:207, 1980.
52. Ziarek S, Deddouche M, Zoubir Y, et al: Tuberculose de la vesicule biliare. *Med Chir* 4:219, 1975.
52a. Scully RE, Mark EJ, McNeely BU: Case records of the Massachusetts General Hospital. *New Engl J Med* 306:349, 1982.
53. Leegard M: Eosinophilic cholecystitis. *Acta Chir Scand* 146:295, 1980.
54. Kerstein MD, Sheahan DG, Gudjonsson B, et al: Eosinophilic cholecystitis. *Am J Gastroenterol* 66:349, 1976.
55. Dawson JC: Clinics in gastroenterology. *Gastroenterology* 2:85, 1973.
56. Wakefield EG, Vickers PM, Walters W: Intestinal obstruction caused by gallstones. *Surgery* 5:670, 1939.
57. Alawneh I: Acute non-calculous cholecystitis in burns. *Br J Surg* 65(4):243, 1978.
58. Ternberg JL, Keating JP: Acute acalculous cholecystitis. *Arch Surg* 110:543, 1975.
59. Petersen SR, Sheldon GR: Acute acalculous cholecystitis. A complication of hyperalimentation. *Am J Surg* 138:814, 1979.
60. Thomas GG Jr, Womack NA: Acute cholecystitis, its pathogenesis and repair. *Arch Surg* 64:590, 1952.
61. Stephenson SE Jr, Nagel CB: Acute cholecystitis: An experimental study. *Ann Surg* 157:687, 1963.
62. Abengowe CU, McManamon PJM: Acute emphysematous cholecystitis. *Can Med Assoc J* 111(10):1112, 1974.
63. May RE, Strong R: Acute emphysematous cholecystitis. *Br J Surg* 58:453, 1971.
64. Campbell EW, Rogers CL: Submucosal gallbladder emphysema. *JAMA* 227:790, 1974.
65. Mentzer RM Jr, Golden GT, Chandler JG, et al: A comparative appraisal of emphysematous cholecystitis. *Am J Surg* 129:10, 1975.
66. Schwartz IS, Mendelow H, Winkler L: Polyarteritis nodosa presenting as acute cholecystitis. *Am J Clin Pathol* 45:468, 1966.
67. Fayemi AO, Ali M, Braun EV: Necrotizing vasculitis of the gallbladder and the appendix: Similarity in the morphology of the rheumatoid arteritis and polyarteritis nodosa. *Am J Gastroenterol* 67(6):608, 1977.
68. Rosen Y, Chen C: Infarction of the gallbladder: A complication of hypertension. *Am J Gastroenterol* 67:249, 1977.
69. Azmy A, Boddy SA, Eckstein HB: Torsion of gallbladder, embedded in an accessory lobe of liver in a neonate with Beckwith syndrome. *Z Kinderchir* 30:277, 1980.
69a. Kohn R: Papillomatosis of the gallbladder in metachromatic leukodystrophy. *Am J Clin Pathol* 52:737, 1969.
70. Amazon K, Rywlin AM: Ceroid granulomas of the gallbladder. *Am J Clin Pathol* 73:123, 1980.
70a. Goodman ZD, Ishak KG: Xanthogranulomatous cholecystitis. *Am J Surg Path* 5:653, 1981.
70b. Hanada M, Tujimura T, Kimura M: Cholecystic granulomas in gallstone disease. A clinicopathologic study of 17 cases. *Acta Pathol Jap* 31:221, 1981.

71. King ESJ, MacCallum P: Cholecystitis glandularis proliferans (cystica). *Br J Surg* 19:310, 1931.
72. Ackerman LV, Rosai J: *Surgical Pathology*, ed 5. St. Louis, Mosby, 1974, p 548.
72a. Esterly JR, Oppenheimer E: Observations in cystic fibrosis of the pancreas. I. The gallbladder. *Johns Hopkins Med J* 110:247, 1962.
73. Laitio M: Melanogenic metaplasia of the gallbladder epithelium. *Acta Chir Scand* 141:57, 1975.
73a. Weedon D, Moore AWE, Graff J: Melanosis of the gallbladder. *Pathology* 12:265, 1980.
74. Curtis LE, Sheahan DG: Heterotopic tissues in the gallbladder. *Arch Pathol* 88:677, 1969.
75. Runge P, Schwartz J, Seigler H, et al: Gallbladder with ectopic gastric mucosa. *Arch Pathol Lab Med* 102:209, 1978.
76. Laitio M: Intestinal, gastric body and antral-type mucosal metaplasia in the gallbladder. *Beitr Pathol* 159:271, 1976.
76a. De Boer WGRM, Ma J, Rees JW, et al: Inappropriate mucin production in gallbladder metaplasia and neoplasia—an immunohistological study. *Histopathology* 5:295, 1981.
77. Lieberman MK: Cirrhosis in ectopic liver tissue. *Arch Pathol* 82:443, 1966.
78. Edmondson HA: Tumors of the gallbladder and extrahepatic bile ducts. *Atlas of Tumor Pathology*. 1967, section 7, pt 26.
79. Foster DR, Foster DEB: Gallbladder polyps in Peutz-Jeghers syndrome. *Postgrad Med J* 56:373, 1980.
80. Arbab AA, Bransfield R: Benign tumors of the gallbladder. *Surgery* 61:535, 1967.
81. Ishii T, Iri H, Yamamoto S, et al: Granular cell myoblastoma of the gallbladder. *Am J Gastroenterol* 68(1):38, 1977.
82. Hussain S, A., English WE, Lytle LH, et al: Pseudolymphoma of the gallbladder. *Am J Gastroenterol* 65:152, 1976.
83. Higgins GA, Turner JA: Mixed tumor of the gallbladder. *Arch Surg* 78:173, 1959.
84. Balaroutsos E, Bastounis E, Karamanakos P, et al: Primary carcinoma of the gallbladder. *Am Surg* 40:605, 1974.
85. Ross FP, Hickock DF: Hernia and gallbladder surgery in patients over 70. *N Engl J Med* 262:501, 1960.
86. Polk HC: Carcinoma and the calcified gallbladder. *Gastroenterology* 50:582, 1966.
87. Parkash OM: On the relationship of cholelithiasis to carcinoma of the gallbladder and on the sex dependency of the carcinoma of the bile ducts. *Digestion* 12:129, 1975.
88. Donaldson LA, Busuttil A: A clinicopathological review of 68 carcinomas of the gallbladder. *Br J Surg* 62:26, 1975.
89. Gray GF, McDivitt RW: *Tumors of the Extrahepatic Biliary System,* Gastrointestinal and Hepatic Pathology Decennial, 1966–1975. New York, Appleton-Century-Crofts, 1975, p 391.
89a. Karasawa T, Itoh K, Komukai M, et al: Squamous cell carcinoma of gallbladder. Report of two cases and review of literature. *Acta Path Jap* 31:299, 1981.
90. Laitio M, Hakkinen I: Intestinal-type carcinoma of gallbladder. *Cancer* 36:1668, 1975.
90a. Albores-Saavedra J, Cruz-Ortiz H, Alcantara Vasquez A: Unusual types of gall bladder carcinoma. A report of 16 cases. *Arch Pathol Lab Med* 105:287, 1981.
91. Do Carmo M, Perpetuo O, Valdivieso M, et al: Natural history study of gallbladder cancer. *Cancer* 42:330, 1978.
92. Nevin JE, Moran TJ, Kay S, et al: Carcinoma of the gallbladder. *Cancer* 37:141, 1976.
93. Hart J, Modan B: Factors affecting survival of patients with gallbladder neoplasms. *Arch Intern Med* 129:931, 1972.
94. Beltz WR, Condon RE: Primary carcinoma of the gallbladder. *Ann Surg* 180(2):180, 1974.
95. Laitio M: Early carcinoma of the gallbladder. *Beitr Pathol Bd* 158:159, 1976.
96. Moossa AR, Anagnost M, Hall AW, et al: The continuing challenge of gallbladder cancer: Survey of thirty years' experience at the University of Chicago. *Am J Surg* 130:57, 1975.
97. Carle G, Lessels AM, Best PV: Malignant melanoma of the gallbladder. A case report. *Cancer* 48:2318, 1981.

98. Hatae Y, Kikuchi M, Segawa M, et al: Malignant melanoma of the gallbladder. *Pathol Res Pract* 163:281, 1978.
99. Christie AC: Three cases illustrating the presence of argentaffin cells in the human gallbladder. *J Clin Pathol* 7:318, 1954.
100. Spence RW, Burns-Cox CJ: ACTH-secreting "apudoma" of gallbladder. *Gut* 16(6):473, 1975.
101. Carpentier Y, Lambilliotte JP: Primary sarcoma of the gallbladder. *Cancer* 32:493, 1973.
102. Mansori S, Cho SY: Malignant mixed tumor of the gallbladder. *Am J Clin Pathol* 73:709, 1980.
103. Higgs WR, Mocega EE, Jordan P Jr: Malignant mixed tumor of the gallbladder. *Cancer* 32:471, 1973.
104. Van Slick EJ, Schumann BM: Lymphocytic lymphosarcoma of the gallbladder. *Cancer* 30:810, 1972.

17
The Bile Ducts

GENERAL APPROACH TO THE SPECIMEN

Persistent cholestasis always raises the possibility of extrahepatic obstruction and, therefore, of a lesion in the biliary tract or pancreas. Adults with severe painless jaundice must be considered to have carcinoma until proven otherwise. This suspicion is strengthened if the gallbladder is markedly dilated (Courvoisier's law) (1) and if there are no gallstones and no history of biliary tract disease. Colicky pain, sometimes with fever and chills in addition to obstructive jaundice, suggests cholelithiasis and passage into the common hepatic duct of a stone. Calculi usually lodge at the notched portion of the common bile duct and can cause cholangitis. However, cholangitis may, rarely, be caused by malignant biliary obstruction (1a). Approximately 15% of patients operated upon for cholelithiasis simultaneously have choledocholithiasis, which occasionally escapes the surgeon's detection. These "retained stones" in the bile ducts may produce major complications such as cholangitis, hepatic abscess, and pancreatitis. Jaundice, abdominal pain and guarding, low-grade fever, elevated serum amylase and lipase, as well as increased urine amylase, suggest pancreatitis. In some of these patients there is a common pancreaticobiliary duct and a stone is impacted within the ampulla. The morphologic changes produced in liver biopsies by extrahepatic obstruction in adults have been described in Chapter 7. Sometimes it is a liver biopsy specimen that gives the first hint that a patient may be suffering from extrahepatic biliary obstruction. In infants the most common obstructive lesion of the biliary tract is extrahepatic atresia. The hepatic lesions produced by extrahepatic obstruction in infants have been described in Chapter 8.

Radiologic investigations and surgical exploration are usually required to localize the lesion responsible for extrahepatic obstruction and pathologic observations, often including frozen sections, are usually necessary to identify the nature of the lesion. Pathologic specimens, usually biopsy specimens of the bile ducts, are seen relatively infrequently in the surgical pathology laboratory. Such specimens do, however, always represent life-threatening lesions and have to be processed with particular care. Because of their different anatomic relationships, lesions of the ampullary region are discussed separately from those of the rest of the biliary tract.

EXTRAHEPATIC BILE DUCTS EXCLUDING THE PERIAMPULLARY REGION

Specimen Handling

Biopsies of extrahepatic bile ducts are generally small and can rarely be oriented grossly. Those that can be oriented are generally obtained at an operation on the extrahepatic biliary system for atresia (2,2a) or in adult extrahepatic obstruction. Since the biliary tract mucosa is so notoriously susceptible to autolysis, it is essential that specimens be submitted immediately, preferably unfixed. If the specimen cannot be dissected at once, the bile ducts should at least be partially opened and the specimen immersed in formalin.

Gross Anatomy, Dissection, and Description

If the normally fairly wide extrahepatic biliary passages of adults can be identified, they should be opened with fine, blunt-tipped scissors. Probing the system is useful, both to straighten the ducts and serve as a guide for the scissors. Probing may not be possible in infants. Considering the many possible variations in length and course of the extrahepatic bile ducts, it is not easy to define the normal anatomy of these passages. However, a normal baseline pattern is generally recognized. This and some of the more significant bile duct anomalies will be described here. For additional details, surgical anatomy texts are available as well as an excellent review (3).

The right and left hepatic ducts emerge from the porta hepatis and usually fuse at about 1 cm from the liver, giving rise to the common hepatic duct. However, the length of these ducts may vary considerably. The junction of the left and right hepatic ducts and even the entire common hepatic duct may be located within the substance of the liver (4). Radiologically, the common hepatic duct averages 0.8 cm in diameter (5). Generally, it extends 1.0–5.0 cm in length from its origin to the cystic duct insertion. At this point, traveling along the free edge of the lesser omentum anterior to the foramen of Winslow, the common hepatic duct becomes the common bile duct. The cystic duct passes from the neck of the gallbladder and, after a series of convoluted bends for 2–4 cm, joins the common hepatic duct at an acute angle. The lumen of the cystic duct is occupied largely by crescentic mucosal folds, the valves of Heister. There is considerably more smooth muscle in its wall than in that of the gallbladder. The common bile duct runs for an average distance of 5 cm in the hepatoduodenal fold. Then it passes behind the first part of the duodenum and pancreas to embed itself in a deep groove on the posterior aspect of the pancreas.

The hepatic artery lies to the left of the common hepatic and common bile ducts. It gives off right and left branches, which pass behind their respective ducts and enter the liver. On its way, the right hepatic artery usually gives off the cystic artery, which passes behind the common hepatic duct and reaches the gallbladder neck. As mentioned above, the pericholedochal lymph nodes draining the gallbladder lie to the right of the common bile duct.

Anomalies of Number, Course and Diameter

Three or more accessory intrahilar ducts may join the two main hepatic ducts when they form the common hepatic duct. This was true in 24% of the anatomic dissections performed by one author (3). Such accessory ducts are generally interpreted as aberrant segmental ducts rather than supernumerary structures. One or both hepatic ducts, or the common hepatic duct, may drain into the gallbladder (6–9). This anomaly may be associated with atresia of the common hepatic duct (9) or common bile duct and drainage of the cystic duct into the second part of the duodenum (9a). The right hepatic duct seems particularly prone to participation in unusual courses and may enter the cystic duct or duodenum directly. Truly accessory hepatic ducts from the right lobe may enter the drainage system at any point. These findings are the results of surgical observations, dissections and injections (3,10,11).

The length of the common bile duct, like that of the common hepatic duct, is a function of the cystic duct insertion, ranging from 1.5–9 cm before joining the pancreatic duct at the ampulla of Vater (3). One of the rare anomalies affecting the course of the common bile duct is a shortening with insertion into the first part of the duodenum. This is often associated with duodenal ulcer (12). Another anomaly is agenesis, generally associated with a common hepatic duct draining into the gallbladder, which in turn, is drained by a long cystic duct into the second part of the duodenum. The common bile duct may also be double barreled (13). Most investigators agree with the division of the common bile duct into two parts: an upper, thin-walled, wide-lumened portion separated from a lower, thicker segment by a notch visible radiologically some 0.2 cm outside the duodenal wall (14). Variations in the thick segment will be discussed below in the section on the periampullary region. With respect to the upper thin-walled portion, the likelihood of pathologic change is in direct proportion to the diameter. In an autopsy study the average diameter of the common bile duct was 0.7 cm and the maximal internal diameter at its entrance into the pancreas 1.3 cm (14a). In an intraoperative cholangiographic study of 252 adults, lesions were most unlikely with internal diameters of the common bile duct below 0.8 cm and occurred in almost 25% at 0.9 cm and in 57% at 1.1 cm. Greater diameters always indicated some abnormality (15).

The cystic duct may be abnormally long and run behind the common bile duct. Cystic and common ducts may be enveloped in a common fibrous sheath; or the two may join externally, yet retain a common inner wall or septum (13).

Preparation of Microscopic Sections

If a specimen is received that can be oriented, it is particularly important not to destroy its continuity when blocks are taken. In extrahepatic atresia a cross section of the proximal end may be taken for frozen section. The specimen is then dissected and pinned to a cork board for fixation (Fig. 1). Cross-sectional blocks of the fixed specimen are taken later (Fig. 2). If the blocks are clearly identified as to origin and a diagram drawn, it will be simple to return to the tissue for appropriate additional blocks.

Most frequently, however, the pathologist is presented only with a small tissue

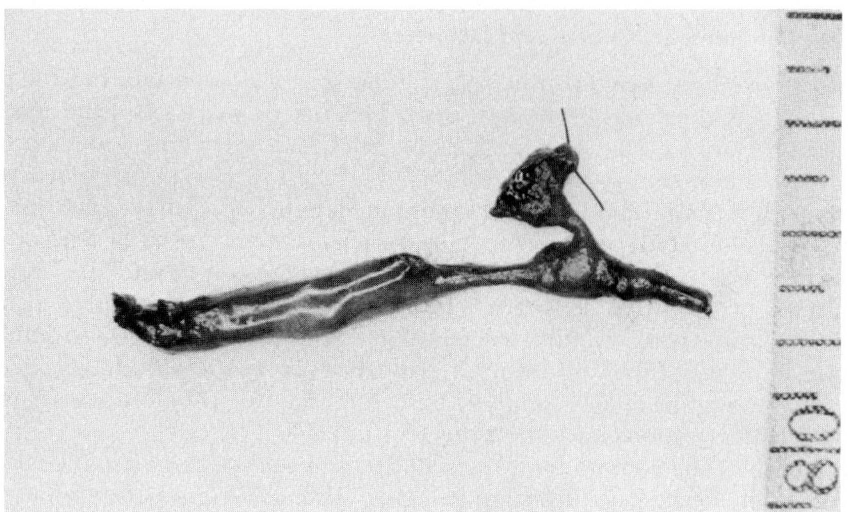

Figure 1. Extrahepatic biliary system removed en bloc at an operation for extrahepatic biliary atresia. (Contributed by M. Kasai, M.D., ref. 2.)

fragment of uncertain anatomic origin and orientation. On this fragment the pathologist is usually requested to perform a frozen section to distinguish between inflammation and neoplasia.

Normal Histology of the Bile Ducts

The bile duct mucosa contains many tiny pits, the sacculi of Beale. Deep to these, in the lamina propria, there are groups of mucous glands (Fig. 3) (16). Some of these are located within the wall of the duct and join the sacculi by short channels, but others are located in the loose outer coat of the ducts, surrounded by concentric layers of connective tissue. Chronic inflammation is so common in this area as to be almost a normal finding. It may cause fibrosis, which entraps some

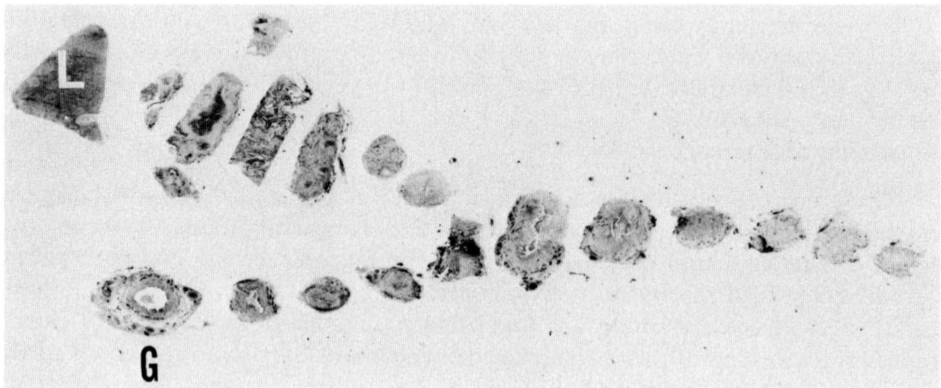

Figure 2. Serial sections of the extrahepatic biliary system shown in Figure 1. L = liver; G = gallbladder. (Contributed by M. Kasai, M.D., ref. 2.)

of the saccules and small mucous glands, and may well lead to distortion or proliferative changes. The presence of a few distorted or atypical glands within abundant collagenous stroma may make the distinction between scarring and well-differentiated scirrhous bile duct carcinoma and pancreatic carcinoma quite difficult (see p. 353).

Stones

Most stones in the extrahepatic bile ducts are probably formed in the gallbladder. Stones are present in the bile ducts of 10–15% of patients with cholelithiasis. They usually lodge at the junction of the thin- and thick-walled segments of the common bile duct proximal to the ampulla of Vater (61). The types of stones found in the bile ducts are essentially identical with those in the gallbladder, except that very large stones cannot enter the bile ducts. However, stones have been found in the bile ducts of patients with agenesis of the gallbladder and cystic duct. The multiple pigment stones found in the intrahepatic bile ducts of Asians with recurrent pyogenic cholangitis (cholangiohepatitis) may also be formed locally (62–62b).

Cholangitis

Acute suppurative cholangitis involving the extrahepatic bile ducts may be associated with cholecystitis, bile duct cysts, strictures, or parasitic infections such as clonorchiasis (63), or much less frequently may be the result of hematogenous or lymphatic spread from neighboring or distant inflammatory lesions. Grossly, there is a variable amount of edema and vascular congestion with modest thickening of the wall. If associated with obstructing calculi, the proximal ductal system will be dilated. Small stones may burrow into the wall. Microscopic findings resemble those seen in acute cholecystitis. There is vascular congestion, hypertrophy of the mucous glands, and an acute inflammatory infiltrate in the lumen as well as in the wall of the bile ducts (64). Should stones be present, the surface mucosa may be eroded or ulcerated. In recurrent cases, fibrosis and chronic inflammation of the submucosa may develop. Recurrent pyogenic cholangitis (cholangiohepatitis) is particularly common among Chinese in Hong Kong (62,62a) but may also be seen in oriental immigrants to Western countries (62b). It is characterized by choledocholithiasis, usually without cholecystolithiasis, but often associated with helminthiasis, biliary strictures and hepatic abscesses.

Extrahepatic Atresia

The etiology of cholestasis in infancy and the differentiation of extra-hepatic atresia from "intrahepatic atresia" and "neonatal hepatitis" by clinical observations and needle biopsy of the liver have already been discussed (Chapter 8). Laparotomy with exploration of the biliary tract is indicated if it is concluded that a mechanical obstruction of the extrahepatic biliary system is probably present.

Most surgeons consider that an obstructing lesion suitable to be bypassed by cholecystenterostomy or choledochoenterostomy can be found in very few of

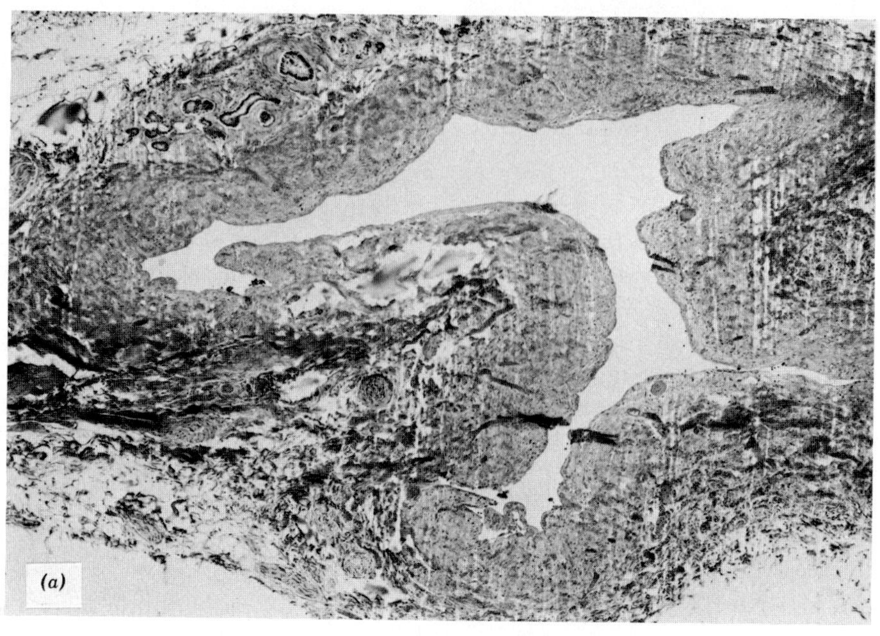

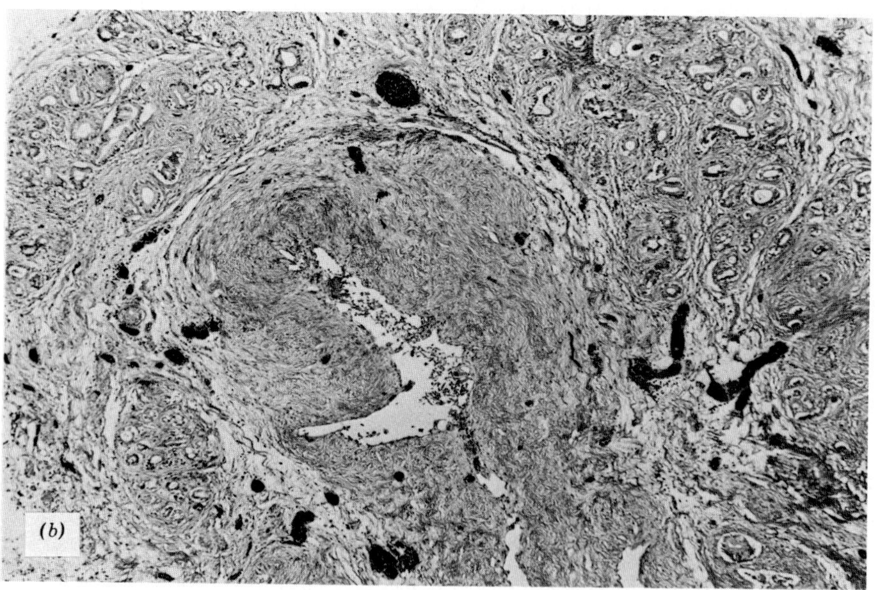

Figure 3. (*a*) Histology of a normal common hepatic duct. (Hematoxylin and eosin, ×40.) (*b*) Histology of a normal cystic duct. (Hematoxylin and eosin, ×40.) (*c*) Histology of a normal common bile duct. (Hematoxylin and eosin, ×100.) Note groups of mucous glands in the walls of these ducts.

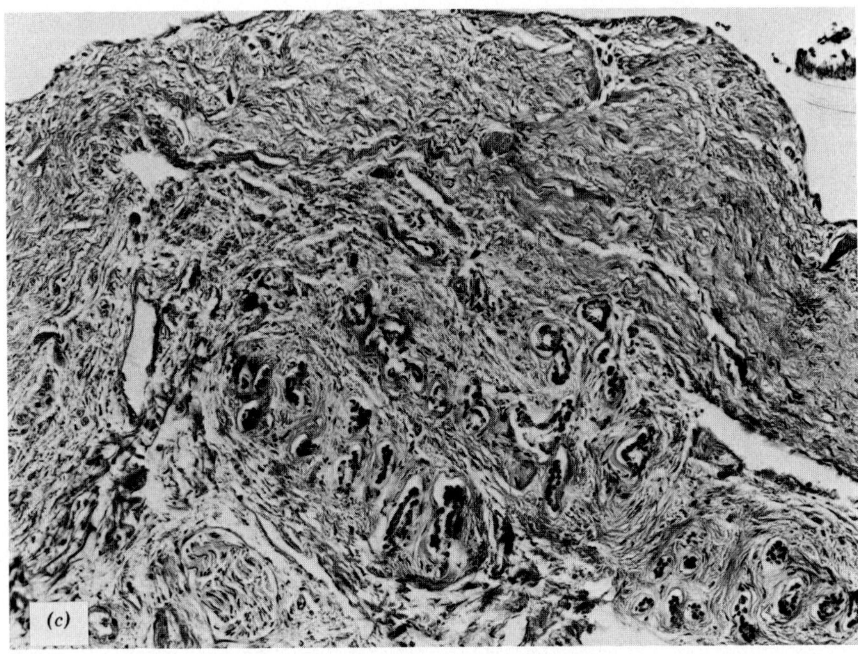

these infants. This very small group of patients is conventionally considered to be surgically correctable. Some recently reported examples of correctable lesions were a case of membranous obstruction at the ampulla of Vater (17) and a partial obstruction of both hepatic ducts by perforated diaphragms, which did not become manifest until adult life (18). A stricture of only the right hepatic duct with unilateral cirrhosis has been identified (22a). Extrahepatic atresia has been investigated intensively in Japan in recent years (19). In one Japanese series (20), about 20% of these infants were considered to be in the correctable category. Kasai (2,2a) has subdivided extrahepatic biliary atresia into type I (atresia of the common bile duct), type II (atresia of the hepatic duct), and type III (atresia of the bile ducts at the portal hepatis (Fig. 4). Kasai distinguishes four subtypes according to the findings in the duct distal to the atresia (Fig. 5). In subtype A, the common bile duct is patent, in B it is fibrotic, and in C it is aplastic. Subtype D consists of all those that cannot be fitted into the first three subtypes. Kasai's subtypes are again divided into subgroups according to the gross appearance of the hepatic radicles at the porta hepatis (Fig. 6). Kasai also classifies most infants with extrahepatic atresia, including all type III cases and some type II cases, as "noncorrectable" surgically. In these infants, the bile ducts at the porta hepatis are replaced by small ductules embedded in fibrous tissue or are entirely absent. It is this group of infants who are candidates for a portoenterostomy operation (2,2a), consisting of anastomosis of the porta hepatis to a loop of intestine.

In a portoenterostomy, the extrahepatic system is excised and then studied pathologically as outlined above. The histologic observations on the excised specimen may be classified according to Chandra and Altman (21). Ductal structures are looked for at the proximal margin of excision (21–26a). Gautier and Eliot (26a) have pointed out that periductal glands must not be confused

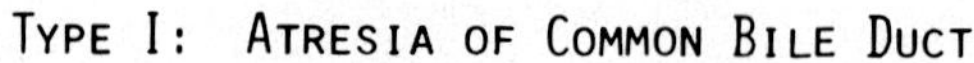

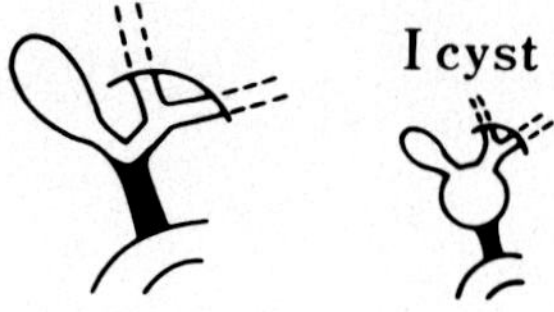

Type II: Atresia of Hepatic Duct

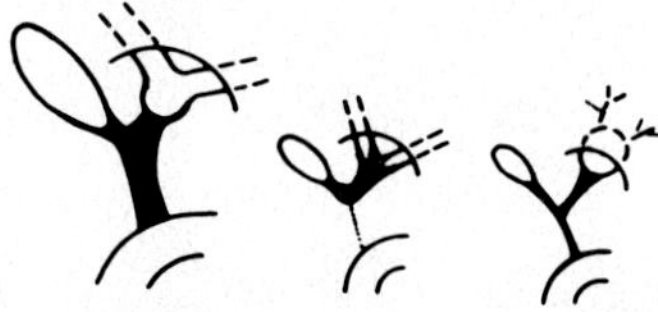

Type III: Atresia of Bile Duct at the Porta Hepatis

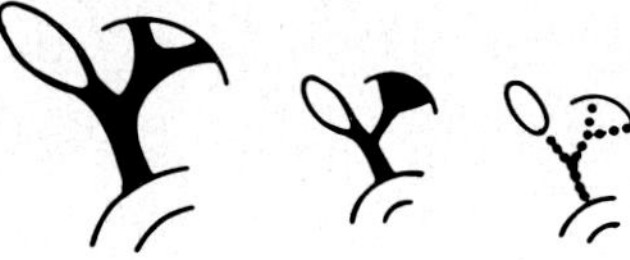

Figure 4. The major types of biliary atresia. (Contributed by M. Kasai, M.D., ref. 2.)

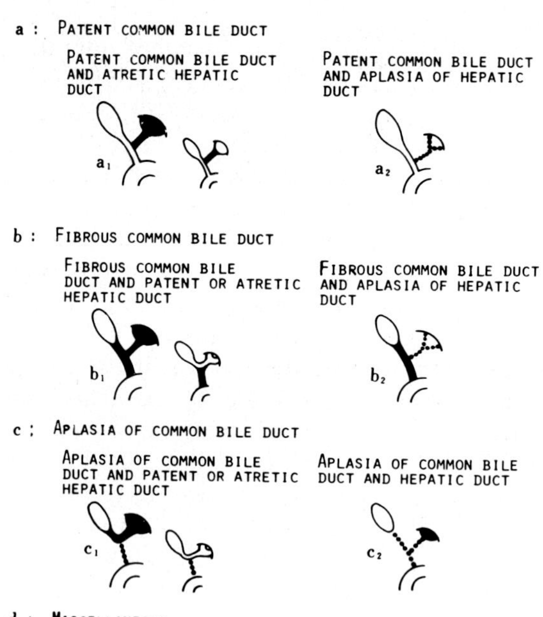

Figure 5. Subtypes of biliary atresia, classified according to the status of the duct distal to the atresia. (Contributed by M. Kasai, M.D., ref. 2.)

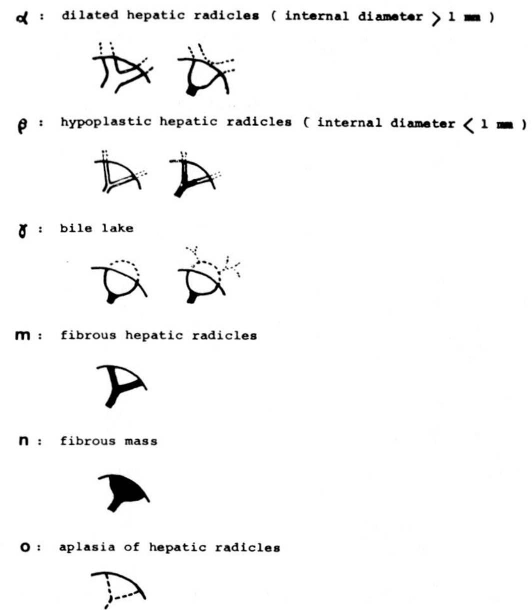

Figure 6. Subgroups of biliary atresia, classified according to the status of the ducts at the porta hepatis. (Contributed by M. Kasai, M.D., ref. 2.)

with ducts. Prognosis may depend on whether bile ducts are found and also on the size of these ducts (21,26a). According to one study (21), the prognosis is good if ducts of 150μm or more are found (Fig. 7). Frozen sections of the proximal end of the biliary system at the time of surgery have been advocated as a guide to the surgeon. If inadequate bile ducts are found, the operation may be extended deeper into the hilum until ductal structures of adequate size are encountered. Immunoglobulin deposits have been detected in the biliary remnants of some of these cases. These findings favor the suggestion that this may be an acquired disease (26b). Other hepatic and intestinal abnormalities, as well as polysplenia, may be found during laparotomy to be associated with extrahepatic atresia (27,28).

Cysts of the Bile Ducts

Cysts of the extrahepatic biliary tree (Fig. 8) are rather rare; they are most frequently found in women in the younger age groups and over one-third of all cases have been reported from Japan (29). Choledochal cyst, the commonest of these anomalies, may be a cause of neonatal jaundice (see Chapter 8). Most authors consider the cysts to be congenital in origin. Choledochal cysts are often associated with an abnormally long common pancreaticobiliary channel (30). Biliary cysts have been classified into five types (31–38), and type I (choledochal cyst proper), the most common type, has been divided into three subtypes (38). In type Ia, the cyst is proximal to a narrowing of the common bile duct and also involves the cystic duct (29,39,40). Type Ib is a segmental dilatation of the common bile duct only; type Ic is a diffuse cylindrical dilatation involving the cystic

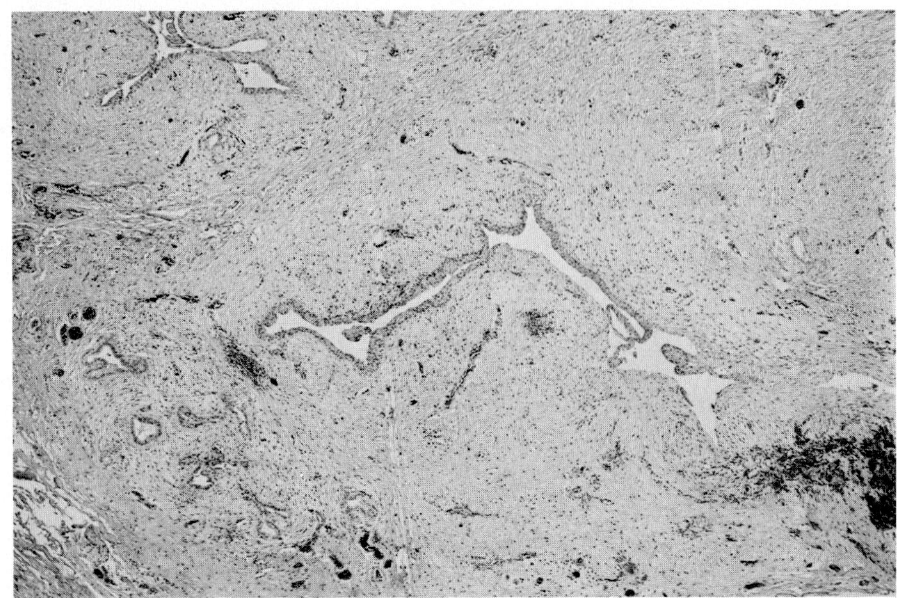

Figure 7. Section of proximal end of extrahepatic biliary system removed at portoenterostomy. Several ductal structures are seen, one measuring 1.5 mm. (Hematoxylin and eosin, ×40.)

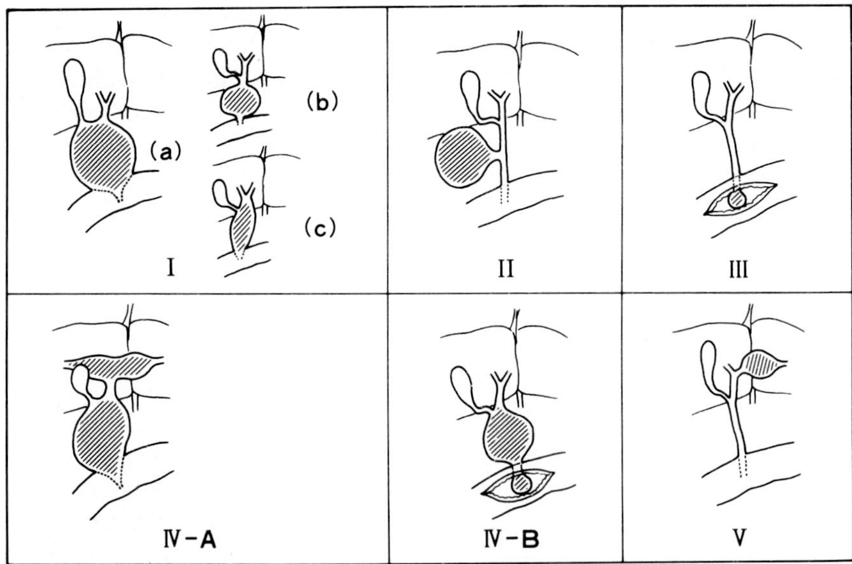

Figure 8. Bile duct cysts, schematic diagram. Ia, Common type; Ib, segmental dilatation; Ic, diffuse dilation; II, diverticulum; III, choledochocele; IVA, Multiple cysts (extra- and intrahepatic); IVB, Multiple extrahepatic cysts; V, Intrahepatic cysts. (Contributed by T. Todani, M.D., ref. 38.)

duct origin. Choledochal cysts are classically associated with jaundice, abdominal mass, and pain. Portal hypertension occasionally develops (41). They may not become symptomatic until adulthood or even old age. Type II is a diverticulum that may be seen in any of the extrahepatic bile ducts and type III, a choledochocele, is a dilatation of the intraduodenal portion of the common bile duct (42,43). Type IV corresponds to Caroli's disease. In type IVa there are multiple cysts of the intra- and extrahepatic ducts, whereas in type IVb there are multiple cysts of the extrahepatic ducts only (38,44,45,45a). Single or multiple intrahepatic bile duct cysts have been classified as type V (60). Bile duct cysts may be associated with other biliary abnormalities, such as Meyenburg's complexes (Chapter 14), congenital hepatic fibrosis, or polycystic disease of the liver (Chapter 13) (47–48a).

Bile duct cysts may be large and contain as much as 5 liters of bile, or may be very small and contain very little; they may be thick or thin-walled and may contain stones (49). The contents of the cyst should be cultured, and multiple cross sections should be obtained to exclude the possibility of carcinoma. When an epithelium is discernible microscopically, the cysts are lined by columnar epithelium that may be stained by bile pigments. The wall consists primarily of dense connective tissue containing collagen and elastic fibers, interspersed with little, if any, smooth muscle. A hamartomatous origin has been suggested for cysts in which the wall contains a variety of solid tissues (50). Cholecystectomy is usually performed in addition to cyst excision or internal drainage. The gallbladder (Chapter 16) and any bile duct removed should be studied by standard methods for the presence of cholangitis which, in association with pancreatitis, is a recognized complication of choledochal cysts (51). Carcinoma, usually adenocarcinoma, but sometimes squamous carcinoma, is another complication reported in 2.5% of biliary cysts by one author (52). However, carcinoma has been recognized more frequently in recent years, not only in choledochal cysts, but also in other anomalies of the biliary system such as polycystic disease of the liver, Meyenburg's complexes, and Caroli's disease (53–60a). It has recently been suggested that Caroli's syndrome may sometimes be an acquired lesion (60b).

Sclerosing Cholangitis

One of the most interesting, yet apparently relatively rare, lesions affecting the biliary tree is sclerosing cholangitis. This may be primary or may be associated with a variety of inflammatory or "autoimmune" diseases, particularly ulcerative colitis (Table 1).

The radiologic findings consist of diffuse and extensive narrowing of the extrahepatic ducts, sometimes with beading. The intrahepatic biliary radicles may be involved and present a "pruned-tree" appearance due to diminished arborization of the intrahepatic ducts (65,66). The differentiation of sclerosing cholangitis from scirrhous carcinoma is important but difficult, since the gross, and sometimes the microscopic, features are strikingly similar. There are occasions when only long-term clinical follow-up will resolve the issue (67).

Grossly, the tissue surrounding the extrahepatic bile ducts appears inflamed and fibrotic. Diffuse rather than localized involvement is the rule. Segmental

Table 1. Etiologic Factors that May Produce the Gross Appearance of Extrahepatic Sclerosing Cholangitis

I. Inflammatory
  A. Biliary tract inflammation
    1. Operative trauma
    2. Choledocholithiasis
    3. Suppurative cholangitis
    4. Strongyloides (146)
    5. Cryptoccus (147)
  B. Inflammatory bowel disease
    1. Chronic ulcerative colitis (78,79,148,149)
    2. Regional enteritis (150)
    3. Eosinophilic gastroenteritis (150b)
  C. Systemic; autoimmune or allergic
    1. Weber-Christian disease (151)
    2. Riedel's thyroiditis (152)
    3. Fibrous retroperitonitis (152,153)
    4. Retractile mesenteritis (154)
    5. Isonicotinic hydrazide (INH) (153)
    6. Porphyria cutanea tarda (146)
II. Neoplastic
  A. Adenocarcinoma, sclerosing
  B. Histiocytosis X (100,100a)

involvement has, however, been described (67a). Regional lymph nodes are enlarged and succulent. The ducts themselves have been variously described as thickened, fibrotic, and rope- or cordlike (68–71). When incised, the mucosa pouts from the cut surface, but is itself normal in appearance. The lumen is markedly compromised by fibrosis and may be difficult if not impossible to probe.

The extrahepatic ducts are characterized microscopically by moderate to pronounced periductal fibrosis. There is some chronic inflammation, which may be focal and unimpressive. Entrapment of ductules and small mucous glands may give a picture resembling infiltrating scirrhous carcinoma. The bile ducts in the portal triads may show similar changes or those of extrahepatic obstruction (Chapter 7). A combination of both types of change may be seen and this may be difficult to interpret. The distinction of sclerosing cholangitis from primary biliary cirrhosis may also be difficult (Chapter 7).

Strictures

Strictures are almost always acquired. Most often they are iatrogenic and occur following cholecystectomy. The gross microscopic findings are essentially those of localized or segmental fibrosis (72). Spontaneous isolated stenosis of the hepatic duct (Mirizzi's syndrome) usually occurs in patients with cholecystitis and cholelithiasis (73). Since effective surgical treatment entails complete excision of these lesions, it is important that the pathologist obtain cross sections of both margins of the specimen in addition to sampling the stricture itself.

Rupture

Actual rupture of the bile ducts with bleeding or leakage of bile into the peritoneal space is distinctly uncommon in the absence of previous surgery or other relatively direct trauma. Nonetheless, spontaneous rupture of bile ducts has been reported in conjunction with calculi and gangrene, infection of the duct, or obstruction at the sphincter of Oddi. Some antecedent inherent duct wall weakness, such as a cyst, is often present (74).

Tumors

Cholangiocarcinoma

Malignant tumors of the bile ducts are usually adenocarcinomas. They are uncommon, though more common than benign tumors. Apart from chronic longstanding ulcerative colitis and cystic dilatation of the bile ducts, few specific etiologic factors have been identified. Choledocholithiasis (75–80) and Crohn's disease (81) are rarely associated with bile duct carcinoma.

Carcinomas may arise from any of the ducts, particularly at bifurcations. The relative frequency of this tumor in different locations of the biliary tract is shown in Figure 9 (81a). When located near the junction of the left and right hepatic

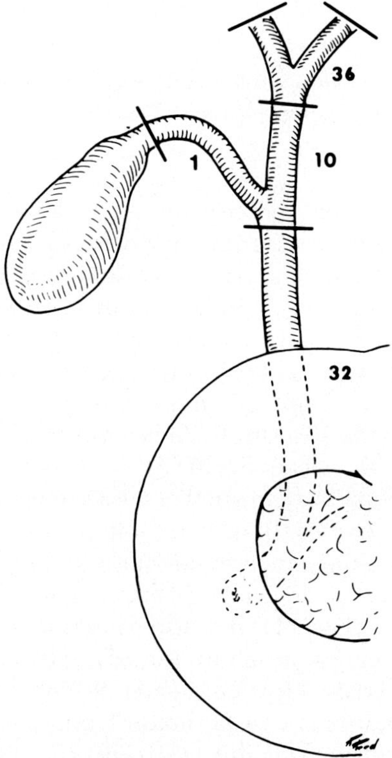

Figure 9. Relative frequency of carcinoma in the different segments of the extrahepatic bile ducts. (Reproduced from C. D. Lees, M.D., ref. 81a.)

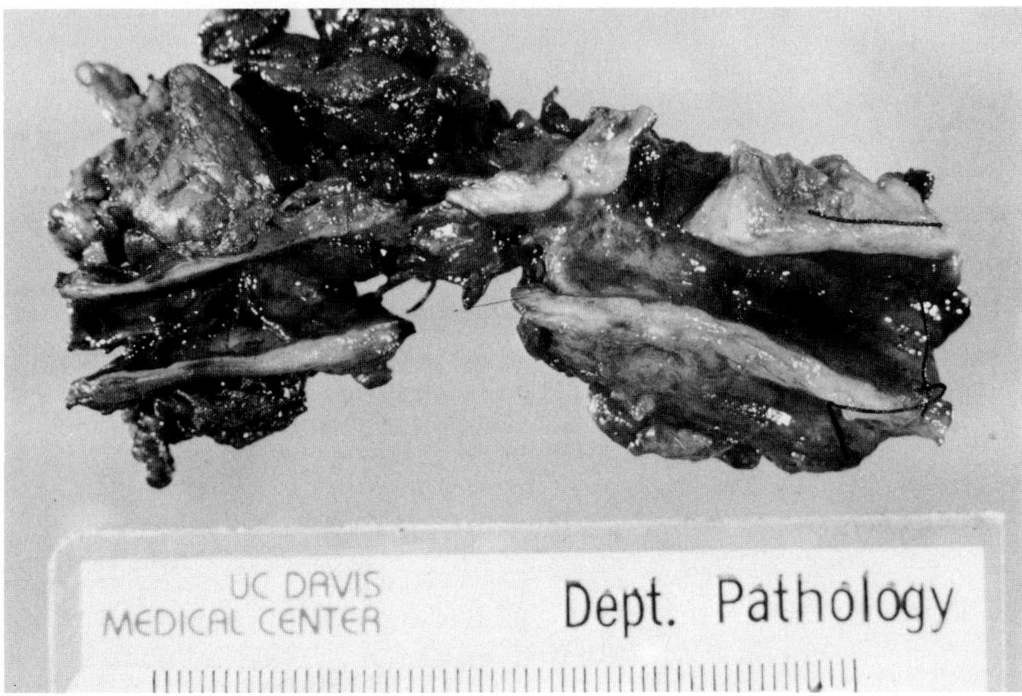

Figure 10. Carcinoma of junction of left and right hepatic ducts (Klatskin tumor). Grossly, only relatively slight thickening of the wall can be seen. (Contributed by R. Cardiff, M.D.)

ducts, these tumors may be inconspicuous at laparotomy (Fig. 10) (82). Adenocarcinomas located in the right and left hepatic ducts or in the common hepatic duct are most frequently scirrhous, constricting, diffusely infiltrating, or nodular and may mimic sclerosing cholangitis or stricture. Tumors of the common bile duct or of the cystic duct are usually fungating adenocarcinomas (83) and may have a better prognosis (84). Carcinomas of the cystic duct are rare. Such patients generally develop abdominal distention and distention of the gallbladder before becoming jaundiced. This diagnosis can be proved only if the neoplasm is restricted to the cystic duct (85).

The pathologist's principal task in such cases is to distinguish between inflammation and carcinoma, frequently in a frozen section. This may be difficult, particularly in small specimens, since an adequate section of bile duct is necessary to show the overall pattern of diffuse invasion diagnostic of well-differentiated, scirrhous adenocarcinoma (Fig. 11). It is also desirable to demonstrate the origin of the tumor from the biliary epithelium (85,86). Histologic and cytologic criteria are similar to those described for pancreatic carcinoma (see p. 353). Occasionally, the diagnosis of carcinoma can be made from a lymph node involved by metastatic tumor or by perineural invasion (Fig. 12). In some cases, diagnosis may have to be deferred until paraffin sections become available. Even then the distinction between inflammation and neoplasia may still be extremely hard. It is

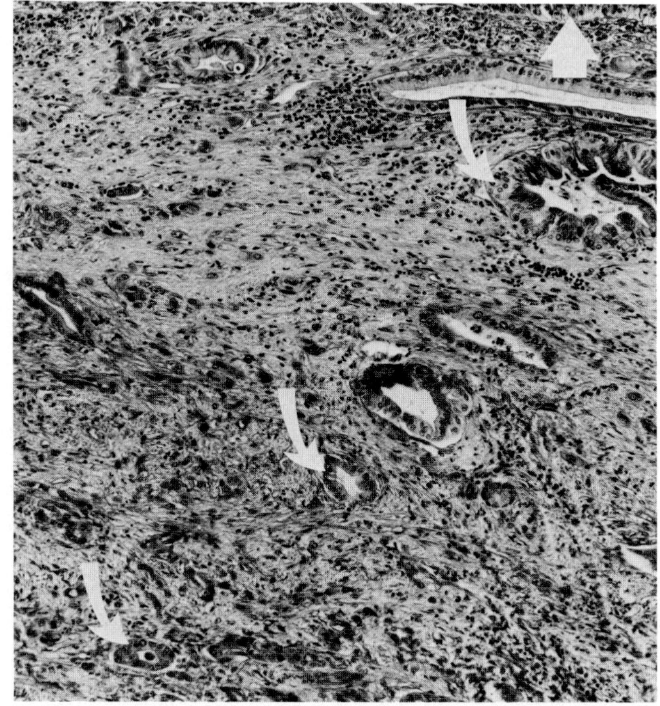

Figure 11. Histologic appearance of thickened area of bile duct shown in Figure 10, exhibiting carcinoma in situ (arrowheads) at the luminal surface as well as infiltrating adenocarcinoma (arrows). (Hematoxylin and eosin, ×85.)

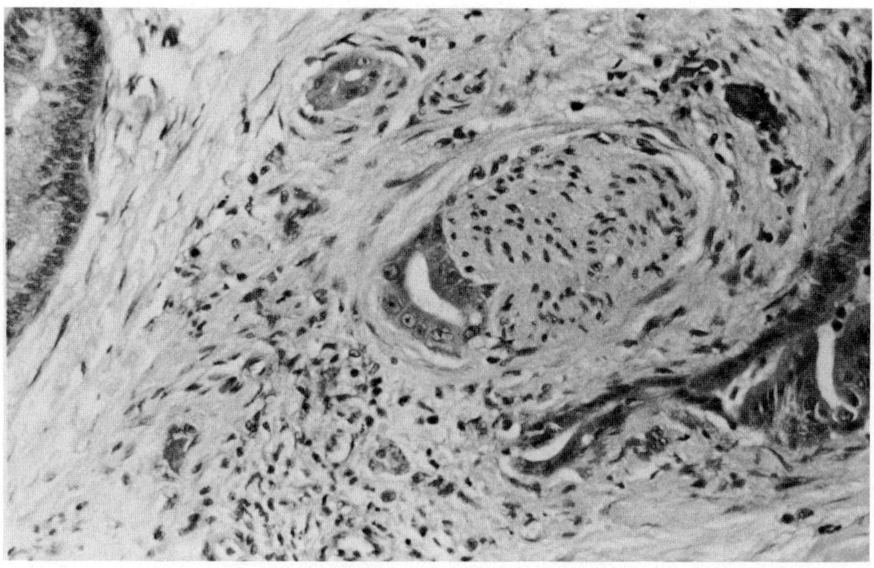

Figure 12. Adenocarcinoma of bile duct. Invasion of perineural space can be clearly seen. (Hematoxylin and eosin, ×215.)

desirable that part of such lesions should be embedded for electron microscopy. This is unlikely to elucidate the differentiation of benign from malignant lesions, but may prove helpful in identifying the type of neoplasm present.

Other Malignant Tumors of the Bile Ducts

Anaplastic and squamous carcinoma have also been observed, although much less commonly than adenocarcinoma (87). Cystadenomas and cystadenocarcinomas (88,89) of the extrahepatic biliary tree are much rarer than hepatic or pancreatic tumors of this type. The problems of distinguishing primary cystadenoma from cystadenocarcinoma have been discussed in Chapter 14. An argyrophilic tumor (apudoma) of the hepatic duct has also been reported (90). Metastatic tumors, particularly breast carcinoma, may also occur in this location and may have similar presenting features (91).

Embryonal rhabdomyosarcoma (sarcoma botryoides) is the most frequently seen malignant tumor of the bile ducts in childhood. Grossly, this is usually a polypoid mass projecting into the lumen. Microscopically, there are closely packed cells, usually just beneath the epithelium. The nuclei are hyperchromatic. The cytoplasm is pink and abundant and may contain cross-striations. Ultrastructural confirmation of this diagnosis is desirable (92–93a). Leiomyosarcoma and carcinosarcoma have also been reported (85).

Benign Tumors

Benign neoplasms occur even less frequently in the extrahepatic biliary system than in the gallbladder. The most common are sessile or stalked papillary adenomas, which may have cystic lobules and usually arise near the ostia or junction of the bile ducts (15a,94). These tumors may be single or multiple and generally produce obstructive symptoms. Malignant transformation has been reported in these lesions (95,96). Benign polypoid bile duct tumors may be associated with simple biliary cysts (96a). Eleven instances of granular cell tumor had been reported up to 1973 in cystic, common bile ducts and common hepatic ducts (97). A more recently described case in the cyst duct was associated with hydrops of the gallbladder (98). Fibroadenomas (15a), leiomyomas (15a,99), a neurilemmoma (15a), histiocytosis X (100,100a), and a granular cell myoblastoma (100b) have also been reported. Postsurgical traumatic or "amputation neuromas," although not neoplastic, may present as mass lesions (95). Also rare are bile duct hamartomas. These are nodules consisting of disorganized mixtures of fibromuscular and bile duct epithelial tissues in variable proportions (15a,54). Heterotopic gastric epithelium in the bile duct has also been observed (100c). A "benign inflammatory tumor" of childhood was described by Stamatakis et al. (101).

INTRADUODENAL BILE DUCT AND PERIAMPULLARY REGION

Specimen Handling

In the intraduodenal bile duct and periampullary region, it is particularly important to identify and preserve the normal anatomic relationships. The surgeon should be asked to submit the specimen unfixed and to instruct the pathologist with respect to the orientation of the specimen in relation to the common bile duct, as well as to the surgical margins. Large resections, such as Whipple's operation for carcinoma of the head of the pancreas (Fig. 16), may include the head of the pancreas as well as the second portion of the duodenum.

Gross Anatomy, Dissection, and Description

The muscular wall of the intrapancreatic common bile duct increases abruptly in thickness about 0.2 cm outside the duodenal wall. A corresponding reduction in luminal caliber also takes place in this location. Radiologically, this junction of proximal (upper) thin-walled and distal (lower) thick-walled common bile duct is seen as a notch (14). It corresponds to Boyden's superior choledochal sphincter. The distal segment, which has a mean length of 1.6 cm, lies within the muscularis propria and submucosa of the duodenum (102).

At some point along the course of the thick lower segment, the main pancreatic duct of Wirsung (1) approaches and the two ducts become invested by a common fibromuscular sheath, their lumens separated only by a mucosal septum. A common channel, the duodenal ampulla or ampulla of Vater, 0.2–0.7 cm in length, is formed in most subjects just before the duodenal papilla or papilla of Vater (1) on the posteromedial aspect of the second part of the duodenum (Figs. 13,14). Since an ampulla is not always present, the term papillary, rather than periampullary region, has been advocated (103). However, the term periampullary has continued in common use. The duodenal papilla is usually found within 12 cm of the pylorus (3,104) and is surrounded by the sphincter of Oddi (1). There is often a triangular mucosal fold covering the papilla and a longitudinal fold emanating from the caudal portion of the base of the ampulla (hood and frenulum, respectively) The most frequent variations are a longer common channel, separate ducts with separate papillae and separate ducts with a single papilla. If separate, the bile duct is almost always anterior or anterolateral to the pancreatic duct. A minor papilla, which may or may not be prominent, is usually present above or cephalad to the major papilla. This represents the opening of the accessory pancreatic duct of Santorini (1). A number of elegant dissections and radiologic studies of the periampullary area have been done (102,103,105–108a).

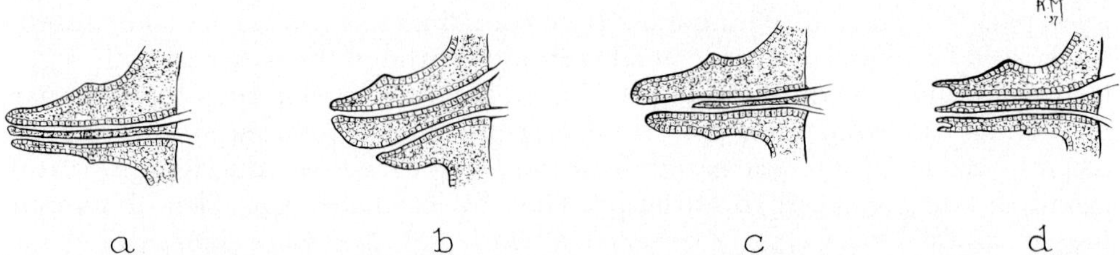

Figure 13. Diagram showing different relationships of the bile duct and pancreatic duct: (*a*) 19 cases, (*b*) two cases, (*c*) 33 cases, (*d*) one case. (Contributed by A. H. Baggenstoss, M.D., ref. 103.)

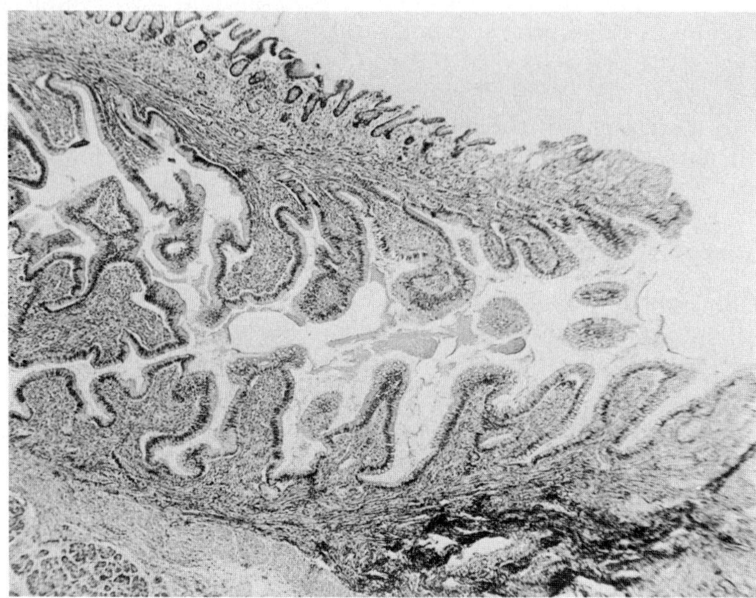

Figure 14. Longitudinal section of the duodenal papilla, showing junction of pancreatic and bile ducts. (×42.) (Contributed by A. H. Baggenstoss, M.D., ref. 103.)

Preparation of Microscopic Sections

We recommend opening immediately the biliary and pancreatic ducts of the fresh, unfixed specimen with fine, blunt-tipped scissors. This will ensure adequate subsequent fixation and will usually delineate the site of origin of a tumor. Photographs should be taken of the fresh gross specimen and a rough sketch made to serve as a key code to the slides when blocks are cut from the fixed material. In this way, one can clearly map the extent of a tumor as well as identify its origin with reasonable assurance. Lymph nodes must be thoroughly dissected from the specimen and their location labeled to assist in staging the lesion.

Normal Histology

The lower intraduodenal segment of the common bile duct, like the upper segment (see above), has mucus secreting glands but lacks sacculi of Beale. The main pancreatic duct of Wirsung has been compared to a fish's "backbone" (109). Enveloped by connective tissue, it runs straight through the pancreas with regularly emerging angled tributaries, the interlobular ducts. It is lined by columnar epithelium with some interspersed goblet cells; small associated mucous glands usually become prominent as the main duct approaches the duodenum. It can usually be distinguished from the bile duct by its smaller size, lack of smooth muscle, and a denser type of connective tissue (85). Accessory pancreatic ducts are commonly observed.

The duodenal papilla (110) is covered by duodenal mucosa, save at its tip, where there are neither intestinal glands nor villi (Fig. 14). Instead, there are a multitude of branched alveolar mucous glands that are often cystic and hyperplastic (85). The underlying ampulla of Vater has been called "a chamber of complicated and variable architecture" (105). Numerous highly vascularized mucosal folds, lined by columnar epithelium and surrounded by abundant smooth muscle, apparently function as a system of valves (111). Simple tubular glands empty into numerous elaborately branched diverticula between the valves. Dense smooth muscle bundles, components of the sphincter of Oddi, are attached to run between these diverticula. This musculature may or may not be independent of the duodenal muscularis propria. In the periampullary tissue, smooth muscle bundles of impressive size run circularly, obliquely, and even longitudinally. However, they do not entirely encircle the duct, and it is a matter of contention whether they function as a true sphincter.

Tumors

Carcinomas of the periampullary region (Fig. 15) include carcinomas of the ampulla and papilla, carcinomas of the duodenum close to these structures, carcinomas of the terminal common bile duct, and carcinomas of the pancreas in the immediate vicinity of the ampulla. In many instances it is impossible to identify the origin of periampullary tumors exactly (112). Even metastatic tumors may occur in this location (113). Some idea as to the relative frequency of the different types of periampullary carcinomas is obtained by a series of 185

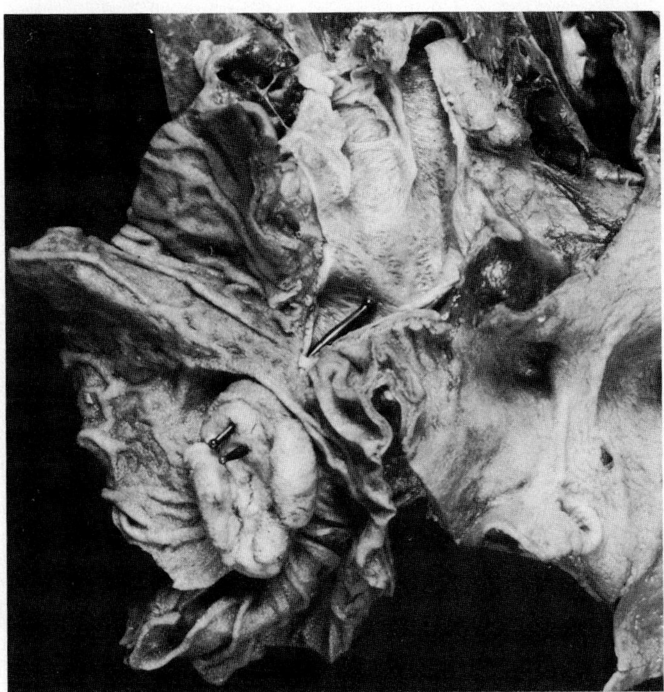

Figure 15. Periampullary carcinoma. (Contributed by A. H. Baggenstoss, M. D., ref. 103.)

patients, 149 of whom had carcinoma of the pancreas, 19 had carcinoma of the papilla or ampulla, and 17 a common bile duct carcinoma (114). Primary carcinoma of the duodenum, excluding the ampulla, is extremely rare, with a reported incidence of 0.035% in half a million autopsies (115). This tumor may also occur in a periampullary location. Every effort should be made to identify the origin of a periampullary carcinoma, since 5-year survivals are significantly better for resectable duodenal and ampullary tumors (40%) than for ductal carcinomas (12%), which tend to be scirrhous and extensive when first diagnosed (116,117), or for carcinomas of the head of the pancreas. Staging and grading of periampullary carcinomas also have prognostic importance (118,118a).

Pancreatic Carcinoma

Pancreatic carcinomas most often arise from ductal epithelium, and in two-thirds of the patients, involve the head of pancreas rather than the body or tail. Grossly, the tumors are ill-defined, and generally consist of a firm gray-white mass (Fig. 16). This appearance may be mimicked closely by chronic pancreatitis. Coexistence of carcinoma with chronic pancreatitis was observed in 10% of one series of pancreatic and ampullary carcinomas. This association clearly compounds the problem of distinguishing scirrhous carcinomas from inflammatory fibrosis (119,120). Since carcinomas in this area have such a poor prognosis and operative mortality is so great, it is imperative that the pathologist be absolutely certain when making a diagnosis of carcinoma, particularly on a frozen section. This can

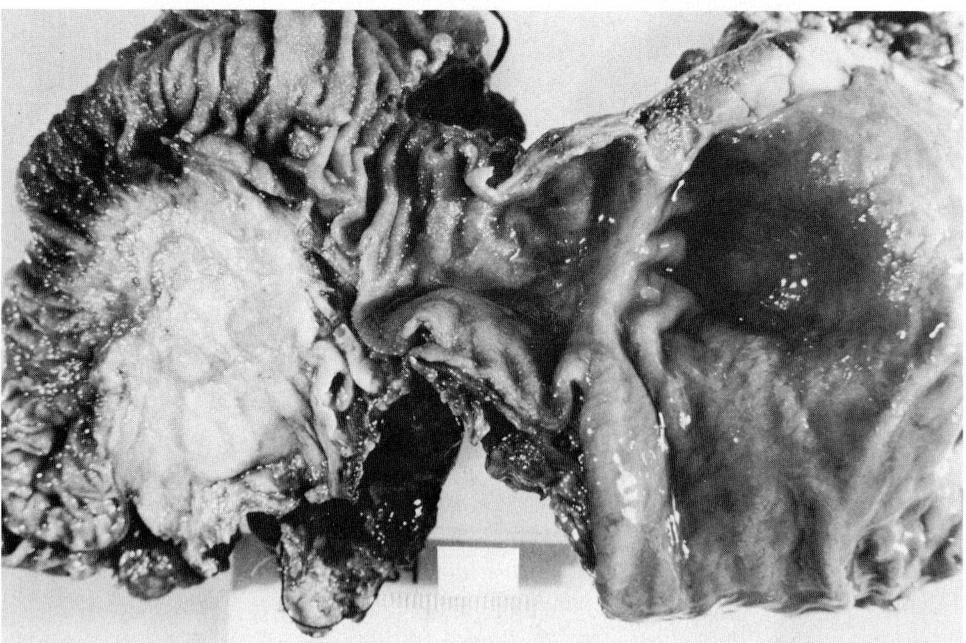

Figure 16. Carcinoma of the head of the pancreas surrounded by the loop of the proximal duodenum. Gross specimen removed at a Whipple operation. (Contributed by R. Edwards, M.D.)

be done with considerable accuracy by experienced pathologists (121). Tumor may fill the duct of origin, but this tissue may not initially be available to the pathologist for frozen section. Cytologic detail is helpful, particularly nuclear size variation of more than 4:1 within a suspicious gland and, less frequently, mitoses and huge irregular nucleoli. Equally important are histologic criteria, such as diffuse infiltration, a cribriform pattern, and perineural invasion. Major and accessory ducts with their mucous glands, metaplastic and entrapped in scars rarely mimic an infiltrative pattern, but do not possess the other criteria. Percutaneous aspiration biopsy of pancreatic lesions with fine needles has been employed successfully by some authors. In one study following radiologic localization, a malignant tumor was correctly dignosed in 83% of 23 patients (122,123). This procedure has the virtue of not requiring frozen sections and allowing the pathologist time for permanent sections with multiple levels through the block, if necessary. It also spares some patients a laparotomy.

The vast majority of pancreatic carcinomas are moderately or well-differentiated ductal adenocarcinomas that are occasionally papillary. Pleomorphic carcinomas are found more frequently in the body and tail than in the head of the pancreas and the male-to-female ratio is higher (4:1) than in adenocarcinoma of the body (2:1) (124). Also observed are giant cell tumors with multinucleate osteoclast-like cells and benign appearing stromal cells, much like giant cell tumors of bone. These may be epithelial in origin (125). Well-differentiated acinar carcinomas are seldom seen.

Well-differentiated, large papillary epithelial neoplasms, probably of pancreatic duct origin, have been reported in children. They are composed of cuboidal to columnar cells with eosinophilic cytoplasm. It seems unclear whether one should view them as papillomas or papillary carcinomas (126,127).

Cystadenocarcinomas of the pancreas, often with areas suggesting antecedent cystadenoma, range from 8 to 30 cm in diameter and may be unilocular or multilocular. Their contents are usually mucoid and the tumor itself is comprised of papillary projections of cuboidal to columnar mucous cells lining the cyst. The distinction between cystadenocarcinoma and cystadenoma is made by cytologic criteria as well as by the presence or absence of invasion and metastases (Chapter 14). Many patients are believed preoperatively to have a pancreatic pseudocyst, since abdominal pain, a palpable mass, and weight loss are the most frequent presenting symptoms (128). Pancreatic pseudocysts and pancreatic duct cysts may also be associated with jaundice (129).

Carcinoma of the Ampulla

Ampullary carcinomas tend to be soft papillary neoplasms occluding the orifice. Criteria of malignancy are similar to those described above for pancreatic carcinoma. These tumors are generally clearly malignant on cytologic grounds and have an infiltrative pattern, including perineural space invasion and lymph node involvement. The superficial aspect of these tumors may be much better differentiated than the base; frozen section material should, therefore, be taken from the deep area at the time of duodenostomy and biopsy (130). The most important feature determining 5-year postresection survival appears to be whether or not regional nodes are involved.

Carcinoma of the Bile Duct

Adenocarcinoma of the distal common bile duct may grossly resemble ampullary carcinoma or be scirrhous in nature, raising the question of sclerosing cholangitis. The diagnosis of malignancy is made cytologically, on the basis of infiltration, and if possible, perineural invasion, as discussed under carcinoma of the pancreas. To identify the origin of the tumor, serial blocks must be carefully taken and the lesion oriented by grossly identifying the major ducts.

Rhabdomyosarcoma

Embryonal rhabdomyosarcomas of the ampulla of Vater have also been reported (131). These contain the characteristic "strap" and "racket" cells, often with cross striations. Electron microscopy is desirable to confirm the identity of these tumors.

Apudomas

Islet cell or carcinoid tumors may pose a problem in histologic diagnosis by morphologically resembling adenocarcinoma. This problem is compounded if the islet cell or carcinoid tumor is not associated with a classical syndrome such as the Zollinger-Ellison or carcinoid syndrome. A recent reappraisal of the clinical, roentgenographic, and endoscopic features of the Zollinger-Ellison syndrome demonstrated that clinical manifestations of gastrinoma are often inconspicuous (132). Of 40 patients, only one-half presented with the picture of idiopathic duodenal ulcer or erosive duodenitis. Serum gastrin and a gastric analysis, particularly in candidates for duodenal ulcer sugery, may well be warranted and would certainly distinguish between gastrinoma and carcinoma. Electron microscopy easily identifies this group of tumors by their characteristic granules, but cannot reliably identify the hormone secreted (133). Immunocytochemical procedures can be performed by the horseradish peroxidase method on formalin-fixed, paraffin-embedded material to demonstrate cells producing insulin, glucagon, gastrin, human pancreatic polypeptide, and vasoactive intestinal polypeptide. Although their clinical symptomatology is usually attributable to a single hormone, islet cell tumors are frequently not uniform with respect to their component cells (134). Carcinoid tumors of the duodenum tend to be nonargentaffin, but argyrophilia may be demonstrated by the Grimelius technique (135). Pancreatic carcinoids are quite rare but have been reported (136).

Benign Tumors

Benign tumors are even less common in the periampullary region than are malignant tumors. Most are mucosal in origin and have been called either papilloma or adenoma (Fig. 17) (115,137). Since a "tubulovillous" microscopic pattern is often found, one could utilize the terminology currently in vogue for colonic polyps. These tumors pose a problem by virtue of their location in the ampulla or terminal bile duct and most patients present with jaundice or symptoms suggestive of cholecystitis. Sizes have varied from 0.4–7.0 cm. Submucosal excision is the procedure of choice provided frozen section fails to disclose invasion. A recent review noted that "in situ" or invasive carcinoma was reported in a high proportion of these lesions (138).

Hypertrophy of one or more of the folds at the orifice of the papilla of Vater

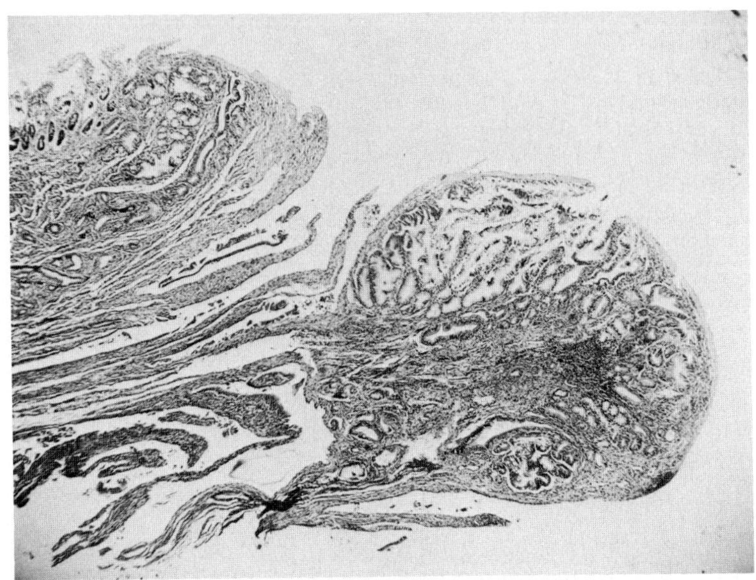

Figure 17. Adenomatous polyp of the duodenal papilla. (×26.) (Contributed by A. H. Baggenstoss, M.D., ref. 103.)

may give rise to polyps. These appear to be generally asymptomatic (85). Fibroadenomatous proliferation of aberrant ducts may cause biliary obstruction. Recognizing this condition requires an adequate understanding of the morphology of the periampullary region (85).

Heterotopic pancreatic tissue in the ampulla of Vater has also been described as a cause of obstructive jaundice (139), as has a membranous obstruction at the ampulla of Vater (21). Congenital anomalies at the ampulla may be responsible for some cases of neonatal obstructive jaundice (140).

Inflammatory Lesions

Chronic inflammation of the papilla of Vater (papillitis) appears to be not uncommon and may occasionally give rise to bile duct stenosis. Usually, this condition is associated with chronic cholecystitis and cholelithiasis or duodenal ulcer (141,142). Chronic pancreatitis also can produce bile duct stenosis and may mimic pancreatic carcinoma grossly (143–143b). The histologic differentiation of inflammation and carcinoma in the periampullary area is notoriously difficult (130) and has been discussed above. Biliary tract obstruction due to tuberculous adenitis has also been described (144). Intrapancreatic compression of the common bile duct has also been reported in cystic fibrosis (145,145a)

REFERENCES

1. Wood M: Eponyms in biliary tract surgery. *Am J Surg* 138:746, 1979.

1a. O'Connor MJ, Schwartz ML, McQuarrie DG: Cholangitis due to malignant obstruction of biliary outflow. *Ann Surg* 193:341, 1981.

2. Kasai M: Treatment of biliary atresia with special reference to hepatic portoenterostomy and its modifications. *Prog Pediatr Surg* 6:5, 1974.

2a. Ohi R, Okamota A, Kasai M: Morphologic studies of extrahepatic ducts in biliary atresia, in cholestasis in infancy. Its pathogenesis, diagnosis and treatment. In Kasai M and Shiraki K (eds): U. of Tokyo Press, 1980, p 157.

3. Dowdy GS, Waldron GW, Brown WG: Surgical anatomy of the pancreaticobiliary system: Observations. *Arch Surg* 84:229, 1962.

4. Linder HH, Green RB: Embryology and surgical anatomy of the extrahepatic biliary tract. *Surg Clin North Am* 44:1273, 1964.

5. Johnson EV, Anson BJ: Variations in the formation of vascular relationships of the bile ducts. *Surg Gynecol Obstet* 94:669, 1952.

6. Paul M: An important anomaly of the right hepatic duct and its bearing on the operation of cholecystectomy. *Br J Surg* 35:383, 1948.

7. Jackson JB, Kelly TR: Cholecystohepatic ducts: Case report. *Ann Surg* 159:581, 1964.

8. Zimmerman GH: Gallbladder inserted in the common hepatic duct: A rare anomaly of the bile ducts. *Chirurg* 48(2):73, 1977.

9. Kihne MJ, Schenken JR, Moor BJ, et al: Persistent cholecystohepatic ducts. *Arch Surg* 115:972, 1980.

9a. Markle GB: Agenesis of the comon bile duct. *Arch Surg* 116:350, 1981.

10. Healey JE, Shroy PC: Anatomy of the biliary ducts within the human liver. *Arch Surg* 66:599, 1953.

11. Hayes MA, Goldberg IS, Bishop CC: The developmental basis for bile duct anomalies. *Surg Gynecol Obstet* 107:447, 1958.

12. Lehmann H, Popken H, Schlaak M: The short choledochus syndrome. Case report and retrograde endoscopic visualization of the biliary system. *Acta Hepatogastroenterol (Stuttg)* 25:158, 1978.

13. Voitk AJ: Double barrelled common bile duct: A threat to biliary surgery. *Am J Surg* 131:611, 1976.

14. Hand BH: An anatomical study of the choledochoduodenal junction. *Br J Surg* 50:486, 1963.

14a. Dowdy GS Jr, Olin WG Jr, Shelton EL Jr, et al: Benign tumors of the extrahepatic bile ducts: Report of 3 cases and review of the literature. *Arch Surg* 85:503, 1962.

15. Persenico SG, Schamaun M: Internal diameter of the common bile duct and its significance in evaluating the biliary tract during surgery. *Helv Chir Acta* 41(5/6):615, 1974.

16. Spitz L, Petropoulos A: The development of the glands of the common bile duct. *J Pathol* 128:213, 1978.

17. Pinter A, Pilaszanovich I, Schafer J, et al: Membraneous obstruction of the common bile duct. *J Pediatr Surg* 10(5):839, 1975.

18. Devanesan J, de Blasi HP, Sable R, et al: Congenital hepatic duct obstruction with perforate diaphragms. *Arch Surg* 113:1452, 1978.

18a. Goldenberg DA, Brooks WS, Galambos JT: Unilateral cirrhosis, bleeding varice, right hepatic duct diaphragm and left hepatic duct atresia.

19. Hays DM, Kimura S: *Biliary Atresia, the Japanese Experience.* Cambridge, Mass, Harvard U. Press, 1980.

20. Kasai M: Results of surgery for biliary atresia, in Javitt N (ed): *Neonatal Hepatitis and Biliary Atresia*, NIH 79-1296. Washington, D.C., US Department of Health, Education, and Welfare, 1977, p 417.

21. Chandra RS, Altman RP: Ductal remnants in extrahepatic biliary atresia: A histopathologic study with clinical correlation. *J Pediatr* 93:196, 1978.

21a. Lawrence D, Howard ER, Tzannato C, et al: Hepatic portoenterostomy for biliary atresia. *Arch Dis Child* 56, 460, 1981.

22. Chiba T, Kasai M, Sasano N: Histopathological studies on intrahepatic bile ducts in the vicinity of porta hepatis in biliary atresia. *Tohuku J Exp Med* 118:199, 1976.

23. Miyano T, Suruga K, Tsuchiya H, et al: A histopathological study of the remnant of extrahepatic bile duct in so-called uncorrectable biliary atresia. *J Pediatr Surg* 12(1):19, 1977.

24. Lawrence D, Howard ER, Tzannatos C, et al: Hepatic portoenterostomy for biliary atresia. *Arch Dis Child* 56:460, 1981.

25. Gautier M, Jehan P, Odièvre M: Histologic study of biliary fibrous remnants in 48 cases of extrahepatic biliary atresia: Correlation with postoperative bile flow restoration. *J Pediatr* 89:704, 1976.

26. Bill AH, Brennom WS, Huseby TL: Biliary atresia. New concepts of pathology, diagnosis and management. *Arch Surg* 109:367, 1974.

26a. Gautier M, Eliot N: Extrahepatic atresia. Morphological study of 98 biliary remnants. *Arch Pathol Lab Med* 105:397, 1981.

26b. Hadchouel M, Hugon RN, Odièvre M: Immunoglobulin deposits in the biliary remnants of extrahepatic biliary atresia: A study by immunoperoxidase staining in 128 infants. *Histopathology* 5:217, 1981.

27. Chandra RS: Biliary atresia and other structural anomalies in the congenital polysplenia syndrome. *J Pediatr* 85(5):649, 1974.

28. Maksem JA: Polysplenia syndrome and splenic hypoplasia associated with extrahepatic biliary atresia. *Arch Pathol Lab Med* 104:212, 1980.

29. Saito S, Ishida M: Congenital choledochal cyst. *Prog Pediatr Surg* 6:63, 1974.

30. Kato T, Hebiguchi T, Kasai M: Etiology of congenital choledochal cyst. *Tohoku J Exp Med* 131:135, 1980.

31. Alonso-Lej F, Rever WB Jr, Pessagno DJ: Congenital choledochal cyst with a report of 2, and an analysis of 94 cases. Collective review. *Int Abst Surg* 10B:1, 1959.

32. Barlow B, Tabor E, Blanc WA, et al: Choledochal cyst: A review of 19 cases. *J Pediatr* 89:934, 1976.

33. Muakkasha K, Obeid S, Slim M: Congenital choledochal cysts. *Arch Surg* 111:1112, 1976.

34. Olbourne NA: Choledochal cysts. A review of the cystic anomalies of the biliary tree. *Ann R Coll Surg Engl* 56:26, 1975.

35. Kimura K, Tsugawa C, Ogawa K, et al: Choledochal cyst. *Arch Surg* 113:159, 1978.

36. Loubeau JM, Steichen FM: Dilatation of intrahepatic bile ducts in choledochal cyst. *Arch Surg* 111:1384, 1976.

37. Matsumoto Y, Uchida K, Nakase A, et al: Clinicopathologic classification of congenital cystic dilatation of the common bile duct. *Am J Surg* 134:569, 1977.

38. Todani T, Watanabe Y, Narusue M, et al: Congenital bile duct cyst. Classification, operative procedures and review of thirty-seven cases including cancer arising from choledochal cyst. *Am J Surg* 134:263, 1977.

39. Scully RE, Galdabini JJ, McNeely BU: Case records of the Massachusetts General Hospital. Presentation of a case—Choledochal cyst. *N Engl J Med* 296:328, 1977.

40. Rangabashyam N, Krishnaraj B, Mohan C, et al: Intrahepatic choledochal cyst. *Am J Gastroenterol* 63:71, 1975.

41. Martin LW, Rowe GA: Portal hypertension secondary to choledochal cyst. *Ann Surg* 190(5):638, 1979.

42. Reiner FZ, Weingarten G: Choledochocele of the common bile duct. *Am J Surg* 132:646, 1976.

43. Hart MJ, White TT: Choledochocele associated with acute hemorrhagic pancreatitis. *West J Med* 133:340, 1980.

44. Norton LW: Caroli's disease: A surgical challenge. *Am Surg* 45(1):70, 1979.

45. Caroli J, Gouinanad C, Soupault R, et al: Une affection nouvelle sans doubte congénitale des voies biliares. La dilatation kystique unilobaire des canaux hépatiques. *Sem Hop Paris* 34:496, 1958.

45a. Schomerus H and Egberts EH: Das Caroli Syndrome. Die fokale Dilatation intrahepatischer Gallenwege. *Ergeb. Inn Med Kinderheilk* 46:1, 1981.

46. Roda E, Sama C, Festi D, et al: Caroli's disease. Description of a rare clinical case with monolobar localization. *Am J Gastroenterol* 71:621, 1979.

47. Barros JL, Polo JR, Sanabia J, et al: Congenital cystic dilation of the intrahepatic bile ducts (Caroli's disease); report of a case and review of the literature. *Surgery* 85:589, 1979.

48. Dusol M Jr, Levi JU, Glasser K, et al: Congenital hepatic fibrosis with dilation of intrahepatic bile ducts. *Gastroenterology* 71(5):839, 1976.

48a. Leong ASY: Segmental biliary ectasia and congenital hepatic fibrosis in a patient with chromosomal abnormality. *Pathology* 12:275, 1980.

49. Mathias K, Waldmann D, Daikeler G, et al: Intrahepatic cystic bile duct dilatations and stone formation: A new case of Caroli's disease. *Acta Hepatogastroenterol* 25:30, 1978.

50. Ansari A, Silvis S, Vennes J, et al: Cystic hamartoma of the left hepatic bile duct: Cause of recurrent jaundice. *JAMA* 235:630, 1976.

51. Cahlin E, Lundholm K, Sahlin O, et al: Choledochal cyst. A case operated upon with excision and anatomical reconstruction. *Acta Chir Scand* 140:161, 1974.

52. Flanigan DP: Biliary cysts. *Ann Surg* 182:635, 1975.

53. Dexter D: Choledochal cyst with carcinoma of the intrahepatic bile ducts and pancreatic ducts. *Br J Cancer* 11:18, 1957.

54. McKenzie AD, Sandy JT, Anderson DO: Choledochus cyst with associated carcinoma. *Can J Surg* 2:88, 1958.

55. Bloustein PA: Association of carcinoma with congenital cystic conditions of the liver and bile ducts. *Am J Gastroenterol* 67:40, 1977.

56. Tsychiya R, Harada N, Ito T, et al: Malignant tumors in choledochal cysts. *Ann Surg* 185:22, 1977.

57. Kagawa Y, Kashihara S, Kuramoto S, et al: Carcinoma rising in a congenitally dilated biliary tract. *Gastroenterology* 74:1286, 1978.

58. Ozawa K, Yamada T, Matsumoto Y, et al: Carcinoma arising in a choledochocele. *Cancer* 45(1):195, 1979.

59. Gallagher PJ, Millis RR, Mitchinson MJ: Congenital dilatation of the intrahepatic bile ducts with cholangiocarcinoma. *J Clin Pathol* 25:804, 1972.

60. Azizah N, Paradinas FJ: Cholangiocarcinoma coexisting with developmental liver cysts. A distinct entity different from liver cystadenocarcinoma. *Histopathology* 4:391, 1980.

60a. Phinney PR, Austin GE, Kadell BM: Cholangiocarcinoma arising in Caroli's disease. *Am J Pathol* 105:194, 1981.

60b. Killer KM, Helwig H, Bertold H: Neonatal HBV hepatitis followed by fatal hepatic cirrhosis. *Med Welt* 32:1482, 1981.

61. George P: Disorders of the extrahepatic bile ducts. *Clin Gastroenterol* 2(1):127, 1973.

62. Johnson LF, Walta DC: Intrahepatic pigment stones: An Asian disease diagnosed with retrograde cholangiography. *Am J Dig Dis* 5:13s, 1978.

62a. Chou S-T, Chan CW: Recurrent pyogenic cholangitis: A necropsy study. *Pathol* 12:415, 1980.

62b. Yellin AE, Donovan AJ: Biliary lithiasis and helminthiasis. *Am J Surg* 142:128, 1981.

63. Sullivan WG, Koep LJ: Common bile duct obstruction and cholangiohepatitis in clonorchiasis. *JAMA* 243(20):2060, 1980.

64. Schein CJ, Mahadevia P: Surgical significance of the histopathology of the common bile duct. *Am J Surg* 137:763, 1979.

65. Albo RJ, Obata WG: Radiologic diagnosis of primary sclerosing cholangitis. *Radiology* 81:123, 1963.

66. Warren KW, Athanassiales S, Monges JI: Primary sclerosing cholangitis. *Am J Surg* 111:23, 1966.

67. Oviedo MA, Volkmer D, Scanlon EF: Primary sclerosing cholangitis. *Arch Surg* 109:747, 1974.

67a. Golematis B, Giannopoulos A, Papchristou DN: Sclerosing cholangitis of the common bile duct. *Am J Gastro* 75:370, 1981.

68. Schwartz SI, Dale WA: Primary sclerosing cholangitis. *Arch Surg* 77:439, 1958.
69. Douglass HO Jr: Idiopathic sclerosing cholangitis. *Am J Surg* 130:82, 1975.
70. Grua OE, McMurrin JA: Sclerosing cholangitis. Review and presentation of an unusual pathologic variant. *Am J Surg* 116:659, 1968.
71. Wiesner RH, La Russo NF: Clinicopathologic features of the syndrome of primary sclerosing cholangitis. *Gastroenterology* 79:200, 1980.
72. McAllister AJ, Hicken NF: Biliary stricture: A continuing study. *Am J Surg* 132:567, 1976.
73. Heil T, Belohlavek D: Mirizzi's syndrome as a special form of obstructive jaundice. *Chirurg* 49(1):57, 1978.
74. Spira IA: Spontaneous rupture of the common bile duct. *Ann Surg* 183:433, 1976.
75. Morowitz DA, Glagov S, Dordal E, et al: Carcinoma of the biliary tract complicating chronic ulcerative colitis. *Cancer* 27:356, 1971.
76. Ross AP, Braasch JW: Ulcerative colitis and carcinoma of the proximal bile ducts. *Gut* 14:94, 1973.
77. Akawari OE, Van Heerden JA, Fould WT, et al: Cancer of the bile ducts associated with ulcerative colitis. *Ann Surg* 181(3):303, 1975.
78. Lupinette M, Mehigan D, Cameron JL: Hepatobiliary complications of ulcerative colitis. *Am J Surg* 139:113, 1980.
79. Dew MJ, Thompson H, Allan RB: The spectrum of hepatic dysfunction in inflammatory bowel disease. *Q J Med* 189:113, 1979.
80. Wanebo HJ, Grimes OF: Cancer of the bile duct: The occult malignancy. *Am J Surg* 130(2):262, 1975.
81. Berman MD, Falchuk KR, Trey C: Carcinoma of the biliary tree complicating Crohn's disease. *Dig Dis Sci* 25:795, 1980.
81a. Lees CD, Zapolanski A, Cooperman AM: Carcinoma of the bile ducts: *Surg Gynecol Obstet* 151:193, 1980.
82. Klatskin G: Adenocarcinoma of the hepatic duct at its bifurcation within the porta hepatis. *Am J Med* 38:241, 1965.
83. Ingis DA, Farmer RG: Adenocarcinoma of the bile ducts. Relationship of anatomic location to clinical features. *Am J Dig Dis* 20:253, 1975.
84. Todoroki T, Okamura T, Fukao K, et al: Gross appearance of carcinoma of the main hepatic duct and its prognosis. *Surg Gynecol Obstet* 150:33, 1980.
85. Edmondson HA: Tumors of the gallbladder and extrahepatic bile ducts. *Atlas of Tumor Pathology*. Washington, D.C., Armed Forces Institute of Pathology, 1967, section 7, p 126.
86. Peck JP, Kern WH, Mikkelsen WP: Sclerosis of the extrahepatic bile ducts. *Arch Surg* 108:798, 1974.
87. Johnson FW, Gilsdorf RB: Carcinoma of the gallbladder and extrahepatic biliary tree. *Surgery* 40(8):456, 1974.
88. Marsh JL, Dahms B, Longmire WP Jr: Cystadenoma and cystadenocarcinoma of the biliary system. *Arch Surg* 109:41, 1974.
89. Ishak KG, Willis GW, Cummins SD, et al: Biliary cystadenoma and cystadenocarcinoma: Report of 14 cases and review of the literature. *Cancer* 39:322, 1977.
90. Judge DM, Dickman PS, Trapukdi S: Nonfunctioning argyrophilic tumor (apudoma) of the hepatic duct. *Am J Clin Pathol* 66:40, 1976.
91. Popp JW, Schapiro RH, Warshaw AL: Extrahepatic biliary obstruction caused by metastatic breast carcinoma. *Ann Intern Med* 91:568, 1979.
92. Kindblom LG, Dalberg K: Sarcoma botryoides of the extrahepatic bile ducts. A light and electron microscopic study of a case. *Pathol Res Pract* 170:258, 1980.
93. Lack E, Perez A, Schuster SR: Botryoid rhabdomyosarcoma of the biliary tract. *Am J Surg Pathol* 5:643, 1981.
94. Cattel RB, Braasch JW, Kahn F: Polypoid epithelial tumors of the bile ducts. *N Engl J Med* 266:57, 1962.

95. Cattel RB, St. Ville J: Amputation neuromas of the biliary tract. *Arch Surg* 83:242, 1961.
96. Neumann RD, LiVolsi VA, Rosenthal NS, et al: Adenocarcinoma in biliary papillomatosis. *Gastroenterology* 70(5):779, 1976.
96a. Austin EH, Mitchell GE, Oliphant M: Solitary hepatic cyst and benign bile duct polyp: A heretofore unheralded association. *Surgery* 89:359, 1981.
97. LiVolsi VA, Perzin KH, Badder EM, et al: Granular cell tumors of the biliary tract. *Arch Pathol Lab Med* 95:13, 1973.
98. Reul GJ, Rubio PA, Berman NL: Granular cell myoblastoma of the cystic duct. *Am J Surg* 129:583, 1975.
99. Kune GA, Polgar V: Leiomyoma of the common bile duct causing obstructive jaundice. *Med J Aust* 1(19):698, 1976.
100. Jones MB, Voet R, Pagani J, et al: Multifocal eosinophilic granuloma involving the common bile duct: Histologic and cholangiographic findings. *Gastroenterology* 80:384, 1981.
100a. LeBlanc A, Hadchouel W, Jehan P, et al: Obstructive jaundice in children with histiocytosis. *Gastroenterology* 80:134, 1981.
100b. Dewar J, Dooley JS, Lindsay J, et al: Granular cell myoblastoma of the common bile duct treated by biliary drainage and surgery. *Gut* 22:70, 1981.
100c. Kalman PG, Stone RM, Phillips MJ: Heterotopic tissue of the bile duct. *Surgery* 89:384, 1981.
101. Stamatakis DD, Howard ER, Williams R: Benign inflammatory tumor of the common bile duct. *Br J Surg* 66:257, 1979.
102. Boyden EA: Anatomy of the choledochoduodenal junction in man. *Surg Gynecol Obstet* 104:641, 1957.
103. Baggenstoss AH: Major duodenal papilla. Variations of pathologic interest and lesions of the mucosa. *Arch Pathol Lab Med* 26:853, 1938.
104. Hand BH: Anatomy and function of the extrahepatic biliary system. *Clin Gastroenterol* 2:3, 1973.
105. Elias H, Sherrick JC: The extrahepatic biliary system, in *Morphology of the Liver*. New York, Academic Press, 1969, p 137.
106. Popper H, Schaffner F: *Liver: Structure and Function.* New York, McGraw-Hill, 1957, p 103.
107. Kune GA: Surgical anatomy of the common bile duct. *Arch Surg* 89:995, 1964.
108. Phillip J, Koch H, Classen M: Variations and anomalies of the papilla of Vater, the pancreas and the biliary duct. *Endoscopy* 6(2):70, 1974.
108a. Nakao I. Changes in morphology of the distal common bile duct associated with aging. *Gastroenterolagia Jap* 16:55, 1981.
109. Ham AW: *Histology*, ed 7. Philadelphia, Lippincott, 1984, p 695.
110. Classen M, Geenen J, Kawai K: *The Papilla Vateri and its Diseases—International Workshop.* Baden-Baden, Witzstrolk, 1979.
111. Tansy MF, Salkin L, Innes DL, et al: The mucosal lining of the intramural common bile duct as a determinant of ductal opening pressure. *Dig Dis* 20:613, 1975.
112. Wise L, Pizzimbono C, Dehner LP: Periampullary cancer. A clinicopathologic study of sixty-two patients. *Am J Surg* 131:141, 1976.
113. Engel JJ, Trujillo Y, Spellberg M: Metastatic carcinoma of the breast: A casue of obstructive jaundice. *Gastroenterology* 78:132, 1980.
114. Aston SJ, Longmire WP: Pancreaticoduodenal resection: Twenty years' experience. *Arch Surg* 106:813, 1973.
115. Kleinerman J, Yardumian K, Tamaki HT: Primary carcinoma of duodenum. *Ann Intern Med* 32:451, 1950.
116. Crane MJ, Gobbel WG, Scott HW: Surgical experience with malignant tumors of the ampulla of Vater and duodenum. *Surg Gynecol Obstet* 137:937, 1973.
117. Spira IA, Ghazi A, Wolfe WI: Primary adenocarcinoma of the duodenum. *Cancer* 39:1721, 1977.

118. Martin ED: Tumors of the Oddian region: Pathological aspects. *Sphincter of Oddi.* Proc. Third Gastroenterology Symposium, Nice 1976, p 95 (Karger, Basel 1977).

118a. Dings HP, Sellner F: Staging and grading of carcinomas of the papilla of Vater. *Wiener Klin Wschr* 93:638, 1981.

119. Gambill EE: Pancreatitis associated with pancreatic carcinoma: A study of 26 cases. *Mayo Clin Proc* 46:174, 1971,

120. Littenberg G, Afroudakis A, Kaplowitz N: Common bile duct stenosis from chronic pancreatitis: A clinical and pathologic spectrum. *Medicine* 58:385, 1979.

121. Hyland C, Kheir SM, Khashlan MB: Frozen section diagnosis of pancreatic carcinoma. A prospective study of 64 biopsies. *Am J Surg Pathol* 5:179, 1981.

122. Dekker A, Lloyd JC: Fine-needle aspiration biopsy in ampullary and pancreatic carcinoma. *Arch Surg* 114:592, 1979.

123. McLoughlin MJ, Ho CS, Langer B, et al: Fine needle aspiration biopsy of malignant lesions in and around the pancreas. *Cancer* 41:2413, 1978.

124. Tschang T-P, Garza-Garza R, Kissane JM: Pleomorphic carcinoma of the pancreas. An analysis of 15 cases. *Cancer* 39(5):2114, 1977.

125. Posen JA: Giant cell tumor of the pancreas of the osteoclastic type associated with a mucus secreting adenocarcinoma. *Hum Pathol* 12:944, 1981.

126. Hamoudi AB, Misugi K, Grosfeld JL, et al: Papillary epithelial neoplasm of pancreas in a child: Report of a case with electron microscopy. *Cancer* 26:1126, 1970.

127. Frable WJ, Still WJS, Kay S: Carcinoma of the pancreas, infantile type. A light and electron microscopic study. *Cancer* 27:667, 1971.

128. Warren KW, Hardy KJ: Cystadenocarcinoma of the pancreas. *Surg Gynecol Obstet* 127:734, 1968.

129. LoLudice A, Jarmolych J, Buhac I: Pancreatic retention cyst: A cause of obstructive jaundice. *JAMA* 238:889, 1977.

130. Ackerman CV, Rosai J: Surgical Pathology. Pancreas and Periampullary Region, ed 5. St. Louis, Mosby, 1974, p 565.

131. Isaacson C: Embryonal rhabdomyosarcoma of the ampulla of Vater. *Cancer* 41:365, 1978.

132. Regan PT, Malagelada J-R: A reappraisal of clinical, roentgenographic, and endoscopic features of the Zollinger-Ellison syndrome. *Mayo Clin Proc* 53:19, 1978.

133. Creutzfeld W, Arnold R, Creutzfeld C, et al: Pathomorphologic, biochemical, and diagnostic aspects of gastrinomas (Zollinger-Ellison syndrome). *Human Pathol* 6(1):47, 1975.

134. Larsson L-I, Schwartz T, Lundquist G, et al: Occurrence of human pancreatic polypeptide in pancreatic endocrine tumors: Possible implication in the watery diarrhea syndrome. *Am J Pathol* 85(3):675, 1976.

135. Wilander E, Portela-Gomes G, Grimelius L, et al: Argentaffin and argyrophil reactions of human gastrointestinal carcinoids. *Gastroenterology* 73:733, 1977.

136. Gordon DL, Chang Lo M, Schwartz MA: Carcinoid of the pancreas. *Am J Med* 51:412, 1971.

137. Ohmori K, Kinoshita H, Shiraha Y, et al: Pancreatic duct obstruction by a benign polypoid adenoma of the ampulla of Vater. *Am J Surg* 132:662, 1976.

138. Perzin KH, Bridge MF: Adenomas of the small intestine: A clinicopathologic review and a study of their relationship to carcinoma. *Cancer* 48:799, 1981.

139. Hocht B, Kuhner U, Gay B, et al: Obstructive jaundice caused by heterotopic pancreatic tissue in the ampulla of Vater. *Z Kinderchir* 22(1):79, 1977.

140. Suda K, Miyano T, Hashimoto K: The choledocho-pancreatico-ductal junction in infantile obstructive jaundice. *Acta Pathol Jpn* 30:187, 1980.

141. Fodisch H-J: The morphology of the papilla of Vater. *Fortschr Med* 93(5):193, 1975.

142. Yvergneaux JP, Bauwens E, Van Ourtyve L, et al: Benign stenosis of the papilla of Vater. *Acta Chirurg Belg* 6:523, 1977.

143. Yadegar J, Williams RA, Passaro E, et al: Common duct stricture from common pancreatitis. *Arch Surg* 115:582, 1980.

143a. Afroudakis A, Kaplowitz N: Liver histopathology in chronic common bile duct stenosis due to chronic alcoholic pancreatitis. *Hepatology* 1:65, 1981.

143b. Gregg JA, Carr Locke DL, Gallagher MM: Importance of common bile duct stricture associated with chronic pancreatitis. *Am J Surg* 141:199, 1981.

144. Murphy TF, Gray GF: Biliary tract obstruction due to tuberculous adenitis. *Am J Med* 68:452, 1980.

145. Vitullo BB, Rochon L, Seemayer TA, et al: Intrapancreatic compression of the common bile duct in cystic fibrosis. *J Pediatr* 93:1060, 1978.

145a. Lambert JR, Cole M, Crozier DN, et al: Intrapancreatic common bile duct compression causing jaundice in an adult with cystic fibrosis. *Gastroenterology* 80:169, 1981.

146. Danzi JT, Makipour H, Farmer RG: Primary sclerosing cholangitis. A report of nine cases and clinical review. *Am J Gastroent* 65:109, 1976.

147. Lefton HB, Farmer RG, Buchwald R, et al: Cryptococcal hepatitis mimicking primary sclerosing cholangitis. *Gstroenterology* 67:511, 1974.

148. Mihas AA, Murad TM, Hirschowitz BI: Sclerosing cholangitis associated with ulcerative colitis. *Am J Gastroenterology* 70:614, 1977.

149. Goldgraber MB, Kirsner JB: Chronic granulomatous cholecystitis and chronic fibrosing choledochitis associated with chronic ulcerative colitis. *Gastroenterology* 38:821, 1960.

150. Atkinson AJ, Carroll WW: Sclerosing cholangitis: Association with regional enteritis. *JAMA* 188:183, 1964.

150b. Murray SM, Woods CJ: Disseminated eosinophilic infiltration of a newborn infant with perforation of the terminal ileum and bile duct obstruction. *Arch Dis Child* 56:66, 1980.

151. Mitchinson MJ: Systemic idiopathic fibrosis: Systemic Weber-Christian disease. *J Clin Pathol* 18:645, 1965.

152. Bartholomew LG, Cain JC, Woolner LB, et al: Sclerosing cholangitis: Its possible association with Riedel's struma and fibrous retroperitonitis. Report of 2 cases. *N Engl J Med* 269:8, 1963.

153. Thompson BW, Read RC: Sclerosing cholangitis and other intra-abdominal fibroses. *Am J Surg* 128(6):777, 1974.

154. Binder SC, Daterling RA Jr, Mahoney SA: Systemic idiopathic fibrosis: Report of a case of the concomitant occurrence of retractile mesenteritis and retroperitoneal fibrosis. *Am J Surg* 124:422, 1972.

Index

Abetalipoproteinemia, 178
Abnormal hepatic storage products, 173–187
  abetalipoproteinemia, 178
  amyloidosis, 184–185
  cerebrotendinous xanthomatosis, 177–178
  cholesterol ester storage disease, 177
  cystinosis, 184
  gangliosidoses, 180–181
  Gaucher's disease, 179
  glycogen disease, 174–176
  hyperlipoproteinemia, 178
  mannosidosis, 183
  mucolipidoses, 183
  mucopolysaccharidoses, 182–183
  Niemann-Pick disease, 178–179
  Tangier disease, 178
Abscess: amebic, 275
  pyogenic, 273–274
Acalculous cholecystitis, 321
Acid-fast bacilli, 85, 91
Actinomycosis, 68–69
Active hepatitis, chronic, 45–49
  biopsy specimen, 36, 43
  bridging necrosis, 39
  cholestatic, 42
  hepatocellular alterations, 34–36
  inflammatory response, 36–39
  massive necrosis, 39–42
Acute cholecystitis, 321
Acute hepatitis, 296–297
Acute intermittent porphyria, 169
Acute suppurative cholangitis, 337
Acute viral hepatitis, 33–43
Adenomyomatosis, 325
Adenovirus infection, 61, 64
Alcoholic hepatitis, 100–101, 223
Alcoholic liver injury, 95–105
  cholestasis and hemosiderosis, 99–100
  cytoplasmic inclusions, 95–98
  fatty change and hydropic swelling, 95
  fetal alcohol syndrome, 104
  fibrosis, 101
  hepatitis, 100–101
  inflammatory response, 98–99
  progression to cirrhosis, 101
Allergic granulomatosis, 90
Alpha-1-antitrypsin deficiency, 9, 12, 26, 157–160
Alpha-fetoprotein, 12
Amanita phalloides, 72, 291
Amebic abscess, 275
Ampulla, carcinoma of, 353
Amyloidosis, 184–185, 204
Anaplastic carcinoma, 348
Anatomic relationships, 5–7
Ancylostoma, 88
Aneurysms, hepatic artery, 205
Anthracosilicosis, 193–194
Antitrypsin deficiency, 224
Apudomas, 354
Arbovirus infection, mosquito-borne, 68
Argentinian hemorrhagic fever, 68
Argyria, 194
Argyrophilic tumor (apudoma), 348
Arteriosclerosis, 204
Arteriovenous fistulae, 204
Arteritis, 203–204
Arthritis, 71
Ascaris, 88
Aspergillosis, 88
Aspergillus flavus, 242
Atresia, extrahepatic, 337–341
Autoimmune disease, 90
Autopsies, histologic differences between biopsies and, 21
Azathioprine, 201

Bacille Calmette Guérin (BCG) immunotherapy, 85
Bacterial infection, 68–69
Banti's syndrome, 214
Benign cavernous hemangioma, 259–260
Benign hepatocellular nodules, 236
Benign mesenchymoma, 267
Benign mesothelioma, 266
Benign neoplasms, 325–326
Benign tumors: bile duct, 348
  periampullary region, 354–355
Bile duct adenomas (bile duct hamartomas, Meyenburg's complexes), 253–254
Bile ducts, 333–362
  carcinomas of, 354
  extrahepatic, excluding periampullary region, 344–348
  general approach to specimen, 333
  intraduodenal and periampullary region, 348–355

Biliary atresia, differential diagnosis between neonatal hepatitis and, 143–146
Biliary cystadenomas, 255
Biliary tract, parasitic infections of, 135
Bilirubin, 4
Biopsies, histologic differences between autopsies and, 21
Blastomycosis, 88
Bolivian hemorrhagic fever, 68
Boutonneuse fever, 68
Bridging necrosis (or submassive confluent), 39
Brucella, 85
Brucellosis, 85
Brushing of tumors, at laparoscopy, 1
Budd-Chiari syndrome, 4, 7, 198, 294
Bush-tea poisoning, 201

Candidiasis of liver, 88
Capillaria hepatica, 81, 84
Caseation, 5
Cerebrotendinous xanthomatosis, 177–178
Ceroid storage disease, 192
Chemical investigations, tissue handling for, 14
Cholangiocarcinoma, 255–258, 345–348
Cholangiolocarcinoma, 258
Cholangitis, 337
  sclerosing, 343–344
Cholecystitis, 318–323
  acalculous, 321
  acute, 321
  chronic, 318
  emphysematous, 321–323
  eosinophilic, 318
Cholestasis, 99–100, 225
  drug-induced hepatic injury, 293–294
  and hyperbilirubinemia, 117–156
Cholestatic hepatitis, 42, 297–298
Cholesterol ester storage disease, 177
Cholesterolosis, 323
Chronic beryllium poisoning, 90
Chronic cholecystitis, 318
Chronic hepatitis, 44–56, 297
  active, 45–49, 224
  biopsy specimen, 48
  carrier of HB_sAg, 52
  hepatocyte with ground-glass cytoplasm, 51
  "hippie," 53–56, 78, 82
  immunopathology, 49–53
  liver of patient, 53
  lobular, 44
  persistent, 44–45
  piecemeal necrosis, 47
  portal triad with inflammatory cells, 49
Chronic inflammation of papilla of Vater (papillitis), 355
Chronic passive congestion, 196–198
Cirrhosis, 216–223
  classification, 216–223
  congestive, 217–219
  definition of, 211–212
  degree of activity, 226
  etiology, 223–226
    alcoholic hepatitis, 223
    cholestasis, 225
    fatty change, 223
    granulomatous hepatitis, 225–226
    hepatic infiltrates, 226
    metabolic disorders, 224–225
    parasites, 225
  focal biliary, 222–223
  hepatic nodules in noncirrhotic liver, 227–229
    nodular transformation, 228–229
    regenerative nodules, 227–228
  hepatocarcinoma with, 299–300
  incomplete septal, 216–217
  Indian childhood, 165
  macronodular, 216, 299
  micronodular, 216
  primary biliary, 221–222
  progression to, 101, 109
  relationship of hepatocarcinoma, 226–227
  secondary biliary, 219–221
  with secondary iron overload, 190
Citrullinaemia, 165
Clinicopathologic correlations, fatty liver, 106–109
Clonorchis sinensis, 135
Coccidioidomycosis, 88, 89
Congenital hepatic fibrosis, 212–214
Congestive cirrhosis, 217–219
Conjugated hyperbilirubinemia, 118
Copper poisoning, 90
Cori's disease (Type III glycogenosis; limit dextrinosis), 175
Coxsackie virus infection, 67
Crigler-Najjar syndrome, 117
Crohn's disease, 90
Cystadenocarcinomas, 255, 348, 353
Cystadenomas, 348
Cystic disease of liver, 214
Cystic lesions, 5
Cystinosis, 184
Cysts, bile ducts, 341–343
Cytomegalovirus infection, 63–67
Cytoplasmic inclusions, 95–98

Dengue forest fever, 68
Donohue's syndrome, 143, 165, 190
Drug-induced hepatic injury, 287–311
  effects of therapy, 300
  general approach, 287
  list of chemicals, 288–291
  predictable (hepatotoxic) reactions, 287–295
  unpredictable (hypersensitivity) reactions, 295–300
Drugs, granulomatous hepatitis, 91
Dubin-Johnson syndrome, 4, 118, 192, 193

Ebola virus, 67
Echinococcosis, 275–277
Eclampsia, 71–72
Embryonal rhabdomyosarcoma (sarcoma botryoides), 348
Embryonal tumors, 252–253
Emphysematous cholecystitis, 321–323
Empyema (gallbladder full of pus), 317
Entamoeba histolytica, 275

Enteric infection, 70
Eosinophilic cholecystitis, 318
Epstein-Barr virus, 63
Erythema nodosum, 90
Erythropoietic protoporphyria, 169
Etiocholanone fever, 90
Excessive lipofuscin deposition, 191–192
Extrahepatic bile ducts (excluding periampullary region), 334–348
  atresia, 337–341
  cholangitis, 337
  cysts, 341
  gross anatomy, dissection, and description, 334
  normal histology, 336–337
  preparation of microscopic sections, 335–336
  rupture, 345
  sclerosing cholangitis, 343–344
  specimen handling, 334
  stones, 337
  tumors, 345–348
  variations and anomalies, 334–335
Extrahepatic blood supply to liver, pathology of, 205
Extrahepatic cholestasis, morphology of, 122–126
Extrahepatic obstruction, neonatal cholestasis and, 146–149

Familial hypofibrinogenemia, 160
Fanconi syndrome, 184
Fasciola hepatica, 135, 318
Fatty change, hydropic swelling and, 95
Fatty liver, 106–116
  clinicopathologic correlations, 106–109
  etiologic factors, 110
  hypervitaminosis A, 113
  large-droplet steatosis, 109–112
    with inflammation, 111–112
  progression to fibrosis and cirrhosis, 109
  small-droplet steatosis, 112–113
  small- and large-droplet, 106
Fetal alcohol syndrome, 104
Fibrosis, 101, 211–216
  congenital hepatic, 212–214
  cystic disease of liver, 214
  definition, 211–212
  etiology, 223–226
    alcoholic hepatitis, 223
    cholestasis, 225
    fatty change, 223
    granulomatous hepatitis, 225–226
    hepatic infiltrates, 226
    metabolic disorders, 224–225
    parasites, 225
  hepatoportal sclerosis, 214–216
  progression to, 109
  see also Cirrhosis
Fibrous tissue, tumors of, 265
Focal biliary cirrhosis, 222–223
Focal fatty change, 238–239
Focal lesions, 4–5
Focal nodular hyperplasia, 239–241
Foreign-body granulomas, 78, 80
Formalin pigment, 193
Fungi, hepatic granulomas, 88

Galactosemia, 162–164
Galactose-1-phosphate uridyl transferase, deficiency of, 162
Gallbladder, 312–332
  abnormalities of content, 316–318
    empyema, 317
    gallstones, 316–317
    hemobilia, 317
    mucocele or hydrops, 317
    parasites, 317–318
  abnormalities of wall, 318–328
    cholecystitis, 318–323
    nodules and tumors, 323–328
    vascular lesions, 323
  general approach to specimen, 312–316
    abnormalities of number, location, and shape, 314–315
    gross anatomy, dissection, and description, 313–314
    handling, 312–313
    normal histology, 315–316
    preparation of microscopic sections, 315
Gallstones, 316–317
Gangliosidoses, 180–181
Gaucher's disease, 179
Gelatin, 10
Giardia lamblig, 318
Gilbert's syndrome, 117
Glucose-6-phosphatase, 11
Glycogen storage disease (glycogenoses), 174–176
Glycosphingolipidosis, 181
GM1 gangliosidosis, 180
Gomori lead salt method, 11
Gomori's trichrome, 9
Graft-versus-host reaction (GVHR), 73
Granulomas, 77–94, 297
  clinical features, 84
  defined, 77
  etiologic factors, 84–92
    autoimmune disease, 90
    drugs, 91
    fungi, 88
    heavy metals, 90
    inflammatory bowel disease, 90
    miscellaneous bacterial infections, 85–88
    mycobacterial infections, 85
    neoplasms, 91
    parasites, 88–90
    Rickettsiae, 88
    sarcoidosis, 87
    systemic granulomatous diseases, 90
    unknown, 92
    viral infections, 87–88
  reported causes (table), 86–87
  significance, 84
  subtypes, 77–84
    foreign-body, 78, 80
    lipogranulomas, 78–84
    tubercles, 78

Granulomatous hepatitis, 225–226
Green staining of cholestasis, 4

Hairy cell leukemia, 202–203
Heavy metals, granulomatous reaction and, 90
Hemangiosarcoma, 262–264
Hemobilia, 317
Hemochromatosis, 189–190
Hemodialysis and transplantation, 73
Hemolytic anemia, 117
Hemosiderosis, 99–100, 188–190
Hepatic congestion, 196–201
  Budd-Chiari syndrome, 198
  chronic passive, 196–198
  periportal sinusoidal congestion, 201
  shock liver, 199
  sickle cell anemia, 199–201
  veno-occlusive disease, 201
Hepatic infiltrates, 226
Hepatic injury, 60–76
  bacterial, 68–70
  eclampsia, 71–72
  graft-versus-host reaction, 73
  hemodialysis and transplantation, 73
  neoplasia, 72–73
  nonspecific reactive hepatitis, 60–61
  protozoal infections, 70
  Q fever, 68
  rheumatic diseases, 71
  thermal, 72
  viral infections, 61–68
    adenovirus, 61, 64
    Coxsackie virus, 67
    cytomegalovirus, 63–67
    herpes, 61–62, 65
    Marburg virus, 67
    miscellaneous, 68
    mononucleosis, 62–63, 66
    yellow fever, 67
Hepatic nodules, noncirrhotic liver, 227–229
Hepatic pathology, 1–32
  principles of description and interpretation, 15–27
    between biopsies and autopsies, 21
    hepatocytes, 25–26
    lobule, 20–21
    morphometry, 27
    nuclear enlargement and inclusions, 23–24
    overall morphology, 16–19
    pigments, 26–27
    portal triads, 19–20
    between surgical wedge and needle biopsy, 21–23
  specimen, 1–12
    anatomic relationships, 5–7
    electron microscopy, 12–13
    focal lesions, 4–5
    general description, 3–4
    general principles of handling, 7–12
    inspection and description, 3–7
    needle biopsy, 1–2
    resection, 3
    tissue handling, 14–15
    wedge biopsy, 2–3
Hepatic pigments, 188–195
  anthracosilicosis, 193–194
  Dubin-Johnson syndrome, 192
  excessive lipofuscin deposition, 191–192
  formalin, 193
  iron overload, 188–191
    cirrhosis with secondary, 190
    hemochromatosis, 189–190
    hemosiderosis, 188–189
  malaria, 193
  polyvinylpyrrolidine, 194
  protoporphyria, 192
  silver, 194
  thorotrast, 194
Hepatic porphyrias, 166–169
  acute intermittent, 169
  erythropoietic, 169
Hepatitis, 33–59
  acute, 33–43, 296–297
    biopsy specimen, 36, 43
    bridging necrosis, 39
    cholestatic, 42
    hepatocellular alterations, 34–36
    inflammatory response, 36–39
    massive necrosis, 39–42
  alcoholic, 100–101
  cholestatic, 297–298
  chronic, 44–56, 297
    active, 45–49
    biopsy specimen, 48
    carrier of HB_sAg, 52
    hepatocyte with ground-glass cytoplasm, 51
    "hippie," 53–56
    immunopathology, 49–53
    liver of patient, 53
    lobular hepatitis, 44
    persistent, 44–45
    piecemeal necrosis, 47
    portal triad with inflammatory cells, 49
  meaning of, 33
Hepatitis A, in infancy, 150
Hepatitis B, 11–12
  in infancy, 150
Hepatocarcinoma, relationship to cirrhosis, 226–227
Hepatocellular adenomas, 236–238
Hepatocellular alterations, in acute viral hepatitis, 34–36
Hepatocellular carcinoma, 241–252
  etiology, 242–243
  gross findings, 245
  microscopic structure, 245–252
  preneoplastic changes, 243–244
  symptoms, 244–245
Hepatocellular degeneration (dystrophic calcification), 26
Hepatocellular necrosis, 291–292
  metabolic diseases, 157–172
    alpha-1-antitrypsin, 157–160
    citrullinaemia, 165
    Donohue's syndrome, 165
    familial hypofibrinogenemia, 160
    galactosemia, 162–164
    hereditary fructose intolerance, 164

Indian childhood cirrhosis, 165
tyrosinemia, hereditary, 164
Wilson's disease, 161–162
Zellweger's cerebrohepatorenal syndrome, 165
Hepatocellular neoplasms, 236–252
Hepatocytes, cytoplasm of, 25–26
Hepatolenticular degeneration (Wilson's disease), 161–162
Hepatoportal sclerosis, 214–216, 294
Hereditary fructose intolerance, 164
Hereditary tyrosinemia, 164
Herpes infection, 4, 61–62, 65
Herpes simplex, 4
Heterotopia, 325
"Hippie hepatitis," 53–56, 78
biopsy specimen, 82
Histochemistry, processing of frozen sections for diagnosis and, 10–11
Hodgkin's disease, 269
Hurler's syndrome (lipochondrodystrophy, dysostosis multiplex, gargoylism), 182–183
Hydropic swelling, 95
Hyperbilirubinemia and cholestasis, 117–156
cholestasis, defined, 118
conjugated, 118
extrahepatic, 122
morphology, 122–126
in infancy, 141–156
cholestatic jaundice, 141–142
differentiation of neonatal hepatitis and biliary atresia, 143–146
etiologic factors, 150
hepatitis A and B, 150
intrahepatic atresia, 150–151
without mechanical obstruction of extrahepatic biliary system, 149–150
miscellaneous cholestatic disorders, 151–152
neonatal cholestasis and extrahepatic obstruction, 146–149
normal liver, 142–143
role of liver biopsy, 142
intrahepatic, 122
morphology, 135–136
suppurative inflammatory lesions, 126–127
morphologic changes, 118–120
parasitic infections, biliary tract, 135
pericholangitis, 134
primary biliary cirrhosis, 127–132
primary sclerosing cholangitis, 134–135
unconjugated, 117, 141
Hyperlipoproteinemia, 178
Hypervitaminosis A, 113
Hypofibrinogenemia, familial, 160

Immunohistology, processing for, 11–12
Immunopathology, of hepatitis, 49–53
Incomplete septal cirrhosis, 216–217
Indian childhood cirrhosis, 165
Infancy, hyperbilirubinemia and cholestasis, 141–156
differentiation of neonatal hepatitis and biliary atresia, 143–146
etiologic factors, 150
hepatitis A and B, 150
intrahepatic atresia, 150–151
jaundice, 141–142
without mechanical obstruction of extrahepatic biliary system, 149–150
miscellaneous cholestatic disorders, 151–152
neonatal cholestasis and extrahepatic obstruction, 146–149
normal liver, 142–143
role of liver biopsy, 142
Infantile hemangioendothelioma, 261–262
Infantile mesenchymal hamartoma, 266–267
Infarction, hepatic, 205–207
Infectious mononucleosis, 62–63, 66
Inferior vena cava, 6
Inflammation, large-droplet steatosis with, 111–112
Inflammatory bowel disease, 90
Inflammatory lesions, space-occupying, 273–277
amebic abscess, 275
echinococcosis, 275–277
pyogenic abscess, 273–274
Inflammatory polyps, 323–325
Inflammatory response: acute hepatocellular injury, 36–39
alcoholic liver injury, 98–99
Injury, hepatic, 60–76
bacterial, 68–70
eclampsia, 71–72
graft-versus-host reaction, 73
hemodialysis and transplantation, 73
neoplasia, 72–73
nonspecific reactive hepatitis, 60–61
protozoal infections, 70
Q fever, 68
rheumatic diseases, 71
thermal, 72
viral infections, 61–68
adenovirus, 61, 64
Coxsackie virus, 67
cytomegalovirus, 63–67
herpes, 61–62, 65
Marburg virus, 67
miscellaneous, 68
mononucleosis, 62–63, 66
yellow fever, 67
Intraduodenal bile duct and periampullary region, 348–355
gross anatomy, dissection, and description, 349
normal histology, 350–351
preparation of microscopic sections, 350
specimen handling, 348–349
tumors, 351–355
Intrahepatic atresia, neonatal cholestasis and, 150–151
Intrahepatic cholestasis, 122
morphology of, 135–136
suppurative inflammatory lesions, biliary tract, 126–127

Iron overload, 188–191
  cirrhosis with secondary, 190
  hemochromatosis, 189–190
  hemosiderosis, 188–189
Islet cell (or carcinoid tumors), 354

Jamaican vomiting sickness, 113
Jaundice, 42, 68

Karnovsky's fixative, 8, 13
Kupffer cells, 21, 27, 36, 44, 70, 71, 72, 78, 119, 146, 173, 177, 181, 184, 185, 188, 190, 194, 205, 226, 300
Kupffer cell sarcoma, 262–264
Kwashiorkor, 106
Kyasanut forest fever, 68

Large-droplet fatty change, 106, 107
  with toxic hepatic necrosis, 292–293
Large-droplet hepatocellular fatty change, 223
Large-droplet steatosis, 109-112
  with inflammation, 111–112
Lassa fever, 68
Left hepatic vein, 6–7
Leishmaniasis, 70–71
Lepromatous leprosy, 85
Leprosy bacilli, 85
Leptospira, 70
Leukemia, 268–272
  and other lymphoreticular neoplasms, 271–273
Lingulatia (tongue worm), 88
Lipofuscin, 27, 191–192
Lipogranulomas, 78–84
Lipomatous tumors, 265–266
Liver: alcoholic injury, 95–105
    cholestasis and hemosiderosis, 99–100
    cytoplasmic inclusions, 95–98
    fatty change and hydropic swelling, 95
    fetal alcohol syndrome, 104
    fibrosis, 101
    hepatitis, 100–101
    inflammatory response, 98–99
    progression to cirrhosis, 101
  biopsies, 60
    in infants with cholestasis, 142
  cystic disease, 214
  fatty change, 106–116
    clinocopathologic correlations, 106–109
    etiologic factors, 110
    hypervitaminosis A, 113
    large-droplet steatosis, 109–112
    progression to fibrosis and cirrhosis, 109
    small-droplet steatosis, 112–113
    small- and large-droplet, 106
  granulomatous diseases, 77–94
    clinical features, 84
    defined, 77
    etiologic factors, 84–92
    reported causes (table), 86–87
    significance, 84
    subtypes, 77–84
  reticulum framework, 20
  space-occupying lesions, 233–286
    general approach, 233–234
    inflammatory, 273–277
    neoplastic, 234–273
  vascular lesions, 196–210
    hepatic congestion, 196–201
    without lobular localization, 205–207
    portal triads, 201–205
Liver injury, drugs and chemicals, 287–311
  effects of therapy, 300
  general approach, 287
  list of chemicals, 288–291
  predictable (hepatotoxic) reactions, 287–295
    Budd-Chiari syndrome, 294
    cholestasis, 293–294
    fatty change, 292–293
    hepatocellular necrosis, 291–292
    hepatoportal sclerosis, 294
    storage phenomena, 294–295
    veno-occlusive disease, 294
  unpredictable (hypersensitivity) reactions, 295–300
    acute hepatitis, 296–297
    cholestatic hepatitis, 297–298
    chronic hepatitis, 297
    granulomas, 297
    hepatitic reactions, 296–298
    hepatocellular neoplasms, 299–300
    mixed reactions, 299
    peliosis hepatis, 299
Lobular hepatitis, chronic, 44
Lobule, 20–21
Lupoid hepatitis, 46
Luschka crypts, 325
Lymphoma, 268–272
  non-Hodgkin's, 269–271
Lymphoreticular neoplasms, 268–272

McDowell's fixative, 8, 13
Macronodular cirrhosis, 216, 219
Malaria, 193
Malignant hemangioendothelioma, 262–264
Malignant mesenchymoma, 267–268
Malignant mixed tumor (carcinosarcoma), 268
Malignant neoplasms, 326–328
Mallory bodies ("alcoholic hyalin"), 95–98
Mannosidosis, 183
Marburg virus, 67
Massive necrosis, 39–42
Menghini needle, 8
Metabolic diseases, hepatocellular necrosis, 157–172
  alpha-1-antitrypsin, 157–160
  citrullinaemia, 165
  Donohue's syndrome, 165
  familial hypofibrinogenemia, 160
  galactosemia, 162–164
  hepatic porphyrias, 166–169
    acute intermittent, 169
    erythropoietic, 169
    PCT (porphyria cutanea tarda), 166–169
  hereditary fructose intolerance, 164
  Indian childhood cirrhosis, 165
  tyrosinemia, hereditary, 164

Wilson's disease, 161–162
Zellweger's cerebrohepatorenal syndrome, 165

Metaplasia, 325
Metastatic tumors, 234–235
Microbiology, tissue handling, 14–15
Micronodular cirrhosis, 216
Microtomy and staining, 9–10
Middle hepatic vein, 6–7
Mononucleosis, infectious, 62–63, 66
Morphometry, 27
Mucocele or hydrops, 317
Mucoepidermoid carcinomas, 258
Mucolipidoses, 183
Mucopolysaccharidoses, 182–183
Mycobacterial infections, 85
Mycobacterium tuberculosis, 85
Myxoma, 266

Needle biopsy, 1–2
histologic differences between surgical wedge and, 21–23
Neonatal cholestasis: extrahepatic obstruction and, 146–149
intrahepatic atresia (paucity of intrahepatic bile ducts), 150–151
without mechanical obstruction of extrahepatic biliary system, 149–150
Neonatal giant cell hepatitis, 46
Neonatal hepatitis: differential diagnosis between biliary atresia and, 143–146
etiologic factors, 150
see also Infancy, hyperbilirubinemia and cholestasis
Neonatal unconjugated hyperbilirubinemia, 141
Neoplasia, 72–73
Neoplasm-like lesions, 236–252
Neoplastic space-occupying lesions, 234–273
benign mesothelioma, 266
combined hepatocellular and cholangiocarcinomas, 258–259
embryonal tumors, 252–253
hepatocellular neoplasms and neoplasm-like lesions, 236–252
infantile mesenchymal hamartoma, 266–267
lipomatous tumors, 265–266
lymphoma, leukemia (other lymphoreticular neoplasms), 268–272
malignant mixed tumor, 268
metastatic tumors, 234–235
myxoma, 266
osteoclastoma, 266
proliferative biliary epithelial lesions, 253–258
proliferative vascular lesions, 259–264
rhabdomyosarcoma, 268
tumors of bone and cartilage, 266
tumors of fibrous tissue, 265
tumors of neural crest origin, 266
tumors of smooth muscle, 265
Niemann-Pick disease, 178–179
Nodules, gallbladder, 323–328
Nonhemolytic hyperbilirubinemia (Gilbert's syndrome), 117
Non-Hodgkin's lymphoma, 269–271
Nonprogressive hepatic fibrosis, 212–216
congenital hepatic, 212–214
cystic disease of liver, 214
definition of, 211, 212
Normal infant liver, 142–143
Nuclei of hepatocytes, 23–24
Nutmeg pattern, 4

Opisthorchis sinensis, 318
Orcein staining method, 9–10
Osler-Weber-Rendu disease, 201–202, 212
Osteoclastoma, 266

Pancreas, cystadenocarcinomas, 353
Pancreatic carcinoma, 352–353
Paraffin blocks, fixation and preparation, 8–9
Parasites, 225
in gallbladder, 317–318
Parasitic infections, foreign-body type granulomas, 88–90
Paratyphoid fever, 70
PCT, *see* Porphyria cutanea tarda
Peliosis hepatis, 205, 206, 299
Pericholangitis, 134
Periodic acid-Schiff (PAS) reaction, 9
Periportal sinusoidal congestion, 201
Perl's stain, 9
Persistent hepatitis, chronic, 44–45
Phrygian cap anomaly, 314–315
"Pick cells," 178–179
Pigments, hepatic, 26–27, 188–195
anthracosilicosis, 193–194
Dubin-Johnson syndrome, 192
excessive lipofuscin deposition, 191–192
formalin, 193
iron overload, 188–191
cirrhosis with secondary, 190
hemochromatosis, 189–190
hemosiderosis, 188–189
malaria, 193
polyvinylpyrrolidine, 194
protoporphyria, 192
silver, 194
thorotrast, 194
Plasma cell hepatitis, 45–46
Plasmodium vivax or *P. falciparum,* 70
Plastic sections, handling, 10
Polyarteritis nodosa of gallbladder, 323
Polymyalgia rheumatica, 71, 90
Polyps, inflammatory, 323–325
Polyvinylpyrrolidine, 194
Pompe's disease (Type II glycogenosis), 175
Porphyria cutanea tarda (PCT), 166–169
Porphyrias, hepatic, 166–169
Porphyria variegata, 4
Portal triads, 19–20
inflammatory response, 36–39
vascular lesions affecting, 201–205
arteriosclerosis and amyloidosis, 204
arteriovenous fistulae, 204

Portal triads, vascular lesions affecting (*continued*)
arteritis, 203–204
extrahepatic portal vein, 205
hairy cell leukemia, 202–203
Osler-Weber-Rendu disease, 201–202
Preeclampsia, 71–72
Pregnancy, fatty liver of, 108
Primary biliary cirrhosis, 90, 127–132, 221–222
Primary hepatic squamous carcinomas, 258
Primary sclerosing cholangitis, 134–135
Proliferative biliary epithelial lesions, 253–258
bileduct adenomas, 253–254
cholangiocarcinoma, 255–258
cystadenocarcinomas, 255
cystadenomas, 255
simple cysts, 254
Proliferative vascular lesions, 259–264
benign cavernous hemangioma, 259–260
hemangiosarcoma, 262–264
infantile hemangioendothelioma, 261–262
Protoporphyria, 192
Protozoal infections, 70–71
Pyogenic abscess, 273–274

Q fever, 68, 84, 88

Rappaport's acinus, 16
Resection, specimen, 3
Reticulin fibers, 20
Reye's syndrome, 106, 113
Rhabdomyosarcoma, 268, 354
Rheumatic diseases, 71
Rickettsia burnetti, 68
Rickettsiae, 88
Rickettsial hepatitis, 68
Riedel's lobe, 5
Rift valley fever, 68
Right hepatic vein, 6–7
Rocky Mountain spotted fever, 68
Rokitansky-Aschoff sinuses, 325
Rotor's syndrome, 118
Round worms (ascaris), 317–318

St. George disease (of cattle), 205
Sandhoff's disease, 181
Sarcoidosis, 80, 87
Schistosoma hematobium, 225
Schistosoma japonicum, 225
Schistosoma mansoni infection, 82, 225
Schistosomiasis, 89
Sclerosing cholangitis, 343–344
etiologic factors, 344
"Sea-blue histiocyte" syndrome, 181
Secondary biliary cirrhosis, 219–221
Shock liver, 199
Sickle cell anemia, 199–201
Silver, 194
Sinusoids, 18, 20–21
Small-droplet fat, 106
Small-droplet steatosis, 112–113
Smooth muscle, tumors of, 265
Space-occupying lesions, 233–286
general approach, 233–234
inflammatory, 273–277
neoplastic, 234–273
Specimen, hepatic pathology, 1–12
anatomic relationships, 5–7
different types of, 1–3
electron microscopy, 12–13
focal lesions, 4–5
general description, 3–4
handling and processing, 7–12
for chemical investigations, 14
fixation and preparation of paraffin blocks, 8–9
frozen sections for diagnosis and histochemistry, 10–11
for immunohistology, 11–12
for microbiology, 14–15
for transmission electron microscopy, 12–13
inspection and description, 3–7
needle biopsy, 1–2
resection, 3
tissue handling, 14–15
wedge biopsy, 2–3
see also Hepatic pathology
Squamous carcinoma, 348
Stones, extrahepatic bile ducts, 337
Storage phenomena, 294–295
"Strawberry" gallbladder, 323
Strictures, bile ducts, 344
Strongyloides, 88
Submassive confluent (or bridging necrosis), 39
Surgical wedge, histologic differences between needle biopsy and, 21–23
Syphilis, 69–70, 85

Tangier disease, 178
Tay-Sachs disease (GM_2 gangliosidosis), 181
Tay Sachs disease with visceral involvement, *see* GM1 gangliosidosis
Temporal arteritis, 71
Teratoma, 267
Tertiary hepatic syphilis, 69, 70
Thermal injury, 72
Thorotrast, 194
Tissue handling: for chemical investigations, 14
for microbiology, 14–15
Toxocara, 88
Treponema pallidum, 69
Tubercles, 78, 79
Tularemia, 85
Tumors: bile ducts, 345–348
of bone and cartilage, 266
fibrous tissue, 265
gallbladder, 323–328
neural crest origin, 266
periampullary region, 351–355
smooth muscle, 265
Type I glycogenosis (von Gierke's disease), 174
Type II glycogenosis (Pompe's disease), 175
Type III glycogenosis (Cori's disease, limit dextrinosis), 175
Type IV glycogenosis (amylopectinosis), 176
Typhoid fever, 70
Tyrosinemia, hereditary, 164

Unconjugated hyperbilirubinemia: hemolysis, 117
  neonatal, 141
Undifferentiated sarcoma, 267–268
"Universal triaditis" of Gall, 39
Urethane, 201

Vascular lesions: gallbladder, 323
  hepatic congestion, 196–201
    Budd-Chiari syndrome, 198
    chronic passive, 196–198
    periportal sinusoidal congestion, 201
    shock liver, 199
    sickle cell anemia, 199–201
    veno-occlusive disease, 201
  of liver, 196–210
  without lobular localization, 205–207
    infarction, 205–207
    peliosis hepatis, 205
  portal triads and, 201–205
    arteriosclerosis and amyloidosis, 204
    arteriovenous fistulae, 204
    arteritis, 203–204
    extrahepatic portal vein, 205
    hairy cell leukemia, 202–203
    Osler-Weber-Rendu disease, 201–202
Veno-occlusive disease, 201, 294
Viral infections: adenovirus, 61, 64
  Coxsackie virus, 67
  cytomegalovirus, 63–67
  granulomatous hepatitis, 87–88
  hepatic lesions, 61–68
  herpes, 61–62, 65
  Marburg virus, 67
  miscellaneous types, 68
  mononucleosis, 62–63, 66
  yellow fever, 67
Von Gierke's disease (Type I glycogenosis), 174

Wedge biopsy, 2–3
Wegener's granuloma, 90
Weil's disease, 70
Whipple's disease, 69
Wilson's disease (hepatolenticular degeneration), 161–162

Xanthomas, 177–178

Yellow fever, 67

Zellweger's cerebrohepatorenal syndrome, 165
Zellweger's syndrome, 143, 190
Ziehl-Nielson's stain, 9